# CARDIAC DYNAMICS

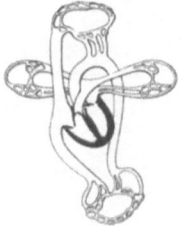

# DEVELOPMENTS IN CARDIOVASCULAR MEDICINE

## VOLUME 2

1. C.T. Lancée. *Echocardiology*. 1979. ISBN 90-247-2209-8.
3. H.J.Th. Thalen, C.C. Meere. *Fundamentals of Cardiac Pacing*, 1979. ISBN 90-247-2245-4.
4. H.E. Kulbertus, H.J.J. Wellens. *Sudden Death*. 1980. ISBN 90-247-2290-X.
5. L.S. Dreifus, A.N. Brest. *Clinical Applications of Cardiovascular Drugs*. 1980. ISBN 90-247-2295-0.

# CARDIAC DYNAMICS

*edited by*

JAN BAAN PH.D.,
ALEXANDER C. ARNTZENIUS M.D.
Leiden University Hospital, Leiden

*and*

EDWARD L. YELLIN PH.D.
Albert Einstein College of Medicine, Bronx, N.Y.

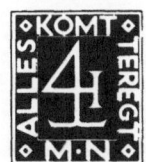

1980
MARTINUS NIJHOFF PUBLISHERS
THE HAGUE/BOSTON/LONDON

The distribution of this book is handled by the following team:

*for the United States and Canada*

Kluwer Boston, Inc.
160 Old Derby Street
Hingham, MA 02043
USA

*for all other countries*

Kluwer Academic Publishers Group
Distribution Center
P.O. Box 322
3300 AH Dordrecht
The Netherlands

Library of Congress Cataloging in Publication Data    CIP

Main entry under title:

Cardiac dynamics.

    (Developments in cardiovascular medicine; v. 2)
    Bibliography: p.
    Includes index.
    1.  Heart–Muscle.  2.  Muscle contraction.
I.  Baan, Jan.  II.  Arntzenius, A. C.  III.  Yellin,
Edward L.  IV.  Series.  [DNLM:  1.  Heart–Physiology.
WL DE997PE v. 2 / WG202 C2645]
QP113.2.C36       612'.171         79-17930

ISBN-13: 978-94-009-8798-2    e-ISBN-13: 978-94-009-8796-8
DOI: 10.1007/978-94-009-8796-8

# TABLE OF CONTENTS

# INTRODUCTION

Cardiac Dynamics is the name of a relatively young field of study, born from the fruitful interaction between branches of two different disciplines: medicine and physics. "Dynamics" is the branch of physics which deals with the action of forces on bodies or particles in motion or at rest. "Cardiac" relates to the clinical field of cardiology but also to cardiophysiology, both of which are specialized branches of medicine. Narrower than the well-established field of Hemodynamics, Cardiac Dynamics is restricted to dynamic phenomena occurring in and around the heart. The mathematical treatment of such phenomena, however, is vastly more complex because of the intricate nature of the mechanisms involved in the cardiac action. Thus, whereas hemodynamics is concerned with predominantly passive (visco-) elastic structures – vessels – containing time-variant flow of viscous fluid – blood –, the mechanical study of the heart requires additional considerations such as: active elastic components representing the contractile mechanism of cardiac muscle, complex geometry and fiber structure in the myocardial wall, autoregulatory mechanisms, and intricate flow patterns associated with valve motion. Viewed in this light it is not surprising that attempts to describe ventricular pump function and to quantify contractile performance have not reached the level of sophistication which is common in e.g. arterial hemodynamics. For the same reason, many of the often simplified approaches to describe ventricular mechanics failed to stand up to more rigorous theoretical, experimental or clinical testing. The heart is a very complex organ, an adequate mechanical description of which still eludes us, even when external neurogenic and metabolic factors are neglected.

This state of affairs is of growing concern to the scientific and clinical community and requires increasing levels of sophistication for both experimental and theoretical studies of the heart in order to deepen our insight into the mechanisms operating in the normal and the diseased state. Persistent input from the basic and the life sciences with intensively stimulated interdisciplinary efforts is mandatory to tackle the problems at hand.

Sharing the essentials of the above reasoning, applied to the entire circulation, about a hundred cardiovascular investigators from different backgrounds have established the Cardiovascular System Dynamics Society, and this book represents its second publication.* The book contains a selection from the proceedings of the Third International Conference of the Society, a three-day single-session meeting held at Leiden University in August of 1978. The theme of the conference was: Basic and Clinical Aspects of Cardiac Dynamics.

While most contributors are Charter Members of the Society, many authors were also invited from outside. The topics presented cover a wide scale of Cardiac Dynamics, starting from the subcellular level of muscle contraction, through dynamic chamber behavior and pump function, ending with the ventricular entrance and exit structures, the valves. In addition, there is a section on methodological assessment of cardiac performance with its important clinical implications. Chapters within the main sections also include renditions of three special lectures established by the Society: the Isaac Starr Lecture given by Jeremy Swan, the Konrad Witzig Memorial Lecture given by Brian Bellhouse, and the Closing Lecture given by Abraham Noordergraaf, president of the Society.

Section 1, *Cardiac muscle mechanics*, is introduced by Jewell who poses some provocative questions to both physiologists and cardiologists. Thus, the wisdom of continuing to use contractility indices, based on muscle models proven to be inadequate, is questioned. More fundamentally, the existence of a separation between inotropic state and preload is doubted. Rather, the basis for the force-length relation is thought to reside in length dependence of activation. In the next chapter, however, Winegrad advocates passive elements of intra- and intercellular structures and connective tissue to account for the different shapes found for the force-length relation. Jewell's theory finds support in the work presented by Ter Keurs. The controversial issue seems to hinge on the ability to quantitate the relation between calcium concentration and developed force.

According to the results reported in the next chapter, preload and contractility are indeed inseparable, but this conclusion is contingent upon the ability of ventricular dp/dt to assess inotropic state in an isovolumic heart. Turning attention to the force and velocity intercepts of the Hill equation, Huntsman shows these contractility parameters to be independent of preload only at muscle lengths larger than 85% of $L_{max}$. Deriving the same parameters from an isovolumically contracting ventricle, the authors of the next chapter conclude that $F_0$ is indicative of active state, being constant during part of systole.

The chapter by Lab reports a dissociation between action potential duration and local muscle shortening behaviour during onset of ischemia,

---

*First publication: Cardiovascular System Dynamics, edited by J. Baan, A. Noordergraaf and J. Raines, (MIT Press, Cambridge, Mass., 1978).

which is thought to be mediated by intracellular calcium distribution. The final chapter deals with measurements of momentary stiffness of skeletal muscle after quick length changes; the findings are explained in terms of behaviour of crossbridges between thick and thin filaments.

Building up from the isolated muscle to the whole heart, Section 2 deals with *Cardiac chamber dynamics*. The section heads off with a chapter by Sagawa who discusses similarities and discrepancies between force-length relations of isolated muscle on the one hand and end-systolic pressure-volume relations of the ventricles on the other. An important point, as yet not settled, is whether or not shortening of cardiac muscle causes de-activation in terms of end-systolic mechanical parameters. In the next chapter, Rankin stresses the importance of the dynamic geometry of the ventricle for its function and behaviour of wall stress. Implications of these findings for ventricular function in patients are discussed in depth.

A chapter by Streeter deals with the intricate anatomy of muscle fibers in the wall and the meaning of the fiber pathways in terms of propagation of the electrical impulse, which is predicted to run a zig-zag course through the wall.

The remaining three chapters represent novel attempts to relate mechanics of the sarcomere to those of the thick-walled left ventricle, using modeling approaches. The chapter by Arts introduces the concept of torsion of the ventricle about its long axis, resulting in realistic predictions of dynamic ventricular geometry.

The next chapter argues that ventricular pressure-volume relations may be "translated" to average sarcomere force-length relations virtually independent of wall thickness. The role of wall thickness to relate cavity volume to sarcomere length is found to be important to relate small variations in length to large changes in volume.

The final chapter represents an approach to relate the dynamics of crossbridge formation to the dynamics of the ejecting left ventricle. Dependence of activation on preload as well as changes in ventricular shape are thought to be essential to explain experimental results.

Section 3 deals with topics related to the *Filling of the left ventricle*. The introductory chapter by Yellin uses a highly invasive but very accurate approach to investigate filling dynamics in the dog. An overview of the following determinants of filling is presented: left ventricular relaxation, left atrial reservoir and booster pump function, diastolic chamber compliance, and mitral valve action. The results of new and interesting approaches toward the study of these factors are presented in the subsequent chapters.

The chapter by Tyberg discusses how the clinically important end-diastolic pressure is influenced by ventricular chamber compliance and venous return. Significant new data are presented which reveal that the pericardium exerts a profound influence on the pressure-volume relation of the left ventricle and that shifts in the P-V curve can occur in patients without changes in ventricular properties.

An exciting study in man, using the non-invasive techniques of Doppler ultrasonography and echocardiography is the topic of the third chapter, and provides new information on blood velocity, flow patterns and valve motion.

The following chapter investigates the relationship between relaxation rate and afterload in the isovolumic rabbit heart. Extrasystoles are used to generate contractions with large changes in afterload and then analyzed with an interesting method employing a normalized phase-plane plot of a contractility index vs. pressure. The negative area of the plot reveals changes in relaxation.

The next chapter is mathematically oriented and describes a finite-element method to compute stress and strain in the myocardium. The highest values for both were found at the endocardium, decreasing toward the epicardium.

An important method to produce shifts in the diastolic pressure-volume relation is the use of nitrates. The sixth chapter presents patient studies showing that venodilation produces preload and afterload reduction with consequent decreased end-diastolic pressure and increased cardiac output.

The next chapter describes an autoregression model to provide the transfer function from diastolic filling period and pressure to aortic pressure amplitude, which is applied to patients with atrial fibrillation.

The final contribution to the section is concerned with the effects of pulmonary emboli in the dog: if left atrial filling is thus impaired, then the "reservoir" will not provide adequate inflow to the left ventricle.

In section 4, *Pump function and ejection – interaction with systemic load and coronary perfusion* are the topics. Four chapters of this section deal with pump function and ejection, another four describe various aspects of coronary circulation.

Undoubtedly our knowledge of the relation between left ventricle and arterial system is still far from complete. Perhaps this is at least partially due to the fact that of the variables: pressure, aortic flow and left ventricular volume, only the first one is easily accessible (at least in clinical situations). It is therefore interesting that in two of the chapters pressure and flow are analyzed and in two other chapters measurements of pressure and left ventricular volume are the starting points to further thoughts.

As regards coronary circulation and its determinants, the clinical situation demands that much research is done in this area, not only to better understand diminished flow through narrowed (atherosclerotic) arteries, but also to explain angiographic findings, myocardial infarction in seemingly normal coronaries and to guide surgical intervention. Results of research presented here include dog experimental studies on evoked transient disappearance of a large coronary artery and mechanisms behind it (ischemia?) are discussed. The techniques to produce experimental partial obstruction of coronaries are improved upon. A study on quantification of extravascular coronary resistance is included and coronary flow determinants such as perfusion pressure, vascular tension and intra-myocardial pressure are studied by simulation.

*Measuring cardiac performance – aims and validity of invasive and non-invasive measurement* is the subject of Section 5. Now that the swing of the pendulum is definitely moving towards non-invasive measurements it is only natural that we demand them to be as accurate as the invasive ones often necessary for clinical assessment and decision making. On the invasive side, the first two chapters of this section deal with the precision of measurements with the balloon flotation catheter, better known as the Swan-Ganz catheter, and with new developments in angiocardiography. The latter ones render them almost non-invasive: only venous injections of small amounts of dye are needed to obtain clearly delineated ventricular contours with the aid of contrast subtraction and digital image processing. These chapters also provide overviews of the complete topic. Of the non-invasive signal, the old and trusted electrocardiogram is still in full swing and the ballistocardiogram may well begin its come-back now that standards from normal males are applied to cardiac patients. Great expectations can be put on two-dimensional echocardiography for the assessment of cardiac function.

Theoretical considerations on what happens in myocardial-infarcted hearts and to the left ventricular center of mass are evaluated in model studies as well as in man. Newer techniques are also presented such as radiocardiography in coronary patients and transcutaneous aortavelography in normal males, while the long advocated and often doubted value of systolic time intervals is revisited. Of particular interest finally is the chapter incorporating advanced thinking on the interrelationship of various parameters during infusion of positive inotropic agents.

The last Section (6) of the book is concerned with *Energy losses – hemodynamics of valves*. The section heads off with a chapter by Bellhouse, describing the role of vortices in natural cardiac valves, prosthetic valves and in a compact membrane lung. In the second chapter, Lee writes with personal delight of the marriage between basic and applied science; between engineers and clinicians.

A mathematical analysis based on model studies of the aortic valve in the chapter by Van Steenhoven is shown to agree with cinematographic observations of the aortic valve and phasic flow measurements in the dog. The importance of the sinus vortices and pressure gradient in aortic valve closure is described analytically and verified in model studies in the fourth chapter. The interested reader may discover differences of opinion regarding the mechanism of aortic valve closure between this approach by Bellhouse and the one by Van Steenhoven, and about the mechanism of mitral valve vortex formation between Bellhouse's first chapter and Yellin's contribution in Section 3.

Aortic stenosis is modeled in the next chapter. Good agreement is found between the model studies and the results predicted by an analysis based on the conservation of energy and momentum.

A less sophisticated approach requiring several simplifying assumptions, next investigates energy losses across prosthetic mitral valves, and discusses the *in-vivo* conditions under which the Gorlin equation gives grossly inaccurate results.

Finally, to end on an optimistic note for the future of noninvasive cardiology, ultrasound is used to measure aortic and intracardiac blood-flow velocities in athletes and in patients with mitral regurgitation and with mitral stenosis. This method holds great promise.

The book concludes with a chapter in which Noordergraaf sums up the material presented at the Conference and puts much of it in a historical perspective. In addition, new considerations are given for the evaluation of myocardial performance using the time-dependent quantity of ventricular compliance.

In conclusion, the contents of this book could not have been produced without the cross-pollenation of the physical and life sciences. Their off-spring called Cardiac Dynamics, is as yet immature and searching for its identity. Though unknown at this stage to which proportions its character, unmistakably present, may grow, its potentials for significant contributions to the scientific world are great, provided the child continues to receive devoted parental guidance and stimulation.

JAN BAAN, PH.D.
*University of Leiden*

ALEXANDER C. ARNTZENIUS, M.D.
*University of Leiden*

EDWARD L. YELLIN, PH.D.
*Albert Einstein College of Medicine*

# ACKNOWLEDGEMENTS

The editors wish to express their gratitude to all who have contributed to the success of the Conference from which this book resulted, and to the realization of the book itself.

In the first place, thanks are due to the chairmen of the conference, who, in addition, were instrumental in the selection and reviewing process of the presented material: Paul Heintzen, Paul Hugenholtz, Brian Jewell, Grant Lee, Scott Rankin, Bob Reneman, Kiichi Sagawa, Wolfgang Schaper, Don Schultz, John Tyberg and Saul Winegrad all did a great job.

Secondly, we would like to thank the special contributors Jeremy Swan, Brian Bellhouse and Bram Noordergraaf who gave the lectures sponsored by the Cardiovascular System Dynamics Conference.

The organization of the conference, nor the publication of this volume, would have been possible without the organizing talents of Ms. Patricia Steen, the continuous assistance of Ms. Joke Vijlbrief and the contributions of Ms. Anke Biemans-Lens, Ms. Corry Korenromp-Roos and Ms. J. Loo-de Bruin.

Finally, we would like to acknowledge the financial support given by the following organizations in the Netherlands:

- ACF Chemiefarma N.V., Maarssen
- Astra Pharmaceutica B.V., Rijswijk
- Ciba Geigy B.V., Arnhem
- Gould Godart B.V., Bilthoven
- Herman Snellen Fund, Leiden
- Hilekes B.V., Bussum
- Hoek Loos B.V., Schiedam
- Hoffman-La Roche B.V., Mijdrecht
- ICI Holland B.V., Rotterdam
- Kooyker N.V., Leiden
- Laméris Instrumenten B.V., Utrecht
- Merck Sharp & Dohme B.V., Haarlem
- Philips Nederland B.V., Eindhoven
- Roussel Laboratoria B.V., Hoevelaken
- Sandoz B.V., Uden
- Siemens Nederlands N.V., Amsterdam
- Skalar Instrumenten B.V., Delft
- Smith Kline & French B.V., Rijswijk
- The Netherlands Heart Foundation, The Hague

*Leiden, October 1979*                                    THE EDITORS

# LIST OF CONTRIBUTORS

Page

Abel, Francis L., M.D., Ph.D.   369
Department of Physiology,
University of South Carolina,
Columbia, SC 29208, USA

Alderman, Edwin L., M.D.   417
Department of Medicine,
Stanford University School of
Medicine, Stanford, CA 94305,
USA

Aouw Jong, Tjong, M.D.   279
Department of Cardiology,
Leiden University Hospital, Leiden.
Netherlands

Arntzenius, Alexander C., M.D.   ix
Department of Cardiology,
Leiden University Hospital,
Leiden, Netherlands

Arts, Theo, Ph.D.   115
Department of Biophysics,
University of Limburg,
Biomedical Centre,
Beeldsnijdersdreef 101, 6126 EA
Maastricht, Netherlands

Baan, Jan, Ph.D.   ix, 123, 279
Clinical Physiology Laboratory,
Department of Pediatrics,
Leiden University Hospital,
Leiden, Netherlands

Bancroft Jr., W.H., M.S.   433
Veterans' Administration
Hospital, Birmingham, AL,
USA

Becker, Ronald M, M.D.   509
Department of Surgery, Albert
Einstein College of Medicine,
Bronx, NY 10461, USA

Bellhouse, Brian, D.Phil.   443, 489
Department of Engineering
Science, University of Oxford,
Parks Road, Oxford OX1 3PJ,
UK

Blangé, T., M.D.   69
Laboratory for Physiology,

University of Amsterdam,
1e Constantijn Huygensstraat 20,
Amsterdam, Netherlands

Bloom, D.S., M.D.   381
Department of Physiology,
Middlesex Hospital, Cleveland
St., London W1, UK

Boom, Herman B.K., Ph.D.   51
Twente Technical University,
P.O. Box 217, Enschede,
Netherlands

Brun, P., M.D.   169
Groupe de Recherche U 138 de
l'INSERM, Service
d'Exploration Fonctionnelle,
Hôpital Henri Mondor, 94 000
Créteil, France

Cherry, G.W., D.Phil.   231
Department of Engineering
Science, Oxford University,
Parks Road, Oxford, UK

Clark, Colin, Ph.D.   497
Department of Engineering
Science, Oxford University,
Parks Road, Oxford OX1 3PJ,
UK

Clay, Tim, M.D.   301
Cardiovascular Research Unit,
Royal Postgraduate Medical
School, Du Cane Rd., London
W 12, UK

Cobo, Julio, M.D.   405
Facultad de Medicina,
Universidad de Granada,
Granada, Spain

Coghlan, H. Cecil, M.D.   395
Department of Surgery,
University of Alabama in
Birmingham, University
Station, Birmingham, AL
35294, USA

Corday, Eliot, M.D.   405
University of California School

of Medicine, Los Angeles, CA,
USA

Dantan, P., Ph.D.                                    169
Laboratoire d'Hydrodynamique
et de Rhéologie, Université
Paris VII, F 75006 Paris,
France

Daughters II, George T., M.S.                        417
Palo Alto Medical Research
Foundation, 860 Bryant Street,
Palo Alto, CA 94301, USA

De Beer, E.L., Ph.D.                                  37
Department of Physiology,
University of Utrecht,
Vondellaan 24, 3521 GG
Utrecht, Netherlands

Denier van der Gon, J.J., Ph.D.                      135
Department of Medical and
Physiological Physics,
University of Utrecht,
Princetonplein 5, 3508 TA
Utrecht, Netherlands

Dinaburg, A.G., M.D.                                 433
Ballistocardiograph Laboratory,
Herrick Hospital, Berkeley, CA,
USA

Doll, Jürgen, Dr.                                    387
Institut für Nuklearmedizin,
Deutsches
Krebsforschungszentrum, Im
Neuenheimer Feld, D 6900
Heidelberg 1, FRG

Eddleman Jr., E.E., M.D.                             433
Veterans' Administration
Hospital, Birmingham, AL,
USA

El-Shuraydeh, Khaled N.B., M.S.
Laboratory for Medical
Physics, University of Utrecht,
De Uithof, Utrecht,
Netherlands

Fich, Sylvan, M.S.                                   355
Department of Electrical
Engineering, Rutgers
University, New Brunswick, NJ,
USA

Folts, John D., Ph.D.                                311
Cardiology Section,
Department of Medicine,
University of Wisconsin,
600 Highland Ave., Madison, WI
53792, USA

Fox, Kim M., M.D.                                    301

Cardiovascular Research Unit,
Royal Postgraduate Medical
School, Du Cane Rd., London
W 12, UK

Frater, Robert W.M., M.D.                    145, 509
Department of Surgery, Albert
Einstein College of Medicine,
Bronx, NY 10461, USA

Gabbay, Shlomo, M.D.                                 509
Department of Surgery, Albert
Einstein College of Medicine,
Bronx, NY 10461, USA

Glantz, Stanton A., Ph.D.                            159
Cardiovasular Research
Institute, 1315 – Moffitt
Hospital, University of
California, San Francisco, San
Francisco, CA 94143, ·USA

Gundel, W.D., M.D.                                   231
Cardiac Department, John
Radcliffe Hospital, Oxford, UK

Heethaar, Robert M.,                                 191
Department of Cardiology,
University Hospital Utrecht,
Utrecht, Netherlands

Heintzen, Paul H., M.D.                              333
Abteilung Kinderkardiologie,
Universität Kiel, Schwanenweg 20,
D-2300 Kiel, FRG

Heng, Ming, M.D.                                     405
University of California School
of Medicine, Los Angeles, CA,
USA

Hoki, Noritake, M.D.                                 293
Department of Medical
Engineering and Systems
Cardiology, Kawasaki Medical
School, Matsushima 577,
Kurashiki 701-01, Japan

Holdefer, Wilfred F., M.D.                           395
Department of Surgery,
University of Alabama in
Birmingham, University
Station, Birmingham, AL
35294, USA

Hugenholtz, Paul G., M.D.                            339
Department of Cardiology,
Thorax Centre, Erasmus
University, P.O. Box 1738,
Rotterdam, Netherlands

Huisman, P.H.,                                       231
Experimental Cardiology
Laboratory, Department of

Cardiology, University of
Leiden Medical School, c/o
Laboratory for Physiology,
Wassenaarseweg 62, Leiden,
Netherlands
Hunter, William C., Ph.D. 123
Clinical Physiology Laboratory,
Department of Pediatrics,
Leiden University Hospital,
Leiden, Netherlands
Huntsman, Lee L., Ph.D. 45
Center for Bioengineering,
University of Washington,
Seattle, WA 98105, USA

Ingels Jr., Neil B., Ph.D. 417
Bioengineering and Physiology
Division, Palo Alto Medical
Research Foundation,
860 Bryant Street, Palo Alto, CA
94301, USA
Inoue, Michitoshi, M.D. 293
the First Department of
Internal Medicine, Osaka
University Medical School,
Fukushima, Osaka, Japan.

Jewell, Brian R., M.D., Ph.D. 3
Department of Physiology,
New Medical and Dental Bldg.,
The University, Leeds LS2
9NQ, UK
Joseph, Daniel S., M.S. 45
Center for Bioengineering,
University of Washington,
Seattle, WA 98105, USA

Kajiya, Fumihiko, M.D. 293
Department of Medical
Engineering and Systems
Cardiology, Kawasaki Medical
School, Matsushima 577,
Kurashiki 701-01, Japan
Kenner, T., M.D. 209, 261
Physiologisches Institut der
Universität Graz A-8010 Graz,
Harrachgasse 21/V, Austria
Kerkhof, Peter L.M., M.S. 279
Clinical Physiology Laboratory,
Department of Pediatrics,
University Hospital, Leiden,
Netherlands
Knapp, Wolfram H., Dr. 387
Institut für Nuklearmedizin,
Deutsches
Krebsforschungszentrum

Heidelberg, FRG
Koops, Jan 279
Department of Cardiology,
Leiden University Hospital,
Leiden, Netherlands
Kresh, J. Yasha, Ph.D. 355
Department of Surgery, Div. of
Cardiothoracic Surgery,
Jefferson Medical College, 1025
Walnut St., Philadelphia, PA
19107, USA
Kübler, Wolfgang, Dr. 387
Med. Univ.-Klinik Heidelberg,
Abt. Innere Medizin III
(Kardiologie), Bergheimer Str. 58,
D 6900 Heidelberg 1, FRG
Kulikowski, Casimir, Ph.D. 355
Mt. Sinai Rutgers Computer,
Health-Care Laboratory,
Rutgers University, New
Brunswick, NJ, USA

Lab, Max J., Ph.D., M.B., B.Ch. 61
Department of Physiology,
Charing Cross Hospital
Medical School, Fulham Palace
Road, London W6 8RF, UK
Laporte, J.P., M.D. 169
Groupe de Recherche U 138 de
l'INSERM, Service
d'Exploration Fonctionnelle,
Hôpital Henri Mondor, 94 000
Créteil, France
Laurent, F., M.D. 169
Groupe de Recherche U 138 de
l'INSERM, Service
d'Exploration Fonctionnelle,
Hôpital Henri Mondor, 94 000
Créteil, France
Lee, Grant de J., M.D. 231, 463
Cardiac Department, John
Radcliffe Hospital, Oxford, UK
Light, L.H. Ph.D. 381
Division of Bioengineering,
Northwick Park Hospital,
Watford Road, Harrow,
Middlesex HA1 3UJ, UK
Llamas, Roberto, M.D. 217
Miami Heart Institute, 4701
North Meridian Avenue,
Miami Beach, FL 33140, USA

Mayrovitz, Harvey N., Ph.D. 217
Miami Heart Institute, 4701 North
Meridian Avenue, Miami Beach,
FL 33140, USA

McQueen, David, Ph.D.                509
   Courant Institute of
   Mathematical Sciences, New
   York University, New York,
   N.Y. 10017, USA
Mead, Carol, B.S.                    417
   Palo Alto Medical Research
   Foundation, 860 Bryant Street,
   Palo Alto, CA 94301, USA
Meerbaum, Samuel, Ph.D.              405
   Cedars-Sinai Medical Center,
   8700 Beverly Blvd., Los
   Angeles, CA 90048, USA
Mehmel, Helmuth C., Dr.              387
   Med. Univ.-Klinik Heidelberg,
   Abt. Innere Medizin III
   (Kardiologie), Bergheimer Str. 58,
   D 6900 Heidelberg 1, FRG
Min, Byoung G., Ph.D.                355
   Department of Electrical
   Engineering, Rutgers
   University, New Brunswick, NJ,
   USA
Misbach, Gregory A., M.D.            159
   Cardiovascular Research
   Institute, 1315-Moffitt Hospital,
   University of California, San
   Francisco, San Francisco, CA
   94143, USA
Moene, Rudolf, J., M.D.              279
   Department of Pediatric
   Cardiology, Free University
   Hospital, Amsterdam,
   Netherlands

Nagelsmit, Michiel, J., M.D.          25
   Experimental Cardiology
   Laboratory, Department of
   Cardiology, Leiden University
   Medical School, c/o Laboratory
   for Physiology,
   Wassenaarseweg 62, Leiden,
   Netherlands
Nelson, Clifford V., Ph.D.           339
   Department of Research, Maine
   Medical Center, Portland, ME
   04102, USA
Neufeld, Henry N., M.D.              197
   Heart Institute, Sheba Tel
   Hashomer Medical Center and
   Sackler School of Medicine, Tel
   Aviv, Israel
Nieuwenhuijs, J.H.M., D.V.M.         183
   Laboratory for Physiology,
   University of Utrecht,
   Vondellaan 24, Utrecht,
   Netherlands

Noordergraaf, Abraham, Ph.D.         531
   Department of Bioengineering
   D2, University of Pennsylvania,
   Philadelphia, PA 19104, USA
Oddou, C., Ph.D.                     169
   Laboratoire d'Hydrodynamique
   et de Rhéologie, Université
   Paris VII, F 75006 Paris,
   France

Parmley, William W., M.D.            159
   Cardiovascular Research
   Institute, 1315-Moffitt Hospital,
   University of California, San
   Francisco, San Francisco, CA
   94143, USA
Perrot, P.                           169
   Laboratoire d'Hydrodynamique
   et de Rhéologie, Université
   Paris VII, F 75006 Paris,
   France
Pfeiffer, K.P., M.A.            209, 261
   Physiologisches Institut der
   Universität Graz, A-8010 Graz,
   Harrachgasse 21/V, Austria

Rabinowitz, Babeth, M.D.             197
   Heart Institute, Sheba Tel
   Hashomer Medical Center and
   Sackler School of Medicine, Tel
   Aviv, Israel
Raines, Jeff, Ph.D.                  217
   Miami Heart Institute, 4701
   North Meridian Avenue,
   Miami Beach, Florida 33140,
   USA
Rajagopalan, B., D.Phil.             231
   Cardiac Department, John
   Radcliffe Hospital, Oxford,
   UK
Rankin, J. Scott, M.D.                95
   Department of Surgery, Duke
   University Medical Center,
   Durham, NC 27710, USA
Reneman, Robert S., M.D.        115, 477
   Department of Physiology,
   University of Limburg
   Biomedical Centre,
   Beeldsnijdersdreef 101, 6216 EA
   Maastricht, Netherlands
Rijnsburger, Wim H., M.S.             25
   Experimental Cardiology
   Laboratory, Department of
   Cardiology, Leiden University
   Medical School, c/o Laboratory
   for Physiology,

Wassenaarseweg 62, Leiden,
Netherlands
Ross, M. Alison, M.A. 107
SM – 42, University of
Washington, Seattle, WA
98195, USA
Sagawa, Kiichi, M.D., Ph.D. 81, 271
Department of Biomedical
Engineering, The Johns
Hopkins University School of
Medicine, Baltimore, Maryland
21205, USA
Sayers, Bruce McA., Ph.D. 395
London, UK
Schaefer, J., M.D. 209
1. Medizinische Klinik, D-23
Kiel, Schittenhelmstr. 12, FRG
Schamhardt, H.C., M.S. 37
Cardiovascular Research
Center, Erasmus University,
P.O. Box 1738, Rotterdam,
Netherlands
Schaper, Wolfgang, M.D. 249
Max-Planck-Institute for
Physiology and Clinical
Research, Parkstrasse 1, D-6350
Bad Nauheim, FRG
Schiereck, Piet, Ph.D. 51
Laboratory for Medical
Physiology, University of
Utrecht, Vondellaan 24,
Utrecht, Netherlands
Schipperheijn, J.J., M.D. 231
Experimental Cardiology
Laboratory, Department of
Cardiology, University of
Leiden Medical School, c/o
Laboratory for Physiology,
Wassenaarseweg 62, Leiden,
Netherlands
Schultz, D.L., D.Phil. 231
Department of Engineering
Science, Oxford University,
Parks Road, Oxford, UK
Selwyn, A.P., M.D. 301
Cardiovascular Research Unit,
Royal Postgraduate Medical
School, Du Cane Rd., London
W12, UK
Sheppard, Louis C., Ph.D. 395
Department of Surgery,
University of Alabama in
Birmingham, University
Station, Birmingham, AL
35294, USA
Sonnenblick, Edmund H., M.D. 145
Department of Medicine, Albert

Einstein College of Medicine,
Bronx, N.Y. 10461, USA
Stienen, G.J.M., M.S. 69
Laboratory for Physiology,
University of Amsterdam, 1e
Constantijn Huygensstraat 20,
Amsterdam, Netherlands
Stinson, Edward B., M.D. 417
Cardiovascular Surgery
Department, Stanford
University School of Medicine,
Stanford, CA 94305, USA
Streeter, Daniel D., Ph.D. 107
Cardiology Division, The
Children's Orthopedic Hospital
and Medical Center, P.O. Box
C-5371, Seattle, WA 98105,
USA
Strom, Joel A., M.D. 509
Department of Medicine, Àlbert
Einstein College of Medicine,
Bronx, N.Y. 10461, USA
Suga, Hiroyuki, M.D., D.M.Sc. 271
Department of Cardiac
Physiology, Research Institute,
National Cardiovascular
Center, Suita, Osaka 565,
Japan
Swan, H.J.C., M.D., Ph.D. 323
Department of Cardiology,
Cedars-Sinai Medical Center,
8700 Beverly Boulevard, Los
Angeles, CA 90048, USA

Tamari, Israel, M.D. 197
Heart Institute, Sheba Tel
Hashomer Medical Center and
Sackler School of Medicine, Tel
Aviv, Israel
Tan, L.B., D.Phil. 231
Department of Engineering
Science, Oxford University,
Parks Road, Oxford, UK
Ter Keurs, Henk E.D.J., M.D. 25
Experimental Cardiology
Laboratory, Department of
Cardiology, Leiden University
Medical School, c/o Laboratory
for Physiology,
Wassenaarseweg 62, Leiden,
Netherlands
Tillmans, Harald, Dr. 387
Med. Univ.-Klinik Heidelberg,
Abt. Innere Medizin III
(Kardiologie), Bergheimer Str. 58,
D 6900 Heidelberg 1, FRG
Tunstall Pedoe, Dan S., M.B.,

D.Phil., FRCP                                      521
  Cardiac Department, St.
  Bartholomews Hospital, West
  Smithfield, London EC1A 7BE, UK

Tyberg, John V., M.D., Ph.D.                       159
  Cardiovascular Research
  Institute, 1315-Moffitt Hospital,
  University of California, San
  Francisco, San Francisco, CA
  94143, USA

Van den Broek, J.H.J.M., Ph.D.                     135
  Department of Medical and
  Physiological Physics, Univer-
  sity of Utrecht, Princetonplein 5,
  3508 TA Utrecht,
  Netherlands

Van der Werf, Tjeerd, M.D.                         191
  Department of Cardiology,
  University Hospital Utrecht,
  Utrecht, Netherlands

Van Dijk, Arjan D., B.S.                           279
  Clinical Physiology Laboratory,
  Department of Pediatrics,
  Leiden University Hospital,
  Leiden, Netherlands

Van Heuningen, Rob                                 25
  Experimental Cardiology
  Laboratory, Department of
  Cardiology, Leiden University
  Medical School, c/o Laboratory
  for Physiology,
  Wassenaarseweg 62, Leiden,
  Netherlands

Van Steenhoven, Anton A., Ph.D.                    477
  Department of Mechanical
  Engineering, Eindhoven
  University of Technology, P.O.
  Box 513, 5600 MB Eindhoven,
  Netherlands

Veenstra, Pieter C., Ph.D.               115, 477
  Department of Mechanical
  Engineering, Eindhoven
  University of Technology, P.O.
  Box 513, 5600 MB Eindhoven,
  Netherlands

Venderink, D.J., M.S.                              183
  Bloemstraat 12, Utrecht,
  Netherlands

Verlaan, Cees W.J.,                                477
  Department of Physiology,
  University of Limburg, P.O.
  Box 616, 6200 ME Maastricht,
  Netherlands

Von Olshausen, Klaus, M.D.                         387
  Med. Univ.-Klinik Heidelberg,
  Abt. Innere Medizin III
  (Kardiologie), Bergheimer Str. 58,
  D 6900 Heidelberg 1, FRG

Welkowitz, Walter, Ph.D.                           355
  Department of Electrical
  Engineering, Rutgers
  University, New Brunswick, NJ,
  USA

Winegrad, Saul, M.D.                               11
  Department of Physiology,
  University of Pennsylvania,
  School of Medicine,
  Philadelphia, PA 19104, USA

Woollard, Keith V., M.B., B.S.,
M.R.C.P.                                           61
  Department of Cardiology,
  Charing Cross Hospital, Fulham
  Palace Road, London W6 8RF,
  UK

Wüsten, Bernd, M.D.                                249
  Zentrum für Innere Medizin
  am Klinikum der Justus-
  Liebig-Universität, Klinikstrasse 36,
  D-6300 Giessen, FRG

Wyatt, H.L., Ph.D.                                 405
  Cedars-Sinai Medical Center,
  8700 Beverly Blvd., Los
  Angeles, CA 90048, USA

Yellin, Edward L., Ph.D.          ix, 145, 509
  Department of Surgery, Albert
  Einstein College of Medicine,
  Bronx, NY 10461, USA

SECTION 1

# CARDIAC MUSCLE MECHANICS: FROM THE FIBER DOWN TO THE SARCOMERE

## 1.1. THE COMING OF AGE OF
## CARDIAC MUSCLE MECHANICS

BRIAN R. JEWELL

When I was invited to make the opening presentation at this conference Dr. Baan suggested that I make some provocative remarks in the hope, I think, that we would have a more interesting and lively session if I could get some adrenaline circulating from the start. It is an honour to be entrusted with this task and perhaps I should begin by pointing out that if this conference had been held four or five years ago there could not have been a session entitled "Cardiac Muscle Mechanics: From the Fibre down to the Sarcomere," as nothing was known at that time about cardiac muscle mechanics at the sarcomere level. I doubt if this could be said of any other of the sessions at this conference!

Over the past four years new and sophisticated techniques have been used to study the properties of isolated preparations of cardiac muscle, and I do not think it is an exaggeration to say that we have entered a new era of cardiac muscle physiology. The state of the art is now such that cardiac muscle mechanics can, and should, cease to be the handmaiden of skeletal muscle mechanics, and I hope we shall soon see this subject "come of age" and emerge as a truly independent field of study.

In the first decade of cardiac muscle mechanics (1958–1968), the conceptual approach and experimental techniques that had been developed by A.V. Hill and others at University College, London, for the study of skeletal muscle were applied to isolated preparations of cardiac muscle. The first work usually quoted in this connection is the 1959 paper by Abbott and Mommaerts (1), but Trendelenburg and Lüllman (2) were in fact on the scene a year before that. However, it was Ed Sonnenblick (3, 4) who really put cardiac muscle on the map and most of the work on cardiac muscle mechanics over those first ten years came from his laboratory or from workers who had been associated with him at one time or another. The finishing touches were added by Dirk Brutsaert (5) who used phase plane techniques to show that a full description of the contractile event in cardiac muscle requires a three-dimensional plot of muscle length, velocity of shortening, and force.

The interpretation of the experimental results obtained during this period depended heavily on the use of analog models of muscle of the kind shown in Figure 1. The essential feature of such models is that the complex

*J. Baan, A.C. Arntzenius, E.L. Yellin (eds.), Cardiac Dynamics, 3–10.*

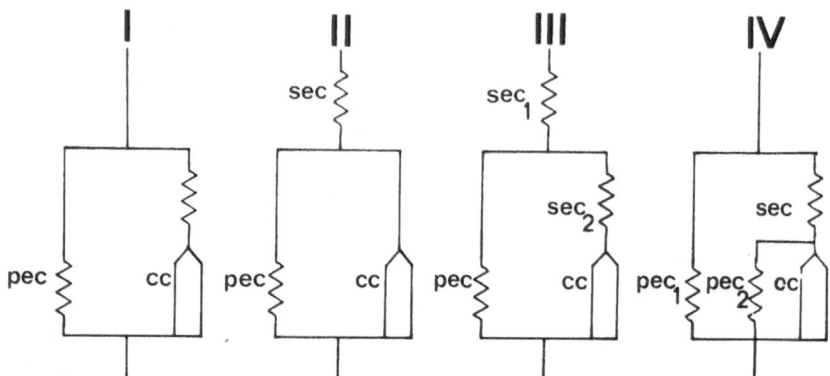

*Figure 1.* Analogs of muscle (6). SEC = series elastic component, PEC = parallel elastic component, CC = contractile component.

mechanical properties of the muscle can be simulated by the interaction of a collection of simple physical elements. These lumped elements are not intended to represent actual structures in the muscle, and the corollary of this is that it is a mistake to look for structures which might have similar properties to elements in the model (7).

From 1958 onwards the classical approach to muscle mechanics was progressively abandoned by skeletal muscle physiologists for reasons that have been reviewed by Simmons and Jewell (8), but a blind eye was turned to this cloud on the horizon by those interested in cardiac muscle. Here I must be careful to avoid any hypocrisy: the papers by Jewell and Wilkie in 1958 and 1960 (9, 10) were the first nails in the coffin of the classical approach to muscle mechanics, yet as late as 1968 (6) and 1972 (11) I was the co-author of reviews of cardiac muscle mechanics in which the continuing use of analog models of the kind shown in Figure 1 was accepted without serious protest. The problem for us, as for everyone else interested in this subject, was that we had no real alternative. The new approach to muscle mechanics that was being vigorously pursued in A.F. Huxley's laboratory (12) and R.J. Podolsky's laboratory (13) seemed out of reach of cardiac muscle physiologists because of the lack of suitable single cell preparations and of techniques for measuring sarcomere length in multicellular preparations such as the cat papillary muscle. So much effort had been expended already in characterizing that particular preparation that people in the field were reluctant to look for other, more suitable, preparations because of the vast amount of groundwork that would have to be done. And so, for want of a viable alternative, the classical approach continued to thrive.

I think it is fair to say that we then lived through several years of stagnation (1969–1974) during which there was consolidation of existing knowledge, but no important new developments in the field of cardiac muscle mechanics. Perhaps it was inevitable that a breakthrough could come only from people who had not been brought up on a diet of cat papillary muscle and classical muscle mechanics. It came from two laboratories: Jerry Pollack's in Seattle and Fred Julian's in Boston. These groups were bold enough to look for new preparations that would be more suitable for mechanical studies at the sarcomere level, and they had the technical knowhow to master the sophisticated technology that such studies entail.

In 1975 full papers were published by both groups (14, 15) on the length-tension relation in rat papillary muscle with measurements of mean sarcomere length instead of simply muscle length, and I regard 1975 as the beginning of the new era referred to earlier. This was also the year in which Alex and Francoise Fabiato (16) published length-tension curves for single rat ventricular muscle fibres which had been mechanically "skinned" (i.e. sarcolemma removed by microdissection). I shall have more to say about these later in my talk.

An example of the new data obtained at this time is given in Figure 2, which is taken from the 1975 paper by Krueger and Pollack (14). The upper panel shows conventional length-tension curves for rat papillary muscle with muscle length as the abscissa. The lower panel shows the mean sarcomere lengths during rest and activity at each muscle length, as determined from the diffraction pattern produced by shining a laser beam through the central (undamaged) region of the preparation.

From the point of view of cardiac muscle mechanics generally, the most crucial point to emerge from studies at sarcomere level was that the extensible series elastic component, which had come to be regarded as a special feature of cardiac muscle, is largely, if not entirely, an artifact of the preparation. Sarcomeres in the central healthy part of the muscle shorten by about 10% because of stretching of the damaged ends, and maximum shortening occurs in contractions on the ascending limb of the length-tension relation, not at $L_{max}$ where maximum tension is developed. While this behaviour could perhaps be reconciled with what might be expected of a Voigt version of the three-component model (analog II or IV in Figure 1), is there any point in struggling to model what is patently artifactual behaviour?

The question this raises for those interested in deriving basic parameters such as $V_{max}$ from measurements on intact ventricles is what should be assumed about series elasticity in *undamaged* muscle. In skeletal muscle the component of series elasticity that cannot be attributed to the tendons at the end of the muscle is now considered to be an integral property of the contractile mechanism. This is incompatible with the classical approach, which treated the series elastic and contractile components as lumped elements with *independent* mechanical properties. Hopefully, answers to important questions about the true nature of series elasticity in cardiac

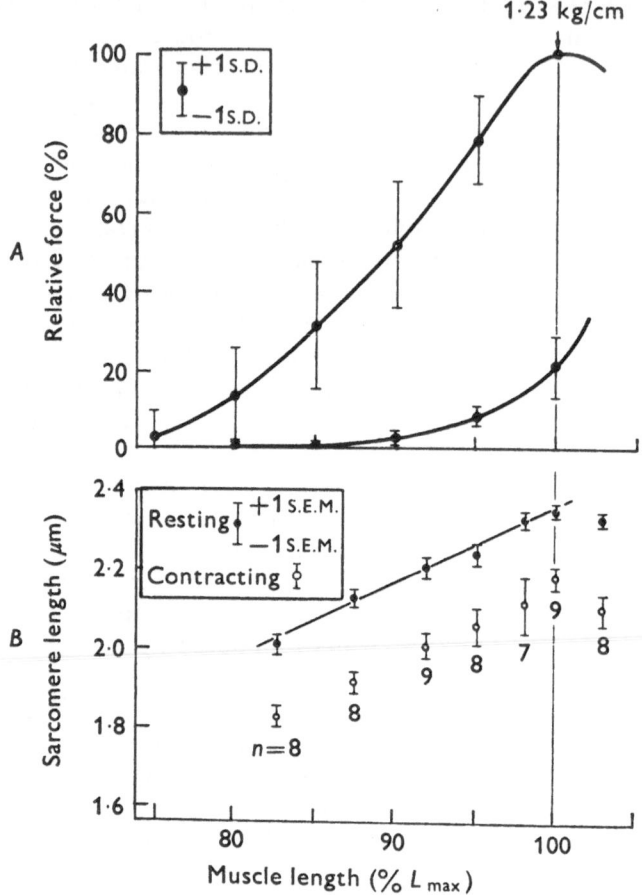

*Figure 2.* Length-tension curves for rat papillary muscle (top panel) with sarcomere lengths during rest and activity at each muscle length (bottom panel). The lower curve in the top panel shows resting tension and the upper curve shows active tension during contractions at each length (14).

muscle will emerge as detailed mechanical studies are carried out on the central undamaged region of isolated preparations with the aid of sarcomere length-clamping techniques.

I should like to turn now to another area of cardiac muscle physiology in which there have been far-reaching advances: this is in our understanding of the chain of events responsible for linking depolarization of the cell membrane to activation of the contractile protein system. The main steps in excitation-contraction are summarized in Figure 3 and the solid brackets on the right show the events that have been generally considered to be

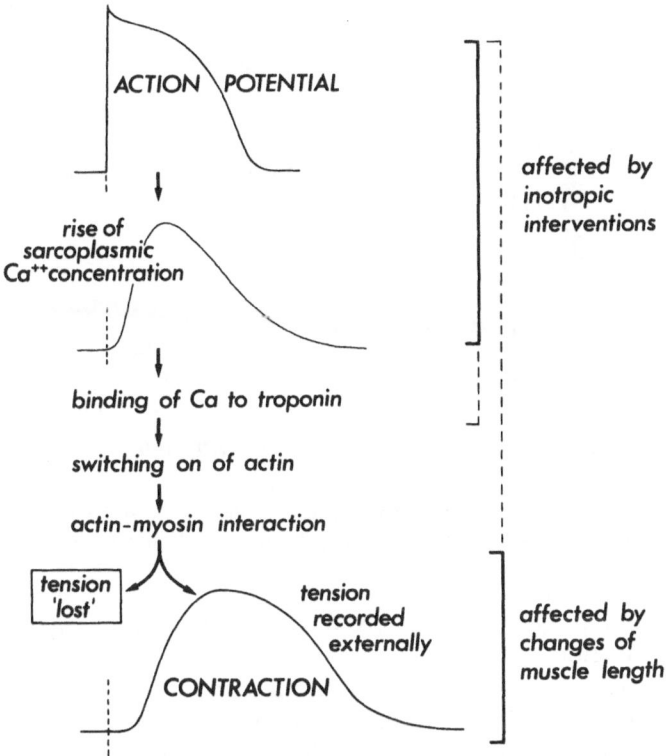

*Figure 3.* Schematic diagram of the main events in excitation-contraction coupling in cardiac muscle (17). The broken lines show how the brackets need to be extended to take account of recent findings.

influenced by inotropic intervention and by changes of muscle length (17). The upper bracket has been extended downwards slightly with a broken line in to include the possibility that inotropic intervention, in addition to increasing the maximum sarcoplasmic $Ca^{++}$ concentration reached in a twitch, may also alter the sensitivity of the system to calcium by affecting the degree of phosphorylation of troponin.

What I should like to focus on is the lower bracket, which has been extended upwards with a broken line to take account of the fact that length-dependence of activation processes seems to be largely responsible for the dependence of tension production on muscle length (and perhaps of myocardial performance on diastolic size in the intact heart). I reviewed some of the evidence for this last year in 1977 (18) and one of the most important arguments advanced was based on a comparison of the length-tension curves obtained for intact and skinned rat ventricular muscle (Figure 4). The curve obtained from sarcolemma-free (i.e. "skinned") muscle

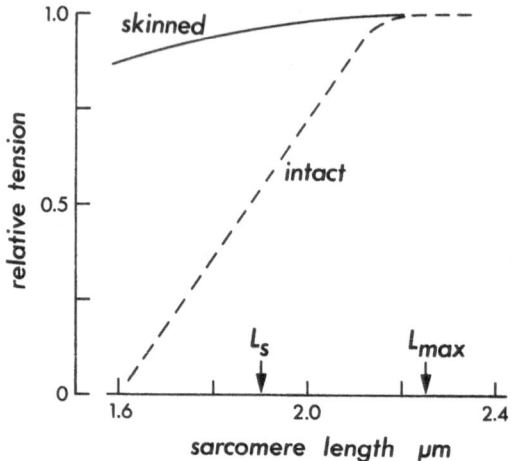

*Figure 4.* Length-tension curves showing the variation of tension production with sarcomere length in intact (19) and skinned (16) rat ventricular muscle: $L_{max}$ shows the *resting* sarcomere length at which maximum tension was developed and $L_s$ indicates the slack length of the muscle (18).

under conditions of maximal activation showed only a small decline of tension production with length over the range of sarcomere lengths covered by the ascending limb of the length-tension relation in intact muscle. This small decline of tension is the same as that observed in skinned and intact frog skeletal muscle fibres under conditions of maximal activation, and it is what would be expected from the sliding filament hypothesis. Some other factor must be responsible for the steep decline of tension production with muscle length observed in the intact muscle and there is now a growing body of evidence in support of the view that this factor is length-dependence of activation (18). According to this hypothesis, tension production declines at shorter muscle lengths because the contractile system is less completely activated. The two most likely possible mechanisms are (1) that the rise in sarcoplasmic $Ca^{++}$ concentration brought about by excitation of the cell is less at short muscle lengths, or (2) the sensitivity of the contractile systems to calcium is length-dependent. There is some evidence for and against each of these explanations (17) but the position should become a good deal clearer if it proves possible to extend the use of the photoprotein aequorin as an intracellular $Ca^{++}$ indicator to mammalian ventricular muscle (20).

I should like to end my introductory remarks for the opening session of this conference by posing six questions. The first three are for cardiac muscle physiologists.

1. What is the nature of series elasticity in undamaged cardiac muscle? Is it an integral part of the contractile mechanism?

2. Do inotropic interventions all work by altering early events in

excitation-contraction coupling, or do some of them modify contractile behaviour itself?

3. What is the underlying mechanism•of length-dependence of activation in cardiac muscle?

The three questions for cardiologists are:

1. Is it reasonable to continue to use any procedures, such as the calculation of $V_{max}$ from the rise in intraventricular pressure, that depend on analog models of the classical kind?

2. Is it reasonable to continue to use, or even to look for, indices of contractility that require the assumption that diastolic size and inotropic state are independent regulators of myocardial performance?

3. If the answer to each of those questions is negative, what is to be done to fill the conceptual vacuum that will be left by abandoning these fundamental ideas in cardiology?

When these questions can be answered entirely from our knowledge of cardiac muscle, rather than by borrowing or extrapolating from what is known about skeletal muscle, then the field of cardiac muscle mechanics will have "come of age." Hopefully, this will be in its twenty-first year, that is, in 1979.

REFERENCES

1. Abbott BC, Mommaerts WFHM: A study of inotropic mechanisms in the papillary muscle preparation. *J Gen Physiol* 42:533–551, 1959.
2. Trendelenburg U, Lüllman H: Über die Messung des "Active State" am Herzmuskel des Frosches. *Biochim Biophys Acta* 29:13–20, 1958.
3. Sonnenblick EH: Force-velocity relations in mammalian heart muscle. *Am J Physiol* 202:931–939, 1962.
4. Sonnenblick EH: In: *The myocardial cell*, SA Briller, HL Conn (eds), Philadelphia, University of Pennsylvania Press, 1966.
5. Brutsaert DL, Sonnenblick EH: Force-velocity-length-time relations of the contractile elements in heart muscle of the cat. *Circ Res* 24:137–149, 1969.
6. Jewell BR, Blinks JR: Drugs and the mechanical properties of heart muscle. *Am Rev Physiol* 8: 113–130, 1968.
7. Pringle JWS: Models of muscle. *Symp Soc Exptl Biol* 14:41–68, 1960.
8. Simmons RM, Jewell BR: Mechanics and models of muscular contraction. *Recent Adv Physiol* 9:87–147, 1974.
9. Jewell BR, Wilkie DR: An analysis of the mechanical components in frog's striated muscle. *J Physiol* 143:515–540, 1958.
10. Jewell BR, Wilkie DR: The mechanical properties of relaxing muscle. *J Physiol* 152:30–47, 1960.
11. Blinks JR, Jewell BR: The meaning and measurement of myocardial contractility. In: *Cardiovascular fluid dynamics*, vol 1, Bergel DH (ed), London, Academic Press, 1972, p 225 ff.
12. Huxley AF, Simmons RM: Mechanical transients and the origin of muscular force. *Cold Spring Harb Symp Quart Biol* 37:669–680, 1973.
13. Podolsky RJ, Nolan AC: Muscle contraction transients, cross-bridge kinetics, and the Fenn effect. *Cold Spring Harb Symp Quart Biol* 37:661–668, 1973.
14. Krueger JW, Pollack GH: Myocardial sarcomere dynamics during isometric contractions. *J Physiol* 251:627–643, 1975.

15. Julian FJ, Sollins MR: Sarcomere length-tension relations in living rat papillary muscle. *Circ Res* 37:299–308, 1975.
16. Fabiato A, Fabiato F: Dependence of the contractile activation of skinned cardiac muscle on the sarcomere length. *Nature* 256:54–56, 1975.
17. Jewell BR: The physiology of cardiac muscle contraction. In: *Developments in cardiovascular medicine*, edited by Dickinson CJ, Marks J (eds), Lancaster, MTP Press, 1978.
18. Jewell BR: A re-examination of the influence of muscle length on myocardial performance. *Circ Res* 40:221–230, 1977.
19. Pollack GH, Krueger JW: Sarcomere dynamics in intact cardiac muscle. *Eur J Cardiol* 4:53–65, 1976.
20. Allen DG, Blinks JR: Calcium transients in aequorin-injected frog cardiac muscle. *Nature* 273:509–513, 1978.

## 1.2. THE IMPORTANCE OF PASSIVE ELEMENTS IN THE CONTRACTION OF THE HEART

SAUL WINEGRAD

## 1. INTRODUCTION

During a single contraction of the heart the diameter of the left ventricle decreases much more than the distance from the base to the apex, the change in orientation of fibres through the thickness of the ventricular wall is not the same for all fibres, and the radii of curvature of different regions of the heart change by different amounts (Figure 1). Not every myocardial cell, therefore, is developing the same force or shortening by the same amount. These geometric changes of the heart are modified with an alteration in the performance. As the activities of the organism change from rest to intense activity, the amount of blood pumped by the heart per minute may increase 500–600%, and in order to meet these needs both the frequency of contraction and the percentage of the end-diastolic volume that is ejected during systole must increase. The time for filling and ejection is decreased (2). Since every cardiac cell normally contracts during every beat, the variable performance of the heart requires each cardiac cell to perform differently as cardiac output increases.

Each cell must possess the capability of independently varying initial length, force, amount of shortening, and rates of shortening and lengthening rapidly in order to produce the changes in end-diastolic volume, filling and systolic emptying that occur. The extent of change is not uniform for all cells. Cells alter their length and force in one region of the heart in a different way from cells in another region in accordance with the changes in wall thickness, radius of curvature, and the extent of systolic shortening.

There are basically only two ways in which differences in contractile performance may be regulated: (1) by modification of the force-generating system (including the electromechanical coupling process), or (2) by the placement of different loads on the individual cardiac cells. There is no indication that amount or the characteristics or the contractile system vary among different regions of the heart, and although the configuration of the action potential varies to some extent over the left ventricle the differences are nowhere near adequate to account for the differences in the contractile performance of individual cells (3). If the diversified performance depends on an intracellular regulatory system, an enormous amount of information

*J. Baan, A.C. Arntzenius, E.L. Yellin (eds.), Cardiac Dynamics, 11–23.*

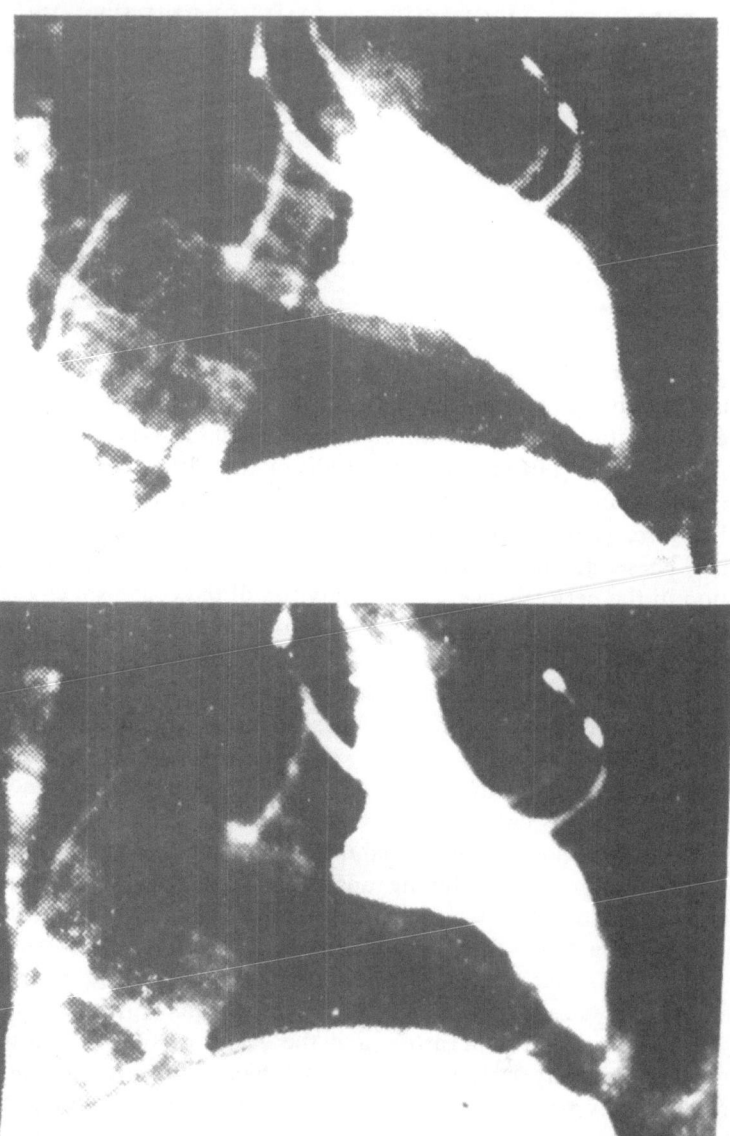

*Figure 1.* Appearance of left ventricular silhouette at end-diastole (above) and end-systole (below) on video monitor, demonstrating electronic recognition of left ventricular chamber borders (18 kg dog under morphine-pentobarbital anaesthesia; heart driven at 110 beats/min; A-V stimulus interval, 80 msec; injection, 1 ml into left ventricle in 0.75 sec). Opacified area has been outlined by electronic assembly which recognizes borders of area of increased roentgen opacity and "brightens" video signal (by increasing the voltage) as each horizontal video line encounters left and leaves right border of area (1).

would have to be communicated to the cardiac cells either for eacn contractile cycle, or, if an elaborate mechanism for the storage of information exists, for each contractile state. Neither type of information transfer has been identified. Although several phosphorylation sites have been identified on contractile proteins, and at least two are dynamic in cardiac muscle (4, 5, 6, 7, 8, 9, 10), only Ca sensitivity (11, 12, 13) has been clearly related to phosphorylation (14, 15).

Passive components of the myocardium built into its structure in the form of tissue loads could provide the mechanism for regulating the cardiac cells and their specific responses to different hemodynamic conditions. The resting length, operational range of length and net force produced by individual cells or groups of cells could be determined by the compliance of tissue loads, and the appropriate nonlinearity in the compliance could account for the different properties of contraction in different hemodynamic conditions. An added advantage of regulation by passive complaint structures is that part of the energy of contraction would be stored during systole and then converted to restoring force that would facilitate ventricular filling during relaxation (16). The more the ventricle emptied, the larger would be the work done against the elastic structures and the greater the energy available for restoring resting length and assisting filling. Most filling normally does occur immediately after systole when the contribution of the elastic force would be greatest, and the shape of the passive filling curve resembles that of a critically damped oscillator returning to its equilibrium point (2).

The tissue loads within the myocardium that are seen by the contractile system can be conveniently divided into intracellular, intercellular, and connective tissue-related components.

## 2. INTRACELLULAR COMPONENTS

The contractile filaments themselves are probably the major intracellular load on the contractile system. The sarcolemma is probably not mechanically important within the physiological range of length (17), since there is very little difference in the passive length-tension relation between intact and mechanically skinned frog skeletal fibres from 100% to 150% of rest length (2.1–3.2 $\mu$m sarcomere length). The viscosity of the myoplasma and other intracellular organelles are unlikely to be significant factors (18), and the mechanical role of the sarcoplasmic reticulum cannot be evaluated in view of the paucity of data.

Four parts of the myofibrils, the thin filaments, the thick filaments, the Z bands, and the M bridges are potential loads. Although movement per se of the thin filaments cannot have a major effect inasmuch as both skinned skeletal and skinned cardiac muscle have significant ranges of length over which maximum developed tension is relatively constant (19, 20, 21) there is resistance to shortening at short sarcomere lengths, where the thin filaments begin to cross the centre of the A band (22, 23, 24). Double overlap of thin filaments has never been clearly demonstrated in skeletal or cardiac muscle cells in the absence of active generation of force (25, 26, 27). Attempts to introduce contralateral thin filaments into a half sarcomere in resting skeletal muscle by embedding the cells in gelatin and compressing the gelatin have failed and resulted only in the production of wavy myofibrils (26). The reason for this resistance to increasing the number of thin filaments in a half sarcomere becomes clear when one examines serial transverse sections through the centre of a sarcomere in an actively shortened myofibril. In order to accommodate the contralateral thin filaments the ipselateral thin filaments move transversely from the trigonal position among three thick filaments to the space between two thick filaments (27) so that there is no apparent structural hindrance of the crossbridge access to thin filaments. The slight bending of the thin filaments that is required for this accommodation of additional thin filaments is no more than 2° and occurs over 100–200 nm, but it requires the performance of work by the contractile system. The resultant configuration resembles that of insect flight muscle, in which the ratio of thin to thick filaments is higher than it is in amphibian or mammalian cardiac muscle (22). The force involved has been estimated from the combination of $Ca^{++}$ necessary to produce double overlap of filaments in fragments of cardiac tissue with mechanically disrupted membranes and the tension generated in isometrically suspended mechanically skinned fibres at this concentration of activator $Ca^{++}$. It is about 5% of maximum force, a small but significant amount (Figure 2). This estimate is consistent with the observation that double overlap of thin filaments reduces maximal isometric tension of a skinned cardiac single cell by only a small amount. It is probably the energy stored in bent thin filaments that re-extends the skinned cardiac cell, whether freely suspended or mounted isometrically, to its original resting sarcomere length when activating Ca ions have been withdrawn as long as shortening has not been excessive. Shortening to sarcomere lengths of less than 1.5 $\mu$m produces irreversible changes in both filament organization and Ca-activated ATPase activity.

As the volume of the filament lattice in intact striated muscle remains constant during shortening (28), the distance between filaments increases and both the M bridges between the thick filaments and the Z band should undergo a strain. The Z band in electron micrographs of short myofibrils appears to be strained, but it has not been possible to evaluate its contribution to the internal load because in skinned fibres, where the relation between the internal load and sarcomere length can be estimated,

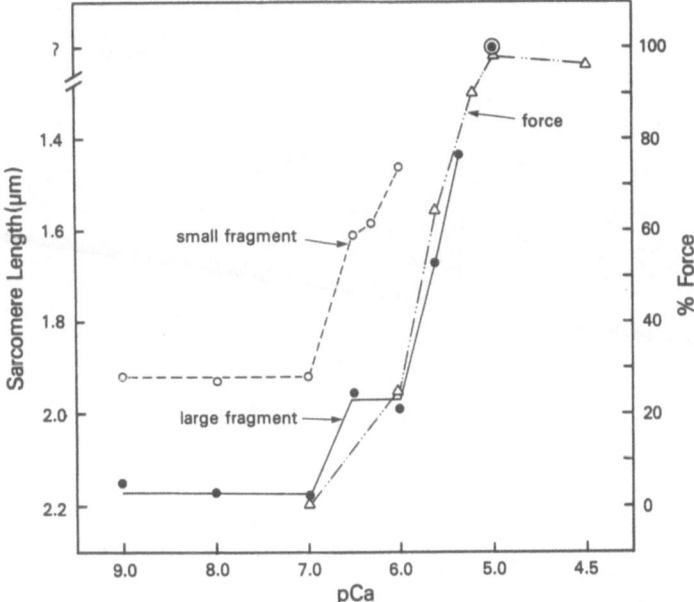

*Figure 2.* The relation between pCa and the sarcomere lengths of large and small fragments of rat ventricular muscle (see Figure 5). Fragments prepared by gentle homogenization allow Ca and other small ions and molecules into the sarcoplasmic from the bathing solution. It is possible to directly activate the contractile proteins with a Ca buffer system that blocks the influence of the Ca pump in the sarcoplasm reticulum. The fragments were freely suspended in the medium and their sarcomere lengths measured by either polarizing or differential interference microscopy. The sarcomere lengths are homogeneous. The larger fragment, which retains more of the tissue organization, has a longer resting, unloaded sarcomere length and a definite step at about the sarcomere length where thin filaments would be expected to cross the centre of sarcomere. The resting, unloaded sarcomere length of the small fragments is about the same as the length at which the step occurs in the larger fragments. The relation between force and pCa for a skinned fibre held isometrically at about 2.2 $\mu$m sarcomere length is included to allow the estimation of force required to produce shortening for small and larger fragments.

the constant volume of the filament lattice is not maintained at different sarcomere lengths (29). The lattice diameter remains constant presumably because the absence of a membrane destroys the Donnan equilibrium that is responsible for the constant volume (29).

## 3. INTERCELLULAR COMPONENTS

In addition to intercalated discs the myocardium has other intercellular connections involving the cell coat, microfilaments that physically resemble

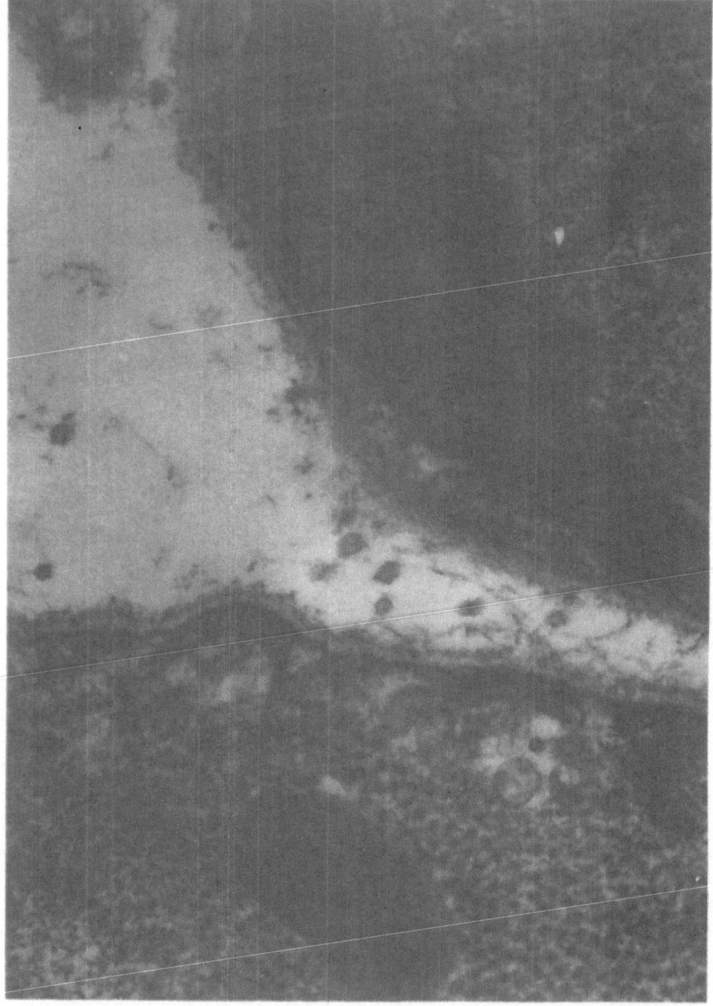

*Figure 3. Electron micrograph of mammalian cardiac muscle showing connections between cells* consisting of microthreads, basement membrane and collagen fibres (30).

tropocollagen, and collagen fibres (Figure 3). These three structures appear in different combinations to produce a variety of intercellular connections. One type involves only microfilaments running between the cell coats of adjacent cells and often connecting with each other to form networks with different organizations and densities. In another type of junction, the cell coats of adjacent cells are attached to collagen fibres in the intercellular space or along the cell coat. A third general type of junction consists of collagen fibres embedded in the matrix of the cell coat of adjacent cells, and it resembles a structure observed in skeletal muscle (31). In view of their morphology one might expect the different types of cell junctions to have diverse elastic properties.

These connections can probably support very large forces. If the in-tercalated discs are opened by treating the tissue with EGTA, normal isometric force can still be transmitted among the cells, and in this state the only visible structures that might provide the necessary mechanical coupling are these intercellular junctions.

## 4. CONNECTIVE TISSUE COMPONENTS

Connective tissue must constitute a significant load for the contractile system even when it is not directly connected to the contracting cells (25). Changes in the dimensions of the individual cardiac cells must be limited by their ability to deform the transverse and longitudinal connective tissue network that forms an elaborate supporting structure for the myocardial cells. This network will define a range of lengths over which individual cells can normally operate since transversely-oriented collagen will be a load for cells that are shortening and the longitudinally-oriented collagen for cells that are lengthening. Inasmuch as the length-tension relation of connective tissue is nonlinear, successive increases in resting length will require progressively greater increments in diastolic pressure, and increases in systolic emptying will need progressively greater contractile force and inotropic state.

The importance of connective tissue as a parallel elasticity and tissue load for cardiac cells can be clearly demonstrated. A contracting cell can extend a relaxed cell in series to a longer sarcomere length than the application of a very large force to the ends of the bundle of fibres (25). In a highly localized contraction, the influence of parallel elasticity should be very small. The geometry of resting fibres is also affected by connective tissue inasmuch as sarcomere length seems to depend on the ratio of transversely-oriented to longitudinally-oriented connective tissue (25), and this dependence disappears as the organization of the connective tissue is mechanically disrupted.

## 5. PHYSIOLOGICAL IMPLICATIONS

In order to evaluate the contributions of intercellular junctions and connective tissue network to the mechanics of contraction, length-dependent properties due to passive rather than active components of the myocardium must be studied during carefully controlled activation. Since activation in intact cells is length-dependent over the physiologically important range of sarcomere lengths from 1.5 to 2.3 $\mu$m, some form of skinned fibre or tissue

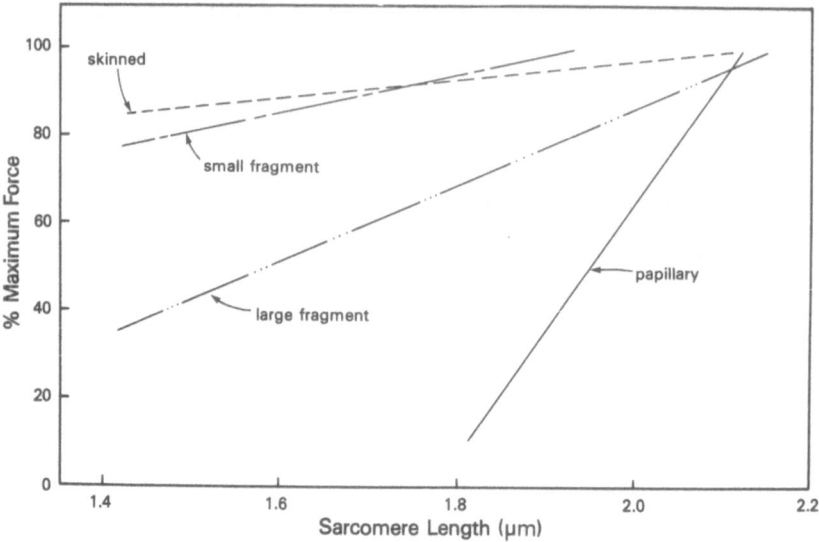

*Figure 4.* The sarcomere length tension relation measured in rat papillary muscle (35), skinned rat single cardiac cells (21), and derived for small and large fragments of rat right ventricle from the sarcomere length-pCa relation and the isometric tension-pCa relation at sarcomere length of 2.2 μm. The small fragment is very similar to a skinned single cell differing only in the fact that in the skinned fibre the disrupted membrane has been mechanically removed. The close similarity of the relation between length and force for the two preparations supports the validity of the derivation for the fragment. The slope of the relation for the larger fragment is about half way between that of the intact papillary muscle and the small fragment. This suggests that tissue organization is a major factor in the decline of net force at shorter sarcomere lengths for intact bundles of cells.

fragment with a disrupted membrane must used to allow direct activation of the contractile proteins. Homogeneity of sarcomere lengths should also exist at rest and during contraction. In freely suspended cell fragments uniformity of sarcomere length is well maintained and although force cannot be measured the relation between sarcomere length and the concentration of activating Ca ions can be used to determine the properties of the internal resistance to shortening. In the steady state at any pCa, length is constant and internal resistance exactly equals shortening force. Since both morphological and biochemical evidence argue against any major impairment of crossbridge access to the thin filament in sarcomeres as short as 1.5 μm, actual shortening force may be deduced from the tension -pCa curve of the isometrically suspended cardiac tissue.

The tissue loads for single cell fragments of both frog and rat ventricle and for multicellular fragments of rat ventricle have been estimated within the physiologically important range of sarcomere lengths (Figures 2, 4, 5).

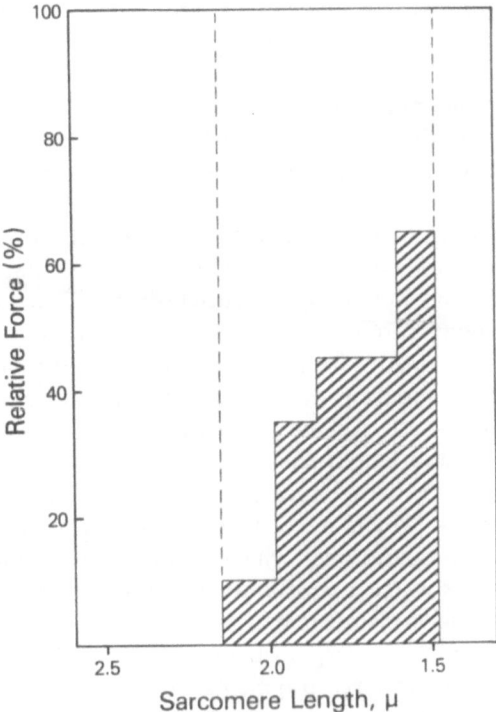

*Figure 5.* The relation between sarcomere length and internal load derived from Figure 2. Only a small amount of internal work is done when the systolic shortening is limited but the total internal work for the maximal shortening seen in normal hearts is about a third of the total work during the contraction.

Internal load increases with decreasing sarcomere length but at a much greater rate in the multicellular than in the unicellular preparations. Since there is no difference in the tension-pCa relation of unicellular and multicellular fragments contracting isometrically at sarcomere lengths about 2.0 $\mu$m, the deficit in shortening of the multicellular fragment cannot be due to the contractile system. The multicellular preparation probably experiences a greater tissue load from intercellular junctions and the connective tissue network that are not preserved in the unicellular fragments. The sharp increase in load in the rat ventricle at about 1.95 $\mu$m probably results from the thin filaments crossing the centre of the sarcomere (27).

A plot of load against sarcomere length indicates the relative amount of internal work done during isotonic contractions with different amounts of shortening (Figure 5). When multicellular fragments, which are the closest model to the intact tissue, shorten by about 10% the internal work is relatively small, but internal work comprises approximately a third of the total work performed during a contraction that produces shortening equivalent to the maximum that occurs in vivo. If this work is done against elastic structures, as the morphology suggests, considerable energy should be available from the contraction for re-extending the fibres during relaxation.

These studies indicate that much of the internal work done during a contraction is against extracellular structures. The importance of this internal work on the net force produced during a contraction can be examined by deriving sarcomere length-tension curves for the unicellular and multicellular fragments from the sarcomere length-pCa and tension-pCa relations and comparing these relations with those for the intact rat ventricular bundle. These are shown in Figure 4. The slope of the rising phase of the sarcomere length-tension curve reflects the size of the tissue load. The rise in force with increasing sarcomere length is small in unicellular preparations, which have a small extracellular load, and large with multicellular preparations, which have greater tissue loads. Since activation and crossbridge accessibility are not length-dependent in the tissue fragments, passive elements that are retained with preservation of the tissue organization must be responsible for most of the decline in net force at shorter lengths in the large fragments. A major portion of the similar decrease in force seen with the intact tissue bundle should also be due to passive elastic elements.

Extracellular elements are also important in determining the resting sarcomere length. The sarcomere lengths of the resting, unloaded cells in the wall of the rat right ventricle increase from approximately 1.9 $\mu$m before fragmentation to about 2.0 $\mu$m after fragmentation, indicating a net force from the passive extracellular elements of the organized tissue. In frog hearts, the resting, unloaded sarcomere length varies from 1.9 to 2.3 $\mu$m in intact tissues but only from 2.15 to 2.20 $\mu$m in unicellular fragments, indicating that the extracellular elements can produce shortening as well as lengthening forces.

## 6. MODEL

Although there are as yet insufficient data for proposing a detailed mechanism of how structural organization might produce the appropriate tissue loads for controlling resting sarcomere length, the amount of shortening, the range of sarcomere length over which the specific cells might operate, the relative movement among the cells and the change in orientation of cells during the contraction, the general principles on which such a

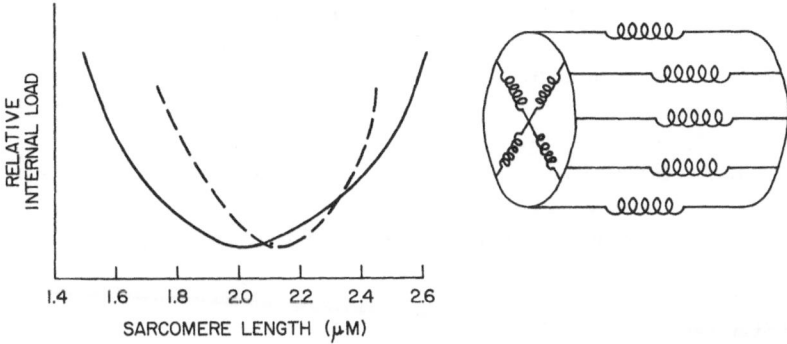

*Figure 6.* A schematic drawing of the way in which tissue elasticity might determine resting, unloaded sarcomere length and the approximate range of length over which cardiac fibres might operate. The relative values for the transverse and longitudinal elasticities would determine resting length and the absolute values would determine the operational range of length.

mechanism might be based are apparent (Figure 6). Resting sarcomere length would be determined by the relative values of transversely-oriented and longitudinally-oriented compliances. The range of length over which the cell normally contracts would be influenced by the absolute value of the two sets of compliances. Relative motion and orientation of cells would depend on the characteristics of their various intercellular junctions.

7. CLINICAL IMPLICATIONS

The importance of passive elements in the normal function of the heart and their contribution to abnormal function in pathological states should be considerable. They should influence diastolic size, change of shape, ejection fraction and diastolic filling of the ventricles by virtue of their effects on resting length, amount of shortening and re-extension of cardiac cells. Acute changes in the dimensions of the heart from dilation or heart failure will distort these junctions and force cells to operate in less favorable ranges of the length-tension relations of these passive elements, and may even disrupt cell linkages. As might be expected, the result should be an alteration in the change of shape, ejection fraction and rate of diastolic filling of the heart, but the extent to which the abnormalities of function are due to modification of passive extracellular elements is not known.

If passive elements are plastic, important adjustments might be necessary following changes in the hemodynamic conditions. There is very little information on this subject except that the amount of connective tissue and its distribution does change with thyrotoxic and valvular heart disease

(32, 33). It is also interesting to note that cells in tissue culture respond to physical stresses with structural changes such as the formation of actin filaments that can bind to membrane proteins (34).

8. ACKNOWLEDGEMENTS

This work is supported by U.S.P.H.S. grants HL 16010, 18900 and 15835.

REFERENCES

1. Tsakiris A, Donald D, Sturm R, Wood E: Volume, ejection fraction and internal dimensions of left ventricle determined by biplane videometry, Fed Proc 28:1358–1367, 1969.
2. Rushmer RF: Structure and function of the cardiovascular system, Philadelphia, Saunders, 1976 (2nd ed).
3. Hoffman BF, Cranefield P: Electrophysiology of the heart. New York, McGraw-Hill, 1960.
4. Perry SV: In: Contraction and relaxation in the myocardium, Nayler W (ed). London, Academic Press, 1975.
5. Cole H, Perry SV: The phosphorylation of troponin I from cardiac muscle. Biochem J 149:525–533, 1975.
6. Frearson N, Perry SV: Phosphorylation of the light chain components of myosin from cardiac and red skeletal muscle. Biochem J 151:99–107, 1975.
7. Frearson N, Solaro RJ, Perry SV: Changes in the phosphorylation of P light chain of myosin in perfused rabbit heart. Nature 264:801–802, 1976.
8. Ray KP, England P: Phosphorylation of the inhibitory subunit of troponin and its effect on the calcium dependence of cardiac myofibril adenosine triphosphatase. FEBS Lett 70:11–16, 1976.
9. Stull JT, Buss J: Phosphorylation of cardiac troponin by cyclic adenosine 3':5'-monophosphate-dependent protein kinase. J Bio Chem 252:851–857, 1977.
10. Ribolow R, Barany M: Phosphorylation of tropomyosin in live frog muscle. Arch Biochem Biophys 179:718–720, 1977.
11. McClellan G, Winegrad S: The regulation of the calcium sensitivity of the contractile system in mammalian cardiac muscle. J Gen Physiol 72:737–764, 1978.
12. Cole H, Frearson N, Moir A, Perry SV, Solaro RJ: Phosphorylation of cardiac myofibrillar proteins. In: Heart function and metabolism, Recent advances in studies of cardiac structure and metabolism 11, Kobayashi T, Saro T, Dhalla N (eds), Baltimore, University Park Press, 1978, p 111–119.
13. Ray KP, England P: Phosphorylation of the inhibitory subunit of troponin and its effect on the calcium dependence of cardiac myofibril adenosine triphosphatase. FEBS Lett 70:11–17, 1976.
14. Ray KP, England P: Correlation between contraction and phosphorylation of the inhibitory subunit of troponin in perfused rat heart. FEBS Lett 50:57–60, 1975.
15. McClellan G, Winegrad S: Abstracts of 1978 meeting of Biophysical Society. J Biophys 21:17a, 1978.
16. Winegrad S: Variable diastolic compliance and variable Ca sensitivity of the contractile system in cardiac muscle. Eur J Cardiol 4:41–46, 1976.
17. Rapoport S: The anisotropic elastic properties of the sarcolemma of the frog semitendinosus muscle fiber. Biophys J 13:14–36, 1973.
18. Ford LE, Huxley AF, Simmons RM: Tension responses to sudden length change in stimulated frog muscle fibers near slack length. J Physiol 269:441–515, 1977.

19. Hellam DC, Podolsky RJ: Force measurements in skinned muscle length. *J Physiol* (London) 200:807–819, 1967.
20. Schoenberg M, Podolsky RJ: Length force relation of calcium activated muscle fibres. *Science* 176:52–54, 1972.
21. Fabiato A, Fabiato F: Dependence of the contractile activation of skinned cardiac cells on the sarcomere length. *Nature* 256:54–56, 1975.
22. Huxley HE: In: *The structure and function of muscle*, vol 1, pt 1, Bourne GH (ed), New York; Academic Press, 1972 (2nd ed).
23. Gordon A, Huxley AF, Julian FJ: The variation of isometric tension with sarcomere length in vertebrate muscle fibres. *J Physiol* 184:170–192, 1966.
24. Robinson TF, Winegrad S: Variation of thin filament length in heart muscle. *Nature* 267:74, 1974.
25. Winegrad S: Resting sarcomere length-tension relation in living frog heart. *J Gen Physiol* 64:343–355, 1974.
26. Brown L, Gonzales-Serratos H, Huxley AF: Electron microscopy of frog muscle fibres in extreme passive shortening. *J Physiol* 208:868, 1970.
27. Robinson TF, Winegrad S: The measurement and dynamic implications of thin filament lengths in heart muscle. *J Physiol*.
28. Elliott GF: X-ray diffraction from living striated muscle during contraction. *Nature* 206:1357–1358, 1965.
29. Elliott GF, Matsubara I: The constant volume behaviour of the myofilament lattice in frog skeletal muscle: studies on skinned and intact single fibres by X-ray and light diffraction. *J Physiol* 88P–89P, 1972.
30. Robinson TF, Winegrad S: Force transmission among heart cells. *J Gen Physiol* 70: 15a, 1977.
31. Luft J: Ruthenium red and violet II. Fine structural localization in animal tissues. *Anat Res* 171:369–416, 1971.
32. Bartosova D, Chvapil M, Korecky B, Puopa O, Rakusan K, Turek Z, Vizek M: The growth of the muscular and collagenous parts of the rat heart in various forms of cardiomegaly. *J Physiol* 200: 285–295, 1969.
33. Buccino RA, Harris E, Spann Jr JF, Sonnenblick EH: Response of myocardial connective tissue to development of experimental hypertrophy. *Am J Physiol* 216:425–428, 1969.
34. Goldman RD, Schloss JA, Starger JM: Organization changes of actin-like microfilaments during animal cell movements, *Cold Spring Harbor Symp Cell Mobility* 1:217, 1976.
35. Krueger JW Pollack GH: Myocardial sarcomere dynamics during isometric contraction. *J Physiol* 251:627–643, 1975.

# 1.3. TENSION DEVELOPMENT AND SARCOMERE LENGTH IN RAT CARDIAC TRABECULAE: EVIDENCE OF LENGTH-DEPENDENT ACTIVATION

HENK E.D.J. TER KEURS, WIM H. RIJNSBURGER,
ROB VAN HEUNINGEN, MICHIEL J. NAGELSMIT

## 1. INTRODUCTION

The slope of the sarcomere length-tension relation in cardiac papillary muscle suggests length-dependent activation of the contractile system (1). However, there are no data on the effect of inotropic interventions on this curve. Only muscle length-tension curves are available, which give conflicting results (1, 2, 3). The purpose of the present study was to examine the effect of varied calcium concentrations on the sarcomere length-tension relationship, using laser diffraction techniques.

We studied long thin trabeculae of the rat heart because they diffract light into a clear diffraction pattern and therefore allow accurate sarcomere length measurements. Preliminary studies (4) indicated that the sarcomere length distribution was uniform throughout most of the specimen, both during rest and during contraction. The mechanical properties of trabeculae are similar to those of papillary muscle preparations.

## 2. METHODS

Trabeculae dissected from the right ventricle of Wistar rats were studied at 25°C and 12 beats per minute at calcium concentrations of 2.5 and 0.5 mM. The muscles were mounted (Figure 1) between a capacitive force transducer and a clamp connected to a servomotor system. The muscle bath was placed on a modified microscope stage and continually perfused with Tyrode solution. The muscle was illuminated by a laser beam. The trabeculae act as a phase grating and diffract the incident light beam into a zeroth-order band and multiple symmetrical pairs of higher-order bands. Spacing between the bands is uniquely related to sarcomere length. The diffracted light was utilized to study the muscle by means of three systems. The central part of the zeroth-order band was used for low-power microscope imaging. The position of each first-order band relative to the zeroth-order band was determined with the aid of two independent detectors which operated on different physical principles. Each first-order diffraction band was deflected by surface mirrors onto a photodetector. The light of these bands passed through Fourier lenses placed between the muscle and the

*J. Baan, A.C. Arntzenius, E.L. Yellin (eds.), Cardiac Dynamics, 25–36.*

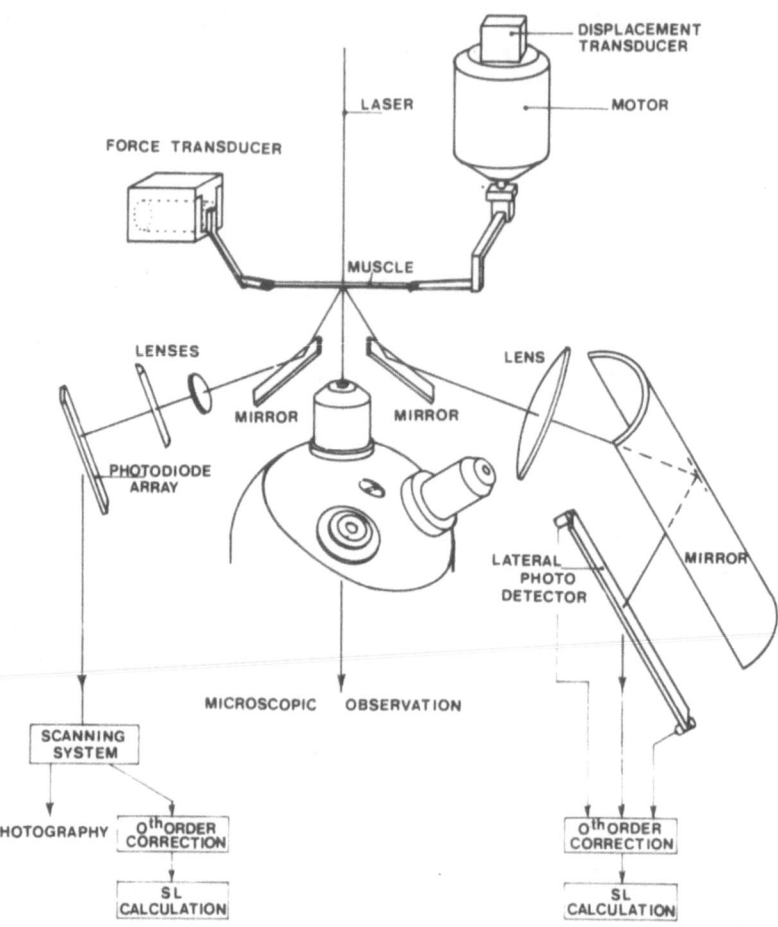

*Figure 1.* Diagram of experimental setup. Muscle and entering laser beam were observed through the microscope. Two surface mirrors deflect the light of the first-order diffraction pattern onto two photodetector systems. The positions of the median and mean of the first-order light-intensity distributions are converted to median and mean sarcomere length respectively. Force is measured with a capacitive force transducer. Muscle length is measured and controlled by a servomotor system with length transducer.

detectors and was converged onto the detectors along the length of the bands using a cylindrical lens and a cylindrical mirror respectively. Assuming the lenses behave as ideal Fourier transformers, the relation between sarcomere length (SL) and distance (d) between zeroth and first order maxima is given by:

$$SL = K\lambda/d$$

where $K$ is a constant and $\lambda$ is the wavelength (0.6328 $\mu$m) of the laser light (5). A considerable spread of light under the principal orders of the diffraction pattern of cardiac tissue occurs, due to scatter by non-contractile elements in the muscle and to non-uniformity of sarcomere lengths. Consequently the first-order straddles on the skirt of the zeroth order. Average sarcomere length was calculated from the distribution of light in the first orders after correcting for contribution of the zeroth-order band.

For the purpose of this study we attempted to eliminate changes in sarcomere length. To achieve this the servomotor system was modified to obtain direct feedback control of sarcomere length. The system thus allowed us to keep either muscle length or sarcomere length constant. Signal levels were adjusted such as to obtain critical damping in any mode of control.

The muscles were stimulated at constant reference length for 10–15 contractions between series of contractions at test lengths. Data on peak force-sarcomere length relations were derived from each third contraction of the test series. Test lengths were chosen in random order. Following a change in calcium concentration in the perfusate measurements were performed after force development was steady.

In two experiments the influence of frequency potentiation was tested. For this purpose the following protocol was used. The muscle was stimulated at intervals of 30 seconds while the potentiation consisted of a train of 20 stimuli given during 4 seconds followed by a single stimulus test. The relation between force developed during such potentiated contractions and sarcomere length was measured from contractions at different test lengths, which were imposed upon the muscle immediately prior to the test. The potentiating stimuli were delivered to the muscle at constant control length.

3. RESULTS

Sarcomeres in the central area of a trabecula such as the one shown in Figure 2 exhibited uniform behaviour. Their length at rest was constant in more than 50% of the region from which diffraction patterns could be obtained. During a twitch these sarcomeres shortened auxotonically by about 16%. The distribution of sarcomere lengths in this region was uniform at the moment of peak twitch force as well. They shortened at the expense of areas close to the clamps holding the muscle. The areas of stretch and those of uniform shortening were usually separated by regions which exhibited relatively little sarcomere length change.

The time course of tension development during muscle isometric contractions exhibited the well-known features: a slow rise of force to a maximum 150 msec after onset of contraction followed by a gradual decay and the relaxation phase.

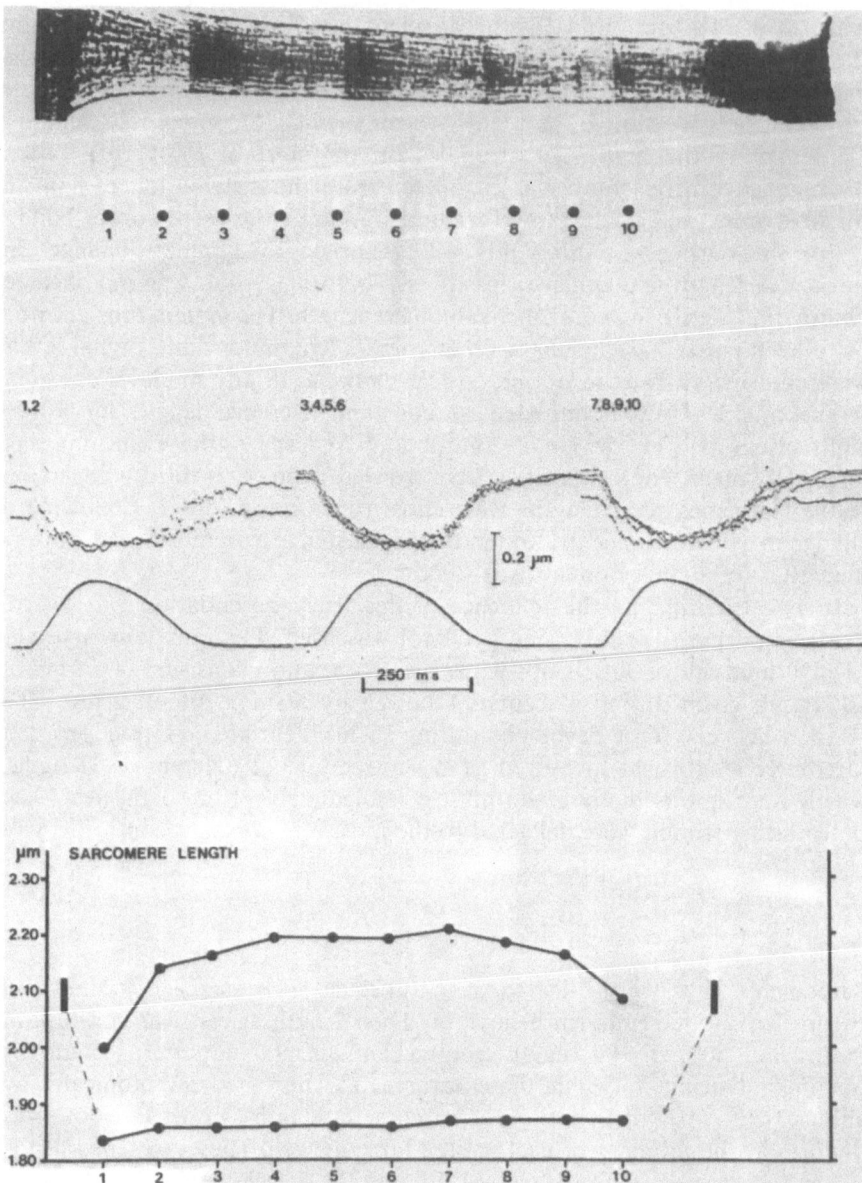

*Figure 2. Upper panel*: composite microphotograph of a trabecula 2300 μm long and 180 μm wide (at region 5). Thickness 90 μm. *Middle panel*: resting sarcomere length and sarcomere length during contractions recorded at positions 1–2, positions 3–6 and 7–10 respectively, together with the force. Length of sarcomeres at rest could be measured closer to the muscle clamps as well. *Lower panel*: observed resting length of the compliant ends (indicated by the bars) and their stretch during contraction (arrows), together with the resting and the active sarcomere length distribution along the fibre.

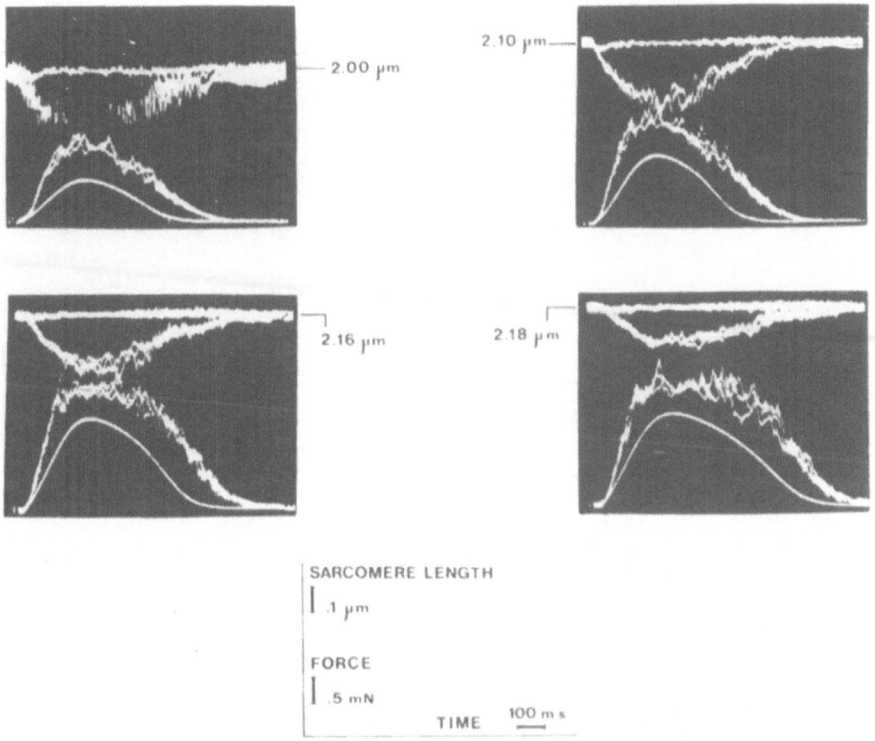

*Figure 3.* Force development during contractions starting at sarcomere lengths of 2.00, 2.10, 2.16 and 2.18 μm. Superimposed are three contractions during which muscle length and three during which sarcomere length are kept constant. Passive force is not shown. Active force developed faster in all contractions when sarcomere length was kept constant.

Tension development at constant muscle length and at constant sarcomere length were compared (Figure 3). Sarcomere shortening could be eliminated completely except for an early transient. When sarcomere shortening was prevented tension rose considerably faster to a maximum which was attained after 60 msec. It remained at a plateau level during 150-200 msec if contraction was elicited at a sarcomere length more than 2.15 μm. Tension then declined slowly and subsequently in an exponential manner. The relations between maximal force developed during twitches and sarcomere length at the moment of maximal force are shown in Figures 4 and 5 for external concentrations of 2.5 and 0.5 mM respectively. Force is expressed as total force minus the passive force borne by the muscle at the sarcomere length existing at peak force. Externally developed force was zero at approximately 1.58 μm and increases continuously with sarcomere length. Obviously the curves neither exhibit a summit nor a plateau or descending limb. The assumption that total tension in muscle isometric

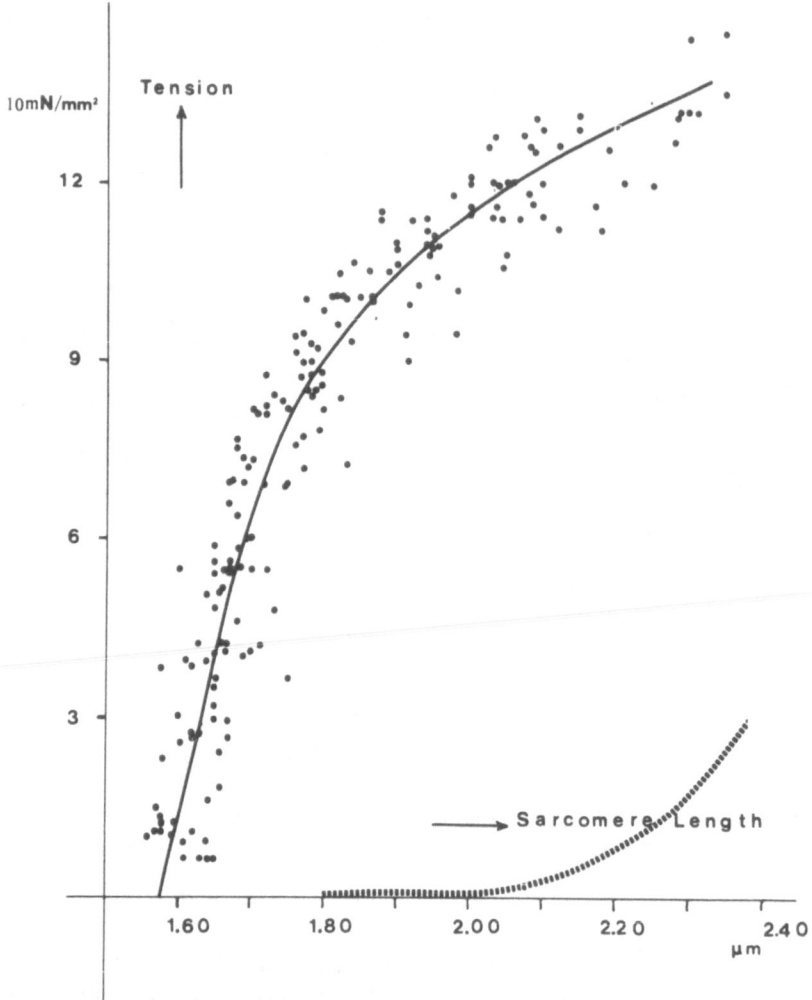

*Figure 4.* The sarcomere length-total tension relation obtained from pooled data derived during muscle isometric contraction of 12 muscles ($[Ca]_0 = 2.5$ mM). Tension is expressed as described in the method section. Passive tension data were averaged. The dotted line going through the average values is drawn only. The line drawn through the total tension data fits an exponential relationship: $T = 25.45$ (1-exp(2.2–1.4 SL)) 10 mN.mm$^{-2}$.

contractions adequately reflects the ability of sarcomeres to develop tension was confirmed by the observation that the length tension relations obtained from muscle-isometric and sarcomere-isometric contractions are identical.

Lowering the calcium concentration of the perfusate at constant stimulation rate caused a reduction of the developed tension. The amount by

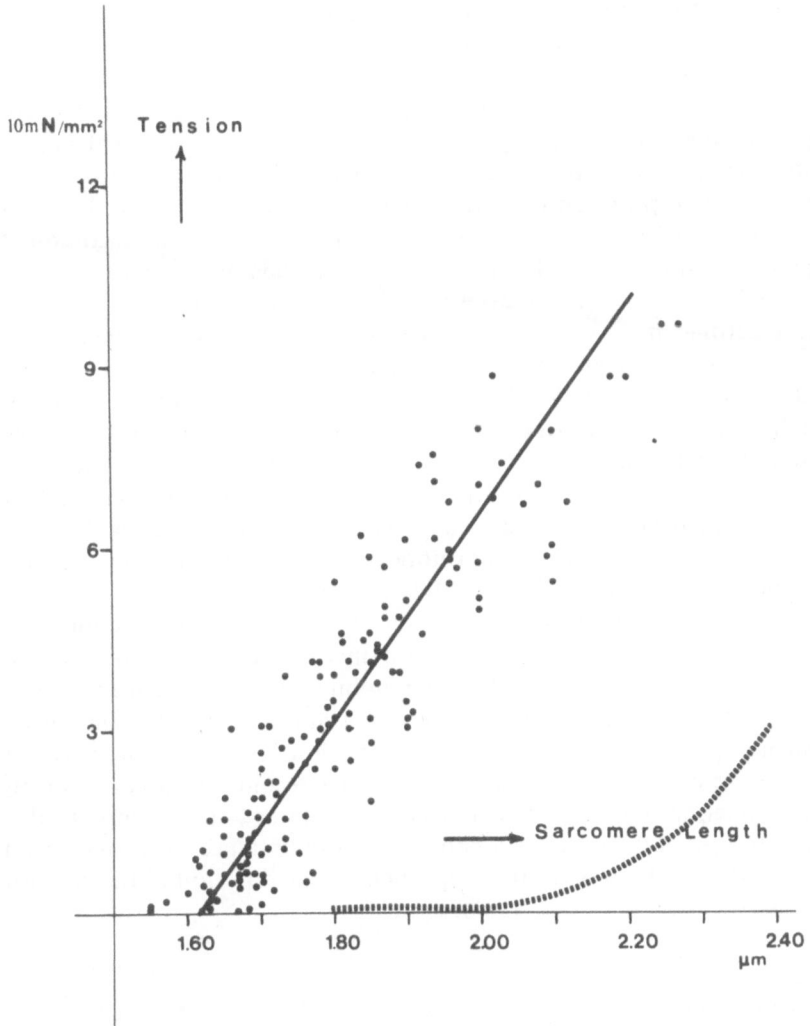

*Figure 5.* The sarcomere length-total tension relation obtained from pooled data derived during muscle isometric contraction of 8 muscles ($[Ca]_0 = 0.5$ mM). Tension is expressed as in Figure 6. Passive tension data were averaged. The dotted line goes through the average values. A straight line fits the total tension data well.

which tension was reduced strongly depended on sarcomere length (cf. Figures 4 and 5). The significant change in shape of the sarcomere length-tension relation as a result of alteration of the external calcium concentration qualitatively corresponds to previously reported changes in shape of the muscle length-tension muscle relation (6). Studying such relations in those preparations it was found that the difference in shape of the curves at high and at low calcium concentrations was more pronounced in the muscle length-tension relation than in the sarcomere length-tension relation. Although they generated less force, the sarcomeres in the central region of the trabeculae appeared to shorten more at low calcium concentrations than at high concentrations. The excess shortening occurred at the moment of peak tension and was accompanied by enhanced stretch of the region in which sarcomere stretch occurred during the relaxation. The apparent compliance of the damaged muscle ends adjacent to the clamps appeared to depend on the external calcium concentration.

Rat cardiac muscle is strongly sensitive to stimulus frequency at low external calcium concentrations(7). This offers a tool to separate the contribution of external calcium concentration to excitation-contraction coupling from the contribution of calcium storage and release processes within the cell. The latter processes are modulated by frequency potentiation, shown in Figure 6. At an external calcium concentration of 2.5 mM, the effect on developed force of a potentiating stimulus series 30 seconds before a test contraction was not noticeable, as has been found previously (7). The sarcomere length-tension relation obtained from such potentiated contractions is identical to the relation obtained from contractions at the same calcium concentration and a stimulus rate of 12 per minute and is independent of the duration of the conditioning interval between 8 and 120 seconds. At low external calcium concentrations (0.5 mM) the effect of frequency potentiation on the test contractions is striking however. The time course of potentiated tension development and the sarcomere length-tension relation of potentiated contractions obtained at an external calcium concentration of 0.5 mM are identical to those obtained at a concentration of 2.5 mM. Likewise, they are independent of the duration of the conditioning interval between 8 and 120 seconds.

4. DISCUSSION

Control of sarcomere length established in this study provides for an accurate description of the time course of activation of force development. The results are in agreement with previous studies of Pollack and Krueger (8). Comparing of the relaxation phase in our data with their results is not possible since their method allowed for control of initial sarcomere length changes only. Qualitative agreement is found with the results of studies on the time course of force development in other species(9, 10). The differences between our data and the results obtained by Brady and by Julian et al. may be due both to species difference and to the different and less direct

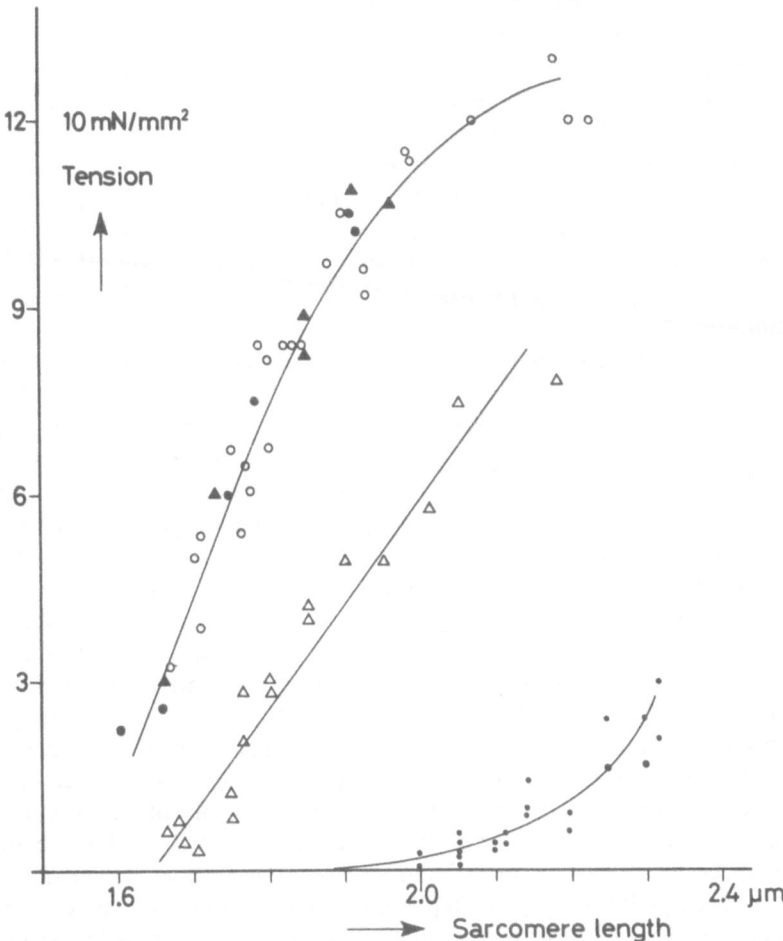

*Figure 6.* The sarcomere length-total tension relation derived from contractions at $[Ca]_0 = 2.5$ mM and 0.5 mM. Open symbols represent tension data measured during muscle isometric contractions, elicited at a regular rate of 0.2 $sec^{-1}$ (circles at $[Ca]_0 = 2.5$ mM, triangles at $[Ca]_0 = 0.5$ mM). Filled symbols represent tensions measured during potentiated muscle isometric contractions both at $[Ca]_0 = 2.5$ mM (circles) and 0.5 mM (triangles). Dots indicate passive tension. The potentiating protocol was as follows: the muscle was kept at reference length and stimulated at a rate of 5 $sec^{-1}$ for 4 seconds, 30 seconds prior to the test contraction. Then the potentiated test contraction was elicited at various test lengths, which were imposed upon the muscle just before the contraction.

method they employed to control length. The rapid rise of activation of force development observed by us agrees well with the desciption of the active state of shortening by Brutsaert and Sonnenblick (11). They are also in keeping with the results of Huntsman and Joseph (this volume), who found that the force-velocity relation of the central region of cardiac muscle preparations is constant rapidly after the onset of contraction.

The influence of different external calcium concentrations on the shape of the sarcomere length-tension relation supports the hypothesis that activation of cardiac muscle is length-dependent(1). It is unlikely that passive restoring forces play a major role in determining the shape of the length-tension relation as their effect should be calcium-dependent in order to explain the observed change of shape with different calcium concentrations.

The similarity of the sarcomere length-tension relations at high and at low external calcium concentrations following frequency potentiation (Figure 6) excludes a direct influence of the external calcium concentration itself. The time course of the effect of potentiation makes it unlikely that variations of the slow inward calcium current as a function of sarcomere length contribute either(7). Therefore, we might conclude that only intracellular processes involved in or linked with storage and release of calcium determine the shape of the sarcomere length-tension relation, especially since it also has been shown(10) that the contractile mechanism is not appreciably affected by sarcomere length changes in the range at which cardiac muscle operates. Reasoning further along these lines, two additional considerations are important: (1) all processes involved in calcium storage during potentiation in this study took place at constant reference length while saturation of the calcium stores is unlikely to occur as reference length was shorter than sarcomere length at which maximal force is developed; (2) complete depletion of the calcium stores by caffeine in skinned fibre studies of Fabiato and Fabiato(12) showed that the available amount of calcium in the stores is independent of sarcomere length in the range at which cardiac muscle operates. In the light of these observations we feel inclined to conclude that the properties of the process of calcium release from cellular stores and/or calcium binding to the myofilaments determine the shape of the sarcomere length-tension relation.

The results suggest the following mechanisms: (1) the release process is triggered by the influx of calcium during the action potential; (2) the amount of calcium released and bound to the myofilaments depends on sarcomere length and on calcium content of the releasable stores; (3) The calcium content of the releasable stores is influenced by external calcium concentration and by frequency potentiation; (4) the calcium content of the releasable stores itself affects the length sensitivity of the calcium release process.

SUMMARY

Sarcomere length-tension relations were derived from contractions at varied external calcium concentrations. The time course of tension development proved to depend on both sarcomere length and external calcium concentration. At all calcium concentrations tension attained during contraction was zero at a sarcomere length of 1.58 $\mu$m and maximal at a sarcomere length of 2.35 $\mu$m. Neither a maximum nor a descending limb was found in the sarcomere length-tension relations. At an external calcium concentration of 0.5 mM, tension increased linearly with sarcomere length, whereas at an external calcium concentration of 2.5 mM it approached maximal tension exponentially with increasing sarcomere length. Sarcomere length-tension relations obtained from contractions at an external calcium concentration of 0.5 mM following frequency potentiation were identical to the sarcomere length-tension relation at an external calcium concentration of 2.5 mM. The results are consistent with the hypothesis that cardiac muscle length affects contractile performance by its influence on excitation-contraction coupling.

ACKNOWLEDGEMENTS

This work is supported by grant numbers 74022 and 77068 of the Netherlands Heart Foundation, of which Dr. ter Keurs is Established Investigator.

REFERENCES

1. Jewell BR: A reexamination of the influence of muscle length on myocardial performance. Circ Res 40:221–230, 1977.
2. Huntsman LL, Stewart DK: Length dependent calcium inotropism in cat papillary muscle. Circ Res 40:366–371, 1977.
3. Sonnenblick EH: Force-velocity relations in mammalian heart muscle. Am J Physiol 202:931–939, 1962.
4. Keurs HEDJ ter: Tension development and sarcomere length in rat heart muscle. In: 7th European congress of cardiology: abstract, vol 1, Amsterdam, 1976, p 57.
5. Goodman JW: Introduction to Fourier optics, New York, McGraw-Hill, 1968.
6. Allen DG, Jewell BR, Murray JW: The contribution of activation processes to the length-tension relation of cardiac muscle. Nature 248:606, 1977.
7. Forester GV, Mainwood GW: Interval dependent inotropic effects in rat myocardium and the effect of calcium. Pflügers Arch 352:189–196, 1974.
8. Pollack GH, Krueger JW: Sarcomere dynamics in intact cardiac muscle. Eur J Cardiol 4:53–65, 1976.
9. Brady AJ: Active state in cardiac muscle. Physiol Rev 48:570–600, 1968.
10. Julian FJ, Sollins MR, Moss RL: Absence of a plateau in length-tension relationship of rabbit papillary muscle when internal shortening is prevented. Nature 260:340–342, 1976.

11. Brutsaert DL, Sonnenblick EH: Force-velocity-length-time relations of the contractile elements in heart muscle of the cat. *Circ Res* 14:137–149, 1969.
12. Fabiato A, Fabiato F: Dependence of the contractile activation of skinned cardiac cells on the sarcomere length. *Nature* 256:54–56, 1975.

# 1.4. INSEPARABILITY BETWEEN PRELOAD AND CONTRACTILITY EFFECTS ON PRESSURE DEVELOPMENT IN THE ISOVOLUMICALLY CONTRACTING ISOLATED RABBIT HEART

H.C. Schamhardt, E.L. de Beer

## 1. introduction

The mechanisms by which the heart adapts its contractile performance after changes in external conditions are usually separated into: (1) changes in muscle load and corresponding fibre length prior to contraction (preload); (2) the load against which the heart has to contract during systole (afterload); (3) intrinsic muscle properties, denoted as contractility. Much effort has been given to quantify contractility with one simple quantity, separated from influences of preload and afterload and preferably easy to derive from hemodynamic measurements (1, 2, 3, 4).

Boom et al. (4) suggested the possibility of discriminating between preload and contractility based on a mathematical description, founded on a sliding filaments model. In their study the slope of the decreasing limb of the plot of isovolumically developed pressure ($P$) versus its time derivative ($dP/dt$), the phase plane plot, was considered as a contractility index, while the preload dependent parameter of the model was a constant ($Q$), multiplied by the crossbridge attachment rate constant ($f$). They assumed $Q, f$ and the crossbridge detachment rate constant $g$ to be time-independent. From their data (4:figure 5), however, it follows that one or more of their assumptions cannot be correct, because neither the phase plane plot as a whole, nor a part of it is linear.

The aim of our study was to extend the model of Boom et al. (4) with a time dependency of the most reliable parameter ($f$) and to quantify the preload and contractility-dependent parameters in the same experimental model.

## 2. materials and methods

The Langendorff-like perfused isolated rabbit heart preparation as described in detail elsewhere (4), was used (Figure 1). The heart was perfused via the aortic trunk with an inorganic solution to which glucose had been added. Perfusion pressure was 7.65 kPa. The contractile state of the heart was altered by changing the calcium content of the perfusate. Preload was

J. Baan, A.C. Arntzenius, E.L. Yellin (eds.), Cardiac Dynamics, 37–43.

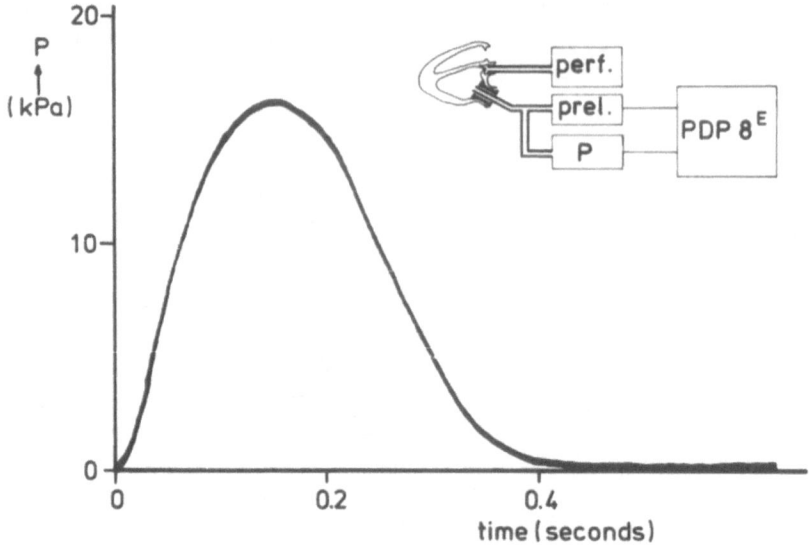

*Figure 1.* Isovolumic pressure tracing of an isolated left ventricle of the rabbit. Inset: experimental setup.

set by controlling end-diastolic pressure. Pressure was measured with a catheter-tip micromanometer, differentiated analogously and digitized on-line with 1000 samples per second by the experiment-controlling PDP8/E computer.

Compared with the original experiments (4) much more care was taken to minimize the time from the removal of the heart to attaching it to the apparatus (<20 sec), thereby avoiding air coming into the coronary system. Another improvement is the on-line sampling of the signals without storage on noise-adding devices like analog magnetic tape.

To check for the absence of aging of the heart the following was required: after each run of eight preload settings (carried out within eight minutes) the developed pressure at preload 0.5 kPa had to be within 3% of the starting value, or else the data were discarded.

Experiments in which the maximum isovolumically developed pressure was below 15 kPa at end-diastolic pressure of 0.5 kPa at a calcium content of the perfusate of 2 mM were also discarded. Only 20% of the hearts could meet both criteria.

As a mathematical description for pressure development the following equation was used (4):

$$dP/dt(t) = Qf - (f+g)P(t) \qquad [1]$$

The basis of this equation in terms of a sliding filaments model and the assumptions needed to transform the force development in a linear muscle to pressure development in an isovolumically contracting heart have been presented before (4). Except activation and deactivation, all time-independent properties of heart muscle, heart geometry and intraventricular volume, including preload, are concentrated in the quantity $Q$. Mathematically $Q$ represents a scale factor which does not affect the time course of the pressure curve; $f$ and $g$ are time constant for crossbridge attachment and detachment, respectively.

The time dependency in the present model is taken into account by assuming $f$ to be a time function, while the crossbridge detachment rate constant $g$ is assumed independent of time. Note that this formalism is usable in any first-order process of force generation and is not necessarily related to a sliding filaments model.

As a mathematical formulation for $f(t)$ the description of Julian (5) was chosen: a multiplication of two exponential functions:

$$f(t) = A(\exp(-(t+T)/D))(1-\exp(-(t+T)/E)) \quad if\ t \leq -T \quad [2]$$
$$f(t) = 0 \quad\quad\quad\quad\quad\quad\quad\quad\quad\quad\quad\quad\quad\quad if\ t \leq -T$$

where $T$ is a time delay and $E$ and $D$ are time constants of increase and decrease of $f(t)$, respectively.

To exclude the influences of the particular form of $f(t)$ on the achieved results, a mathematically totally different formula was used: a solution of a one-dimensional diffusion equation, describing the diffusion of calcium from the internal stores via the sarcomeres to a sink. The time course of the calcium concentration at the sarcomeres is then:

$$f(t) = K t^{-1/2}(exp(-B/t) - exp(-C/t)). \quad\quad\quad [3]$$

Experimental data and these model equations were fed into a computer program that returned the parameter values at optimum fit of model and experiment. (Least sum of squared differences, steepest gradient method (6)).

## 3. RESULTS

Rising limbs of developed pressure tracings as sampled from an experiment are shown in Figure 2 for three preloads and two values of the calcium concentration of the perfusion fluid ($[Ca^{++}]$). All curves show nearly the same shape, which is clear after normalizing them to their maximum developed pressure ($P_{max}$), as indicated in Figure 2. In contrast with previous results (4) it is not possible to find unique influences in the shapes of the curves after preload or contractility interventions. This implies that the straight line fitting procedure used previously (4) does not result in an

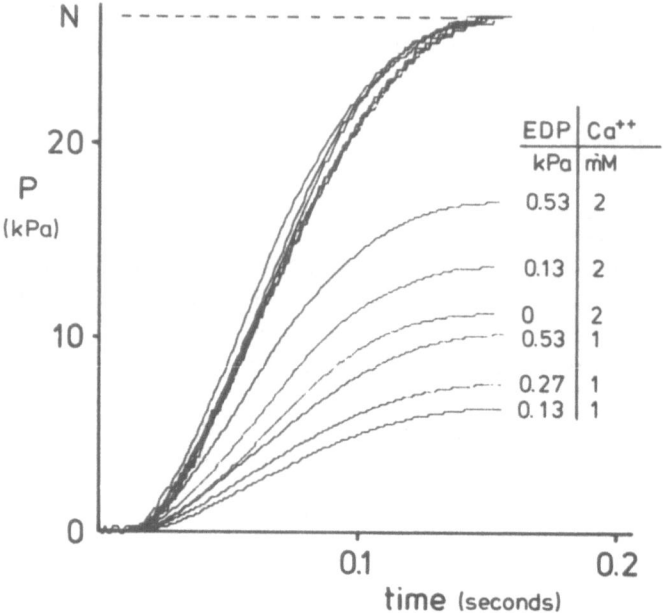

| EDP | Ca$^{++}$ |
| --- | --- |
| kPa | mM |
| 0.53 | 2 |
| 0.13 | 2 |
| 0 | 2 |
| 0.53 | 1 |
| 0.27 | 1 |
| 0.13 | 1 |

*Figure 2.* Rising limbs of isovolumic pressure as a function of time. Preload is indicated as end-diastolic pressure in kPa; contractility as calcium content of the perfusion fluid. The curves indicated with N are the same tracings after normalization to their maximum developed pressures.

unique relation between the slope and contractility or preload, which we verified.

The model fitting procedure did not result either in quantification of the separated preload and contractility parameters. The fit of model and experimentally measured data was quite good (Figure 3). The parameters $g$, $T$ and $D[1,2]$ could be quantified well but $E$ tended to become infinite, thereby decreasing the amplitude of $f(t)$ to zero. The time course remained identical for all pressure data sets, independent of preload or [Ca$^{++}$]. Preload and contractility changes only resulted in changes in the amplitude of the term $Qf(t)$. Therefore, it proved impossible to estimate two parameters which were uniquely dependent on contractility or preload.

The use of [3] instead of [2] led to the same observation: the amplitude of $f(t)$ vanished as compared with $g$, leading again to coupling between preload and contractility.

## 4. DISCUSSION

The separation between the contributions of preload and contractility to the developed pressure in the heart does not seem to be perfect, as many

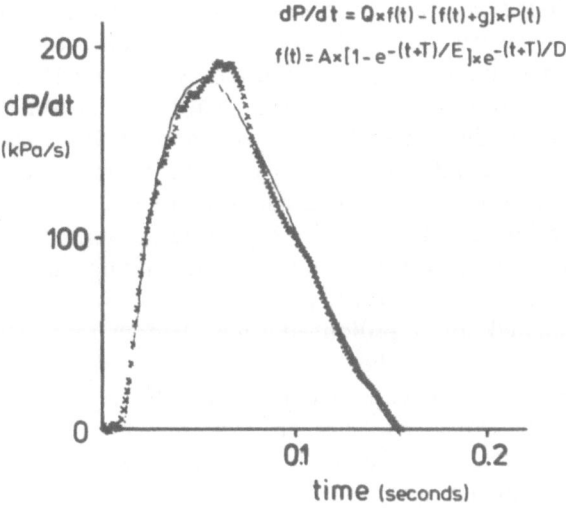

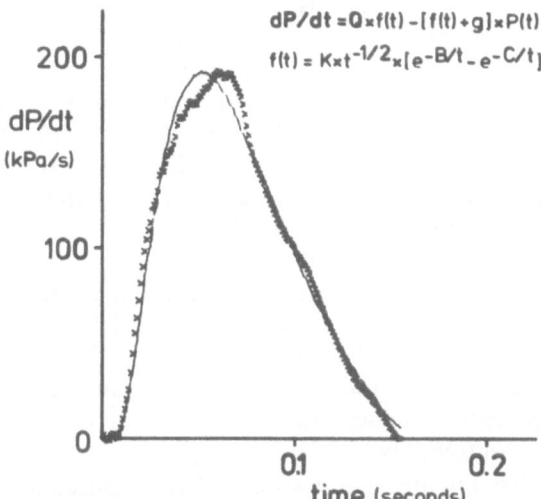

Figure 3. Fit of model and experiment using [1] and [2], upper, and [1] and [3], lower. Experimental data are shown by crosses; the continuous line indicates the computed fit.

investigators reported influences from preload on contractility indices and vice versa (1, 2, 3). Using the model of pressure generation described before (4), our study was aimed at obtaining preload and contractily parameters separated as much as practically possible after modifying the model with a time-dependent activation function.

As experimental model we used the same isovolumically contracting isolated rabbit left ventricle because of its simplicity of handling and its reproducibility. Hearts were selected on contractile performance, as reflected by a maximum developed pressure ranging from 15 up to 24 kPa at an end-diastolic pressure of 0.5 kPa and $[Ca^{++}]$ of 2 mM.

Most significant differences between our and previous experiments are the more stringent conditions under which the hearts were examined, the minimization of added noise and oscillations to the recorded signals, and the better care for repeatability of pressure development. The most ready explanation for the differences between our findings after preload and contractility interventions and the previous results (4) might be that hearts, after being isolated for a prolonged time, demonstrate responses which differ from those of the same heart in a "younger" stage.

The main result of our experiments is that shapes of the rising limb of isovolumically developed pressure are independent of preload and contractility. This finding seems to conflict with the previous report (4), finding slight differences in the time course of the pressure tracings.

The analysis of the data carried out by Boom et al. (4) might also be questioned. The computation of the slope of the (curved) phase plane plot depends largely on the data points near the maxima of $P$ and $dP/dt$. The experimental data showing a curve (4) conflict with the presumed constancy of the quantity $f$ especially. If $f$ is considered to be dependent on time, the formula describing the slope of the phase plane is extended with a term containing $Q$ and the partial time derivatives of $f$ and $P$, instead of being the negative sum of $f$ and $g$. The deviation from $-(f+g)$ is maximal at the maxima of $dP/dt$ and $P$. The data points in this region, however, mainly influence the slope. The previously used analysis therefore may not be permitted on mathematical grounds.

The shape identity between all pressure tracings, regardless of their history, implies that every pressure curve can be derived from another by linear multiplication of all data points. This is also true for the time derivatives of pressure. As a consequence, contractility indices based on the shapes of the pressure tracing, their derivatives, or combinations of both cannot quantify contractility.

The remarkable finding that $f \ll g$ is hardly acceptable in a sliding filaments model is which $f$ and $g$ are considered as rate constants, whether time-dependent or not. Another possibility to add time dependency to the model would be to localize it in the number of possible crossbridge sites, *in casu* in $Q$ as proposed by Grood and Mates (7). The final formula in their model is identical with [1], after $f(t)$ has been neglected as compared with $g$ and the recall of the constant $f+g$ to $g'$. A consequence of such a model is the explicit impossibility of separating the effects of preload and contractility to developed pressure. This result is in accordance with our findings.

Finally, an attractive hypothesis to which our findings might be related is a fibre-length-dependent release of calcium, which has been advocated for skeletal and papillary muscle (8) and for cardiac muscle by ter Keurs et al. (this volume). A change in preload results then in a change in the amount of calcium contributing to the contractile processes.

Until this last hypothesis has been verified extensively, a useful, albeit preload-dependent index of myocardial contractility will be the maximum isovolumically developed pressure at known preload. The maximum of its first time derivative, commonly reached in situ before ejection occurs, will be of the same value.

SUMMARY

In an attempt to separate preload and contractility contributions to pressure development in the isovolumically contracting isolated rabbit heart, shapes of pressure tracings were investigated after interventions in preload and inotropism.

The shapes of the pressure curves were identical, independent of the kind of the intervention. The fit with a mathematical model in which amplitude and time course of the pressure curve were explicitly separated did not result in identifying parameters related to preload or contractility separately. Both interventions exhibit their influences on the pressure curves indistinguishably. It is concluded that contractility indices based on the shape of isovolumic pressure and/or its time derivative must be used with great caution.

REFERENCES

1. Bos GC, van den, Elzinga G, Westerhof N, Noble MIM: Problems in the use of indices of myocardial contractility. *Cardiovasc Res* 7:834–848, 1973.
2. Parmley WW, Chuck L, Yeatman L: Comparative evaluation of the specificity and sensitivity of isometric indices of contractility. *Am J Physiol* 228(2):506–510, 1975.
3. Mahler F, Ross Jr J, O'Rourke RA, Covell JW: Effects of changes in preload, afterload and inotropic state on ejection and isovolumic phase measures of contractility in the conscious dog. *Am J Cardiol* 35:626–634, 1975.
4. Boom HBK, Denier van der Gon JJ, Nieuwenhuijs JHM, Schiereck P: Cardiac contractility: actin-myosin interaction as measured from the left ventricular pressure curve. *Eur J Cardiol* 1:217–224, 1973.
5. Julian FJ: Activation in a skeletal muscle contraction model with a modification for insect fibrilar muscle. *Biophys J* 9:547–570, 1969.
6. Fletcher R, Powell MJD: A rapid descent method for minimization. *Computer J* 6(2):163–168, 1963.
7. Grood ES, Mates RE: Influence of crossbridge compliance on the force-velocity relation of muscle. *Am J Physiol* 228(1):244–249, 1975.
8. Jewell BR: A reexamination of the influence of muscle length on myocardial performance. *Circ Res* 40:221–230, 1977.

# 1.5. FORCE-VELOCITY-LENGTH RELATIONS IN CARDIAC MUSCLE SEGMENTS

LEE L. HUNTSMAN, DANIEL S. JOSEPH

## 1. INTRODUCTION

Extensive study of the mechanical properties of cardiac muscle over the past two decades has led to a fairly well-established view of the way in which the primary variables, force, length and velocity, are interrelated. Developed force is observed to fall rapidly with decreasing fibre length below the optimum length ($L_{max}$) approaching zero in the vicinity of 80% $L_{max}$ (1, 2, 3). The relationship of force and velocity is highly dependent on the method of measurement, but is often not well described by the Hill equation since linear regions and maximum velocities at non-zero forces sometimes occur (4, 5, 6). The dependence of velocity on length has not been extensively studied but recent work by Brutsaert has shown unloaded shortening velocity to be independent of length above about 87% $L_{max}$, falling with length below that region (7). It has also been shown that the muscle's capability for maximal velocity is developed very early after stimulation, as contrasted to the capability for force development, which builds nearly as slowly as the twitch force (7, 8).

These results have proved troublesome, however, not only because there have been larger-than-expected variations between laboratories and species, but also because there are significant and unexplained differences from observations made on skeletal muscle. Recently, additional concern has arisen about the adequacy of isolated cardiac muscle preparations. Damaged end regions have been found to be much more compliant than expected, so that major deviations from isometric behaviour occur in central regions of the preparation even though the whole muscle is held at constant length (9, 10).

Now, newly developed techniques have made it possible to make mechanical measurements on the undamaged, central segments of isolated cardiac muscle. One such method has been developed in our laboratory, and early results have shown that the mechanical properties of segments are substantially misrepresented by whole-muscle measurements (11).

A surprising example of this is the observation that the force-velocity relation is essentially invariant from very early after-stimulation (< 50 msec at $L_{max}$, faster at shorter lengths) to the time of peak developed force (12).

*J. Baan, A.C. Arntzenius, E.L. Yellin (eds.), Cardiac Dynamics, 45–50.*

Consequently, mechanical activation appears to rise rapidly and maintain a plateau over this period – at least under the experimental conditions employed. In the present study, we have taken advantage of the constancy of activation and used data obtained all during the rising phase of the twitch to establish the interrelationships between force, velocity and length.

## 2. METHODS

Right ventricular papillary muscles isolated from the hearts of ferrets and cats were studied at 30°C, 12 beats per minute, with an extracellular calcium concentration of 2.25mM. After determination of $L_{max}$, each muscle was equilibrated at that length for at least one hour.

Segment length was measured from a chosen central segment using a magnetic induction technique (11). A flexible sense coil was fitted to each muscle, and the segment length recorded when muscle length equalled $L_{max}$ was defined as $SL_{max}$. Measurement and/or control of the mechanical variables was accomplished using an apparatus which has been previously described (13). Force, muscle length and segment length were sampled at 5 msec intervals using a PDP-12 computer. Velocity was computed by digital differentiation of segment length.

## 3. RESULTS

When muscle length is held constant, central segments undergo auxotonic contractions, exhibiting appreciable shortening (9, 11). If muscle length is not changed, the muscle stabilizes with reproducible amounts of developed force and segmental shortening over long periods. All the results reported here were obtained with muscles contracting stably at $L_{max}$ prior to the test protocol. Perturbations of loading conditions were imposed only transiently and re-equilibration was established before subsequent perturbations.

Load clamps were imposed at various times during the rising phase of contraction. Very little elastic recoil occurs in central segments with the transition from muscle length control to force control, most of the compliance being in the end regions. Rather, segmental shortening velocity is rapidly altered. Velocity and force were measured immediately after the stabilization of force ($\sim 10$ msec) and the data pairs were used to define a force-velocity relation. The data points in Figure 1 are an example of such results. As we have reported elsewhere, the relationship is remarkably independent of time from early in the twitch to nearly the time of peak force (12).

The Hill equation has been fitted to these data using a linearized form of the equation and least squares error minimization (14). Standard error of

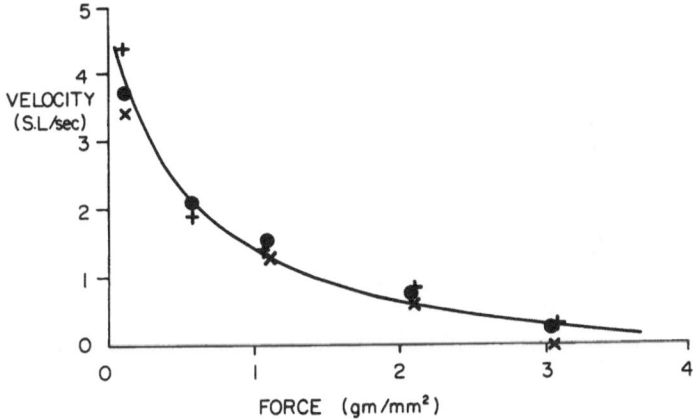

*Figure 1.* Force-velocity data determined with load clamps early (10 msec, +), midway (~100 msec, spots) and late (~200 msec, ×) in the rising phase of contraction for a representative ferret muscle. The solid line is the Hill equation curve fit to the data.

this fit is 0.08 SL/sec and the correlation coefficient is 0.98. The resultant curve is indicated by the line in Figure 1. Hill equation parameters $a$ and $b$ are 0.592 and 0.585, respectively. The force-axis intercept, $P_0$, has a value of 4.78 g/mm² while the velocity-intercept, $V_{max}$, is 4.73 $SL$/sec.

Since the load clamps applied at different instants during the twitch are also applied from different segment lengths, the invariance of the force-velocity relation indicates that there is no segment length-dependence over the range studied. However, segment shortening during muscle isometric contractions at $L_{max}$ seldom exceeds 10–15%, and the observation of a constant force-velocity relation is thus limited to above 85% $SL_{max}$.

To measure force and velocity at shorter segment lengths, transient changes of muscle length have been employed. Following equilibration at $L_{max}$, muscle length was reduced coincident with the stimulus and the time course of force, segment length and velocity were measured in the third contraction following the length change. Our observation has been that the third beat still exhibits a level of activation equal to that of the $L_{max}$ equilibration phase, yet the rapid change of passive force is largely completed. Examples of the trajectories of the rising phase of such contractions in the force-velocity plane are shown by the solid lines in Figure 2. These curves exhibit an envelope which has approximately the same shape and position as the force-velocity relation determined from load clamps (upper dashed line).

Using the fitted Hill equation, $P_0$ and $V_{max}$ values were determined for each segment length and these are plotted in Figure 3. Because $a$ and $b$ happen to be nearly equal for this muscle, $P_0$ and $V_{max}$ have almost the same

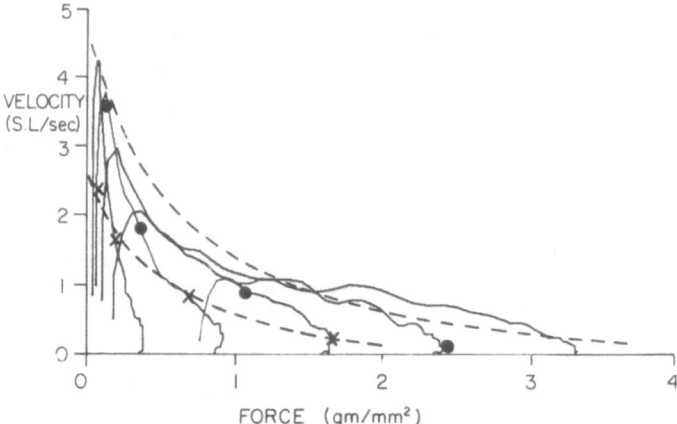

*Figure 2.* Force-velocity trajectories of segment auxotonic contractions at muscle lengths of 80, 84, 88, 92, 96 and 100% $L_{max}$ (solid lines, rising phase only). Representative values illustrating depression of the force-velocity relation at short segment lengths are shown for 83% (●) and 78% (×) $SL_{max}$. For comparison, the Hill curve from Figure 1 is reproduced by the upper dashed line. The lower dashed line is the scaled Hill equation curve (same *a* and *b* as the upper curve) which best fits the 78% $SL_{max}$ points.

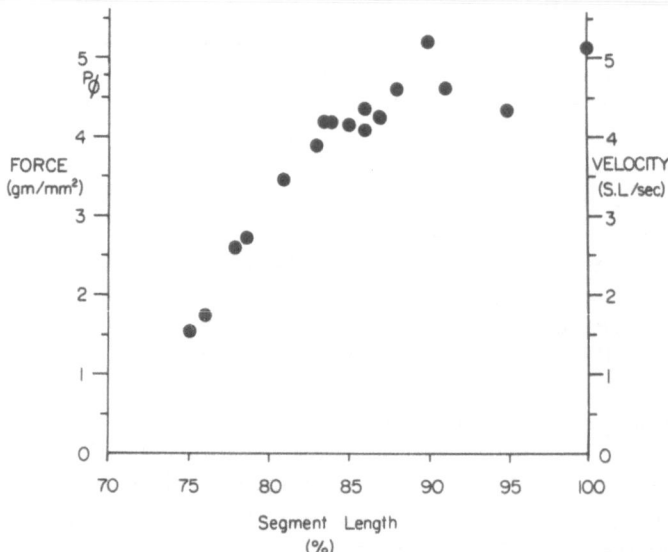

*Figure 3.* Hill equation force and velocity intercepts as a function of segment length. The intercepts for a best fit scaled Hill equation are shown. The data falls linearly below 85% ($r = 0.98$).

numerical values. Linear regression analysis of the points below 85% $SL_{max}$ yields a line ($r = 0.98$) which intercepts the $SL$ axis at 69% $SL_{max}$ and reaches the load $P_0$ value (4.78 g/mm$^2$) at 86% $SL_{max}$.

Sarcomere length measurements by other investigators suggest that resting sarcomere length at $L_{max}$ is probably about 2.35 $\mu$m (2). Assuming this value, the line fit to the data below 85% $SL_{max}$ has an $SL$ axis intercept of 1.63 $\mu$m and reaches the value of $P_0$ at 2.03 $\mu$m.

## 4. DISCUSSION

The results of this study suggest the following properties of undamaged cardiac muscle segments: (1) force and velocity are related in a manner which is well described by the Hill equation; (2) this relation appears to be independent of segment length above about 85% $SL_{max}$; (3) below 85% $SL_{max}$ the force-velocity relation is described by a scaled Hill equation with $P_0$ and $V_{max}$ decreasing linearly with segment length.

These findings are at variance with the characterization of cardiac muscle mechanics which has developed from studies of whole papillary muscles. Some aspects of the results – for example the $P_0$-segment length relationship – are more reminiscent of skeletal muscle behaviour than of previous cardiac muscle measurements. Yet, corroboration of these results is also to be found in earlier cardiac muscle studies. Whole-muscle measurements which might be expected to be least affected by compliant end regions include the unloaded velocity studies of Brutsaert (7) and the cardiac tetanus investigation of Foreman and colleagues (15). Brutsaert noted that unloaded shortening velocity was independent of muscle length above 87% $L_{max}$ and fell with length below that value (7). This is in accord with our estimates of $V_{max}$ (Figure 3). Foreman et al. found force-velocity relations in tetanized cardiac muscles to be well described by the Hill equation, with roughly equal $a$ and $b$ values, which were independent of length, while $P_0$ and $V_{max}$ fell linearly with length below 90% $L_{max}$ (15). Direct observation of sarcomeres and single cells has also yielded results which are generally in agreement with those reported here as oposed to the bulk of the whole-muscle data (9, 16).

The description of cardiac mechanics which is emerging from these studies emphasizes the need to measure undamaged portions of the muscle, avoiding the artificial effects of the end regions. It is also a description which appears to remove some of the unexplained differences between skeletal and cardiac mechanics. Hopefully, the variability and complexity which has characterized results from different laboratories and species will also be reduced by further measurements of this sort.

SUMMARY

The force-velocity relationship has been measured in central segments of isolated cardiac muscles using a new technique. Maximum force potential and unloaded shortening velocity have been determined by extrapolation of a Hill equation curve which describes the data well. The characteristics, and the entire force-velocity relation, are independent of segment length above about 85% $SL_{max}$. Below this range, the capability for developed force and active shortening falls in proportion to segment length reductions, approaching zero at about 68% $SL_{max}$.

ACKNOWLEDGEMENTS

This work was supported by grants from the U.S.P.H.S. (HL 20613 and HL 00344) and from the American Heart Association, with funds contributed in part by the American Heart Association of Washington.

REFERENCES

1. *The physiological basis of Starling's law of the heart*, CIBA symposia 24, Amsterdam, Elsevier, 1974.
2. Jewell BR: A reexamination of the influence of muscle length on myocardial performance. *Circ Res* 40:221–230, 1977.
3. Sonnenblick EH, Skelton CL: Reconsideration of the ultrastructural basis of cardiac length-tension relations. *Circ Res* 35:517 ff, 1974.
4. Blinks JR, Jewell BR: The meaning and measurement of myocardial contractility. In: *Cardiovascular fluid dynamics*, vol 1, Bergel DH (ed), London, Academic Press, 1972, p 225ff.
5. Edman KAP, Nilsson E: The mechanical parameters of myocardial contraction studied at a constant length of the contractile element. *Acta Physiol Scand* 72:205–219, 1968.
6. Noble MIM, Bowen TE, Hefner LL: Force-velocity relationships of cat cardiac muscle, studied by isotonic quick-release techniques. *Circ Res* 24:821ff, 1969.
7. Brutsaert DL: The force-velocity-length-time interrelation of cardiac muscle. In: *The physiological basis of Starling's law of the heart*, CIBA Symposia 24, Amsterdam, Elsevier, 1974, p 155ff.
8. Brady AJ: Active state in cardiac muscle. *Physiol Rev* 48:570–600, 1968.
9. Krueger JW, Pollack GH: Myocardial sarcomere dynamics during isometric contraction. *J Physiol* 251:627–643, 1975.
10. Huntsman LL, Day SR, Stewart DK: Nonuniform contraction in the isolated cat papillary muscle. *Am J Physiol* 233:H613, 1977.
11. Huntsman LL, Joseph DS, Oiye MY, Nichols GL: Auxotonic contractions in cardiac muscle segments. (Submitted.)
12. Joseph DS, Huntsman LL: Cardiac activation rises rapidly to a plateau. (Submitted.)
13. Hunstman LL, Stewart DK: Length-dependent calcium intropism in cat papillary muscle. *Circ Res* 40:366, 1977.
14. Edman KAP, Mulieri LA, Scubon-Mulieri B: Non-hyperbolic force-velocity relationships in single muscle fibres. *Acta Physiol Scand* 98:143, 1976.
15. Foreman R, Ford LE, Sonnenblick EH: Effect of muscle length on the force-velocity relationship of tetanized cardiac muscle. *Circ Res* 31:195, 1972.
16. Fabiato A, Fabiato F: Dependence of the contractile activation of skinned cardiac cells on the sarcomere length. *Nature* 256:54–56, 1975.

## 1.6. THEORETICAL AND EXPERIMENTAL FORCE-VELOCITY RELATIONS OF THE VENTRICULAR MYOCARDIUM

PIET SCHIERCK, HERMAN B.K. BOOM

## 1. INTRODUCTION

Striated muscle has been demonstrated to develop active force ($F$) in an inverse relationship to the velocity of shortening ($v$) it is allowed to attain. At a constant level of activation this relationship is fairly well approximated by Hill's equation (1, 2, 3, 4):

$$(F + a)(v + b) = (F_0 + a)b \qquad [1]$$

The constants $a$ and $b$ appearing in this equation suffer from lack of physiological interpretability; they are mere empirical constants obtained from fitting the force-velocity hyperbolic relation to experimental force and velocity data.

When dealing with skeletal muscle the significance of the Hill equation is clear due to the fact that force and shortening velocity can be readily measured in the functioning muscular organ. The validity of the force-velocity relation for cardiac muscle, in contrast, is more difficult to appreciate since myocardial wall force and myocardial fibre shortening have a more distant relationship to circulatory variables such as pressure and flow. One would like to have a cardiac or ventricular equivalent of the force-velocity relation in terms of ventricular pressure and volume.

The study that is presented in this paper was aimed at deriving such an equation, followed by designing and carrying out experiments enabling an evaluation of its validity. It was found that the Hill equation can very well describe the phenomena measured in the experiments.

## 2. METHODS

### 2.1. Theory

In order to arrive at a ventricular equivalent of the force-velocity relation some basic assumptions had to be made. They were based on physiological and anatomical considerations but inevitably contain appreciable simplifications.

*J. Baan, A.C. Arntzenius, E.L. Yellin (eds.), Cardiac Dynamics, 51–59.*

First, the contractile elements within the ventricular wall, postulated to obey the Hill equation, were assumed to shorten by extending a series elastic element even when total fibre length, or in this case ventricular volume, remained constant. It was also assumed that the force-extension relation of the series elastic element is exponential, giving rise to a linear stiffness-force relation:

$$\frac{dF}{dx} = c_1 F + c_2 \qquad [2]$$

where $x$ is the series elastic element length, $F$ is fibre force and $c_1$ and $c_2$ are constants. Stiffness $dF/dx$ may be replaced by: $dF/dx = dF/dt \cdot dt/dx$. This gives rise to:

$$\frac{dF}{dt} = v(c_1 F + c_2) \qquad [3]$$

Series elastic extension velocity $v$ appearing in [3] is identical to contractile element shortening velocity in [1] if total length of the fibre under consideration is unchanging. Consequently this quantity may be eliminated from [1] and [3] yielding:

$$\frac{dF}{dt} = c_1 b \cdot \frac{(F_0 - F)(F + c_3)}{a + F} \qquad [4]$$

with $c_3 = c_2/c_1$.

This equation has the advantage that the original two mechanical time-dependent variables: force and shortening velocity, have been replaced by one variable and its time derivative: $F$ and $dF/dt$.

For simplicity it was assumed in the following that the ventricle may be represented by a thin-walled sphere with a circular homogeneously distributed fibre orientation. A thick-walled sphere could have been used with more exertions but essentially the same result. For the thin-walled sphere a simple proportionality exists between wall force and intracavity pressure: $F_{wall} = \pi r^2 p$ where $r$ denotes ventricular radius and $p$ intraventricular pressure. Total equatorial wall force $F_{wall}$ may be identified with muscle force, and [4] is transformed into

$$\frac{dp}{dt} = c_1 b \frac{(p_0 - p)(p + c_3')}{a' + p} \qquad [5]$$

with $c_3' = c_3/\pi r^2$ and $a' = a/\pi r^2$. In analogy with the definition of $F_0$, $p_0$ is the maximally developed pressure under zero shortening velocity conditions.

This equation predicts a unique relationship between pressure $p$ and rate of pressure development $dp/dt$ as long as muscle fibre length and, thus, $r$ is constant. This condition is approximately met if ventricular contraction is isovolumic. If $p$ is sufficiently large, $a'/p$ and $c'_3/p$ will be negligible with regard to 1, leaving a linear relationship between $dp/dt$ and $p$ with negative slope: for smaller $p$ values $dp/dt$ will be larger. At sufficiently small pressures, however, $dp/dt$ should level off and eventually decrease, giving rise to a maximum in the $dp/dt$ versus $p$ curve.

It was not permissible to apply [5] to the time course of ventricular pressure itself, since it is not known beforehand that $a$, $b$ and particularly $p_0$ are independent of time. Therefore, [5] had to be tested at fixed instants, i.e. at one moment at a time during the cardiac cycle.

## 2.2. Experiment

Since the ventricle generates pressure through spontaneous internal processes its value at one instant of the contraction cycle is fixed. However, [5] can only be tested by realizing a number of pressure values, and measuring the accompanying $dp/dt$. Therefore, some kind of intervention was required. Instantaneous pressure may be changed by slightly, though rapidly, altering volume (5, 6, 7). This was realized by using a pump (Figure 1).

Isolated left ventricles of rabbits were perfused by connecting the aortic root to a perfusing system supplying an inorganic salt solution. Intraventricular pressure was measured with a small catheter-tip micromanometer, allowing the measurement of very fast pressure changes. The value $dp/dt$ was determined by analog differentiation ($\omega_0 = 1000$ rad/s). The ventricle was stimulated artificially with large silver electrode plates. By preventing ejection, end-diastolic volume was kept constant until the moment of measurement.

Various volume changes of up to 10% of ventricular end-diastolic volume were effected within 5 msec by a small electrically driven, computer controlled pump connected to a special cannula fitting snugly into the mitral orifice. Series of volume disturbances were applied during consecutive contractions, all at the same instant relative to the cardiac cycle. During such series pump stroke volume was gradually increased. Im-

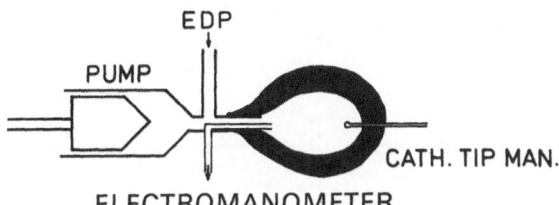

*Figure 1.* The principle of rapidly induced pumping. The ventricle is connected to a pump via a tube ligated in the mitral orifice. Additional branches enable setting of end-diastolic pressure and measurement of intra-ventricular pressure.

mediately following each pump stroke $p$ and $dp/dt$ were measured. Series were carried out at a number of chosen instants in order to investigate the influence of time on the $dp/dt$ versus $p$ relation.

Although contractions before and after the pump stroke continued to be isovolumic, this was naturally not the case during the pump stroke. Volume decreased somewhat giving rise to a slight decrease of $r$ in [5]. This effect was corrected for by making use of the assumed spherical geometry. A new $r$ value was computed from the old one and the known pump stroke volume.

Pre-pumping volume was estimated from diastolic pressure by arresting the ventricle through injection of 10% KCl solution and measuring diastolic pressure at different volumes as changed by means of a syringe.

Experiment and theory were compared by fitting [5] to the experimental data obtained using a least-squares error criterion for the remaining difference between measured and calculated $dp/dt$ at all measured $p$ values.

### 3. RESULTS

Examples of pressure and $dp/dt$ tracings obtained have been presented elsewhere (7). Experimental $dp/dt$ versus $p$ relations at one instant, for two different diastolic pressures and, hence, volume are given in Figure 2. Note

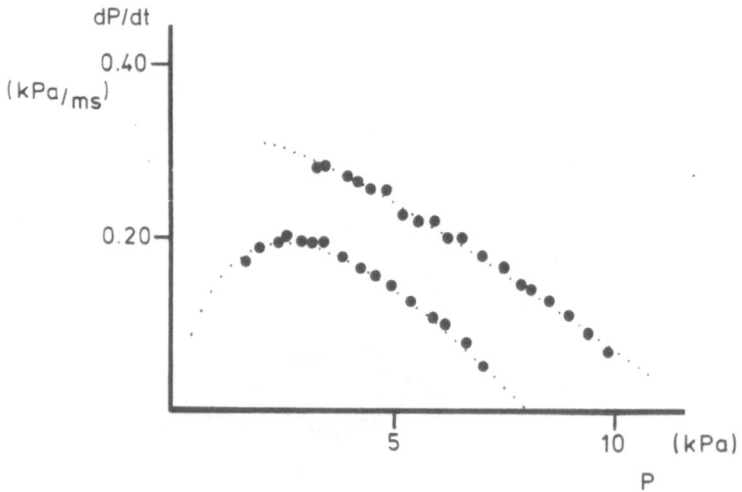

*Figure 2.* Instantaneous $dp/dt$ versus $p$ relations for two settings of end-diastolic pressure (EDP), $dp/dt$ is approximately linearly related to instantaneous pressure with negative slope. Below pressure values of 3 kPa $dp/dt$ decreases with decreasing instantaneous pressure.

that the right-hand sides of the graphs indeed approximate linearity as indicated by [5]. The curves do not intersect the $p$-axis since $dp/dt$ is not zero in the absence of a pump stroke, but equal to the undisturbed value found by taking the slope of the pressure-time curve at that instant.

Following the interpretation of [5], the increase of $dp/dt$ when $p$ is decreasing arises from the fact that lower pressure implies lower muscle force which enables a larger shortening velocity. Although series-elastic stiffness has decreased according to [2], this does not compensate for the increased shortening velocity, resulting in augmented $dp/dt$. However, if the volume disturbance results in very lower ventricular pressure, stiffness has decreased progressively, due to the exponential series-elastic force-length relation used. In such cases increased shortening velocity does not compensate for decreased stiffness, resulting in a net decrease of $dp/dt$.

Fitting of [5] to experimental data as shown in Figure 2 always resulted in excelent correspondence. This is also illustrated in the figure by the broken lines. Experimental $dp/dt$ versus $p$ relations, though always similar in shape in one heart, varied considerably between different hearts, the variable location of the maximum being particularly noticeable. In some hearts it occurred at halfway the undisturbed pressure, sometimes it could not be observed at all. In all cases however, the same close theoretical fit could be obtained. These observations were considered sufficient evidence that [5] could be used as a working hypothesis.

Data obtained from 30 hearts were fitted by theory. This resulted in values of the parameters occurring in [5]. For purposes of comparison the Hill constant $a$ was calculated as its value relative with respect to $F_0$: $a/F_0 = a'/p_0$. This parameter showed a good amount of scatter, which is in agreement with the literature (8, 9, 10). Values found ranged from 0.001 to 1.3. The scatter is obviously associated with the variable location of the $dp/dt$ maximum. The Hill constant $b$ cannot be estimated directly from these experiments since, in [5], it occurs multiplied by the first stiffness constant $c_1$. The product $c_1 \cdot b$ assumed values more consistent than those of $a$: $7$–$49$ $s^{-1}$.

Of more physiological interest was the possibility of obtaining data for $F_0 = \pi r^2 p_0$ since it represents total myocardial force extrapolated for zero shortening velocity. This is a quantity that has been long assumed to represent active state (1). Results on this will be discussed below.

The experimental technique of rapid pumping is especially suited to study influences of time or time-related factors on various contraction parameters, since this method itself yields virtually instantaneous values. Figure 3 illustrates a family of $dp/dt$ versus $p$ curves obtained by repeating series of pump strokes at a number of instants during the ascending limb of the isovolumic contraction cycle. These curves are examples of cases which did not exhibit a maximum. They were fitted well by [5] as demonstrated by the

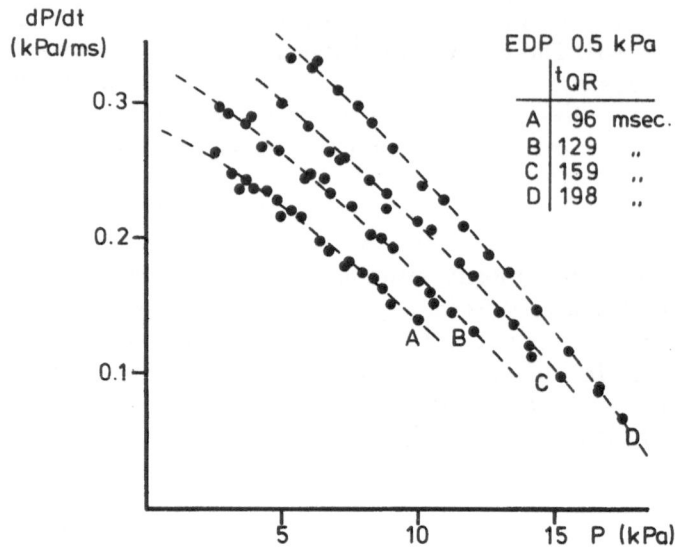

*Figure 3.* Instantaneous *dp/dt* versus *p* relations for four different instants during the ascending limb of the isovolumic pressure curve. Extrapolated intercepts with the *p*-axis represent pressure at which myocardial fibre-shortening velocity would be zero ($p_0$). This figure is independent of time for the later moment, implying a plateau in the "active state" of the myocardium.

broken lines. Although starting points (A, B, C, D) were clearly distinct, the curves are similar. This suggests that the state of the myocardium in these instances is not as different as suggested by the values of the starting pressures. The suggestion is enhanced by the convergence of the *dp/dt* versus *p* relations towards the *p*-axis. Intersection with this axis corresponds with $p_0$, which is the pressure that would be measured in the ventricle at zero myocardial shortening velocity. The value of $p_0$ appears to be fairly constant during part of the isovolumic pressure curve. Since $F_0$ represents the ability of the myocardium to develop active force under isometric conditions, this parameter may be considered as active state, which apparently is fairly constant throughout an appreciable part of ventricular systole.

A more extensive exploration of the ventricular pressure curves of one ventricle than corresponding to five instants proved difficult. Redevelopment rate of pressure after rapid pumping appeared to be very sensitive to various external or internal conditions and henceforth seems a good index for myocardial contractile quality. After five series usually the state of the myocardium was slightly but definitely changed with consequent loss of reproducibility. Combining data from a number of hearts one obtains the results shown in Figure 4. Here the influence of increasing end-diastolic

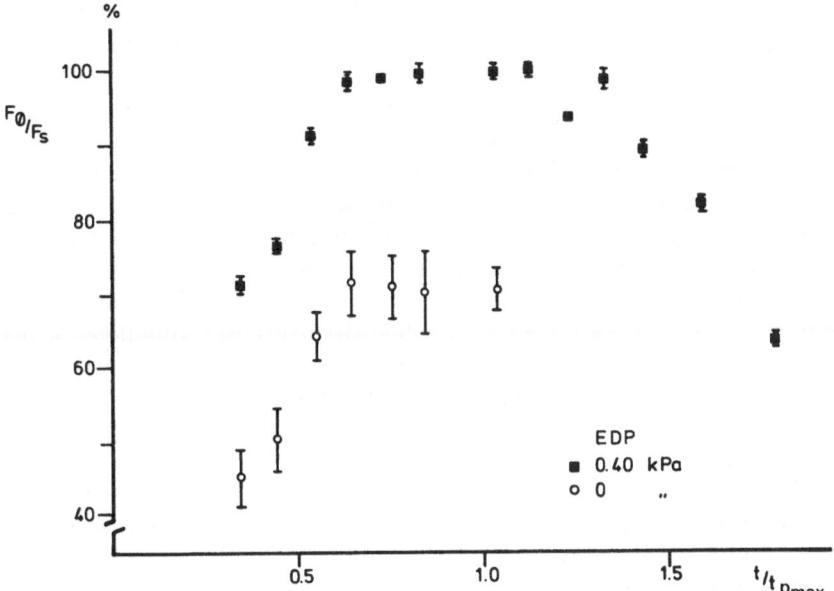

*Figure 4.* Averaged time course of $p_0$ (myocardial active state) at two EDP values: $p_0$ values of each heart were taken relative to maximal $p_0$ at an EDP of 0.4 kPa (3 mmHg). Time coordinates were normalized to time of maximal pressure in each heart ($t_{p_{max}}$). A plateau in "active state" is clearly visible at both EDP values, which extended from 0.6 to 1.0 $t_{p_{max}}$.

pressure, which shifted the level of the curve upward, is also shown. This corresponds to the classical Frank-Starling mechanism. In order to allow the combining of results for different hearts which, in general, exhibited slightly different rates of pressure developments, time scales had to be normalized. For each contraction, time of maximal pressure was taken as a point of reference. Time coordinates were rounded off to integer multiples of 0.1. Additionally, $F_0$ values were taken relative to the $F_0$ value each heart developed at an end-diastolic pressure of 0.4 kPa. From the composite plot of Figure 4 a fairly constant value of $F_0$ is evident from 0.6 to 1.0 $t_{p_{max}}$.

4. DISCUSSION

The results presented indicate that, if pressure development by the ventricle during the rising limb of the pressure-time curve is interpreted as a process during which the contractile element is allowed to shorten at the expense of a series elastic element, the instantaneous relation between $dp/dt$ and $p$ is predicted correctly. An interesting aspect is that the extent to which a true series elastic elasticity is active in the ventricular wall is presently almost completely unknown. Direct evidence as to the presence and the properties of the series-elastic element originates from papillary muscle experiments (11, 12, 13, 14). These experiments are now disputed because of the procedure-induced necrotic endings which made up for nearly all of the series-elastic compliance, leaving at most one percent rapid elastic extensibility of such muscle tissue (15, 16, 17). In the intact ventricle more possible sources for series-elastic extensibility are present. Endocardial structures and changes in shape of the ventricles could contribute. In the preparation used in this study influences of bulging valves, aortic trunk, and so on, were eliminated as much as possible (7), while the heart was stimulated synchronously. Nevertheless the possibility exists that part of the required series-elasticity is the result of shape changes that take place during isovolumic contractions.

While values for the constants $a$ and $b$ as found in this study have only physiological significance as far as one accepts the applicability of the Hill equation for the ventricular myocardium, this is less stringently the case for results found on $F_0$. Any model that allows for the possibility of muscle shortening during isovolumic contraction and in which developed muscle force depends inversely on contractile element-shortening velocity will probably yield the same result, whenever, it fits the data equally well. Therefore, conclusions regarding the time course of "active state" $F_0$ seem to be of fairly general validity. In this respect it is of interest that the concept of a more or less constant "active state" during part of systole, although originally rejected (18) has received renewed support in recent years (17, 19). In the study by Ter Keurs et al. a nearly constant $F_0$ was demonstrated in isolated trabecular fibres of rats under truly isometric conditions (17). It seems therefore that the constant $F_0$ level found for the intact ventricle in this study is a reflection of a comparable phenomenon inherent to the functional microscopic constituents of heart muscle.

SUMMARY

A theoretical relation between rate of rise of ventricular pressure $dp/dt$ and pressure $p$ was derived starting from the Hill equation and using a simple thin-walled spherical model for the left ventricle. An approximately linear relation was predicted between $dp/dt$ and $p$ for high and moderate pressure and a maximum in $dp/dt$ at a small $p$ value. This relation was tested experimentally by disturbing ventricular pressure instantaneously by rapidly induced pumping of the ventricle. Rapid small decreases in ventricular volume resulted in large decreases of pressure. Immediately following each pump stroke, pressure redeveloped and $dp/dt$ could be measured. This value was related to pressure measured at the same instant. Experimental $dp/dt$ relations obtained in this way could be fitted by the theoretical relation with a high degree of correspondence. From the fitting procedure the parameters of the Hill equation could be estimated. The following values were found: $a/F_0 = 0.001 - 1.3$ and $c_1 \cdot b = 7 - 49\ s^{-1}$. Influence of time was examined by changing the timing of volume changes in the contraction cycle. It was found that $F_0$ reached a plateau of 0.6 $t_{p_{max}}$ which continued to 1.0 $t_{p_{max}}$. This was considered as evidence for a phase of constant "active state" during myocardial contraction.

REFERENCES

1. Hill AV: The heat of shortening and the dynamic constants of muscle. *Proc R Soc Lond* B126:136–195, 1939.
2. Sonnenblick EH: Force-velocity relations in mammalian heart muscle. *Am. J. Physiol* 202: 931–939, 1962.
3. Edman KAP, Nilsson E: Relationships between force and velocity of shortening in rabbit papillary muscle. *Acta Physiol Scand* 85:488–500, 1972.
4. Brutsaert DL, Sonnenblick EH: Nature of the force-velocity relation in heart muscle. *Cardiovasc Res* (suppl 1): 18–33, 1971.
5. Covell JW, Taylor RR, Sonnenblick EH, Ross Jr J: Series elasticity of the Hill model for muscle to the intact left ventricle. *Pflügers Arch* 357:225–236, 1975.
6. Templeton GH, Ecker PR, Mitchell JH: Left ventricular stiffness during diastole and systole; the influence of changes is volume and inotropic state. *Cardiovasc Res* 6:95–100, 1972.
7. Schiereck P, Boom HBK: Left ventricular active stiffness: dependency on time and inotropic state. *Pflügers Arch* 374:135–143, 1978.
8. Edman KAP, Mattiazzi A, Nilsson E: The influence of temperature on the force-velocity relationship in rabbit papillary muscle. *Acta Physiol Scand* 90:750–756, 1974.
9. Brutsaert DL, Sonnenblick EH: Force-velocity-length-time relations of the contractile elements in heart muscle of the cat. *Circ Res* 24:137–149, 1969.
10. Brutsaert DL, Parmley WW, Sonnenblick EH: Effects of various inotropic interventions on the dynamic properties of the contractile elements in heart muscle of the cat. *Circ Res* 27:513–522, 1970.
11. Sonnenblick EH: Series elastic and contractile elements in heart muscle: changes in muscle length. *Am J Physiol* 207:1330–1338, 1964.
12. Meiss RA, Sonnenblick EH: Dynamic elasticity of cardiac muscle as measured by controlled length changes. *Am J Physiol* 226:1370–1381, 1974.
13. Parmley WW, Sonnenblick EH: Series elasticity in heart muscle: its relation to contractile element velocity and proposed muscle models. *Circ Res* 20:112–123, 1967.
14. Pollack GH, Huntsman LL, Verdugo P: Cardiac muscle models: an overextension of series elasticity? *Circ Res* 31:569–579, 1972.
15. Krueger JW, Pollack GH: Myocardial sarcomere dynamics during isometric contraction. *J Physiol* 251:627–643, 1975.
16. Pollack GH, Krueger JW: Sarcomere dynamics in intact cardiac muscle. *Eur J Cardiol* 4: 53–65, 1976.
17. Keurs HEDJ Ter, Bloot R, Rijnsburger WH, Nagelsmit MJ: The influence of sarcomere length on tension development in rat heart muscle. *Biophys J* 21:86a, 1978.
18. Edman KAP, Nilsson E: The mechanical parameters of myocardial contraction studied at a constant length of the contractile element. *Acta Physiol Scand* 72:205–219, 1968.
19. Joseph DS, Huntsman LL: Force-velocity relations in cardiac muscle. *Biophys J* 21:55a, 1978.

## 1.7. TIME COURSE OF CHANGES IN ACTION POTENTIAL DURATION AND EJECTION SHORTENING DURING REGIONAL TRANSIENT ISCHAEMIA OF PIG VENTRICLE IN SITU

MAX J. LAB, KEITH V. WOOLLARD

### 1. INTRODUCTION

The duration of the action potential is normally one of the determinants of the strength of contraction of cardiac muscle. The longer the cardiac cell membrane is depolarized per unit time the greater the inward calcium current and the greater the tension (1). When cardiac muscle is made ischaemic the action potential duration (APD) shortens (2), and this will contribute to the deterioration in contraction during ischaemia (3). Some evidence has also been presented suggesting that the time course of mechanical recovery from oxygen deprivation may be related to changes in APD (4). To our knowledge no systematic study has been carried out in the intact heart correlating action potential duration measurements and myocardial dynamics during regional ischaemia. The object of this study is therefore to determine the time course of these electromechanical measurements on a beat-to-beat basis during transient occlusion of small branches of the coronary arteries in pig hearts, and to see if they may be causally related.

### 2. METHODS

Pigs of about 25 kg were anaesthetized with 1% halothane and a mixture of nitrous oxide and oxygen (1:1). The animals were ventilated and, during the experimental phase, the halothane was discontinued and a 1% solution of chloralose administered intravenously as necessary.

The chest was opened and a pericardial cradle was fashioned to support the heart. A catheter was inserted through the apex of the ventricle and intraventricular pressure was measured. Arterial pressure was measured via a catheter inserted into the proximal aorta. A small branch of the left anterior descending branch of the left coronary artery was selected so that when a catgut snare was tightened around the vessel a cyanotic area about 1.5 cm × 2.5 cm was produced.

A tripodal device (5) was attached, by vacuum through the legs, to the area of epicardium to be made ischaemic. This device provided three

*J. Baan, A.C. Arntzenius, E.L. Yellin (eds.), Cardiac Dynamics, 61–67.*

outputs due to strains on gauges attached to the legs. The distance between each leg and the central point of the triangle they formed was about 7 mm. The movement of the legs along the axes from the centre to the corners of the base plane was recorded and taken to represent length changes in the underlying segments of epicardium. This assumption depends on the compliance of the instrument which was about 0.1 mm/g along the axis of movement of each leg. Little movement was possible in any other direction. Even though the device was somewhat stiffer than mercury-in-silastic gauges (6) our results are similar to those obtained with these gauges and also to the results obtained from ultrasonic crystals (7). In particular, marked elongation during isovolumic contraction was not observed.

The three outputs from the legs of the tripod, representing length changes in three directions over a small area, were fed into an analog computer for on-line analysis (8). Briefly, this first involved continuous arithmetical summing of the three outputs to produce a "summed segment length" which was used to represent the behaviour of the underlying area of epicardium. The aortic and ventricular pressure signals were used to define the phases of the cardiac cycle, and the instantaneous values for pre-ejection length (PEL), segment length at the beginning, and end-ejection length (EEL), segment length at the end of the ejection period, were displayed. The difference between these two values represents the length change during systole (ejection shortening).

A monophasic action potential (9) was obtained with a suction electrode which was capable of following changes in duration due to ischaemia (5). The indifferent electrode consisted of a thin wick of cotton wool which completely surrounded the suction electrode and from which the epicardial ECG was also recorded. The monophasic action potential and epicardial ECG were obtained either using one of the legs of the tripod as an electrode or from an area as close to the tripodal device as possible.

All the signals were passed to a Devices M19 pen recorder, displayed on paper and on a Tektronix storage oscilloscope. The signals were also stored on magnetic tape for later analysis. The action potential duration could be automatically measured with a device constructed for this purpose (10).

## 3. RESULTS

Figure 1 is an example of a mechanical recording (ejection shortening) during an episode of transient regional ischaemia, as obtained with the tripodal device. The outputs of the changes in each direction of movement of the legs of the tripod have been summed to provide an indication of the mechanical behaviour of the underlying myocardium. The changes observed were seen to be in keeping with those obtained with other techniques

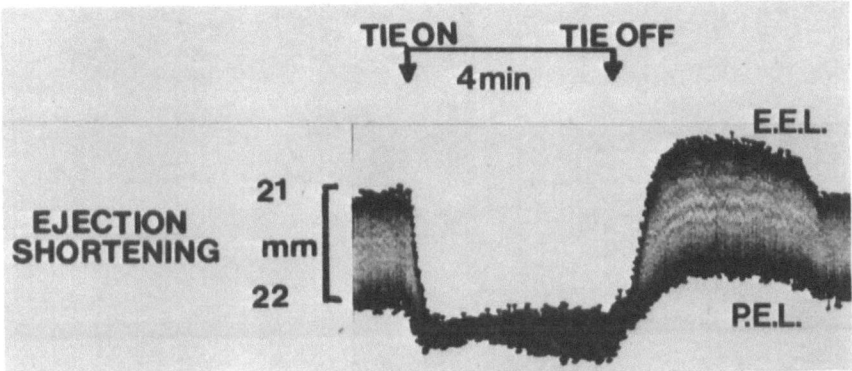

*Figure 1.* Continuous display of instantaneous segment length at the beginning (PEL) and end (EEL) of the ejection phase during a period of ischaemia. The width of the band represents the magnitude of the shortening during the ejection phase. On occluding the artery a reduction in ejection shortening may be detected within a few beats. The rapid mechanical deterioration is nearly complete in 30 sec. With reperfusion ejection shortening recovers over a minute reaching values greater than control, for several minutes, before pre-ischaemic levels are reattained.

and during ischaemia the area showed early systolic expansion and reduced overall shortening.

A rapid reduction in inward calcium current could conceivably explain the rapid loss of the ability of the myocardium to contract during the onset of ischaemia. An abbreviation in action potential duration (APD) could be a cause of the reduction and it was pertinent to follow the time course of changes in APD from this area on a beat-to-beat basis. On occlusion the APD actually slightly increased transiently and we could not detect a significant reduction in APD until two minutes after the tie (Figure 2). Apart from the increase in APD, there was no change in action potential amplitude or configuration during this period. The duration and amplitude thereafter steadily declined.

There was a close relationship between the action potential duration and the T wave of the epicardial ECG. As the action potential shortened the T wave became more positive (inset of Figure 2), and correspondingly, lengthening of the action potential was associated with increasing negativity of the T wave. The S-T segment however did not alter in a biphasic manner. Some elevation could be detected within the first minute and it slowly increased over the next 3–4 minutes.

The question now arose as to the precise relationship between the time course of the mechanical deterioration and the APD alterations. This relationship is clearly seen in Figure 2 where ejection shortening and APD were plotted during transient ischaemia. The early, rapid reduction in ejection shortening corresponds in time to the slight transient increase in

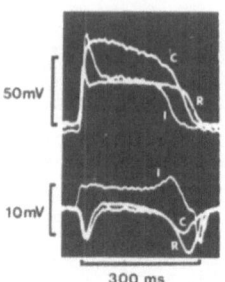

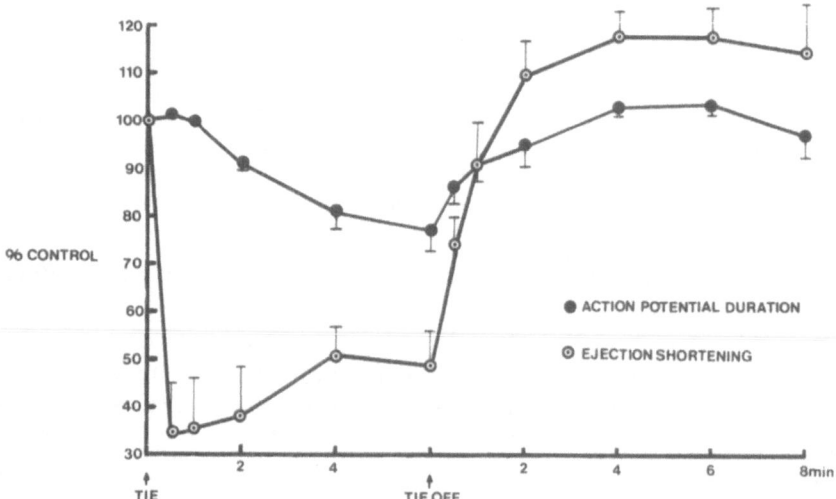

*Figure 2.* Graphs to show time course of changes, produced by ischaemia and reperfusion, in ejection period shortening and action potential duration (mean $\pm$ S.E., $n = 15$). Ejection shortening deteriorates much more rapidly than the action potential duration which actually first increases over the first minute ($P < 0.05$). There is a transient improvement in ejection shortening 2–4 minutes after the tie, which is also not accompanied by a comparable electrical change. However, on reperfusion electrical and mechanical changes recover at a similar rate and both exceed control values for a short period. *Inset*: Effects of ischaemia on monophasic action potentials (upper traces) and epicardial electrocardiograms (lower traces). Compared to the control situation (C), ischaemia (I) produces a reduction in duration of action potentials and a raised S-T segment. The base-lines of the epicardial ECG are superimposed. There is in fact significant T-Q depression. The sharp downward deflection at the end of T-waves are conducted atrial pacing spikes. (they are not detected in the action potential).

APD. Thereafter the ejection shortening showed some improvement, although the APD now steadily declined, and this improvement was a consistent finding with the type of preparation we have studied. The action potential rarely disappeared with these small ischaemic areas. However, with longer or larger infarcts, areas could easily be found with the suction electrode that were electrically quiescent, but where the epicardial ECG was completely monophasic in character, showing a marked S-T elevation (5).

We wished to answer three questions concerning reperfusion. First, do the electromechanical changes follow the same time course, during recovery as on occlusion? On removing the occlusion, electrophysiological measurements and the mechanical measurements show a rapid parallel recovery towards control values contrasting with the opposite biphasic behaviour at the onset of ischaemia. The next question was whether we could observe values of ejection shortening greater than control, during the reperfusion period, as previously reported for other mechanical measurements and preparations (4, 11). Such an overshoot is clearly demonstrated in both Figures 1 and 2. Finally, we wished to see whether in the intact heart in situ an increase in APD above control levels occurred in parallel with this ejection shortening overshoot. An overshoot above control values was observed in the electrophysiological as well as the mechanical recordings, both having roughly the same time course (Figure 2).

4. DISCUSSION

Correlations between epicardial electrocardiograms, action potentials, and mechanical performance in intact hearts in situ have not been studied before. Part of the difficulty in attempting to correlate mechanical changes and alterations in APD in epicardial segments during ischaemia and reperfusion on a beat-to-beat basis lies in the continuous recording of action potentials with microelectrodes while normal mechanical changes are unhindered. Recording with microelectrodes alone without measuring mechanical change is difficult enough, frequently necessitating immobilization of the area studied. However, the immobilization itself may influence the recorded potentials (12, 13). Monophasic action potentials obtained with suction electrodes can overcome some of the difficulties and give an indication of transmembrane events, particularly the time course of repolarization. Action potentials thus obtained may show the same changes in duration observed with microelectrodes during anoxia (5).

On release of the tie after 5 to 10 minutes of ischaemia, there was a dramatic restoration of contraction and action potential duration over approximately the same time course. During this period of reperfusion ejection shortening was greater than control and there was also a transient increase in action potential duration above control values. These observations on epicardial segments support those on isolated perfused preparations in which there was a prolongation in tension (particularly a delayed relaxation on re-oxygenation) (4, 11).

Simultaneous microelectrode and mechanical studies have previously shown an increase in action potential duration above control on reoxygenation (4) although this has not been confirmed by others (11). These supranormal mechanical and electrical changes could be causally related in that a prolongation in action potential duration by electrical means can increase tension development in isolated muscle (1). The increase in tension is thought to be mediated by an increase in calcium-inward current (14). However if this mechanism operates it may only be part of the explanation. Figure 2 shows that recovery of the ejection shortening is slightly faster than the recovery of the APD and, furthermore, the overshoot in ejection shortening lasts a little longer than the overshoot in APD.

Although electromechanical recovery during reperfusion is rapid and parallel in time, and the changes in APD and segment shortening may be causally related, our results clearly show that no such relationship exists during the onset of acute ischaemia. The mechanical deterioration is faster than the change in APD. It is thus unlikely that the rapid reduction in contractility is mediated via a reduced inward calcium current and thus a fall in contractile dependent calcium. However, the interruption of the energy-dependent chain governing intracellular $Ca^{++}$ has a sound basis (3) and this mechanism probably operates later. A small but consistent and hence potentially significant observation is that the action potential duration actually increased over the period of rapid mechanical deterioration. Cooling of the myocardium can prolong the APD (5, 15) and qualitatively this change is in the right direction. However, we feel that this is not the explanation because our temperature measurements from the centre of the small ischaemic zones show very small reductions ($0.1°C$). Furthermore, other electrophysiological measurements during the first 2 min of ischaemia have been known to follow a biphasic pattern similar in time course to the changes in APD observed here (16).

What common denominator could exist between the increase in APD and reduction in contractility? One interesting possibility is the calcium ion, for it has been suggested that an increase in internal calcium may increase the outward current which would reduce the APD (17). If, therefore, the reduction in contraction is due to a reduction in available free intracellular calcium in the case under discussion, it would be associated with a reduction in outward current and thus a prolongation in APD. It is thus conceivable that the electromechanical changes during ischaemia and reperfusion may both be calcium-mediated, but with different mechanisms.

ACKNOWLEDGEMENTS

K.V. Woollard is in receipt of Trustee Fellowships of Charing Cross Hospital (Clinical Research Committee). We thank Mr. R. Price for constructing the tripodal device and Mrs. R. Kingaby for her technical assistance.

REFERENCES

1. Antoni H, Jacob R, Kaufmann R: Mechanische Reaktion – des Frosch- und Säuge-Tiermyokard bei Veränderung der Aktions-potential-Daur durch konstante Gleichstromimpulse. *Pflügers Arch* 306:33–57, 1969.
2. Samson WE, Sher AM: Mechanism of S-T segment alteration during acute myocardial injury. *Circ Res* 8:780–787, 1960.
3. Coraboeuf E, Deroubaix E, Hoerter J: Control of ionic permeabilities in normal and ischaemic heart. *Circ Res* Suppl 1:92–98, 1976.
4. Trautwein W, Dudel J: Aktionspotential und Kontraktion des Herzmuskels im Sauerstoffmangel. *Pflügers Arch* 263:23–32, 1956.
5. Lab MJ, Woollard KV: Monophasic action potentials, electrocardiograms and mechanical performance in normal and ischaemic segments of pig ventricle in situ. *Cardiovasc Res* 12:555–565, 1978.
6. Tyberg JV, Forrester JS, Wyatt HL, Goldner SJ, Parmley, WW, Swan, HJC: An analysis of segmental ischaemic dysfunction utilizing the pressure-length loop. *Circulation* 69:748–754, 1974.
7. Bugge-Asperheim B, Leraand S, Kiil F: Local dimensional changes of the myocardium measured by ultrasonic technique. *Scand J Clin Lab Invest* 24:361–371, 1969.
8. Child RO, Colley NOD, Gartside IB, Lab MJ, Woollard, KV: The use of analogue circuits for measurement and calculation in cardiac physiology. *J Physiol* 289:10P, 1979.
9. Hoffman SF, Cranfield PF, Lepeschkin, E, Surawicz B, Herrlich HC: Comparison of cardiac monophasic action potentials recorded by intra-cellular and suction electrodes. *Am J Physiol* 196:1296–1301, 1959.
10. Lab MJ, Child RO: A fully automatic cardiac action potential duration meter. *Am J Physiol* 236:H183.H188, 1979.
11. Brooks WW, Sturckow B, Bing HL: Myocardial hypoxia and reoxygenation: electrophysiologic and mechanical correlates. *Am J Physiol* 226:523–527, 1974.
12. Kaufmann R, Lab MJ, Hennekes R, Krause H: Feedback interaction of mechanical and electrical events in the isolated ventricular myocardium (cat papillary muscle). *Pflügers Arch* 324:100–123, 1971.
13. Lab MJ: Mechanically dependent changes in action potentials recorded from intact frog ventricle. *Circ Res* 42:519–528, 1978.
14. Wood EH, Heppner RL, Weidmann S: Inotropic effects of electric currents or current impulses applied during cardiac action potentials II: hypothesis: calcium movements excitation-contraction coupling and inotropic effects. *Circ Res* 24:409–445, 1969.
15. Toyoshima H, Prinzmetal M, Haribu M, Kobayashi T, Mizuno Y, Nakayama R, Yamada K: The nature of normal and abnormal electrocardiograms. *Arch Intern Med* 115:4–16, 1965.
16. Elharrar V, Zipes DP: Cardiac electrophysiologic alterations during myocardial ischemia. *Am J Physiol* 233:H329–H345, 1977.
17. Bassingthwaighte JB, Fry CH, McGuigan JAS: Relationship between internal calcium and outward current in mammalian ventricular muscle: a mechanism for the control of action potential duration? *J Physiol* 262:15–38, 1976.

## 1.8. A QUANTITATIVE ANALYSIS OF THE FORCE TRANSIENTS OF SKELETAL MUSCLE IN RESPONSE TO QUICK CHANGES IN LENGTH

G.J.M. Stienen, T. Blangé

### 1. INTRODUCTION

Recently, adaptations of the sliding filament model (1) have been proposed as a description of the dynamic properties of the contractile mechanism which provide an explanation of the transient force response after a quick change in length in which data of the ultrastructure and the biochemical reactions are taken into account (2, 3, 4). The present experiments were undertaken as a contribution to the identification of the reaction steps of the kinetic scheme (5) in the transient force response. In a preceding study attention was focused on the early parts of the tension response of frog sartorius muscle (6). From these experiments it was concluded that the initial fall in tension during a fast shortening can be described in terms of a visco-elastic element. Furthermore, it was found that in the metabolically inhibited muscle in which the ATP concentration was lowered by repeated stimulation, the early phases of the tension recovery are depressed.

The results described here concern the force responses to rapid shortenings as well as to rapid lengthenings completed within 4 msec and an analysis of the slow recovery. Furthermore, changes in stiffness during the transients were determined.

### 2. METHODS

Changes in muscle length were induced by means of a position servo system (6). Position changes of one end of the muscle up to 60 $\mu$m could be imposed with a rise time from 5% to 95% of 0.15 msec. Larger changes were performed in the shape of a ramp with an acceleration and deceleration phase of 0.15 msec. During the series of experiments the maximum velocity was increased from 0.25 to 0.35 m/s. For the registration of the force responses a strain gauge transducer was used with a resonance frequency of 7 kHz and a sensitivity of 0.15 V/N (7).

The sartorius muscle of the frog (*Rana esculenta*) was dissected free together with part of the os pubis. This part was tied to the displacement system and the tibial tendon was fixed to the force transducer. This last

*J. Baan, A.C. Arntzenius, E.L. Yellin (eds.), Cardiac Dynamics, 69–78.*

connection was glued in order to minimize the influence of the tendon. The muscle was mounted horizontally in the tissue chamber at resting length ($L_0$). The muscle was stimulated electrically by means of two silver wires running alongside. The oxygenated bathing solution contained (in mM): NaCl, 115; KCl, 2.5; $CaCl_2$, 1.8, d-tubocurarine chloride (10 mg/l) and a sodium phosphate buffer (pH = 7.3). The temperature was kept at about 0°C, except where otherwise stated.

## 3. RESULTS

Ramp-shaped length changes with a maximum duration of 4 msec were applied to isometrically contracting frog sartorius muscle. The general features of the tension responses to shortenings as well as to lengthenings of different amplitudes are shown in Figure 1. In accordance with the results

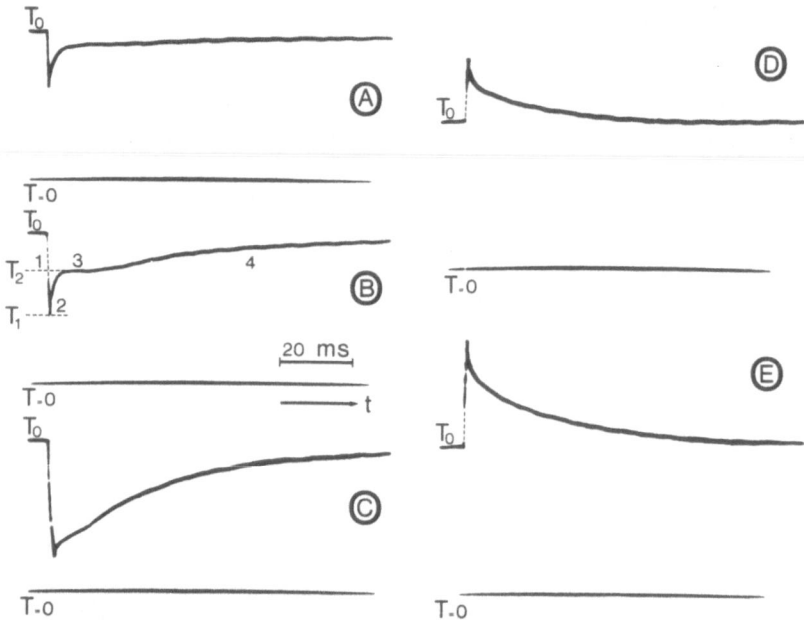

*Figure 1.* Tension responses of isometrically tetanized frog sartorius muscle at resting length to ramp-shaped changes in length. *Left*: responses to shortenings of 4.3 (A), 8.5 (B) and 17 nm/half-sarcomere (C); *right*: responses to lengthenings of 4.3 (D) and 8.5 nm/half-sarcomere (E). Displacement rate per half-sarcomere: 8.5 nm/msec. The tension response to a shortening can be divided in a decrease in tension during the ramp (1) followed by fast recovery (2), plateau phase (3) and slow recovery (4). *Experimental conditions*: muscle resting length ($L_0$) = 24.5 mm, sarcomere length ($s_0$) = 2.2 μm, isometric tetanic tension ($T_0$) = 2.2 × 10⁵ N/m², temperature = 2°C.

derived from other preparations (8) the transient force response to a quick shortening consists of 4 distinct phases as indicated in Figure 1. The force response to a quick lengthening can be divided into an increase in tension during the length change followed by a tension recovery to the isometric tension level in an exponential fashion. In some of the experiments, the tension course showed a slight undershoot in tension about 50 msec after the lengthening.

The $T_1$ and $T_2$ data derived from this type of responses are shown in Figure 2. $T_1$ is defined after Huxley and Simmons (9) as the extreme in tension reached during the ramp (B in Figure 1). The definition of $T_2$ is based on the practice introduced by Ford, Huxley and Simmons (8). In case of shortening $T_2$ is defined as the intersection of the extrapolated "plateau" in the transient tension response and the initial fall in tension. (B in Figure 1). In case of lengthening the minimum of the undershoot in tension is given as $T_2$. Figure 2 shows that, if the rate of shortening is increased, the minimum in tension $T_1$ is found at a lower value while the maximum in tension $T_1$ resulting from a lengthening is found at a higher value. The $T_2$ curve was found to be independent of the rate of the displacement.

Analysis of the time course of the slow recovery after a shortening was carried out in the following way. The recorded responses were sampled with a frequency of 8 kHz, and in search of an exponential, the tension recovery after the plateau phase was plotted semi-logarithmically starting at about 25 msec after the displacement. The tension level reached 250 msec after the shortening was chosen as a point of departure for the estimation of the base line. A semi-logarithmic plot as good as that shown in Figure 3 could always be obtained when allowance was made for differences within 5% of this level. These curves suggest that the slow recovery can be fitted adequately with one exponential only. The time constant of this exponential was calculated from the mean slope of the semi-logarithmic plot during the first 75 msec. After about 100 msec the measurements start to deviate from the calculated curve. This deviation is small and was not investigated in detail. In A of Figure 4 the force response and the exponential fit are compared. The time constant is independent (within 5%) of the amplitude of the shortening. The time constant obtained from 8 experiments was $37 \pm 2$ msec (mean $\pm$ S.E.M.). In two experiments the temperature was varied in the range from 0 to 15°C. The time constant was found to decrease with increasing temperature from 38 msec at 0°C to 8.5 msec at 15°C, corresponding with a $Q_{10}$ value[1] of 2.7 and the relative $T_1$ value was found to increase with a $Q_{10}$ of about 1.2. The "amplitude" of the exponential ($A$) was determined by extrapolating backwards to the moment at which the

---

[1] In this case $Q_{10}$ is taken as the ratio by which the time constant changes for a 10°C temperature change.

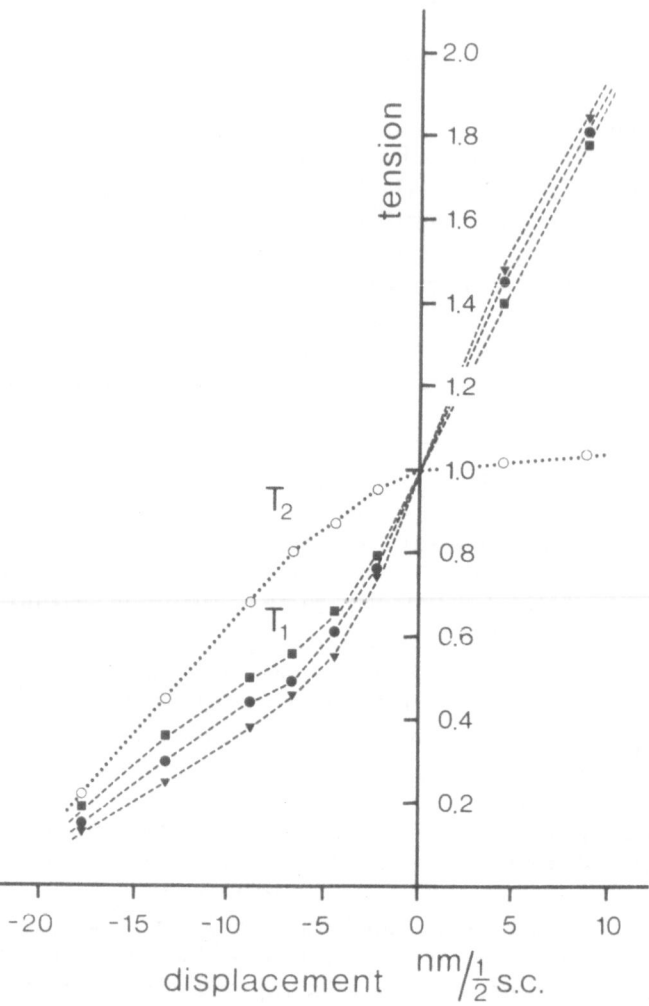

*Figure 2.* $T_1$ and $T_2$ curves at different displacement rates of 4.4 (squares), 8.8 (spots) and 13.2 (triangles) nm/msec per half-sarcomere. The $T_1$ values (filled symbols) denote the extreme in tension reached during the ramp, normalized to $T_0$. The $T_2$ values (circles) denote the plateau in the responses relative to $T_0$. The $T_1$ values clearly depend on the displacement rate, in contrast to the $T_2$ values which superimpose at the different velocities of the ramps. *Experimental conditions:* $L_0 = 27$ mm, $s_0 = 2.4$ $\mu$m, $T_0 = 2.1 \times 10^5$ N/m$^2$, temperature $= 2$°C.

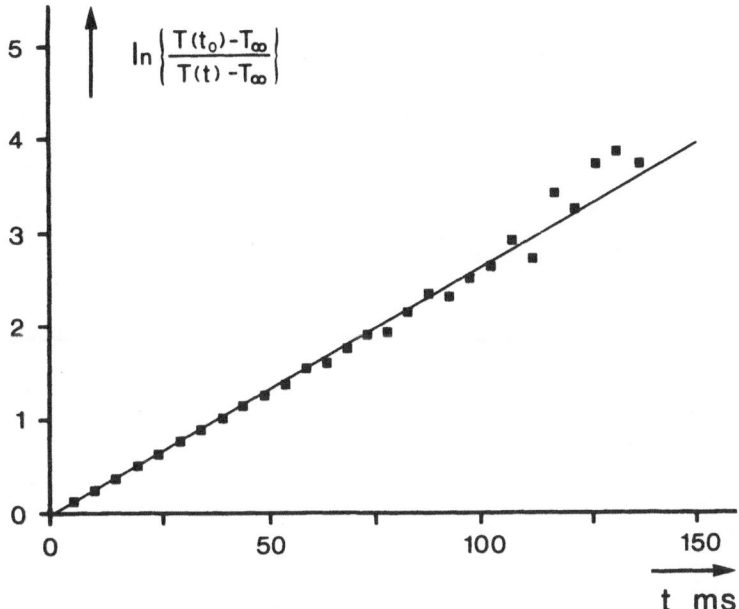

*Figure 3.* Semi-logarithmic plot of the slow recovery after a shortening of 17.6 nm/half-sarcomere. In this figure $T_\infty$ denotes the base line tension level. The starting point ($t_0$) of the slow recovery at 25 msec after the change in the displacement is taken as the origin of the horizontal axis. *Experimental conditions*: identical to those of Figure 2.

minimum in tension $T_1$ occurred (A in Figure 4). The amplitude $A$ varied with the amplitude of the displacement change according to B in Figure 4.

The stiffness during the transient force change was determined by applying a second "test" length change at different times after the initial one. As an example one registration is shown by A in Figure 5. The relative momentary stiffness ($S'$) is obtained by dividing the amplitude of the change in force due to the test length change by the amplitude of the change due to a similar length change when the initial one was omitted (starting at the isometric tetanic tension level). In doing so two problems arise. Firstly, the momentary stiffness depends on the amplitude of the test length change. This can be seen in B in Figure 5, where the amplitude of the change in force is plotted as a function of the amplitude of the test length change. It is evident that the slope, i.e. stiffness, decreases at larger shortenings. For test stretches the change in the slope is smaller. These features arise consistently at every instant during the transient force change. Secondly, because of the duration of the test length change the tension recovery during, for example, a test shortening could lead to underestimation of the momentary stiffness after an initial shortening and to over-estimation after an initial lengthen-

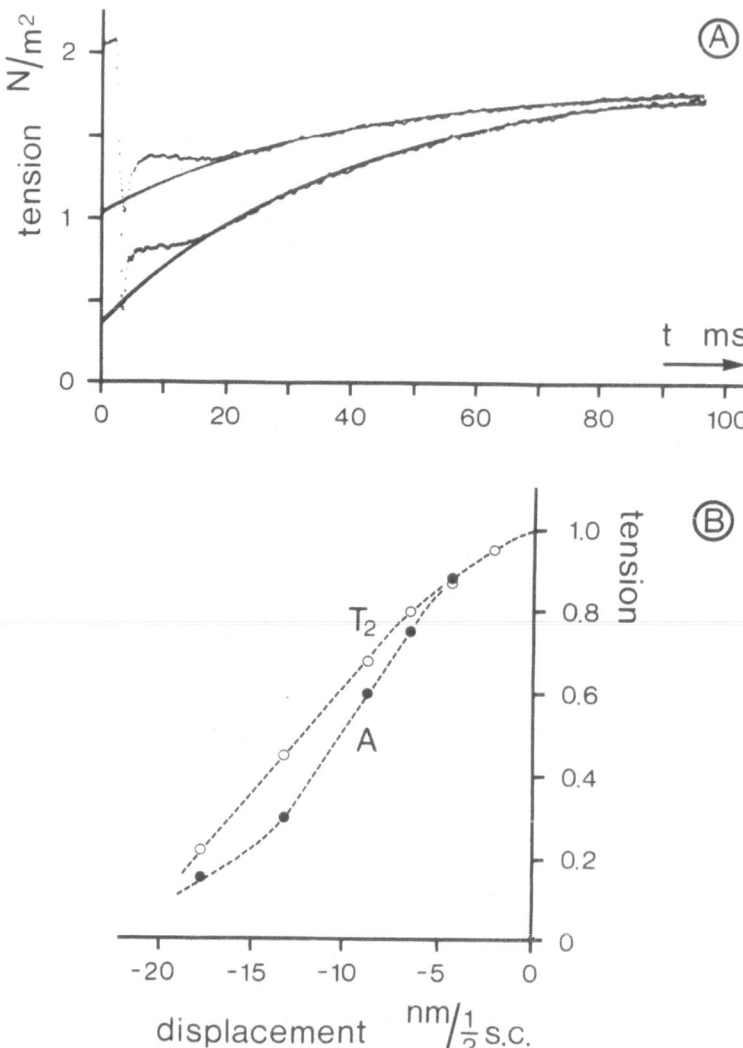

*Figure* 4. A: Comparison of the tension responses to shortenings of 8.8 and 13.2 nm/half-sarcomere and the calculated exponential fit of the slow recovery. Time constant: 38 msec; B: Amplitude dependence (*A*) of the exponential fit of the slow recovery as a function of the amplitude of the displacement. *A* was determined by extrapolating the calculated curve to the moment at which the minimum in tension $T_1$ occurred. The amplitude dependence of the fit resembles the $T_2$ curve (circles). *Experimental conditions*: identical to those of Figure 2.

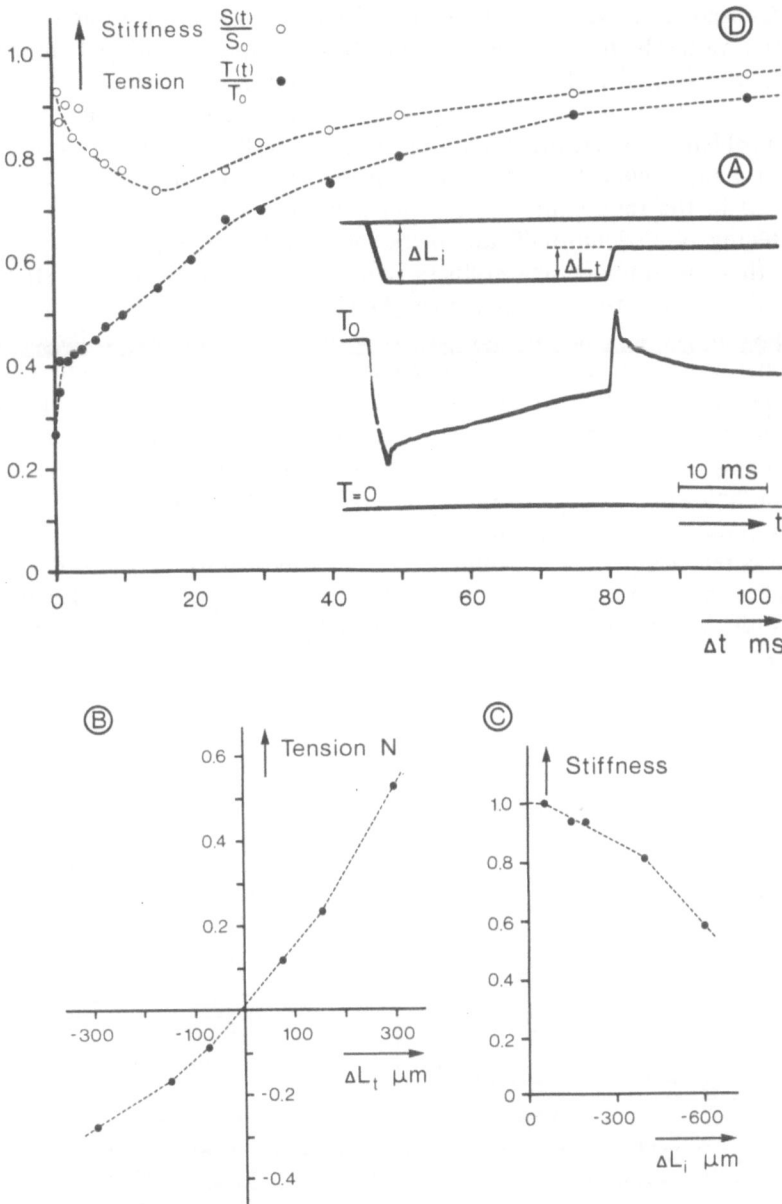

*Figure 5.* Momentary stiffness after shortening determined by a test displacement ($\Delta L_t$) after an initial displacement ($\Delta L_i$): A: typical example of the resulting tension course; B: force versus test displacement at 15 msec after an initial shortening of 12.3 nm/half-sarcomere. The test displacements were completed in 1 msec; C: normalized momentary stiffness at 15 msec as a function of the initial displacement; D: time course of the momentary stiffness normalized to the isometric stiffness (circles) compared with the relative tension (spots)—$\Delta L_i = 17.2$ nm/half sarcomere, $\Delta L_t = 8.6$ nm/half-sarcomere. *Experimental conditions:* $T_0 = 2.0 \times 10^5$ N/m², $s_0 = 2.5$ μm, $L_0 = 30$ mm, temperature = 2°C.

ing. Consequently, the ordinate of B in Figure 5 is intersected at a slightly positive value. If the test change in length is completed within 1 msec this effect, however, only plays a role in the determination of $S'$ during the first 2 or 3 msec after completion of the initial change in length. In view of these two problems, changes in force due to small test lengthenings completed within 1 msec were taken as a measure of the momentary stiffness. This resulted in the time course of the normalized momentary stiffness after a shortening of 17.2 nm/half-sarcomere shown by D in Figure 5. It can be seen that the momentary stiffness, compared to the isometric stiffness, decreases during the plateau phase. During the slow recovery phase the stiffness recovers. It can also be seen that the relative stiffness is larger than the relative tension. The minimum in stiffness is reached about 15 msec after the start of the initial shortening, that is, at the end of the plateau phase. The momentary stiffness at 15 msec depends on the amplitude of the initial shortening according to C of Figure 5. After an initial shortening of about 22 nm/half-sarcomere corresponding with a displacement of $-500$ $\mu$m, which reduces the $T_2$ value to zero (cf Figure 2) the minimum in the relative stiffness reaches a value of about 0.7. After lengthening on the other hand the momentary stiffness is increased, as is illustrated in Figure 6. Even after 250 msec when the tension was nearly reduced to its isometric level the stiffness was still found to be clearly increased.

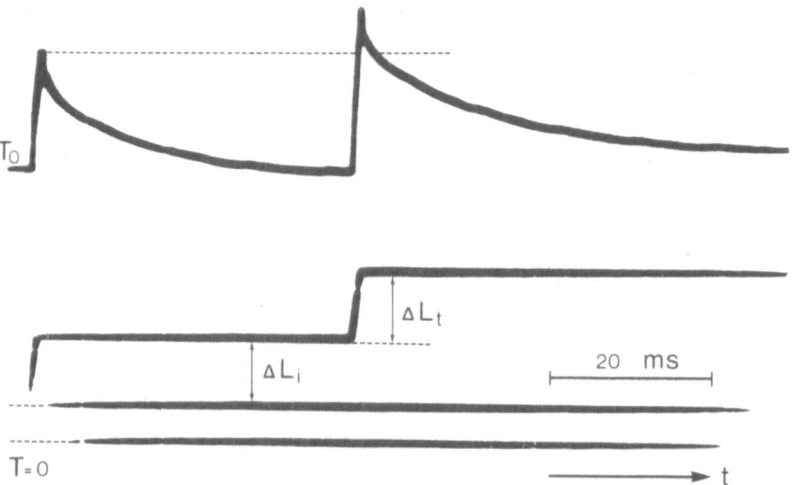

*Figure 6.* An initial stretch of 5.3 nm/half-sarcomere followed by a similar test lengthening and the resulting tension response. The interrupted line indicates the maximum ($T_1$) of the initial tension response. The amplitude of the response due to the test lengthening is considerably larger, indicating that the momentary stiffness is increased. *Experimental conditions:* $T_0 = 2.1 \times 10^5$ N/m$^2$, $s_0 = 2.1$ $\mu$m, $L_0 = 27$ mm, temperature $= 1°$C.

## 4. DISCUSSION

The tension responses to ramp-shaped length changes shown in Figure 1 have many features in common with the responses of single fibre preparations (8, 10). Furthermore the dependence of $T_1$ on the velocity of the ramp lengthenings is in accordance with the results of ramp shortenings (6).

The slow recovery after a shortening is dominated by one exponential only and, as shown by A in Figure 4, the amplitude dependence of the fit shows correspondence to the amplitude dependence of the $T_2$ level. These results indicate that the slow recovery is determined by the amplitude of the shortening alone in contrast with the early tension recovery which also depends on the velocity of the ramp.

Extending earlier results of pulse measurements (6) it is found that the decrease in momentary stiffness after a shortening already takes place during the plateau phase. Assuming that the momentary stiffness is a measure of the number of attached crossbridges (10) this implies that detachment of crossbridges already takes place during the plateau phase. The inaccuracy of our measurements during the fast recovery phase does not allow us to mark a starting point for the decrease in stiffness. The difference between relative tension and relative momentary stiffness indicates that, during the plateau phase, rather rapid detachment of crossbridges at low strain prevails while during the slow recovery the formation of crossbridges at high strain prevails. From their measurements during isotonic transients Julian and Sollins (10) derived that stiffness measured by small sinusoidal length changes depends on the tension level. A comparable effect (stiffness versus initial shortening) is shown by C in Figure 5. The increase in the momentary stiffness after a lengthening, however, is more difficult to interpret. The concept of proportionality of stiffness and the amount of attached crossbridges would require an increase in the amount of attached crossbridges after stretch. According to these measurements this amount should remain increased, although the tension recovers towards the isometric level. Moreover, the increased stiffness after a small rapid stretch might be related to the stretch activation phenomena (12) which have been shown to occur in various preparations, including glycerinated frog sartorius muscle.

### SUMMARY

The dynamic properties of the contractile mechanism were investigated in electrically stimulated sartorius muscle of the frog. The force transients to ramp-shaped length changes at different rates of displacement were recorded and the momentary stiffness during the transients was determined. The time course of the momentary stiffness after a shortening suggests that during the plateau phase in the tension response, detachment of crossbridges at low strain prevails and that during the slow recovery phase crossbridges formed at high strain are in majority. After a lengthening, the momentary stiffness was increased considerably.

ACKNOWLEDGEMENTS

We are very much indebted to Prof. J.Th.F. Boeles and Prof. L.H. van der Tweel for encouragement and valuable discussions, to Miss M. Zethof for general assistance, and to Mr. P. Broekhuijsen and the electronics department for technical assistance. This study was supported in part by a grant from the Netherlands Organization for the Advancement of Pure Research (ZWO).

REFERENCES

1. Huxley AF: Muscle structure and theories of contraction. In: *Progress in biophysics and Biophysical Chemistry*, vol 7, Butler AV, Katz B (eds), Oxford, Pergamon, 1957, p 255–318.
2. Abbott RH: The relationship between biochemical and mechanical properties. In: *Insect flight muscle*, Tregear RT (ed), Amsterdam, North-Holland, 1977, p 269–273.
3. Huxley AF: Muscular contraction, review lecture. *J Physiol* 243:1–43, 1974.
4. Julian FJ, Sollins KR, Sollins MR: A model for the transient and steady-state mechanical behaviour of contracting muscle. *Biophys J* 14:546–562, 1974.
5. Lymn RW, Taylor EW: Mechanism of adenosine triphosphate hydrolysis by actomyosin. *Biochemistry* 10:4617–4624, 1971.
6. Stienen GJM, Blangé T, Schnerr M: Tension responses of frog sartorius muscle to quick ramp-shaped shortenings and some effects of metabolic inhibition. *Pflügers Arch* 376:97–104, 1978.
7. Blangé T, Karemaker JM, Kramer AEJL: Elasticity as an expression of cross-bridge activity in rat muscle. *Pflügers Arch* 336:277–288, 1972.
8. Ford LE, Huxley AF, Simmons RM: Tension responses to sudden length changes in stimulated frog muscle fibres near slack length. *J Physiol* 269:441–515, 1977.
9. Huxley AF, Simmons RM: Proposed mechanism of force generation in striated muscle. *Nature* 233:533–538, 1971.
10. Julian FJ, Sollins MR: Variation of muscle stiffness with force at increasing speeds of shortening *J Gen Physiol* 66:287–302, 1975.
11. Ford LE, Huxley AF, Simmons RM: Mechanism of early tension recovery after a quick release in tetanized muscle fibres. *J Physiol* 240:42–43P, 1974.
12. Pringle JWS: Stretch activation of muscle: function and mechanism. *Proc R Soc Lond* B201:197–130, 1978.

SECTION 2

# CARDIAC CHAMBER DYNAMICS: FROM THE FIBER UP TO THE MYOCARDIUM

## 2.1. A FUNDAMENTAL SIMILARITY BETWEEN ISOLATED MUSCLE MECHANICS AND CARDIAC CHAMBER DYNAMICS

KIICHI SAGAWA

### 1. INTRODUCTION

The fundamental similarity that I want to discuss here is that which becomes evident when one compares the pressure-volume relation in the ventricular chamber against the force-length relation of isolated heart muscle. Perhaps no one will doubt that there is a close correspondence between ventricular pressure $P(t)$ and myocardial force $F(t)$ and an even closer interrelation between ventricular lumen $V(t)$ and muscle length $L(t)$. At the same time, no one will doubt that an accurate translation of ventricular $P$-$V$ variables into muscle $F$-$L$ variables is a formidable task for many reasons such as the complex shape and non-uniform thickness of the ventricular wall, the complex fibre course, and complex patterns of propagation of excitation and relaxation waves. The inverse path, that is, from one-dimensional muscle mechanics to the three-dimensional world has been fairly well beaten by modellers who assumed simple geometry, homogeneous wall, isotropic material property. Even this conceptual path is considerably bumpy to most cardiologists. Under the circumstances it is justifiable and it may even be wise to pursue entirely separate models, one for ventricular contraction and another for myocardial contraction. Nevertheless, a number of able researchers have challenged various aspects of the difficult task of unifying the two and some of them are presenting here the able consequences of their attempts. In the following I will review examples of parallelism between ventricular pressure-volume relationship and myocardial force-length relationship.

### 2. VENTRICULAR PRESSURE-VOLUME RELATIONSHIP

Primarily for the sake of mathematical simplicity earlier investigators of cardiovascular system dynamics (1, 2, 3, 4, 5) proposed to model contractions of cardiac chambers by a time-varying volume elastance, $E(t)$. That is, they proposed, to relate instantaneous intraventricular pressure $P(t)$ to instantaneous ventricular lumen volume $V(t)$ simply by

$$P(t) = E(t) \cdot V(t) \qquad [1]$$

J. Baan, A.C. Arntzenius, E.L. Yellin (eds.), Cardiac Dynamics, 81–94.

Under an assumption that $E(t)$ is independent of loading conditions, the model could easily handle either isovolumic or any ejecting contractions under a variety of conditions.

This equation has been considered an oversimplification by those who remembered the classical concept that was shaped first by Frank (6) and confirmed later by Reichel and Kapal (7). Frank concluded his famous thesis (6) by stating:

a simple *a priori* relation between length and tension does not exist in cardiac muscle for every moment of its action. The mechanical conditions under which muscle has functioned before this instant have a decisive influence.

One of the bases of this statement is shown in A in Figure 1 (8) which indicates two end-systolic $P$-$V$ relationship curves, one observed at the end of isovolumic systole (designated as "isometrische Maximakurve") and another at the end of isobaric ejecting systole (labelled "Isot. Max."). He stressed how similar these findings are to those in skeletal muscle. Reproduced for comparison are end-systolic force-length relation curves obtained by Buchthal and Kaiser (9) in a single fibre preparation of frog's skeletal muscle.

What people might have forgotten is that Frank based his thesis on the findings from *frogs'* ventricles and skeletal muscle. That the end-systolic $P$-$V$ relationship is considerably different in the mammalian left ventricle became apparent only in the 1960's. Three families of $P$-$V$ trajectories (10, 11, 12) are collected in Figure 2 which indicate that in contradiction to Frank-Reichel's concept, end-systolic points of those $P$-$V$ trajectories appear to fall on the same pressure-volume relation line whether they contracted from large or small volume, isovolumically or ejecting under increasing pressure or about the same pressure. The slope of the solid line represents $E_{es}$, the end-systolic value of the volume elastance $E(t)$ in [1]. In parallel with these findings in the ventricle there was a finding in cat papillary muscle (13) which indicated a perfect correspondence (D in Figure 2). The end-systolic force-length relation was nonlinear, but all the contractions studied ended on or very nearly on this single curve regardless of the mode of contraction and initial length.

From a large number of $P(t)$-$V(t)$ relations determined in canine ventricles in vivo (12) and in vitro (14), we arrived at an empirical description of the relation which is similar to [1].

$$E(t) = P(t)/[V(t) - V_d(t)] \hspace{4cm} [2]$$

At an instant of time $t_i$ during systole, the pressure $P(t_i)$ was linearly correlated with the simultaneous volume $V(t_i)$ in disregard of end-diastolic volume and mode of contraction (Figure 3). $E(t_i)$ is the slope of this linear $P$-$V$ relation line. The volume axis intercept of the regression line is

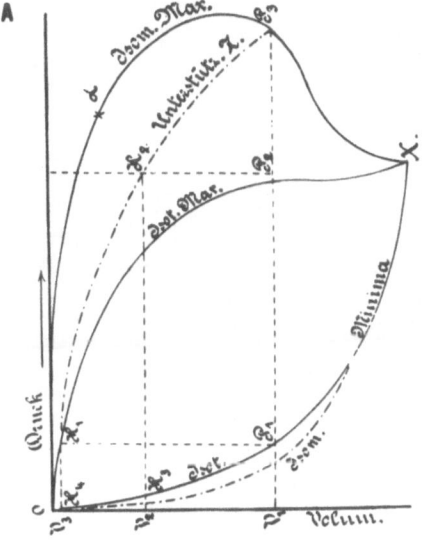

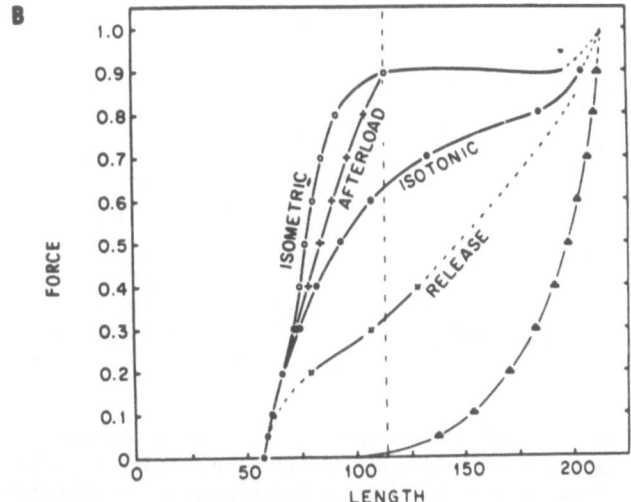

*Figure 1.* A: Frank's schematic pressure-volume diagram in the frog ventricle. Reproduced from Frank O: Die Grundform des arteriellen Pulses. *Z Biol* 37:483–526, 1898, with the permission of Urban and Schwarzenberg. B: Force-length relationship in a single skeletal muscle fibre in different modes (isometric, isotonic and afterloaded isotonic) of contractins. Reproduced from Buchthal and Kaiser (9), with permission of the authors and the Danish Academy of Letters and Science.

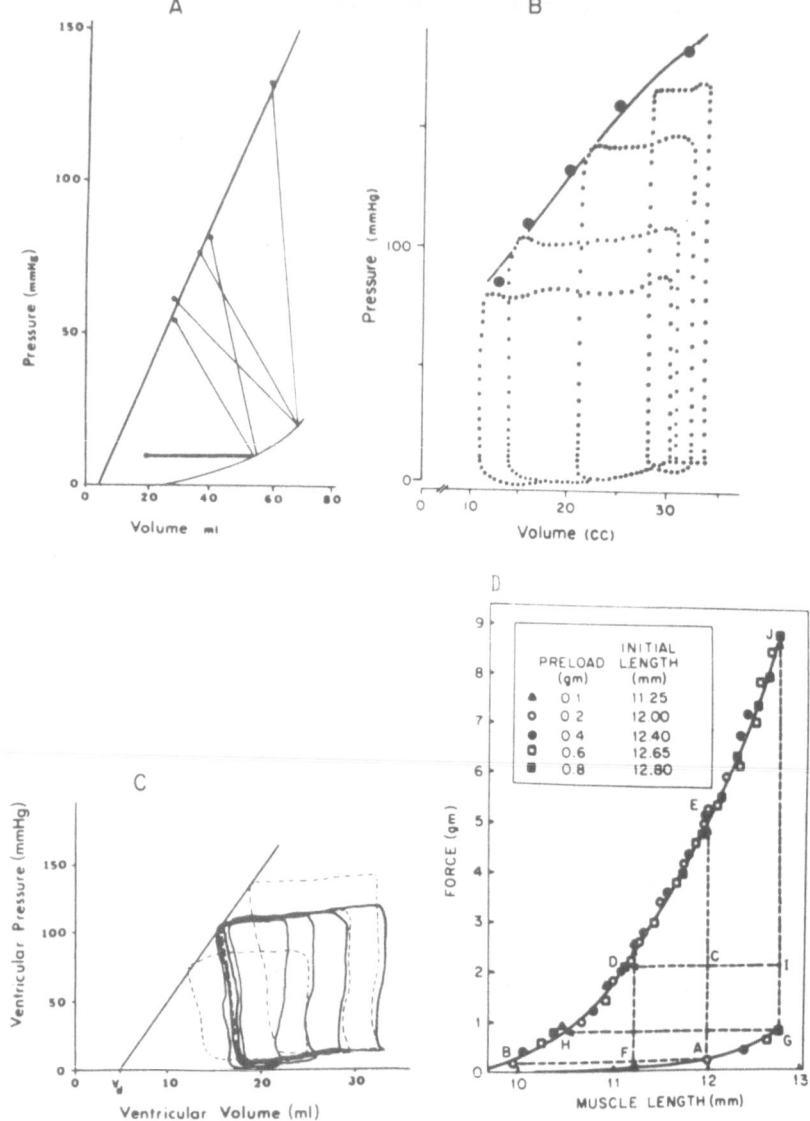

*Figure 2.* Some more recent pressure-volume diagrams in canine ventricles. A: *P-V* diagram obtained in an isolated left ventricle which was filled with air and connected with an air chamber. The ventricle compressed air during systole. Reproduced from Monroe et al. (10) by the courtesy of the authors and with the permission of the American Heart Association, Inc. B: *P-V* diagram obtained in an isolated left ventricle which ejected liquid against a hydraulic servo-controlled loading system. The large circles near the solid line represent the peak isovolumic pressures at various volumes. Reproduced from Weber et al. (11) by courtesy of the authors and permission of the American Physiological Society. C: *P-V* diagram obtained in a left ventricle ejecting blood. Volume was measured by a cardiometer while venting the right ventricles. Modified from a figure published in Suga et al. (12) with the permission of the American Heart Association, Inc. D: Force-length relation of cat's papillary muscle. Note that no distinct end-systolic relationship curves resulted from different modes of contractions (such as isometric, isotonic and afterloaded isotonic contractions) in heart muscle. Reproduced from Downing and Sonnenblick (13) with the courtesy of the authors and the permission of the American Physiological Society.

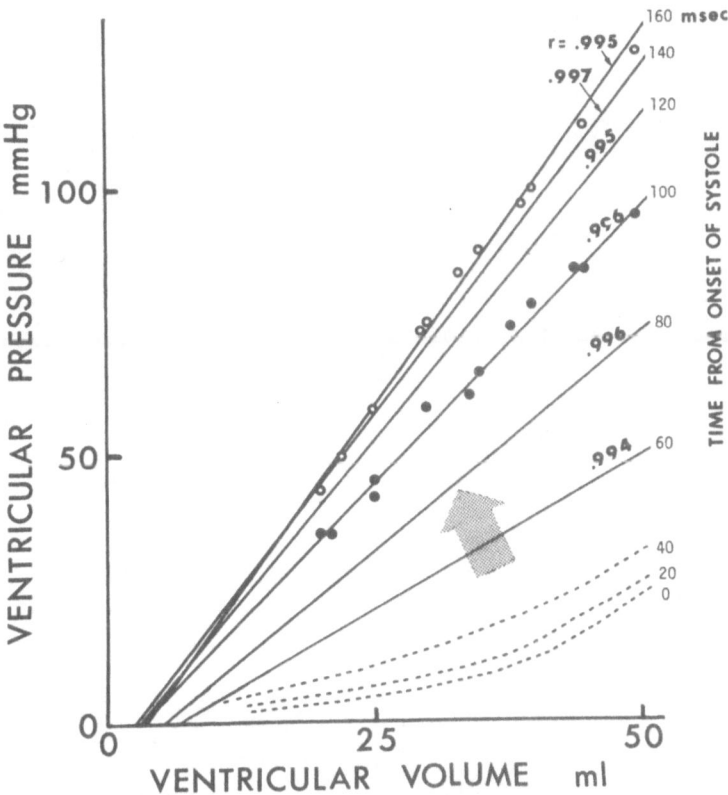

*Figure 3.* Instantaneous relationship between pressure and volume (isochrons). Regression analysis was applied to multiple sets of isochronal *P-V* data points obtained from isovolumic and ejecting beats in a ventricle. The shaded arrow indicates that the *P-V* regression line increases its slope, *E(t)*, with time during systole. Reproduced from Sagawa et al. End-systolic pressure/volume ratio: A new index of ventricular contractility. *Am J Cardiol* 40:748–753, 1977 with permission of the American College of Cardiology.

designated dead volume ($V_d$) because it is a fraction of ventricular lumen which does not contribute to generation of active pressure in systole. The magnitude of $V_d$ varied slightly with time reaching a minimum at the end of systole (Figure 3).

In a ventricle contracting under a constant contractility the difference between $E(t)$ calculated from isovolumic contractions and $E(t)$ from ejecting contractions was very small. This is shown in A in Figure 4. In fact, there is no statistically significant difference between the systolic portions of the two $E(t)$ curves in most ventricles. However, a careful inspection will reveal that the time to $E_{max}$ ($T_{max}$) is slightly shorter for the isovolumic $E(t)$ curve than for the ejecting $E(t)$ curve. In addition, there is a significant difference during the diastolic phase; $E(t)$ decays much faster after ejecting systole than after isovolumic systole. This corresponds to the well-known fact (15) that the peak

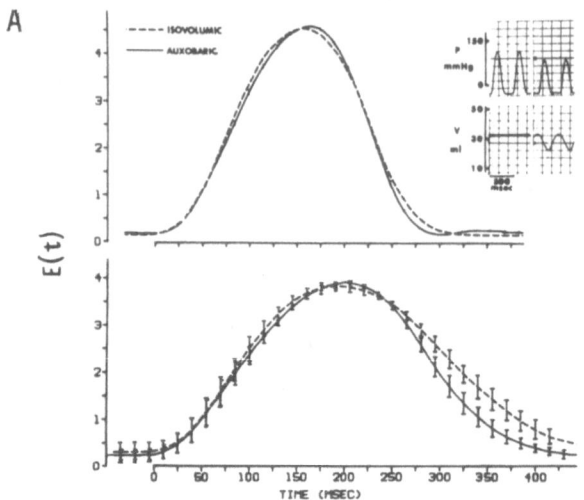

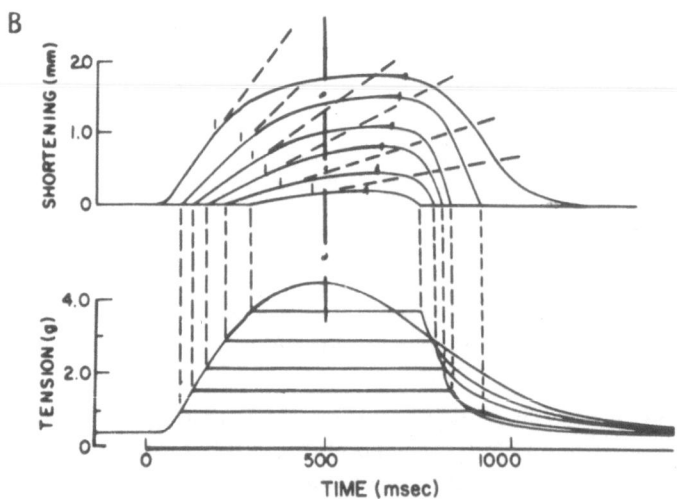

*Figure 4.* A: top shows two $E(t)$ curves (see [2]), one from an isovolumic contraction and the other from ejecting contraction of a left ventricle. Bottom shows the mean and standard deviation of five $E(t)$ curves obtained from isovolumic (broken line) and ejecting (solid line) beats. Note that the peak values are similar but the peak of the $E(t)$ curve occurs earlier and the relaxation process is slower in the isovolumic $E(t)$ curve. Reproduced from Suga and Sagawa (14) with the permission of the American Heart Association, Inc. B: top shows a family of isotonic shortening curves at various afterloads. Bottom shows the force curves. Note that the peak of isometric curve occurs earlier and the relaxation process of isometric contraction is slower. Reproduced from Sonnenblick (15) with the permission of the author and the Federation of the American Societies of Experimental Biology.

force time of isometric muscle contraction occurs earlier than the time of maximum shortening, and that the relaxation process proceeds faster after shortening than after isometric contraction (B in Figure 4). It will be discussed later that [2] is valid only for the systolic portion of the ventricular contractions, with an ejection fraction below 50%, which was the case with those ventricles which ejected against a cyclinder load system.

A recent study (16) on the right ventricular $P(t)$-$V(t)$ relationship also yielded essentially the same result (Figure 5). As expected, however, the $E_{max}$ value was about 2.5 mmHg·ml$^{-1}$, or 50 to 70% of the left ventricular $E_{max}$. On the other hand the $V_d(t)$ value for the right ventricle was larger and varied more extensively with time than the left ventricular $V_d(t)$. Besides in most right ventricles the end-systolic $P$-$V$ relation line from ejecting beats was clearly separated from the isovolumic $P$-$V$ relation line.

When epinephrine, isoproterenol, or Ca$^{++}$, was infused into the coronary artery, either left or right ventricular $E_{max}$ markedly increased while $T_{max}$ (time to $E_{max}$) shortened significantly. An example of the inotropic change in left ventricular $E_{max}$ and $T_{max}$ is shown in Figure 6.

In summary, systolic pressure-volume relationship in the canine ventricle can be closely approximated, as long as the ejection fraction does not exceed 50%, by a simple time-varying elastance $E(t)$ as early modellers had assumed for mathematical convenience. There is a piece of evidence that heart muscle behaves in the same manner. The classical concept offered by

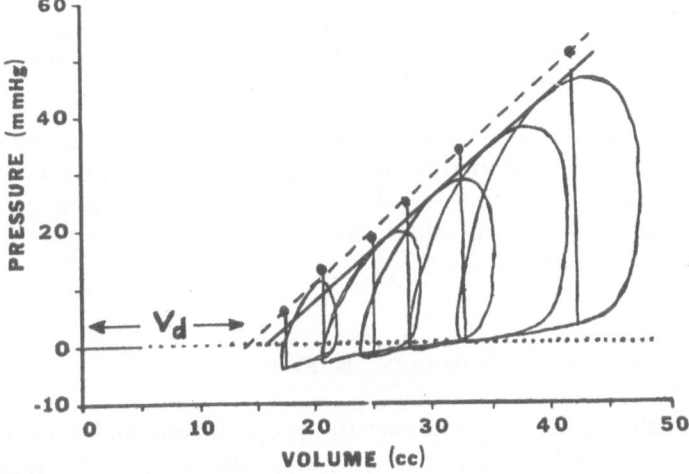

*Figure 5.* Pressure-volume loop diagram of the right ventricle of an isolated canine heart. The broken slant line connects the end-systolic points of several isometric contractions. Note the small difference of this line from the solid line which connects the shoulders of several *P-V* loops obtained in the same ventricle. Reproduced from Maughan et al. (16) with the permission of the American Heart Association, Inc.

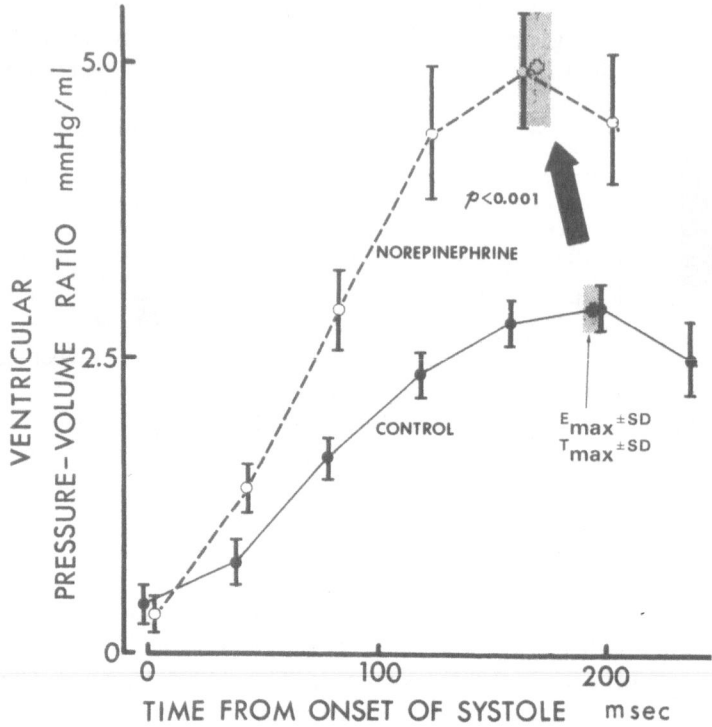

*Figure 6.* Shift of mean *E(t)* curve of the left ventricle caused by norepinephrine (0.2 mg·min⁻¹) infusion into the coronary artery. The vertical bars represent the standard deviations. By the courtesy of Dr. Hiroyuki Suga.

the Munich school based on frogs' ventricular behaviour left an exaggerated impression of the history-dependent aspect for the end-systolic *P-V* relation of the mammalian ventricle. What happens if the ventricle ejects a large fraction of its end-diastolic volume and if heart muscle shortens to a large extent? This issue will be discussed next.

## 3. FORCE-LENGTH RELATIONSHIP OF HEART MUSCLE

It is probably inappropriate to refer to the contracting and relaxing phase of twitch of isolated heart muscle as systole and diastole. Because of the lack of better words, however, I would use end-systole to mean the peak of contractile activity whether it is measured in force generation, shortening or some function of both.

As mentioned earlier, Downing and Sonnenblick (13) found that, under a constant contractile state, the history of contractile event during the same systole did not affect the end-systolic *F-L* relation curve, which therefore uniquely represented the state of heart muscle (D in Figure 2). When epinephrine was added to the muscle the slope of the curve markedly increased without a significant change in the intercept of this curve with the length axis (13). I would call this intercept dead length ($L_d$), because it is a portion of muscle length which does not participate in the active force generation and is strongly analogous to $V_d$, dead volume, of the ventricle. The lack of the effect of loading conditions on end-systolic $F$-$L$ relation, the sensitivity of the relation to changes in inotropism, and the relative constancy of $L_d$ are all similar to the properties of $E_{max}$ and $V_d$ parameters of the end-systolic $P$-$V$ relation line of the left or right ventricle. That the end-systolic $F$-$L$ relation for the muscle is curvilinear is geometrically consistent with the rectilinear $P$-$V$ relation for ventricular chamber (17).

Furthermore, it is suggested in a recent report by Pollack and Krueger (18) that the relative insensitivity of end-systolic $F$-$L$ relation to history of contractile event may exist even at the sarcomere level. These investigators determined an end-systolic force sarcomere length relation curve with a servo control of sarcomere length and the other relationship curve from ordinary isometric contraction data. They could not distinguish the two curves. If these findings were further borne out, they would indicate very strongly the fundamental similarity between ventricular end-systolic $P$-$V$ relation and end-systolic $F$-$L$ relation of muscle and of sarcomere.

There are reports (19, 20, 21, 22, 23) on the history-dependence of heart muscle. These investigators found evidence that in general isotonic or afterloaded isotonic contraction produces an end-systolic $F$-$L$ relation curve which is situated lower than the end-systolic $F$-$L$ relation curve obtained from isometric contractions. One example from Brady's study (20) on rabbits' papillary muscle is shown in Figure 7, which indicates that the

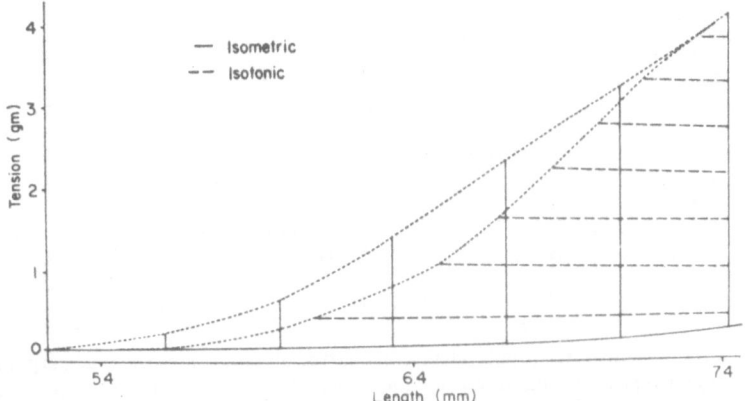

*Figure 7.* End-systolic relation curves from isometric and afterloaded isotonic contractions in a rabbit papillary muscle. Reproduced from Brady (20) by courtesy of the author and the permission of the American Society of Zoologists.

greater the extent (and/or rate) of shortening, the greater the deficit of end-systolic force. If a sudden and large extent of shortening of a very brief duration (a few msec) was imposed on muscle while it is contracting isometrically, the force development thereafter will be seriously hampered (24). This is a clear example of the deactivation effect of shortening. As a whole, these latter findings suggest that the end-systolic *F-L* relationship in mammalian heart muscles is more clearly history-dependent than the *P-V* relation of canine ventricle.

How about the instantaneous force-length relation of heart muscle? There exists a meagre amount of information in this respect. Plotted in Figure 8 are two sets of instantaneous $F(t)$-$L(t)$ relationship data from cat papillary muscle (25). One set of data (filled circles) is from isometric contractions at various lengths and another set (open circles) from isotonic contractions. In either set $F(t)$-$L(t)$ data were collected at 135, 270, 405 and 540 msec after the onset of contractions and the isochronous data points are connected by broken lines. Thus at 135 msec the set of isometric force-length data labelled 135 was obtained, whereas during isotonic contractions the end-systolic *F-L* relation line proceeded at the same instant of time only to those points represented by the right-handmost set of open circles. If the model of simple time-varying elastance were valid for muscle, these two broken lines should coincide. Instead the isotonic relation line appears to

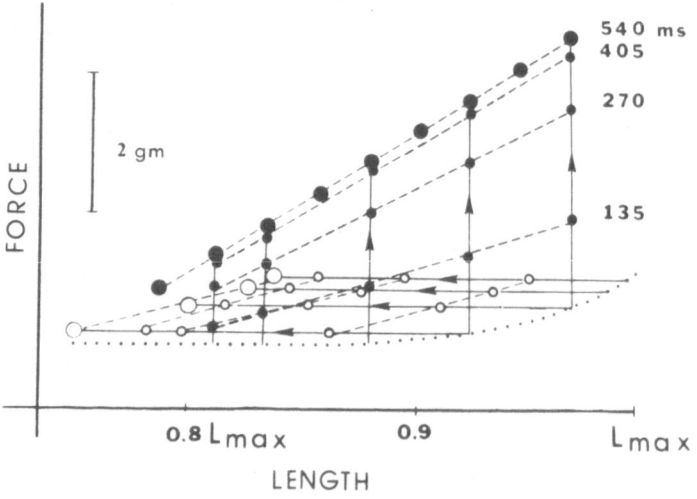

*Figure 8.* Instantaneous force-length relationship curves obtained in a cat's papillary muscle. The solid circles represent data at various times after the onset of isometric contraction at various muscle lengths. The open circles represent data at the same instants of time during isotonic contractions from various lengths. Reproduced from Sagawa (26) with the permission of the American Heart Association, Inc.

lag behind the isometric relation line, and this lag can never be recovered by the end-systole. As mentioned earlier (B in Figure 4), (1) the end of systole of isotonic or afterloaded isotonic contraction occurs later than the end of systole of isometric contraction at the same initial length, but (2) the relaxation process proceeds faster in the isotonic contraction than in isometric contraction. These suggest the possibility that even though the amount of $Ca^{++}$ released from the source and available for the contractile machine might be the same at the beginning of the two modes of contraction, sliding of myofilaments takes time as any motion will do and also because binding and unbinding of crossbridges proceed at a finite rate, and this reduces the amount of $Ca^{++}$ bound to the contractile machine at the same length during systole. Thus, the active transport of $Ca^{++}$ back into the storage site may begin before the contractile machine can develop the full potential force at that length, resulting in a force deficit relative to the isometric force.

I would conclude this review with a brief comparison of two recent findings both obtained in the canine heart. In one study (23) we measured the transient and steady-state contraction force achieved by an in vivo papillary muscle after it was suddenly switched from isometric contraction at a given length to isotonic shortening to the same length and compared them with the steady-state isometric force recorded at the identical end-systolic length. The average results are shown in Figure 9. The difference between the transient and steady-state deficit is quite large. In either case however the force deficit increased with increase in the extent of shortening. The steady-state force deficit amounted to as much as 40% when muscle

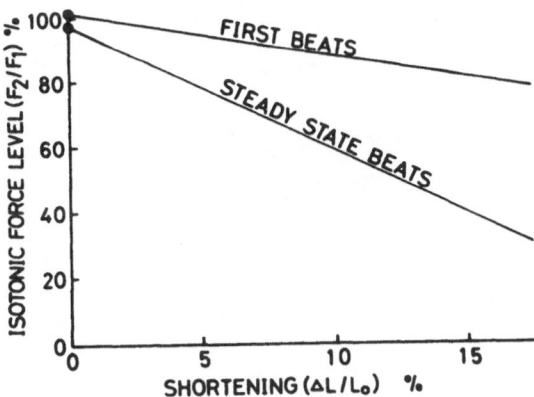

*Figure 9.* Mean relation between the extent of shortening and the deficit of end-systolic force attained by afterloaded isotonic contractions compared with the isometric force developed by the same in vivo muscles at the same end-systolic length. Reproduced from Suga et al. (23) with the permission of the American Physiological Society.

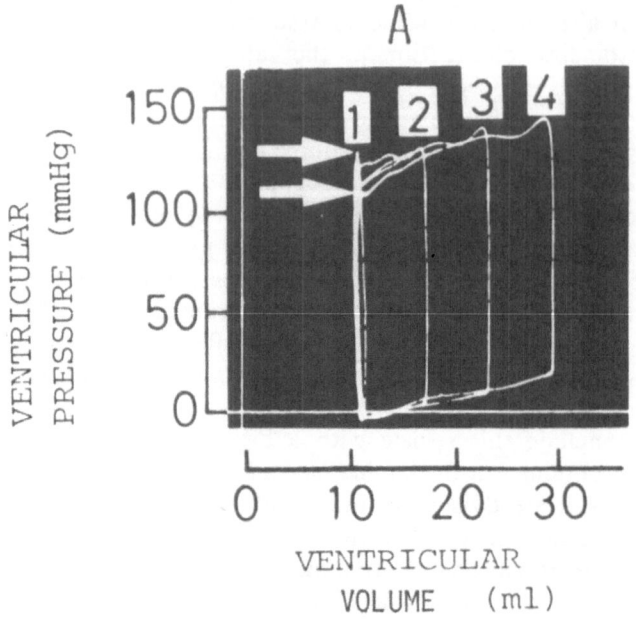

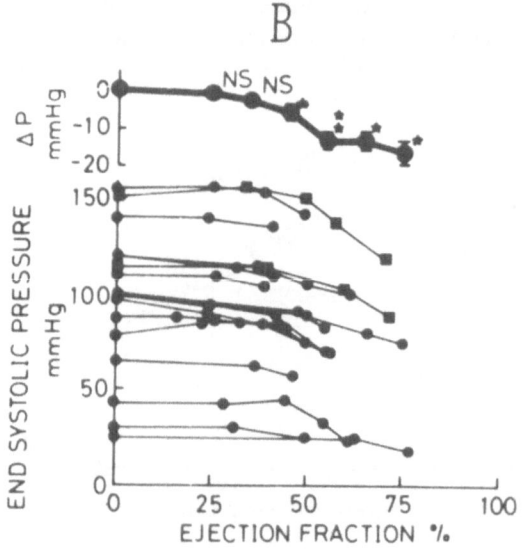

*Figure 10.* Relationship between the extent of ejection and the pressure deficit compared with isovolumic end-systolic pressure in a canine left ventricle. By the courtesy of Dr. Hiroyuki Suga.

shortened 10% of its original length. In another study (this volume) we clamped end-systolic volume of an isolated ventricle much more rigorously than possible before in order to determine the effects of ejection fraction on end-systolic pressure. There were steady-state deficits of 10 to 20% compared with isometric end-systolic pressure when the ejection fraction exceeded 40% (Figure 10).

SUMMARY

Frank showed in the frog's ventricle that just like the F-L relation of skeletal muscle, the P-V relationship at the end of systole depends heavily on the prior mechanical event during the same systole. More recent studies including ours, however, showed that in the canine ventricle the history-dependence was not significant. By contrast, the F-L relation of mammalian papillary muscle was found history-dependent by most investigators, and we verified this in canine in vivo papillary muscle. Therefore, we returned to the canine ventricle for reinvestigation and found that when ejection fraction was greater than 40%, the end-systolic pressure-volume relation clearly depended on the magnitude of ejection fraction. Thus, we rediscovered the fundamental similarity that Frank perceived between the frog's ventricle and frog's skeletal muscle, this time between the canine ventricle and canine papillary muscle.

REFERENCES

1. Warner HR: The use of an analog computer for analysis of control mechanisms in circulation. *Proc of IRE* 47:1913–1916, 1959.
2. Beneken JEW: Investigation on the regulatory system of the blood circulation. In: *Circulatory analog computers*, Noordergraaf A, Jager GN, Westerhof N (eds), Amsterdam, North-Holland, 1963, 16–44.
3. Robinson DA: Ventricular dynamics and the cardiac representation problem. In: *Circulatory analog computers*, Noordergraaf A, Jager GN, Westerhof N (eds), Amsterdam, North-Holland, 1963, p 16–28.
4. DeFares JG, Hara HH, Osborne JJ, McLeon J: Theoretical analysis and computer simulation of the circulation with special reference to the Starling properties of the ventricles. In: *Circulatory analog computers*, Noordergraaf A, Jager GN, Westerhof N (eds), Amsterdam, North-Holland, 1963, p 91–121.
5. Snyder MF, Rideout VC, Hillestad RJ: Computer modelling of the human systemic arterial tree. *J Biomech* 1:341–353, 1968.
6. Frank O: Zur Dynamik des Herzmuskels. *Z Biol* 32:370–447, 1895. (Chapman CB, Wasserman E (trans), *Am Heart J* 58:282–317, 467–477, 1958.)
7. Reichel H, Kapal E: Die Mechanik des Herzens bei Aenderung des arteriellen Drucks. *Z Biol* 99:581–589, 1939.
8. Frank O: Die Grundform des arteriellen Pulses. *Z. Biol* 37:483–526, 1898.
9. Buchthal F, Kaiser E: Rheology of cross striated muscle fiber. *Dan Biol Medd* 21:1–318, 1951.

10. Monroe RG, French GN: Left ventricular pressure-volume relationships and myocardial oxygen consumption in the isolated heart. *Circ Res* 9:362–374, 1961.
11. Weber KT, Janicki JS, Hefner LL: Left ventricular force-length relations of isovolumic and ejecting contractions. *Am J Physiol* 231:337–343, 1976.
12. Suga H, Sagawa K, Shoukas AA: Load independence of the instantaneous pressure-volume ratio of the canine left ventricle and effects of epinephrine and heart rate on the ratio. *Circ Res* 32:314–322, 1973.
13. Downing SE, Sonnenblick EH: Cardiac muscle mechanics and ventricular performance: force and time parameters. *Am J Physiol* 207:705–715, 1964.
14. Suga H, Sagawa K: Instantaneous pressure-volume relationships and their ratio in the excised, supported canine left ventricle. *Circ Res* 117–126, 1974.
15. Sonnenblick EH: Implications of muscle mechanics in the heart. *Fed Proc* 21:975–990, 1962.
16. Maughan L, Shoukas AA, Sagawa K, Weisfeldt ML: Instantaneous pressure-volume relationship of the canine right ventricle. *Circ Res* 1978 44:309–315, 1979.
17. Suga H, Sagawa K: Mathematical relationship between instantaneous ventricular pressure-volume ratio and myocardial force-velocity relation. *Annals Biomed Engr* 1:160–181, 1972.
18. Pollack GH, Krueger JH: Sarcomere dynamics in intact cardiac muscle. *Eur J Cardiol* 4:53–65, 1976.
19. Brady AJ: Time and displacement dependence of cardiac contractility: problems in defining the active state and force-velocity relations. *Fed Proc* 24:1410–1420, 1965.
20. Brady AJ: Length-tension relations in cardiac muscle. *Am Zoologist* 7:603–610, 1967.
21. Taylor RR: Active length-tension relations compared in isometric, afterload and isotonic contractions of cat papillary muscle. *Circ Res* 26:279–288, 1970.
22. Meiss RA, Sonnenblick EH: Controlled shortening in heart muscle: velocity-force and active state properties. *Am J Physiol* 222:630–639, 1972.
23. Suga H, Saeki Y, Sagawa K: End-systolic force-length relationship of non-excised canine papillary muscle. *Am J Physiol* 233, H711-H717, 1977.
24. Bodem R, Sonnenblick EH: Deactivation of contraction by quick releases in the isolated papillary muscle of the cat. *Circ Res* 34:214–225, 1975.
25. Nakayama K, Sagawa K, Shoukas AA: Force-length-time relations in heart muscle under various mechanical loadings (abstract). *Fed Proc* 34:412, 1975.
26. Sagawa K: Ventricular pressure-volume diagram revisited. *Circ Res* 43:677–687, 1978.

## 2.2. THE CHAMBER DYNAMICS OF THE INTACT LEFT VENTRICLE

J. SCOTT RANKIN

### 1. INTRODUCTION

Inquiry into the dynamics of cardiac function has been of central importance to the development of cardiac physiology. This area of investigation not only has furthered our basic understanding of myocardial performance but also has improved the care of patients with cardiac disease. Much of the current therapy of cardiac disorders is based on scientific principles painstakingly unravelled in physiology laboratories over the past century.

### 2. HISTORICAL PERSPECTIVE

Although speculation on the function of the heart can be traced to the ancients (1), our current understanding of cardiac chamber dynamics began with William Harvey (2). Using careful scientific methods, Harvey observed that "the heart at the moment it acts becomes constricted all over, thicker in its walls and smaller in its ventricles, in order to expel its content of blood. It contracts all over, but particularly to the sides, so that it looks narrower and longer". This lucid description of ventricular geometry can scarcely be improved three-and-a-half centuries later. Harvey also first proposed the passive nature of diastole and described the dynamics of ventricular filling and ejection. His contributions established the foundation for all subsequent research in this field.

The dynamic volume characteristics of the ventricles originally were measured with plethysmographic cardiometers (3, 4, 5). In Henderson's classic 1906 treatise (5), previous hypotheses were reviewed, and then the author described the first detailed measurements of ventricular chamber dynamics (Figure 1). Henderson characterized the three phases of filling, the passive nature of diastole, and the effects of respiration and heart rate on ventricular volume. Using similar techniques, Patterson et al. (6) defined the interrelationships between systolic loading, end-diastolic fibre length, and cardiac output. Within the next decade, Wiggers and Katz (7) published their meticulous study of the factors that affect the contour of the ventricular volume curve. In this paper, it was clearly demonstrated that the atrial contribution to ventricular filling was variable, becoming more pronounced as ventricular volume decreased.

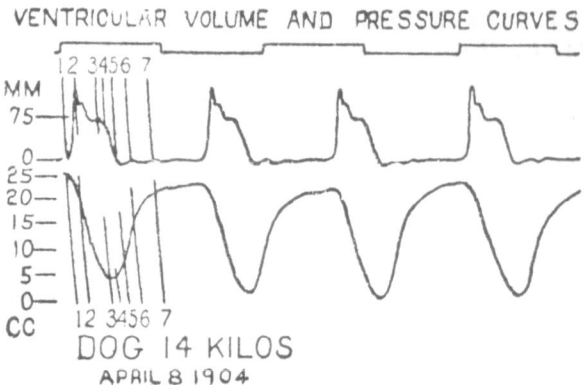

Figure 1. The first detailed measurements of the volume curve of the ventricles published by Henderson in 1906(5).

## 3. GEOMETRY OF LEFT VENTRICULAR CONTRACTION

In the early 1950s, Rushmer et al. (8, 9, 10) began a series of experiments designed to measure the pattern of ventricular contraction and filling. These investigators soon discovered that the chamber dynamics of the left ventricle were more complex than had been appreciated previously. With the use of strain gauge length transducers (10), Rushmer showed that during isovolumic contraction the minor axis diameter of the left ventricle expanded, and the major axis shortened, a shape change that was termed *sphericalization*. These findings were confirmed by Hawthorne (11) who developed the hypothesis illustrated in Figure 2. During isovolumic contraction, the minor axis diameter increased, the major axis diameter decreased, and the ventricle became more spherical. During ejection, the minor axis diameter shortened more than the major axis diameter, and the chamber became more elliptical. During isovolumic relaxation, there was a further ellipticalization; during filling, the largest dimensional change was in the minor axis diameter, and the ventricle became more spherical.

Over the next decade, several investigators published results that were inconsistent with the foregoing hypothesis. The first report was by Rushmer et al. (12), in their classic description of pulse-transit sonomicrometry. In this study, shortening of the minor axis diameter was observed during isovolumic contraction in the awake dog. The authors suggested that this pattern of contraction could have been related to the larger ventricular volumes present in the conscious state. McDonald (13) confirmed this finding in studies of conscious humans, utilizing surgically implanted radiopaque epicardial markers. In virtually all of the patients examined, shortening of the minor axis diameter was noted during isovolumic con-

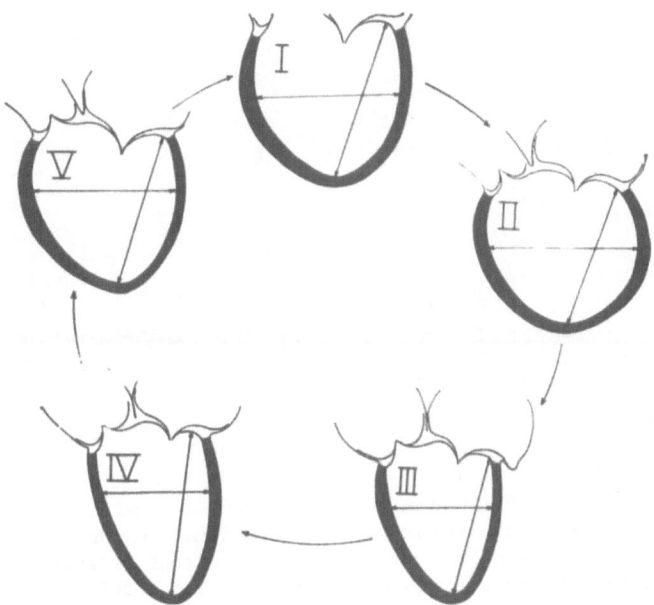

*Figure 2.* The dynamic geometry of the left ventricle as hypothesized by Hawthorne (11): I is end-diastole, II is the beginning of ejection, III is the end of ejection, IV is the beginning of rapid filling, and V is diastasis.

traction. On the basis of these data, Hawthorne concluded that the chamber dynamics of the left ventricle remained controversial (14).

Our group examined this problem in conscious dogs, chronically instrumented with pulse-transit ultrasonic dimension transducers (15). The orientation of the transducers allowed the measurement of minor axis diameter, major axis diameter, and equatorial wall thickness. Assuming ellipsoidal geometry, left ventricular cavity volume could be calculated from the dimension data and correlated well with direct measurements obtained with a saline-filled intracavitary balloon (15). The dogs were studied in the conscious state seven to ten days after implantation. Left ventricular and intrapleural pressures were obtained with high-fidelity micromanometers. Aortic blood flow was measured with implanted electromagnetic flow probes. Ellipticalization of the left ventricular chamber, with shortening of the minor axis and lengthening of the major axis, usually was observed during isovolumic contraction in the conscious state (A in Figure 3). During isovolumic relaxation, the opposite shape change occurred. However, as ventricular volume was decreased by balloon occlusion of the venae cavae, the isovolumic contraction pattern gradually changed. At smaller volumes (B), the ventricle began to sphericalize during isovolumic contraction and

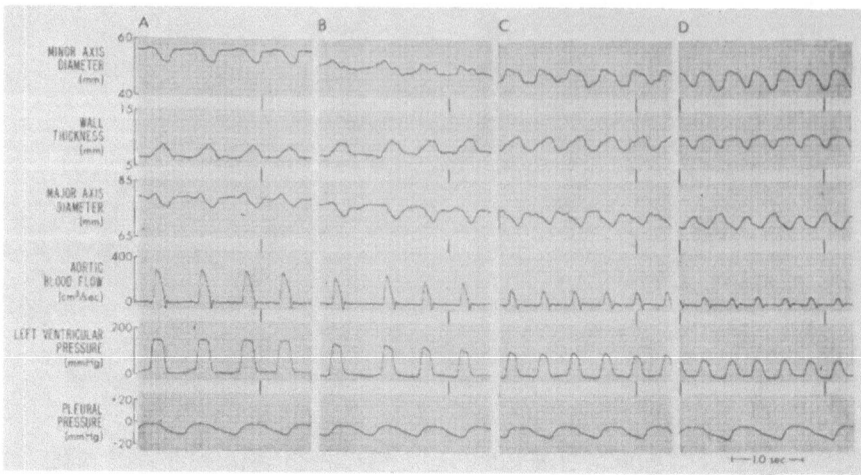

*Figure 3.* Measurements of left ventricular geometry, aortic flow, and left ventricular pressure obtained in the conscious dog as chamber volume was varied over the entire physiological range by inflation of vena-caval occluders. Panel A represents control conditions, panels B and C represent progressive phases in the vena-caval occlusion, and panel D represents maximum vena-caval occlusion.

ellipticalize during isovolumic relaxation. At maximum vena-caval occlusion (D) isovolumic rearrangements in geometry constituted the major change in all three of the dimensions throughout the cardiac cycle. Thus, the contraction pattern of the left ventricle seemed to be related to chamber volume, a finding that resolved many of the conflicting results of previous experiments. Similar observations recently have been made in man using pulse-transit ultrasonic transducers implanted on the left ventricle at the time of open heart surgery (Chitwood WR, Wechsler AS, personal communication, 1978).

The dynamic chamber geometry of the left ventricle as described above has been represented mathematically by relating midwall chamber eccentricity to cavity volume (16). Midwall eccentricity (*e*) was calculated from the three-dimensional measurements of left ventricular geometry in the conscious dog, using the equation:

$$e = \frac{\sqrt{(a-0.55h)^2-(b-h)^2}}{a-0.55h},$$ [1]

where *a* is the external major axis diameter, *b* is the external minor axis diameter, and *h* is the equatorial wall thickness. Cavity volume (*V*) was calculated from the formula:

$$V = \pi/6(b-2h)^2(a-1.1h).$$ [2]

The entire physiological range of ventricular volumes was analyzed from

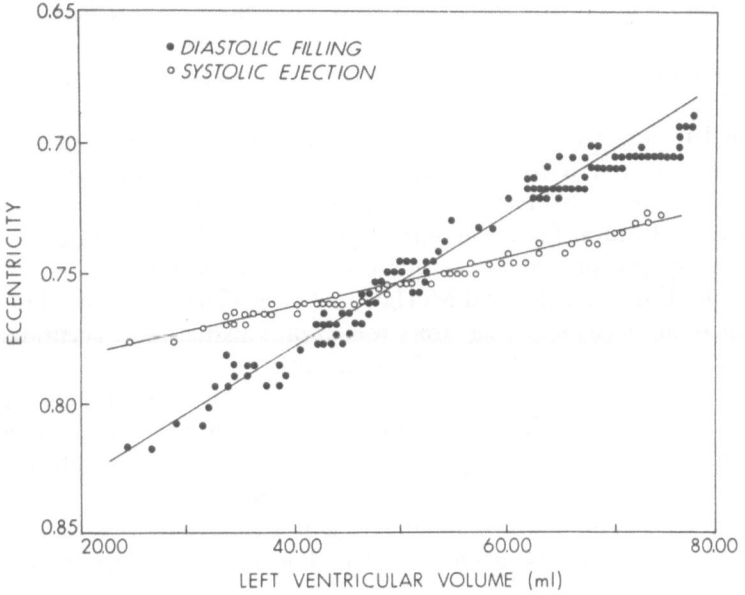

*Figure 4.* Comparison of chamber eccentricity (*e*) and cavity volume of the left ventricle. An *e* value of 0.85 is more elliptical and 0.65 is more spherical. Diastolic data are represented as filled circles and ejection-phase data as open circles. The wide range of volumes was obtained during transient vena-caval occlusion in the conscious dog.

data obtained during vena-caval occlusion. During diastolic filling, a linear relationship was observed between eccentricity and ventricular volume (Figure 4), with the chamber becoming considerably more spherical as volume increased. During ejection, a different linear relationship was obtained, and the ventricle became only slightly more elliptical as volume decreased (i.e. the dimensional changes during ejection were fairly concentric). As shown in Figure 4, the diastolic and ejection phase relationships consistently intersected. Because of this crossing of the curves, the transition from the diastolic to the ejection-phase curve during isovolumic contraction produced an ellipticalization of the chamber when the volume was large and a sphericalization when the volume was small. The basic relationships between eccentricity and volume were not changed significantly by positive inotropic interventions or by increasing systolic loading by inflation of aortic occluders (16). These relationships thus appeared to reflect structural properties of the left ventricular wall. It has been proposed (16) that the diastolic geometry of the left ventricle is determined primarily by the anisotropic three-dimensional stress-strain properties of the myocardium. The ejection-phase geometry, however, is probably related more to the fibre orientation within the wall which has a fairly uniform distribution (17).

## 4. EFFECTS OF CHAMBER GEOMETRY ON LEFT VENTRICULAR FUNCTION

The geometry of the left ventricular chamber is a major determinant of overall cardiac function. Woods (18) first proposed that the force within the wall of the left ventricle is proportional both to the distending pressure within the chamber and to the radius of curvature. This principle was verified experimentally by Hefner et al. (19), who demonstrated that the directly measured mural force was linearly proportional to the product of the intracavitary pressure and the square of the radius. Burns et al. (20) later reproduced these results, and McHale and Greenfield (21) showed that the experimentally measured wall stress was approximated most accurately with the use of a thin-walled ellipsoidal shell theory.

In our studies of left ventricular geometry in conscious dogs (16), it was observed that equatorial radius of curvature and wall thickness were related in a linear inverse manner (Figure 5). Similar findings have been published by Sasayama et al. (22). Interestingly, the relationship for diastole was not the same as for ejection, a finding that again points out differences in diastolic and ejection-phase geometry. The linear relationship between

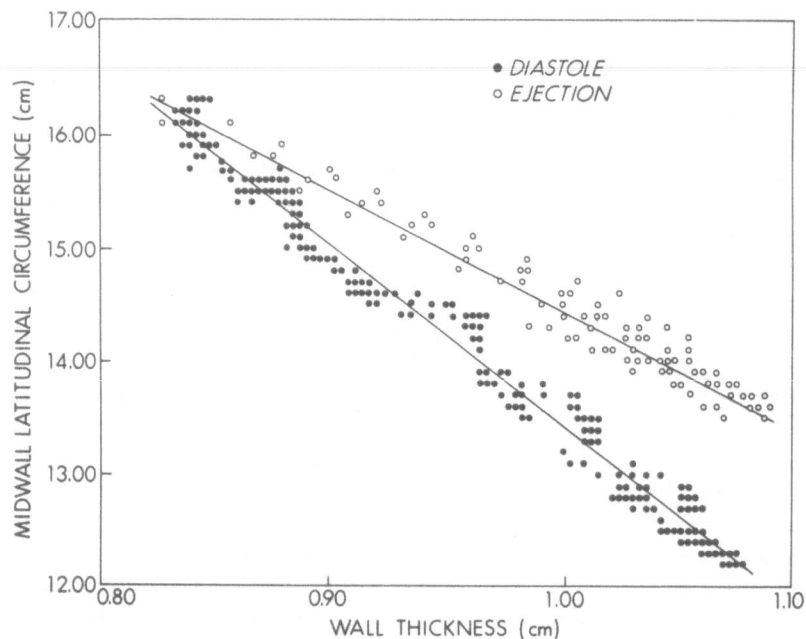

*Figure 5.* The relationship observed between diastolic (filled circles) and ejection-phase (open circles) midwall minor-axis circumference and wall thickness. Circumference is proportional to midwall radius. The wide range of data was obtained during transient vena-caval occlusion in the conscious dog.

radius and wall thickness may be fundamentally important to the calculation of wall force. Most stress theories are modifications of LaPlace's law:

$$\sigma \propto P \cdot r/h, \qquad\qquad\qquad [3]$$

where $\sigma$ is the mean tensile stress, $P$ is the transmural pressure, $r$ is the radius of curvature, and $h$ is the wall thickness. Since the radius and wall thickness are related linearly, the slope of the $r/h$ relationship is a constant that determines the relationship between transmural pressure and wall stress. Indeed, the diastolic stress calculated from ellipsoidal shell theory has been found experimentally to be a linear function of diastolic transmural pressure (16). Thus, the major effect of ventricular geometry on cardiac function is to determine this relationship between distending pressure and wall force.

## 5. CHAMBER GEOMETRY IN CARDIAC DISEASE

Hypertrophy is a long-term adaptive reserve of the heart that is capable of altering ventricular geometry to compensate for abnormal hemodynamic loads. This hypothesis originally was proposed by Linzbach (23) who postulated that the mural force in a ventricle subjected to chronic pressure overload was equivalent to normal because of hypertrophy and wall thickening. Hood et al. (24) experimentally tested this hypothesis in the catheterization laboratory and observed that the peak mural stress in patients with compensated pressure overload and volume overload was not different from the normal values. These findings suggested that wall thickening had maintained mural force within the normal range. Similar data have been published by Grossman and associates (25). Sasayama et al. (26) studied pressure overload in conscious dogs by chronically inflating implanted aortic occluders to increase left ventricular pressure above 200 mm Hg. After an initial slight increase in the minor axis diameter and thinning of the wall, the process of hypertrophy rapidly increased the wall thickness, so that after three weeks, the systolic wall stress had returned toward normal. This change in geometry could be characterized as a shift of the radius-wall thickness relationship (Figure 6) and seemed to be a means of adaptation to the high cavity pressures.

Gunther and Grossman (27) recently studied ventricular geometry in patients with chronic pressure overload from aortic stenosis. These authors found an inverse relationship between ejection fraction and mean ejection stress in these patients (Figure 7). Subjects with low ejection fractions seemed to have inordinately high wall stress values, possibly because of inadequate hypertrophy and wall thickening. Gunther concluded that ventricular function in aortic stenosis is closely correlated with circumferential

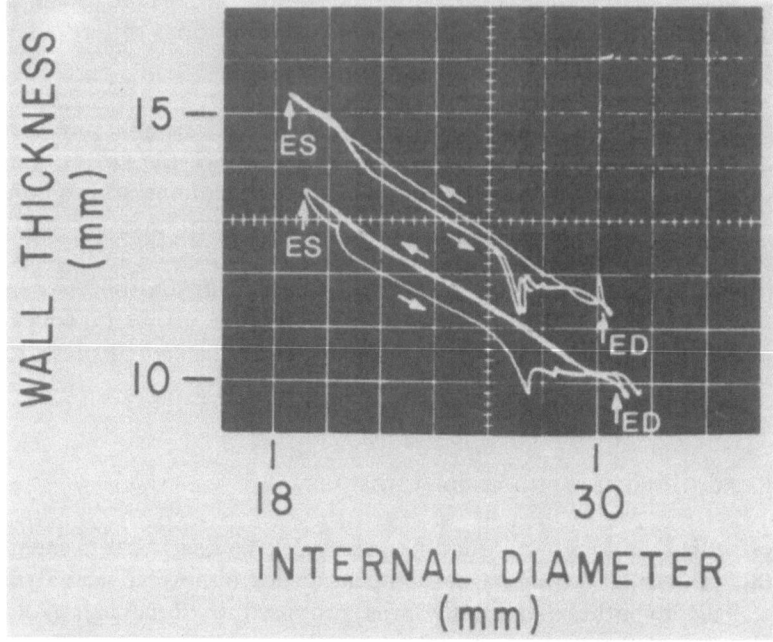

*Figure 6.* Relationship observed between the internal diameter and wall thickness of the left ventricle in the control state (lower curve) and after chamber hypertrophy induced by chronic pressure overload (upper curve). Data were obtained in the awake dog with the use of chronically implanted ultrasonic dimension transducers (26).

wall stress and chamber geometry. Thus, impaired cardiac performance may be related to inadequate geometric adaptation to altered loading rather than to a depression of intrinsic myocardial function.

Chamber geometry may also be important in chronic volume overload. Our group tested this hypothesis in a chronically instrumented dog model of infrarenal aortocaval shunt (28). After one week of volume overload, we observed a marked increase in the major and minor ventricular diameters and wall thickness implying significant chamber dilatation and hypertrophy. The radius-wall thickness relationship was shifted upward and to the right by the dilatation and hypertrophy (Figure 8: top). However, the wall thickening appeared to be proportional to the dilatation, and the control relationship between diastolic pressure and stress was maintained relatively constant by the hypertrophy (Figure 8: bottom).

Gaasch et al. (29) recently studied left ventricular geometry in chronic volume overload in a series of patients undergoing aortic valve replacement for aortic regurgitation. Echo ultrasonic techniques were used to measure left ventricular diameter and wall thickness before and serially after correction of regurgitation. The typical response after aortic valve replacement

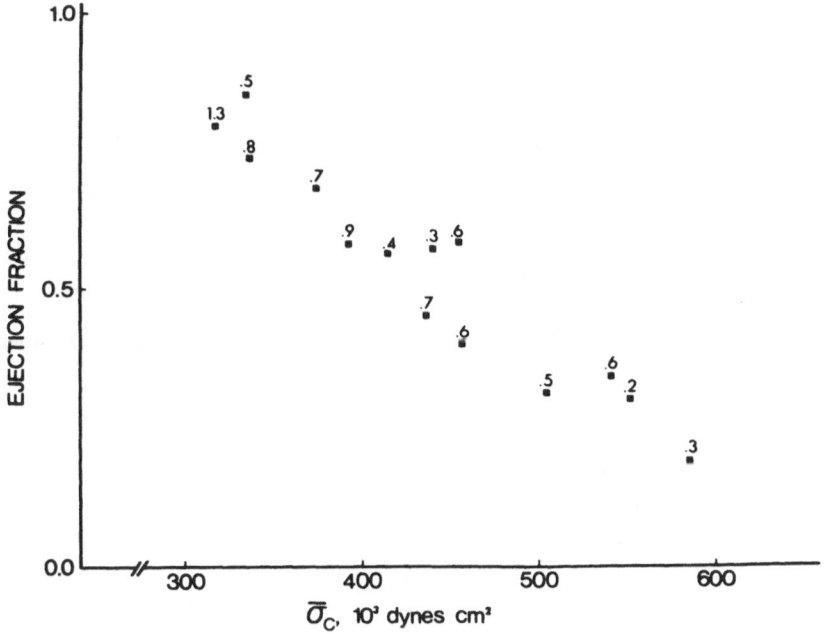

*Figure 7.* Data from the work of Gunther and Grossman (27) in patients with chronic pressure overload. Each square represents data from an individual patient obtained during resting conditions.

was an immediate reduction in diameter and an increase in wall thickness, consistent with a decrease in end-diastolic volume. Then over several months, there was a further reduction in diameter and a decrease in wall thickness, characteristic of regression of hypertrophy. This pattern of improved ventricular function was seen in all but four patients. In these patients, ventricular dilatation continued, hypertrophy persisted, and congestive heart failure worsened despite a successful surgical procedure. When preoperative indices of ventricular function were examined, there was no difference between the groups of patients in terms of end-diastolic diameter, wall thickness, left ventricular mass, cardiac output, or ejection fraction. The only parameter that distinguished the group of patients that did not benefit from surgery was the preoperative ratio of radius to wall thickness. When the *r/h* ratio was greater than 4.0, the long-term hemodynamic result was suboptimal. This finding may reflect inadequate hypertrophy or inappropriate geometric adaptation to the volume overload in these patients. Thus, measurements of chamber geometry may be of some utility in the selection of patients for surgery in valvular heart disease.

In recent years, basic and clinical physiologists have made significant advances in the search for clinically useful methods of measuring cardiac

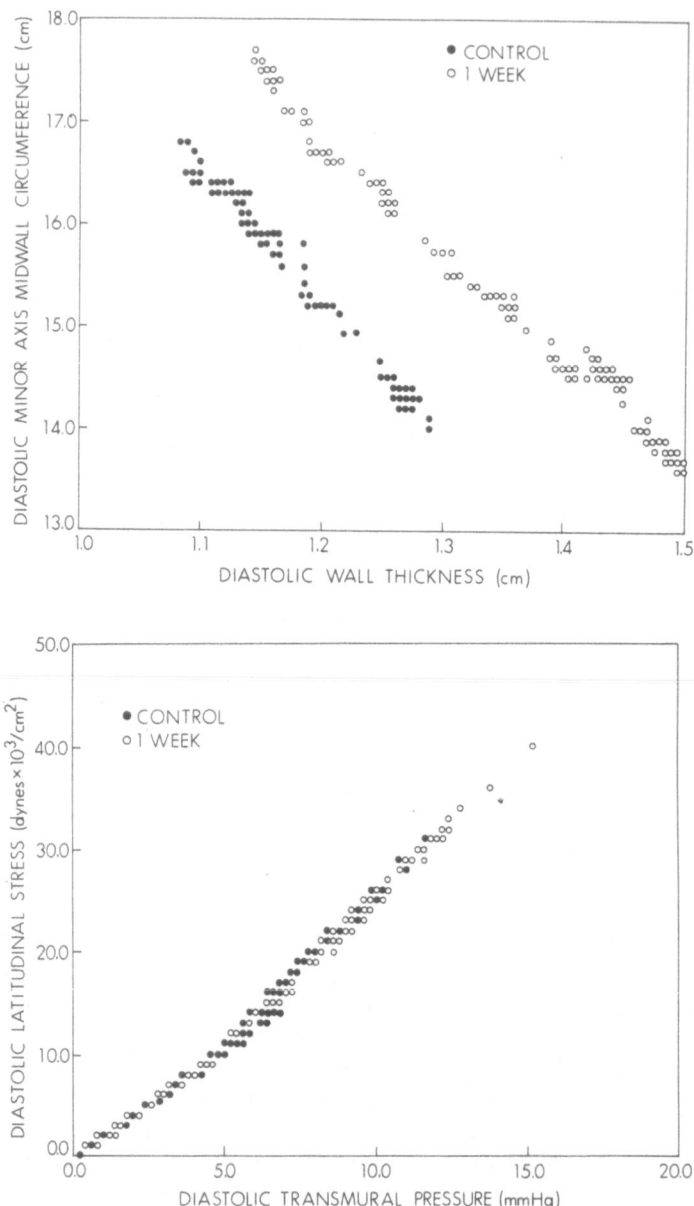

*Figure 8. Top*: the relationship between minor axis circumference and wall thickness observed in instrumented conscious dogs in the control state (filled circles) and after a period of chronic volume overload (open circles). The data represent diastolic measurements obtained over the entire physiological range during vena-caval occlusion. *Bottom*: effects of chronic volume overload on the relationship between diastolic transmural pressure and calculated equatorial tensile stress. Symbols are the same as in the top panel.

function. The potential for improving the care of patients with cardiac disorders is great. Because most chronic cardiac diseases produce major alterations in the structure of the ventricular wall, analysis of dynamic chamber geometry may prove to be particularly useful in the assessment of myocardial function in man.

SUMMARY

The chamber dynamics of the left ventricle have been studied intensively in recent years. Several investigators have shown that complicated changes in ventricular geometry occur during diastolic filling, ejection, and the isovolumic phases of the cardiac cycle. In the dog, these shape changes have been represented mathematically as distinct linear relationships between eccentricity and cavity volume during diastole and ejection. Similar observations have been made in man using a number of measurement techniques. These relationships were not altered by changes in loading or inotropism and appear to reflect structural properties of the left ventricular wall. The geometry of the ventricular chamber is a major determinant of overall cardiac function. It has been shown that the radius of curvature ($r$) and the thickness of the ventricular wall ($h$) are related in an inverse linear manner. Therefore, the slope of the $r/h$ relationship is a geometric constant that determines the mural force at any given transmural pressure. Chronic chamber dilatation changes the geometric slope constant and increases the mural force resisting ejection. In either volume overload or pressure overload, hypertrophy affects the geometric interrelationships to return systolic mural force toward normal. It is possible that primary alterations in ventricular geometry associated with inadequate hypertrophy could adversely affect overall cardiac function. Recent studies in patients with chronic volume overload have shown that the $r/h$ relationship may be of value in distinguishing between reversible and irreversible impairment of myocardial performance. There are also data which suggest that chamber geometry is a critical determinant of ventricular function in patients with pressure overload. Because most chronic cardiac diseases produce major alterations in the structure of the ventricular wall, analysis of dynamic chamber geometry may prove to be of prognostic value in the assessment of myocardial function in man.

REFERENCES

1. Fleming D: Galen on the motions of the blood in the heart and lungs. *Isis* 46:14–21, 1955.
2. Harvey W: *Exercitatio anatomica de motu cordis et sanguinis in animalibus*, Leake CD (trans), Springfield, Illinois, Thomas, 1928.
3. Françoise–Franck M: Nouvelles recherches sur les effets de la systole des oreillettes, *Archives de Physiologie Normale et Pathologique* 2 (series 5): 395–410, 1890.

4. Roy CS, Adami JG: Contributions to the physiology and pathology of the mammalian heart. *Philosophical Transactions* 183B:199–298, 1893.
5. Henderson Y: The volume curve of the ventricles of the mammalian heart, and the significance of this curve in respect to the mechanics of the heart beat and the filling of the ventricles. *Am J Physiol* 16:325–367, 1906.
6. Patterson SW, Piper H, Starling EH: The regulation of the heart beat. *J Physiol* 48:465–513, 1914.
7. Wiggers CJ, Katz LN: The contour of the ventricular volume curves under different conditions. *Am J Physiol* 58:439–475, 1921.
8. Rushmer RF, Crystal DK: Changes in configuration of the ventricular chambers during the cardiac cycle. *Circulation* 4:211–218, 1951.
9. Rushmer RF, Crystal DK, Wagner, C, Ellis RM, Hendron JA: Continuous measurements of left ventricular dimensions in intact, unanesthetized dogs. *Circ Res* 2:14–22, 1954.
10. Rushmer RF: Initial phase of ventricular systole; asynchronous contraction. *Am J Physiol* 184:188–194, 1956.
11. Hawthorne EW: Instantaneous dimensional changes in the left ventricle in dogs. *Circ Res* 9:110–119, 1961.
12. Rushmer RF, Franklin DL, Ellis RM: Left ventricular dimensions recorded by sonocardiometry. *Circ Res* 4:684–688, 1956.
13. McDonald IG: The shape and movements of the human left ventricle during systole. *Am J Cardiol* 26:221–230, 1970.
14. Hawthorne EW: The contractile behaviour of the heart: introduction to section III. In: *Factors influencing myocardial contractility*, Tanz RD et al (eds), New York, Academic Press, 1967, p 137–140.
15. Rankin JS, McHale PA, Arentzen CE, Ling D, Greenfield Jr JC, Anderson RW: The three-dimensional dynamic geometry of the left ventricle in the conscious dog. *Circ Res* 39:304–313, 1976.
16. Rankin JS, Arentzen CE, Ring WS, McHale PA, Anderson RW: The deformational characteristics of the left ventricle in the conscious dog. *Circ Res* (in press).
17. Streeter Jr DD, Spotnitz HM, Patel DJ, Ross Jr J, Sonnenblick EH: Fiber orientation in the canine left ventricle during diastole and systole. *Circ Res* 24:339–347, 1969.
18. Woods RH: A few applications of a physical theorem to membranes in the human body in a state of tension. *J Anat Physiol* 26:362–370, 1892.
19. Hefner LL, Sheffield LT, Cobbs GC, Klip W: Relation between mural force and pressure in the left ventricle of the dog. *Circ Res* 11:654–663, 1962.
20. Burns JW, Covell JW, Myers R, Ross Jr J: Comparison of directly measured left ventricular wall stress and stress calculated from geometric reference figures. *Circ Res* 28:611–621, 1971.
21. McHale PA, Greenfield Jr JC: Evaluation of several geometric models for estimation of left ventricular circumferential wall stress. *Circ Res* 33:303–312, 1973.
22. Sasayama S, Franklin D, Ross Jr J, Kemper WS, McKown D: Dynamic changes in left ventricular wall thickness and their use in analyzing cardiac function in the conscious dog. *Am J Cardiol* 38:870–878, 1976.
23. Linzbach AJ: Heart failure from the point of view of quantitative anatomy. *Am J Cardiol* 5:370–382, 1960.
24. Hood Jr WP, Rackley CE, Rolett EL: Wall stress in the normal and hypertrophied human left ventricle. *Am J Physiol* 22:550–558, 1968.
25. Grossman W, Jones D, McLaurin LP: Wall stress and patterns of hypertrophy in the human left ventricle. *J Clin Invest* 56:56–64, 1975.
26. Sasayama S, Ross Jr J, Franklin D, Bloor CM, Bishop S, Dilley RB: Adaptations of the left ventricle to chronic pressure overload. *Circ Res* 38:172–178, 1976.
27. Gunther S, Grossman W: Critical role of left ventricular wall thickness and geometry as determinants of performance in patients with aortic stenosis. *Circulation* (II) 56:450, 1977.
28. Rankin JS, Ring WS, Arentzen CE, Ling D, Anderson RW: The functional reserves of the left ventricle in chronic volume overload. *Circulation* (II) 56:906, 1977.
29. Gaasch WH, Andrias CW, Levine HJ: Chronic aortic regurgitation: the effect of aortic valve replacement on left ventricular volume, mass, and function. *Circulation* (in press).

## 2.3. LV WALL FIBRE PATHWAYS FOR IMPULSE PROPAGATION

DANIEL D. STREETER, JR., M. ALISON ROSS

### 1. BACKGROUND

Pathways for depolarization in the heart wall tend to follow the principal muscle fibre pathways that imbricate gently through the wall in a figure of eight (1, 2, 3). Each pathway is remarkably close to a geodesic, as described by Clairaut's theorem (4). All pathways in the LV wall lie in nested sets of toroidal shells that are crescentic in longitudinal section (5, 6).

Our understanding of these pathways has come slowly. The long history of dissections by Lower (7), Gerdy (8), Weber (9), Ludwig (10), Pettigrew (11), and Krehl (12), extending from 1669 to 1891, belongs to the European school. Their dissections showed left ventricular fibre pathways as partial or full figures of eight that wind from epicardium to endocardium and back. Our preferred representation of these figures shows them inscribed on surfaces resembling double sets of double cones, one set inside the other, with bases joined epicardially and endocardially at the equator, and tips truncated basally and apically to make cusps joining the truncated portions of the double cones (5:fig. 9.2; 6:fig. 11). These anatomists recognized that fibrepaths in the figure of eight were continuous at the base as well as at the apex, not necessarily inserting into the valve ring. They also acknowledged the smooth transition of helix angle of the fibre path from epicardium to endocardium. The classic sketches of Krehl (12) reveal his deep understanding of the toroidal shell structure of the left ventricular (LV) wall. His *Triebwerk* illustration showed the outermost of the toroidal shells that extends from base to the vicinity of the apex without closing it. In other words, he recognized the apical orifice that is as intrinsic as the basal to the LV fibre structure. Unfortunately, Krehl provided no quantitative data or protocol for dissection to support his *Triebwerk* concept. As with many artists, he was ahead of his time.

The scene next shifted across the Atlantic. At the turn of the century a new school of blunt dissection was started with MacCallum (13) and continued with Mall (14), Flett (15), Shaner (16), Thomas (17) and Robb and Robb (18). MacCallum tried to demonstrate the simple truth that was conceptualized in the previous century: that fibre pathways through the papillary muscles have continuity with those that run exteriorly. Wanting to

J. Baan, A.C. Arntzenius, E.L. Yellin (eds.), Cardiac Dynamics, 107–113.

show that they constitute a structural system, he separated large masses of muscle tissue from neighbouring masses by "unrolling", a procedure necessitating ripping of fibres. But a fibre is just an end-to-end sequence of muscle cells. He did not realize that the cardiac muscle "fibre" was like a sausage joined at either end to one, two, or three other sausages, and so on, really having no definition because a large number of fibre directions could be derived from one starting point, depending upon the protocol or "bias" for ripping.

A rigid, formal terminology ensued from this: *bulbospiral* and *sinospiral* describing supposed deep and superficial bands of muscle.

In 1956 Lev and Simkins (19) questioned the validity of the ripping procedure (noting the syncytial character of myocardium), followed by Hort (20), Grant (21), Streeter and Bassett (22), and Torrent-Guasp (23, 24). The separate bundles and layers of muscle were shown to be artificial.

To bring out the figure-of-eight fibre paths hidden within LV myocardium, Torrent-Guasp (23, 24) developed a novel dissection technique that revealed only the individual pathways that were in the principal fibre direction. Thus a dissectable fibre was defined for the first time (as a statistical entity) and a rigorous protocol for dissections followed. If a principal fibre direction conflicted with the fibre directions in nearby myocardium, the nearby myocardium was cleared away so that the principal fibre direction could be further pursued. Such dissections were done fibre by fibre, so that adjacent fibre courses appeared roughly parallel, giving the surface a raked appearance. The surfaces revealed rarely coincided with the shape of the epicardial surface. They were toroidal, and crescentic in longitudinal section when basal and apical halves of the LV were put together.

Despite the careful definition of Torrent-Guasp's procedures, it was necessary to obtain other indications that such procedures were correct. How could correctness be verified? Unknown to Torrent-Guasp, Hort (20, 25, 26) was working on this problem. He studied the fibre shape and organization, showing that the fibre retains its approximately circular cross-section during its length change from the dilated to the contracted state. He showed that a through-wall block of myocardium has a significantly greater cell count radially when in the contracted state than in the dilated. In other words, during dilation of the ventricle, the cells interdigitate (between anastomoses). He also showed that such motion is facilitated by pinnation, the regular arrangement of lamellar zones that are poor in anastomoses. This led Streeter et al. (27) to conclude that the muscle fibre, being free to roll or slide over its neighbor during the cardiac cycle, carries only axial tension (like a rope) and that it assumes a geodesic configuration. Using the theorem of Clairaut (4), Streeter et al. (5) showed that the locus of a geodesic path in the LV wall is the toroid. The profile in longitudinal section of a nested set of toroids was reconstructed from helix angle and radius measurements in the LV wall of the macaque and the dog. These profiles possessed the same features as those observed in the dissections.

Still, despite the observed similarity of features between the geodesic path and the dissection paths, it might be asked whether such paths have actually been measured in their three-dimensional orientation in the LV wall. The reply is again yes. By the rotated sections method of histological measurement of two fibre-angle components in through-wall blocks of macaque myocardium fibre-path profiles in a longitudinal section of the LV wall were reconstructed (5, 6). This reconstruction has also been made with histological measurements on rotated sections from the cadaver LV wall (6). In each instance the reconstructions possessed the same toroidal features as those observed in the dissections.

Because of these confirmations, the probability is high that Torrent-Guasp's dissection protocol is correct and that Hort's interdigitating muscle fibres are geodesic. The three-dimensional fibre orientation obtained by the rotated sections method is, necessarily, the sine qua non.

Krehl's foresight (12) is also vindicated by these confirmations. One might say that MacCallum and his successors have taken us on a trip. But another could argue that it was necessary; MacCallum broke the philosophical hold that the European school had on heart research and established a new school based on systematic dissection.

This demonstrated, by elimination of alternative procedures, that all myocardial dissection is artifact, but that such an artifact is reproducible and meaningful when the principal fibre pathway is the sole arbiter of the dissection protocol.

## 2. PATHWAYS FOR IMPULSE PROPAGATION

Because of the confirmations above it is unimportant whether the fibre pathways chosen for impulse propagation are those determined by (1) dissection, (2) the geodesic criterion, or (3) the rotated sections method. We chose the geodesic criterion for the distended cadaver LV wall.

### 2.1. Methods

We used five non-pathologic cadaver left ventricles in the unfixed state (6). These were cannulated in the two coronary ostia and perfused with a buffer to promote muscle relaxation. A rubber balloon was inserted into the LV cavity and inflated by water, distending the ventricle to $52.4 \pm 11.4$ (SD) ml. The hearts were fixed in half-strength Karnovsky's glutaraldehyde fixative (28).

The procedure used to obtain through-wall blocks, serially section at 5 $\mu$m in paraffin, stain with hematoxylin and eosin, measure helix angles $\alpha_1$, measure epicardial wall radius and wall thickness, apply Clairaut's theorem, plot the orthogonal grid of points in a longitudinal section of the wall, construct fibre-path contours in the $X$-$Y$ plot, measure declination angles $\alpha_2$, calculate traverse angles $\alpha_3$ as a function of latitude, recalculate smoothed values of $\alpha_2$, prepare the matrix of points $(r, z)$ for contours of constant $K$ in the wall, calculate fibre-path length (as a half figure of eight from epi- to endocardium), calculate the angle of wrap of the fibre path about the LV $Z$ axis, and estimate the $l/d$ ratio for the typical distended ventricular-wall muscle cell where $l$ is the length between anastomoses and $d$ is the cell diameter, has already been documented [6].

## 2.2. Results and discussion

The measured data appear in Streeter (6): (figs. 33, 34, 45–50; tables 1, 2, 5). We measured the lengths of the geodesic paths at the equator, at 30° and at 60° of latitude as approximately 14.5, 8.9 and 3.7 cm. The angle of wrap was approximately 275, 225, and 165° about the axis of LV symmetry. In the living human heart, with greater cavity volumes than those obtained by distending these cadaver ventricles, the fibre-path length (but not the angle of wrap) will be greater by approximately the cube root of the cavity volume.

Assuming an extremely low resistance across the intercalated disc, the flow of an impulse will proceed not only forward but retrograde into an adjacent cell. The extreme of the retrograde mode of propagation would be perpendicular to the geodesic, a continuously retrograde pathway zigzagging from one end of the first cell to the far end of the next, and so on, back and forth, across the entire wall radially and laterally instead of by the figure of eight. A 50–50 choice of mode presents itself at each bifurcation. By mapping both choices one can sequentially map the whole event of depolarization.

We can estimate the length of the through-wall zigzag path as $l/d$ times the wall thickness. If $l$ is cell length, then by one source $l/d = 5.3$ in the myocardial cell of the rat heart, both normal and hypertrophied, where sarcomere lengths average 1.8 $\mu$m (29). Supposing, as an extreme case, sarcomere lengths to average 2.25 $\mu$m in a ventricle during excitation, $l/d = 7.4$. Thus longitudinal propagation is possible at a rate sevenfold faster than transverse propagation, which measures about 0.3 m/sec through the wall. This brings it to the order of magnitude of impulse velocity in the right and left bundles. It is difficult to reconcile this observation with the measured 0.75 m/sec in trabecular strands (2), unless the compact arrangement of near-parallel cells in the wall facilitates such a propagation velocity, or unless the width of extracellular space exceeds the cell diameter.

We estimate the lengths of the zigzag pathways at latitudes 0, 30, and 60° as approximately 7.5, 6.2, and 4.7 cm. Thus the zigzag route is shorter (and faster) than the geodesic everywhere except near the apex.

Assuming a longitudinal propagation velocity of 2.0 m/sec, the time for the wall thickness to be penetrated along the geodesic route is 73 msec (for 79% of the circumference), starting at the equator. At latitudes 30 and 60° the figure-of-eight geodesic pathways take 45 and 19 msec (for 62 and 46% of the circumference).

Contrast this performance with that on the zigzag path. At latitudes 0, 30 and 60°, the timing is 38, 31 and 24 msec. The 60° path with left bundle branch block would actually depolarize the LV free wall endocardium by a geodesic route before the LV septal endocardium at that latitude. Data, from implanted mural electrodes in the dog heart, are available for comparison with these observations (30, 31).

A computer-graphic programming of the time sequence of depolarization of the LV wall would display the combined increments of geodesic and zigzag paths at each bifurcation reached by the wave front By trial and error, the velocity of travel can be more accurately estimated when the computer-graphic displays are compared with electrode data.

The rationale for attempting the computer-graphic display, fibre by fibre and msec by msec lies in the powerful logic of the geodesic path as one of the modes and the zigzag path as the orthogonal mode by which the wave of depolarization may spread. It is now possible, timely, and appropriate to do such mapping. The authors will be glad to help those who wish to start.

SUMMARY

Pathways of depolarization in the heart wall tend to follow principal muscle fibre pathways that imbricate gently through the wall in a figure of eight. Each pathway is geodesic and lies on a toroidal shell that is crescentic in longitudinal section.

We used five normal cadaver left ventricles (LV) fixed in a pressure-distended state to $52.4 + 11.4$ (SD) ml, after coronary perfusion with a buffer to promote muscle relaxation. Windows were cut into the LV walls totalling eight at the equator and nine elsewhere. The excised blocks were sectioned serially in paraffin at 5 microns parallel to the epicardium. Helix angle ($\alpha_1$) and radius ($r$) measured at a sequence of sections permitted us to reconstruct the geodesic fibre pathways in a composite LV wall by Clairaut's theorem.

We measured the lengths of the geodesic paths at the equator, at 30° and at 60° of latitude as approximately 14.5, 8.9, and 3.7 cm. The angle of wrap was roughly 275, 225, and 165° about the axis of LV symmetry. Assuming extremely low resistance across the intercalated disc, the flow of an impulse will proceed not only forward but retrograde into an adjacent cell. The extreme of the retrograde mode of propagation would be perpendicular to the geodesic, a continuously retrograde pathway zigzagging from one end of the first cell to the far end of the next and so on, back and forth, across the entire wall radially and laterally instead of by the figure of eight. A 50-50 choice of mode presents itself at each intercalated disc. By mapping both choices one can sequentially map the whole event of depolarization.

From estimates of cell length ($l$) to thickness ($d$) in the distended LV wall, we estimate the velocity of propagation along the cell to be $l/d$ times the usual 0.3 m/sec through the wall. This brings it near to the 2.0 m/sec in the right and left bundles.

We estimate the length of the through-wall zigzag pathway as $l/d$ times the wall thickness. At latitudes 0, 30, and 60 these lengths are approximately 7.5, 6.2, and 4.7 cm. Thus the zigzag route is faster than the geodesic everywhere except near the apex. In a left bundle branch block, however, depolarization of the LV endocardium will depend upon geodesic pathways everywhere except in the neighbourhood of the septum, where the zigzag mode can relay the right bundle signal more directly.

ACKNOWLEDGEMENTS

This research was supported by the U.S. P.H.S. grants HL 13517 and HL 20883.

REFERENCES

1. Weidmann S: The functional significance of the intercalated disc. In: *International symposium on the electrophysiology of the heart*, Taccardi B, Marchett G (eds), New York, Pergamon, 1965, p 149–152.
2. Weidmann S: Electrical constants of trabecular muscle from mammalian heart. *J Physiol* 210:1041–1054, 1970.
3. Woodbury JW, Crill WE: On the problem of impulse conduction in the atrium. In: *Nervous inhibition*, Florey E (ed), New York, Pergamon, 1965, p 124–135.
4. Struik DJ: *Lectures on classical differential geometry*, Reading, Mass, Addison-Wesley, 1950 (2nd ed 1961), p 134.
5. Streeter Jr DD, Powers WE, Ross MA, Torrent-Guasp F: Three-dimensional fiber orientation in the mammalian left ventricular wall. In: *Cardiovascular system dynamics*, Baan J, Noordergraaf A, Raines J (eds), Cambridge, Mass, MIT Press, 1978, p 73–84.
6. Streeter Jr DD: Gross morphology and fiber geometry of the heart. In: *The heart*, Berne RM, Sperelakis N (eds). *Handbook of Physiology, The Cardiovascular System*, vol 1, Bethesda, Maryland: American Physiological Society, 1979, p 61–112.
7. Lower R: *Tractatus de corde*, London, 1669. (Franklin K, trans, London, Oxford University Press, 1932.)
8. Gerdy PN: Recherches, discussions et propositions d'anatomie. Thesis, Paris, 1823. Cited by Mall (14).
9. Weber EH: Das Herz. In: *Hildebrandts Handbuch der Anatomie des Menschen*, Brunswick, Schulbuchhandlung, 1831, p 124–168.

10 Ludwig C: Ueber den Bau und die Bewegungen der Herzventrikel. *Z Ration Med* 7:189–220, 1849.
11. Pettigrew J: On the arrangement of the muscular fibres of the ventricular portion of the heart of the mammal. *Proc Roy Soc* 10:433–440, 1860.
12. Krehl L: Kenntnis der Füllung und Entleerung des Herzens. *Abhandl K S Gesellsch Wissensch* 29:341–362, 1891.
13. MacCallum JB: On the muscular architecture and growth of the ventricles of the heart. *Johns Hopkins Hosp Rep* 9:309–335, 1900.
14. Mall FP: On the muscular architecture of the ventricles of the human heart. *Am J Anat* 11:211–266, 1911.
15. Flett RL: The musculature of the heart, with its application to physiology, and a note on heart rupture. *J Anat* 62:439–475, 1927.
16. Shaner RF: The development of the muscular architecture of ventricles of the pig's heart, with a review of the adult heart and a note on two abnormal mammalian hearts. *Anat Record* 39:1–35, 1928.
17. Thomas CE: The muscular architecture of the ventricles of hog and dog hearts. *Am J Anat* 101:17–57, 1957.
18. Robb JS, Robb RC: The normal heart: anatomy and physiology of the structural units. *Am Heart J* 23:455–467, 1942.
19. Lev M, Simkins CS: Architecture of the human ventricular myocardium: technic for study using a modification of the Mall-MacCallum method. *Lab Invest* 5:396–409, 1956.
20. Hort W: Makroskopische und mikrometrische Untersuchungen am Myokard verschieden stark gefüllter linker Kammern. *Virchows Arch Pathol Anat Physiol Klin Med* 333:523–564, 1960.
21. Grant RP: Notes on the muscular architecture of the left ventricle. *Circulation* 32:301–308, 1965.
22. Streeter Jr DD, Bassett DL: Engineering analysis of myocardial fiber orientation in pig's left ventricle in systole. *Anat Record* 155:503–511, 1966.
23. Torrent-Guasp F: *The electrical circulation*, Marqués de Campo 21, Denia (Alicante), Spain, 1970.
24. Torrent-Guasp F: *The cardiac muscle*, Madrid, Fundacion Juan March, 1973.
25. Hort W: Untersuchungen über die Muskelfaserdehnung und das Gefüge des Myokards in der rechten Herzkammerwand des Meerschweinchens, *Virchows Arch Pathol Anat Physiol Klin Med* 329:694–731, 1957.
26. Hort W: Mikrometrische Untersuchungen an verschieden weiten Meerschweinchenherzen. *Verhandl Deut Ges Kreislaufforsch* 23:343–346, 1957.
27. Streeter Jr DD, Vaishnav RN, Patel DJ, Spotnitz HM, Ross Jr J, Sonnenblick EH: Stress distribution in the canine left ventricle during diastole and systole. *Biophys J* 10:345–363, 1970.
28. Karnovsky MJ: A formaldehyde-glutaraldehyde fixative of high osmolarity for use in electron microscopy: abstract *J Cell Biol* 27:137A–138A, 1965.
29. Koreky B, Rakusan K: Normal and hypertrophic growth of the rat heart: changes in cell dimensions and number. *Am J Physiol* 234:H 123–H 128, 1978.
30. Scher AM: Electrical correlates of the cardiac cycle. In: *Physiology and biophysics*. Ruch TC, Patton HD (eds), Philadelphia, Saunders, 1965, p 565–599.
31. Becker RA, Scher AM, Erickson RV: Ventricular excitation in experimental left bundle branch block. *Am Heart J* 55:547–556, 1958.

# 2.4. TRANSMURAL COURSE OF STRESS AND SARCOMERE LENGTH IN THE LEFT VENTRICLE UNDER NORMAL HEMODYNAMIC CIRCUMSTANCES

THEO ARTS, PIETER C. VEENSTRA,
ROBERT S. RENEMAN

## 1. INTRODUCTION

In this paper the dynamic behaviour of mechanical stresses and strains in the wall of the left ventricle is described. Though several investigators are rather optimistic (1), direct determination of stresses in the wall of the left ventricle is difficult and unreliable (2). A better approach is calculation of these stresses by the use of a mathematical model of the mechanics of the left ventricle (3). Following this principle, several investigators (2, 4, 5) have computed wall stress from left ventricular pressure, assuming a certain geometry of the left ventricle and certain mechanical properties of the wall. However, none of these models can be used to study the dynamic behaviour of the stresses in the wall of the left ventricle since these models are based on unrealistic approximations, such as isotropic myocardial material or inadequate geometry, while usually fibre orientation in the wall of the left ventricle and physiological contractile behaviour of the myocardial material are not taken into account. Therefore, a new model was developed in which all of these factors are considered (3).

## 2. DESIGN OF THE MATHEMATICAL MODEL OF THE LEFT VENTRICLE

In designing a mathematical model of the mechanics of the left ventricle, simplifications concerning the characteristics of the heart are required. Each simplification is a compromise between accuracy and simplicity. Following this principle the following simplifications were made.
- Only the left ventricle was simulated.
- The left ventricle is a thick-walled cylinder composed of eight concentric cylindrical shells (Figure 1). The relation between left ventricular pressure and wall stress is most realistically described by an ellipsoidal geometry. Cylindrical geometry, however, approximates the realistic relation closely, i.e. within 10%, and better than if spherical geometry is assumed (3).
- The muscle material is taken to be anisotropic, because experiments have shown that assuming isotropic properties of the myocardial wall, unrealistic findings are obtained (3,6). Anisotropy is introduced by assuming

*J. Baan, A.C. Arntzenius, E.L. Yellin (eds.), Cardiac Dynamics, 115–122.*

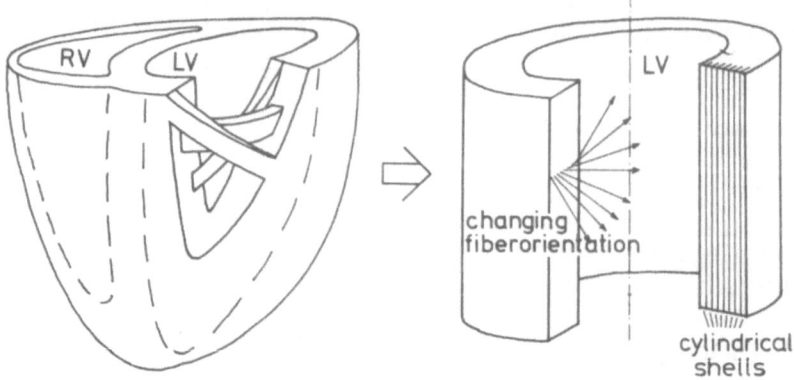

*Figure 1.* Schematic representation of the geometry of the left ventricle. The ventricle is simulated by a cylinder. Subdivision of the thick-walled cylinder in a number of cylindrical shells and changing fibre orientation are indicated.

that the myocardial tissue consists of a contractile fibre structure embedded in a soft, incompressible material (6).
- The contractile properties of the fibre structure were derived from experimental data on papillary muscle (7, 8). These properties were simplified in a mathematical model which calculates the velocity of sarcomere shortening from the instantaneous state of activation and the tensile stress borne by the fibre structure (3).
- The fibre orientation changes across the ventricular wall according to the findings of Streeter and Hanna (9).
- Spread of onset of muscle contraction across the wall is assumed to occur only in a radial direction, and is based on the electrical activation pattern found by Durrer et al. (10).
- The aortic valve and aortic input impedance were simplified to a network (11) which is represented diagrammatically in Figure 2.
The mathematical basis of the model is a system of differential equations.

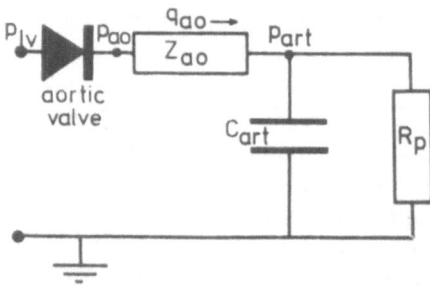

*Figure 2.* Network which represents the aortic input impedance including the aortic valve.

Thus the time derivatives of a number of characteristic quantities were calculated, so that the increment of these quantities during the following increment in time could be computed. In this way the values of the characteristic quantities were computed at intervals of 2 msec. All quantities of physiological interest incorporated in the model were derived from the set of characteristic quantities.

The instantaneous state of deformation of the myocardial material was calculated from the volume of the inner cavity and the cylindrical shells and from the height and torsion angle of the cylinder. The height of the cylinder (Figure 3) represents the base-to-apex distance. The torsion angle is defined as the angle over which the upper cross-sectional surface of the cylinder is rotated around the axis with respect to its lower cross-sectional surface (Figure 3). This angle represents the angle of rotation of the base with respect to the apex around the axis of the left ventricle (3). The height and torsion angle are calculated from equilibria of forces and torques in the upper cross-sectional surface of the cylinder. The axial force exerted by the left ventricular pressure is in equilibrium with the total force due to axial stresses in the wall of the cylinder. The torques acting in the upper surface of the cylinder due to tangential shear stresses are in equilibrium too. Both equilibria result in a set of two equations, that can be solved for height and torsion angle.

### 3. SIMULATION OF A CARDIAC CYCLE

In order to simulate a cardiac cycle, values of several parameters had to be substituted in the mathematical relations describing the model. Values of many parameters were obtained from experimental results described in the

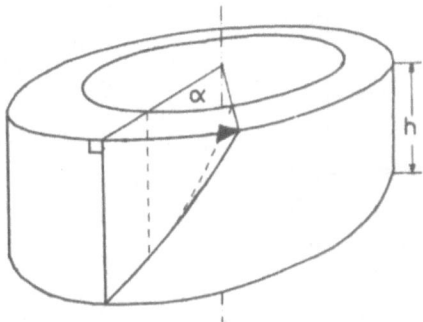

*Figure 3.* Definition of the height *h* and torsion angle α of the cylinder. The arrow denotes the rotation of the upper surface over an angle α due to the deformation of the cylinder.

literature such as end-diastolic ratios of left ventricular wall thickness and height to internal radius (12), transmural distribution of fibre orientation (9), sarcomere length (9) and sequence of depolarization (10) and, finally, contractile properties of cardiac muscle (7, 8). To be able to compare the simulation with an animal experiment, the values of several parameters, such as heart weight, aortic input impedance, end-diastolic left ventricular pressure, and heart rate, were obtained from the findings in that particular experiment.

A simulation of a normal cardiac cycle is shown graphically in Figure 4. The time course of left ventricular and aortic pressure and aortic volume flow agree fairly well with results obtained from animal experiments under comparable circumstances (Figure 5). In the simulation the cylinder lengthens 2.3% and the inner radius shortens 1.1% during the isovolumic contraction phase. During ejection, height and radius decrease 6.3% and 23%, respectively (Figure 4).

At the beginning of the isovolumic contraction phase, the torsion angle decreases. Just before opening of the aortic valve, the torsion angle reaches a minimum and subsequently increases approximately linearly during ejection. The angle reaches a maximum during the relaxation phase whereupon it decreases rather rapidly until the diastolic level is reached. It is remarkable that no discontinuities in the time course of the torsion angle are present when the aortic valve opens or closes.

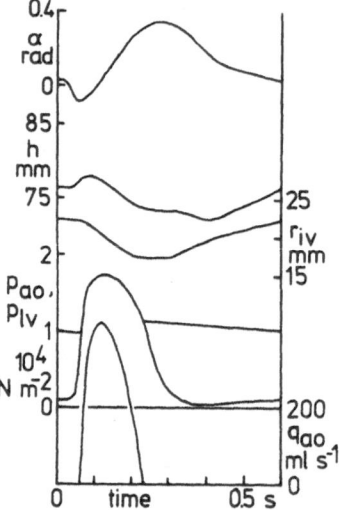
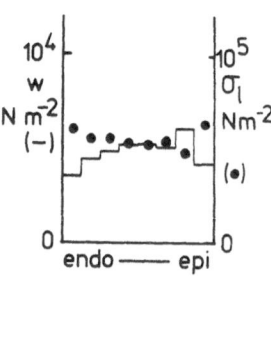

*Figure 4.* Results of a simulation of a normal cardiac cycle: $p_{ao}$ = aortic pressure; $p_{lv}$ = left ventricular pressure; $q_{ao}$ = aortic volume flow; $h$ = height of the cylinder; $r_{iv}$ = inner radius of the cylinder; $\alpha$ = torsion angle of the cylinder; $\sigma_1$ = tensile muscle stress ($t$ = 120 msec); $w$ = generated mechanical energy per unit of volume per beat.

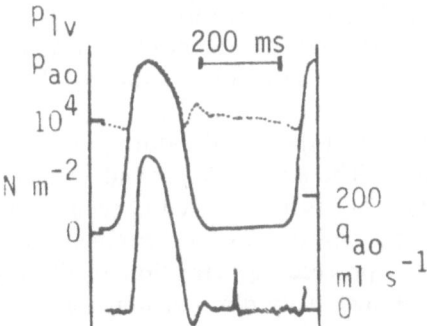

*Figure 5.* Experimental results of a normal cardiac cycle (dog 25 kg).

Quantitative data concerning the time course of base to apex distance and radius are available from animal experiments of Rankin et al. (Figure 6). In their experiments the increase of the base-to-apex distance during the isovolumic contraction phase was 2.1%. During ejection this distance and the inner radius decreased 6.2% and 22%, respectively. These findings are in excellent agreement with the results obtained from the model, in which the height and inner radius of the cylinder, respectively, represent the base-to-apex distance and the inner radius of the left ventricle. The behaviour of the torsion angle in the model cannot be evaluated since to our knowledge no information is available about the torsion angle in animal experiments.

From the model several physical mechanisms can be understood. Since

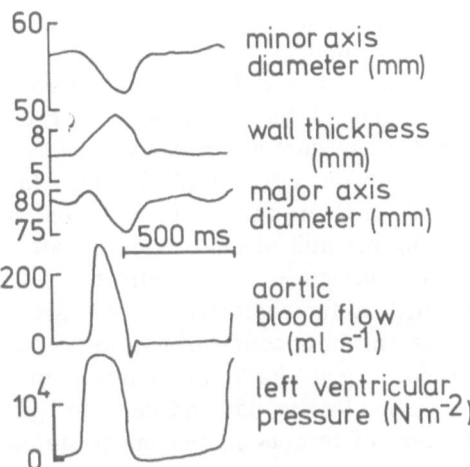

*Figure 6.* Time course of dimensions of the heart, aortic volume flow and left ventricular pressure in a normal cardiac cycle, as measured by Rankin et al. (13).

the results of the model agree fairly well with several findings in animal experiments, some of the underlying mechanisms of the model may be extrapolated to the in vivo situation. Examples of such mechanisms are described below.

Changes in dimensions of the cylinder during isovolumic contraction can be explained as follows. The innermost subendocardial layers are activated first. The fibres in these layers are directed in such a way that the influences of axial and tangential stresses on the geometry are approximately in equilibrium. However, proceeding activation of the myocardium involves contraction of more tangentially directed fibres, resulting in a decrease of inner radius and concomitant lengthening of the cylinder during the isovolumic contraction phase.

Because of the spiral course of the subendocardial muscle fibres around the ventricular cavity, early shortening of the subendocardial sarcomeres in the model causes twisting of the ventricle around its axis early in the isovolumic contraction phase. This is shown by a decrease of the torsion angle. Due to a reverse spiral course of the subepicardial muscle fibres, those fibres are stretched by this twisting. Later in the isovolumic contraction phase contraction of the subepicardial layers has developed to such an extent that the stresses generated by these layers are large enough to prevent further twisting. Then the torsion angle reaches a minimum. Without torsion, subendocardial sarcomere shortening during ejection would be much larger than subepicardial sarcomere shortening because of the thick-walled behaviour of the cylinder. An increase of the torsion angle without ejection lengthens subendocardial sarcomeres and shortens subepicardial sarcomeres. In the model, the torsion angle appears to increase during ejection in such a way that both effects cancel and transmural differences in velocity of sarcomere shortening are small.

In the simulation transmural differences in tensile stress as well as sarcomere length are small at the beginning of the ejection phase. The differences in tensile stress (Figure 4) and velocity of sarcomere shortening remain small throughout the ejection phase. Therefore, at the end of ejection transmural differences in sarcomere length and generated mechanical energy of shortening per unit of muscle volume are small too.

The small differences in tensile muscle stress across the wall during systole can be explained by the character of the transmural course of the fibre orientation. The transmural course of tensile muscle stress is mainly a result of equilibria of forces and torques in the upper surface of the cylinder. Layers with a fibre angle close to 45° and close to −45° counterbalance through the equilibrium of torques in the upper surface of the cylinder. Layers with mainly axially and tangentially directed fibres counterbalance through the equilibrium of axial forces in the upper surface of the cylinder. Extrapolated to the real ventricle this means that the layers between the center and subepicardium counterbalance with the subendocardial layers through the equilibrium of torques, whereas the center layers counterbalance the subepicardial layers through the equilibrium of axial forces. The transmural course of the fibre orientation determines the thickness of the layers, which are involved in these equilibria, and thus determines the transmural distribution of tensile muscle stress. Since the transmural course of the fibre angle changes to a minor degree during the cardiac cycle, tensile stress remains uniformly distributed during the whole systolic period.

SUMMARY

In a mathematical model of the dynamics of the left ventricle, the ventricle is simulated by a thick-walled cylinder composed of eight concentric subcylinders. The orientation and the sequential activation of the muscle fibres across the ventricular wall are considered per subcylinder. The relation between tensile muscle stress, sarcomere length, velocity of sarcomere shortening, and time are derived from experimental data.

In the model, contraction starts in the subendocardial layers. Because of the spiral course of the subendocardial fibres around the left ventricular cavity, torsion of the left ventricle around its axis and stretching of the subepicardial muscle fibres occur during the isovolumic phase of contraction.

Transmural differences in quantities which are closely related to the state of mechanical loading of myocardial material, such as tensile stress, sarcomere length, velocity of sarcomere shortening and generated mechanical energy per unit of volume are small. Hence, the heart seems to be optimally designed, as far as the process of contraction is concerned.

The validity of the model is demonstrated by the good agreement between the model and animal experiments as far as left ventricular pressure, aortic pressure and volume flow and left ventricular dimensions are concerned. A general conclusion is, that the present model is a useful tool in understanding the dynamic behaviour of the mechanics of the left ventricle.

ACKNOWLEDGEMENTS

This work was supported by a grant from the Foundation for Medical Research FUNGO.

REFERENCES

1. Feigl EO, Simon GA, Fry DL: Auxotonic and isometric cardiac force transducers. J Appl Physiol 23:597–600, 1967.
2. Huismans RM: Forces in the wall of the left ventricle. Thesis, Free University of Amsterdam, The Netherlands, 1977.
3. Arts MGJ: A mathematical model of the dynamics of the left ventricle and the coronary circulation. Thesis, University of Limburg, Maastricht, The Netherlands, 1978.

4. Woods RH: A few applications of a physical theorem to membranes in the human body in a state of tension. J Anat Physiol 26:362–370, 1892.
5. Back L: Left ventricular wall and fluid dynamics of cardiac contraction. *Math Biosc* 36:257–297, 1977.
6. Arts T, Reneman RS: Analysis of intramyocardial pressure (IMP): a model study: 9th European Conference on Microcirculation, Antwerp, 1976. *Bibl Anat* 15:103–107, 1977.
7. Brutsaert DL, Sonnenblick EH: Nature of the force-velocity relation in heart muscle. *Cardiovasc Res* 1:18–33, 1971.
8. Pollack GH, Krueger JW: Sarcomere dynamics in intact cardiac muscle. *Eur J Cardiol* 4:53–65, 1976.
9. Streeter Jr DD, Hanna WT: Engineering mechanics for successive states in canine left ventricular myocardium: II: fiberangle and sarcomere length. *Circ Res* 33:656–664, 1973.
10. Durrer D, Dam RT van, Freud GE, Janse MJ, Meyler FL, Arzbaecher RC: Total excitation of the isolated human heart. *Circulation* 1:899–912, 1970.
11. Westerhof N, Enzinga G, Bos GC van den: Influence of central and peripheral changes on the hydraulic input impedance of the systemic arterial tree. *Med Biol Eng* 710–722, 1973.
12. Streeter Jr DD, Hanna WT: Engineering mechanics for successive states in canine left ventricular myocardium: I. cavity and wall geometry. *Circ Res* 33:639–655, 1973.
13. Rankin JS, McHale P, Arentzen CE, Ling D, Greenfield JC, Anderson RW: The three-dimensional dynamic geometry of the left ventricle in the conscious dog. *Circ Res* 39:304–313, 976.

## 2.5. THE ROLE OF WALL THICKNESS IN THE RELATION BETWEEN SARCOMERE DYNAMICS AND VENTRICULAR DYNAMICS

WILLIAM C. HUNTER, JAN BAAN

### 1. INTRODUCTION

In his article Rankin (this volume) noted that William Harvey was one of the first to stress that the "heart becomes thicker in its walls" during a contraction. Measurements in conscious dogs and man (1, 2) indicate that wall thickness near the equator normally increases 10–50% during systole. Despite this considerable change, we aim to argue in this chapter that the thickening of the wall during systole is not a significant phenomenon for relating the average behaviour of sarcomeres in the wall to the dynamics of the whole left ventricle.

Other contributors to this book have presented detailed studies which explicitly included differences in fibre dynamics at different locations in the ventricular wall. Our approach, on the other hand, has sought to study an average behaviour representative of all the fibres in the wall. For this reason we have selected the equatorial region as most representative and assumed rotational symmetry to eliminate variations around the equator. Finally, we have averaged together differences across the wall from endocardium to epicardium.

In previous work (3) we have been studying the fibre to ventricle transformation with a thin-walled model. The natural question arose: What does wall thickness contribute? At first we focused on one half of the fibre-ventricle transformation, namely, relating the average force borne by the fibres to ventricular pressure, volume, shape, and wall thickness. Later we studied how the average sarcomere length varied with changes in ventricular geometry. Some preliminary results were reported earlier (4).

### 2. AVERAGE FORCE

The problem that first confronts any study of force in the ventricular wall is how best to define this force. Viewing the myocardium as a continuum, many have calculated wall stress, that is, force per instantaneous area. Stress does not seem appropriate, however, when considering that the myocardium is composed of discrete fibres rather than being a continuum. A fibre's force-generating capacity depends on the number of sarcomeres

J. Baan, A.C. Arntzenius, E.L. Yellin (eds.), Cardiac Dynamics, 123–134.

acting in parallel and not their area. During contraction, cross-sectional area increases, and it could be misleading to include this area change in "stress" calculations when the number of sarcomeres remains constant. This intuitive reasoning suggests that systolic changes of ventricular wall thickness should be ignored in calculating the force per fibre in the wall.

To relate pressure to wall dynamics it is therefore necessary to use the total force generated by a segment of the wall rather than stress. Total force is simply the sum of the parallel components of force exerted by fibres from all layers of the myocardium. At the equator total force is resolved into two components: one acting circumferentially around the equator, the other acting longitudinally in the direction of the axis. If the segment contains a constant number of fibres, then the total force generated by the segment is proportional to the average force per fibre. Thus, to express the average force we chose to calculate the force per angular sector. We define an angular sector so that it subtends a constant wall volume, which in turn contains a constant number of fibres.

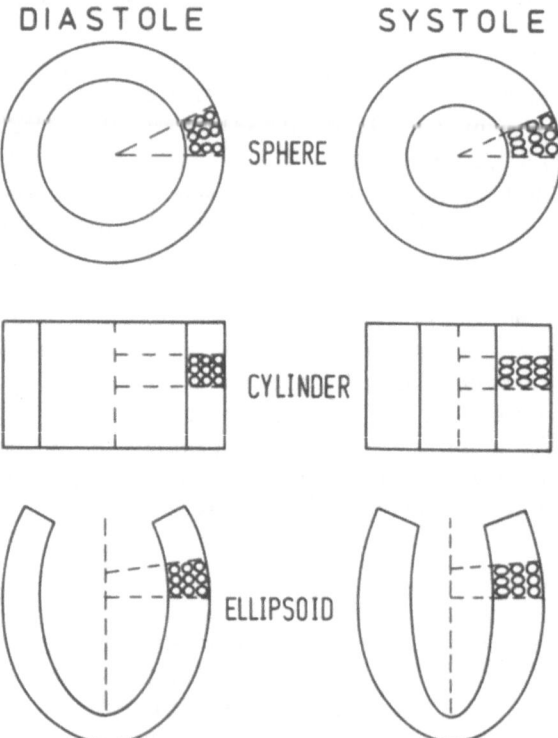

*Figure 1.* Angular sectors from differently shaped ventricles. Despite ejection and wall thickening, the volume of each sector and the number of fibres within a sector remain constant. Small circles or ovals represent fibre cross-sections, whose area increases at shorter fibre lengths.

Figure 1 illustrates angular sectors taken near the equator for ventricles of different shapes. As the cavity shrinks from diastole to systole, the wall thickens; but the wall volume contained within the angular sectors indicated remains constant. Consequently, the number of fibres will also be constant provided the orientation of the fibres does not change significantly, a reasonable assumption (5).

To define more precisely the angular sectors in a symmetric ellipsoid of revolution, consider Figure 2 (top). In the equatorial plane the polar angle

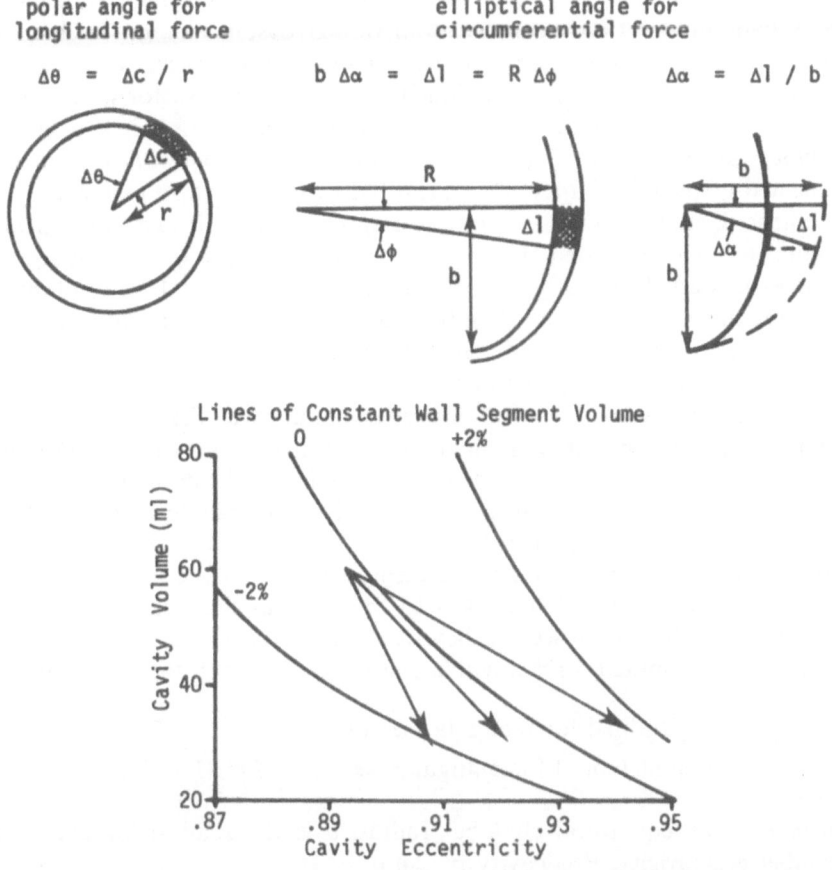

*Figure 2. Top:* definition of an angular sector near the equator of a symmetrical ellipsoidal ventricle. Left is the equatorial plane with circular cross-section; right is a meridional plane with elliptical cross-section. Stippled area indicates the wall sectors intersected by angles $\Delta\theta$ and $\Delta\alpha$. *Bottom:* contour lines showing variations in volume of a small sector of the wall when cavity volume and shape change. From a typical end-diastolic volume and shape, the cavity contracts to a smaller volume and more elliptical shape with increased eccentricity (arrows indicate possible end-systolic points), but wall-segment volume remains practically constant ($\pm$ 2%).

($\Delta\theta$) follows the standard definition, which selects a constant fraction of the equatorial circumference at the inside of the wall. In the longitudinal plane a definition is more difficult because the radius of curvature ($R$) varies greatly with shape changes. Instead of the conventional angle ($\Delta\phi$) we elected to define an "elliptical angle" ($\Delta\alpha$), which selects a portion ($\Delta l$) of the elliptical circumference which is a constant fraction of the elliptical semi-major axis ($b$). For angles near the equator, this definition is equivalent to the angle of longitude used in an elliptical coordinate system (Figure 2, right panel), as suggested by Streeter and Hanna (6).

It is required that the polar and elliptical angles produce an angular sector containing a nearly constant wall volume despite changes in chamber volume or shape. For either spherical or cylindrical shapes with uniform wall thickness, the definitions obviously lead to constant sector wall volume because a constant fraction of the total circumference and height is always included in the sector. We also computed the sector wall volume for truncated ellipsoidal shapes. The epicardial surface was also assumed to be an ellipsoid, confocal with the endocardial (chamber) ellipsoid. Streeter and Hanna (6) have suggested this as a first approximation for describing the changes in wall thickness from base to apex. Because total wall volume is constant during changes in chamber volume and in eccentricity, the wall volume contained within the angular sector could be calculated (see Appendix). The bottom panel of Figure 2 shows that the change in sector wall volume is within 2% of its average volume over the whole range of chamber volumes and shapes encountered normally in a canine ventricle.

Now that an angular sector has been defined with the desired property of constant wall volume, the forces borne by this sector can be examined. Wall forces in both the longitudinal (base-apex) direction and circumferential direction combine to balance the pressure exerted on the inner surface of the sector. This force balance leads to the same equilibrium equations as Falsetti et al. (7) used; however, they went on to compute stress (force/area) whereas we computed force/angular sector. As shown in the appendix:

$$\text{longitudinal force/angular sector} = \tfrac{1}{2}\, Pr^2$$
$$\text{circumferential force/angular sector} = \tfrac{1}{2}\, Pr^2\, (1 + e^2)\, b/r$$

where $r$ is the equatorial chamber radius; $b$ is the semi-major axis; $e$ is chamber eccentricity; $P$ is cavity pressure.

The most pertinent conclusion from these force equations is the fact that wall thickness does not enter as a factor. This confirms the intuitive argument presented earlier. Note that if we had computed stress, as Falsetti et al. (7) did, wall thickness would have remained; however, when multiplying stress by the area of the angular sector to compute force/sector, thickness factors in area cancel those in stress (see Appendix). Falsetti et al.

also attempted to compute force per fibre ("fibre-corrected stress"), but their correction did not completely cancel wall thickness because of an erroneous assumption about area changes (see Appendix).

## 3. AVERAGE SARCOMERE LENGTH

The second component of the transformation between fibre and ventricle relates the average fibre length to the volume and shape of the ventricle. We will focus here on lengths in the circumferential direction averaged across the wall. Sarcomere lengths are likely to vary across the wall even at end-diastole; more importantly, during ejection the circumferential shortening of inner fibres is proportionally greater than that of outer ones because of the thick wall. Thus, we were again faced with the question of how to define an average value. To guarantee that the force-sarcomere length relations would be identical for both the individual fibres and the average behaviour across the wall, we defined the average sarcomere length as the length at which a fibre would exert the average force.

Figure 3 illustrates the process of computing an average sarcomere length in our model study. First, the distribution of sarcomere lengths across the wall was calculated for each particular chamber diameter (assuming an initial wall thickness and an initial distribution of lengths in a typical end-diastolic state). For a particular form of the force-length relation, the force contributed by each fibre was summed and the average force calculated. Then, using the same force-length relation as used for the individual fibres, the average sarcomere length was found. More important than the average length itself, however, was the layer in the wall where the fibre having the average length was located. This layer was defined so that length changes in it were proportional to the length changes of the average sarcomere.

The results of this study of average sarcomere length are summarized in Figure 4. The average length was found to be located at a layer in the wall that surrounded an almost constant fraction (35–40%) of wall volume over the entire normal range of chamber diameters. This finding held not only for simple models – left panel: cylinder or sphere with linear force-length function and homogeneous wall – but it also held when complicating factors present in the real ventricle were introduced – right panel: two hypothetical nonlinear force-length functions, realistic variations in fibre angles across the wall (5), and realistic non-uniform initial sarcomere lengths (8). This conclusion could obviously be challenged during the spread of activation across the wall; however, this should not be a severe restriction because activation is normally completed before ejection begins.

That the average length should lie near the centre of the wall is intuitively clear. For assessing the influence of changes in wall thickness, however, the

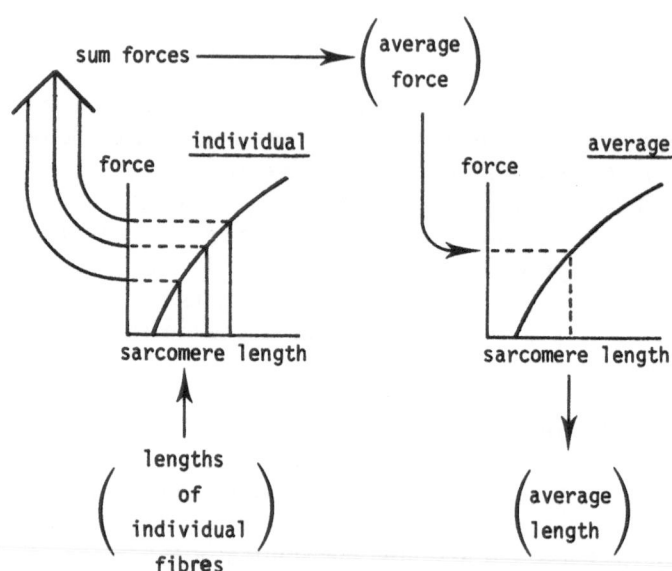

*Figure 3.* The process of computing the average sarcomere length from a distribution of sarcomere lengths across the wall.

observation that a nearly constant volume of the wall is included within the layer where the average length is located has a significant consequence: wall thickening during systole proves to be an insignificant factor in locating the average length. We have only to add to the cavity volume a constant quantity representing the wall volume within the "average-length" layer; systolic variations in wall thickness have once again dropped out of the picture.

A simple model based on these results concerning average force and average length is shown in Figure 5. The average length-layer surrounds 40% of the total wall volume (assumed 90 ml), so that the average sarcomere length is calculated from a cylinder containing 36 ml more than the cavity volume. This leads to a realistic range of cavity volumes for a canine left ventricle (10–70 ml) corresponding to the physiological range of sarcomere lengths (1.7 to 2.3 $\mu$). In contrast, if a thin-walled model had been chosen, the same range of sarcomere lengths would span only one third of the volume range (15–35 ml). It is here that the difference between thick-walled and thin-walled models is most pronounced.

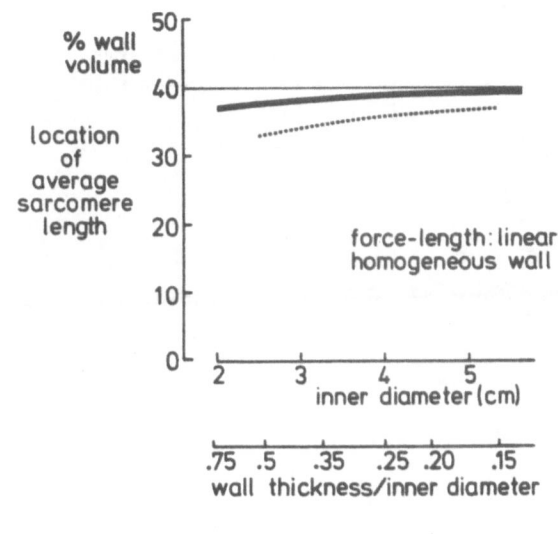

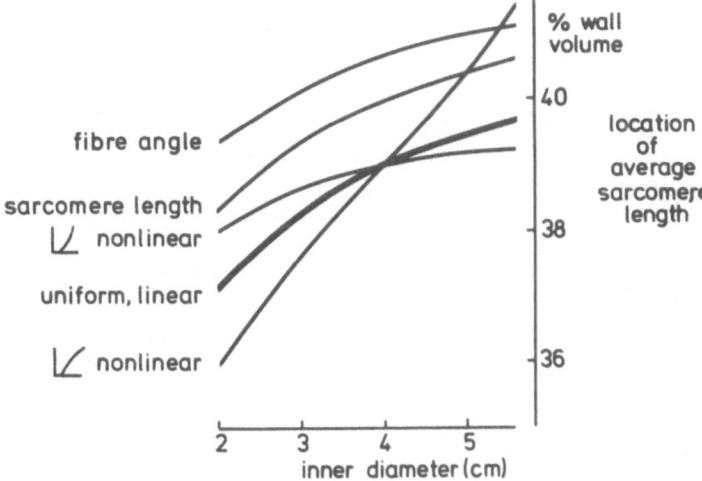

*Figure 4. Left:* location of the average circumferential sarcomere length, expressed as the fraction of wall volume lying within the layer containing the average length, plotted as a function of cavity diameter. Thick line: – cylindrical model; dotted line: – spherical model. Both had linear force-length functions and no variations across the wall in end-diastolic length or fibre angle. *Right:* same relationship (on an expanded vertical scale) for cylindrical models containing complicating phenomena: variations of fibre angles across the wall, non-uniform end-diastolic sarcomere lengths, nonlinear force-length functions.

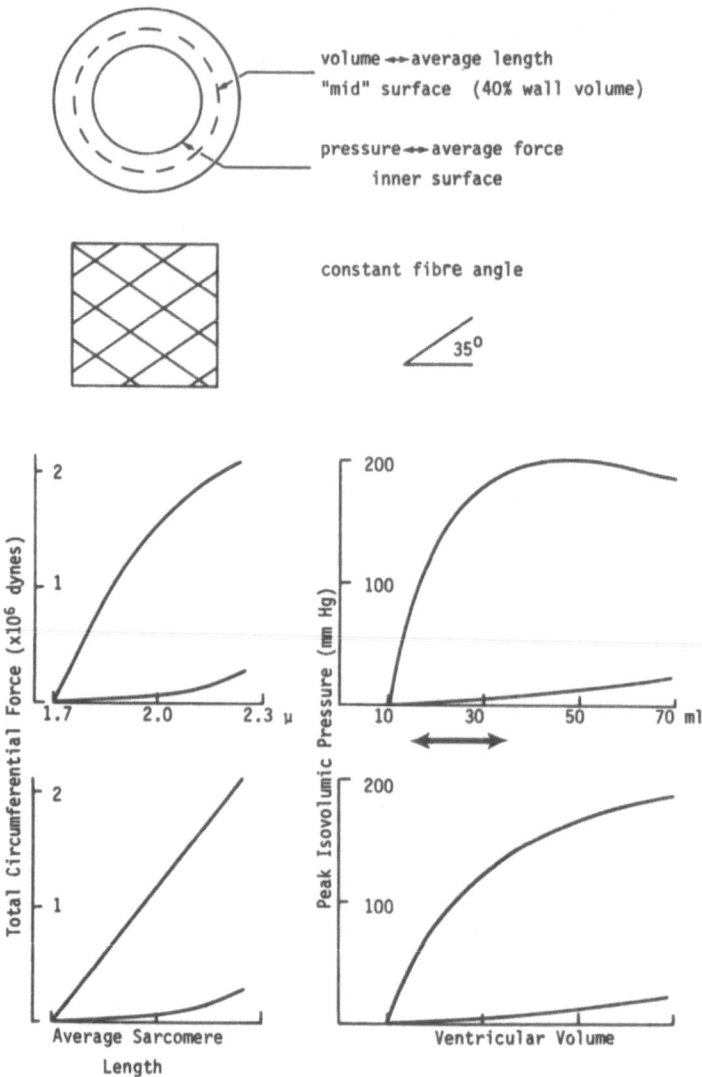

*Figure 5.* Using a cylindrical model (above), two sets of hypothetical force-length relations (nonlinear: top, linear: bottom) were transformed into ventricular pressure-volume relations (below). Both systolic and diastolic relations are shown. The shape of the cylindrical fibre layer near mid-wall (40% wall volume) was assumed to be constant, so the fibre angle was constant at 35°. Total wall force balanced the pressure on the inner wall surface. If a thin-walled model had been used, the severely limited range of chamber volumes for the same range of sarcomere lengths is indicated by the heavy arrow (right).

A second phenomenon to note in Figure 5 is the curvature in the plots of peak isovolumic pressure versus volume. These model calculations were based on patterns of peak force as a function of sarcomere length following recent measurements by ter Keurs et al. (this volume). The corresponding pressures show a tendency to plateau at higher volumes, even when force shows no tendency to plateau. Similar curvature in the pressure-volume relationship has also been measured recently in our laboratory (Kerkhof et al., this volume).

## 4. CONCLUSION

These studies on uniformly contracting model ventricles suggest that systolic wall thickening has no effect on either (1) the average force borne by the sarcomeres, or (2) the average length of the sarcomeres. The wall thickening appears to be only a corollary of sarcomere shortening with constant fibre volume. This does not imply that wall thickness plays no role. On the contrary, a thin-walled model cannot span the normal range of cavity volumes with a physiological variation of sarcomere lengths. Thus, the thick wall cannot be omitted from the relation between sarcomere length and ventricular geometry.

Measurements of wall thickness also contain other important information. Chronic changes in thickness follow chronic changes in the number of fibres (hypertrophy), so one measurement of thickness during a standard, reproducible physiological state could serve to estimate the number of fibres. Furthermore, non-uniform changes in thickness could act as quantitative markers of poorly contracting regions (9, 10).

## 5. APPENDIX

### 5.1. *Volume of wall sector*

Examining the stippled wall sector in Figure 2:

$$\Delta \text{ volume} = \int_0^h (R+x)\Delta\phi \ (r+x)\Delta\theta \ dx$$

where $x$ represents the distance from the inner wall to various shells within the wall, and $dx$ gives the thickness of each shell. The remaining factors give the area of each shell. $R$, $r$, $\Delta\theta$, and $\Delta\phi$ are constant for all layers in the wall. Straightforward integration yields:

$$\Delta \text{ volume} = \Delta\theta \ \Delta\phi \ \{Rrh + (R+r)h^2/2 + h^3/3\}.$$

Using $\Delta\phi = \Delta\alpha \ (b/R)$, the volume expression was rewritten:

$$\Delta \text{ volume} = \Delta\theta \ \Delta\alpha \ \{brh + (1+r/R)bh^2/2 + (b/R)h^3/3].$$

A sector is defined by constant values for $\Delta\theta$ and $\Delta\alpha$. Thus, the expression within brackets was computed to examine the constancy of sector wall volume with changes in chamber size and shape.

### 5.2. Computation of forces per angular sector

Across a plane cut through the ellipsoidal model ventricle at the equator, the longitudinal force exerted by the fibres must balance the force from cavity pressure:

$$\text{total longitudinal force} = P\pi r^2$$

Because the total polar angle is $2\pi$, there results:

$$\text{longitudinal force/polar angle} = T_{\text{long}} = \tfrac{1}{2} \ P \ r^2$$

The circumferential force is computed by balancing forces on the small angular sector of the wall (Figure 2). The radially directed force of cavity pressure ($P \cdot$ inner wall area) is balanced by the radial components of the forces acting in the circumferential ($\Delta F_{\text{circ}}$) and longitudinal ($\Delta F_{\text{long}}$) directions on the faces of the wall sector:

$$P(r \ \Delta\theta)(R \ \Delta\phi) = \Delta F_{\text{long}} \sin \Delta\phi + \Delta F_{\text{circ}} \sin \Delta\theta$$

The radii of curvature ($r$, $R$) and angles ($\Delta\theta$, $\Delta\phi$) are shown in Figure 2. The forces per angular sector are defined by:

$$\text{longitudinal force/polar angle} = T_{\text{long}} = \Delta F_{\text{long}}/\Delta\theta$$
$$\text{circumferential force/elliptical angle} = T_{\text{circ}} = \Delta F_{\text{circ}}/\Delta\alpha$$

where the elliptical angle ($\Delta\alpha$) is given by (Figure 2):

$$\Delta\alpha = (R/b) \ \Delta\phi$$

For small angles the sine equals the angle itself, so that the force balance can be rewritten:

$$PrR\Delta\theta \ \Delta\phi = T_{\text{long}} \ \Delta\theta \ \Delta\phi + T_{\text{circ}}(R/b) \ \Delta\theta \ \Delta\phi$$

Cancelling the angles and solving for $T_{\text{circ}}$:

$$T_{\text{circ}} = Prb - (b/R) \ T_{\text{long}}$$

Substituting the expression computed above for $T_{\text{long}}$ and rewriting:

$$T_{\text{circ}} = \tfrac{1}{2}Prb(2 - r/R)$$

The expression $(2-r/R)$ can be related to the eccentricity $(e)$ of the chamber:

$$T_{circ} = \tfrac{1}{2} Pr^2(1+e^2) \quad (b/r)$$

Falsetti et al. (7) derived stresses from the same force balance. Their equations can be rewritten in the following form:

$$\frac{\text{mean circumferential stress}}{\text{mean longitudinal stress}} = \frac{(1+e^2)(1+h/d)}{1+(h/d)(1-e^2)}$$

where $h$ is equatorial wall thickness and $d$ is chamber diameter $(d=2r)$. To compare this expression with the forces/angle computed above, we examined the ratio of cross-sectional areas intersected by the wall sector:

$$\frac{\text{area of circumferential fibres}}{\text{area of longitudinal fibres}} = \frac{\Delta l_{mid}\ h}{\Delta c_{mid}\ h}$$

where $\Delta l_{mid}$ and $\Delta c_{mid}$ are the mid-wall lengths corresponding to $\Delta l$ and $\Delta c$ in Figure 2. Applying the same definition of angles to the mid-wall and taking the case that circumferential and longitudinal angles are equal:

$$\frac{\Delta l_{mid}}{\Delta c_{mid}} = \frac{\Delta\alpha\ b_{mid}}{\Delta\theta\ r_{mid}} = \frac{b_{mid}/b}{r_{mid}/r} \quad (b/r)$$

where $b_{mid}$ and $r_{mid}$ are the semi-major axes of the mid-wall ellipsoid. The ratios of mid-wall to inner-wall axes can be expressed in terms of wall thickness and chamber shape. The derivation is straightforward for $r_{mid}/r$, and an expression accurate within 2% can also be derived for $b_{mid}/b$. Thus:

$$\frac{\text{area of circumferential fibres}}{\text{area of longitudinal fibres}} = \frac{1+(h/d)(1-e^2)}{1+(h/d)} \quad (b/r)$$

When this expression for area ratio is multiplied by the expression for stress ratio derived from Falsetti et al. (7) the result is the ratio of circumferential to longitudinal forces per angular sector. All terms containing wall thickness $(h)$ cancel. Falsetti et al. incorrectly assumed the area ratio to be constant in their attempt to compute forces per fibre.

SUMMARY

The relation between left ventricular pressure, volume and shape on the one hand, and myocardial fibre force and length on the other hand, was investigated especially regarding the role played by wall thickness. Using a new definition of average force borne by the muscle fibres and defining an average sarcomere length of a fibre exerting this force, it was found that the instantaneous changes in wall thickness occurring during the cardiac cycle are not significant in the transformation between ventricular and fibre dynamics. Various complications such as nonlinear force-length relations, variation of fibre angle and sarcomere length across the wall were taken into account.

An important implication of these findings is that realistic sarcomere length variations result in a wide volume range over which the ventricle is able to operate, both during diastole and systole. It is concluded that the proposed analysis may give a better approximation of the actual situation than ventricular models used before.

ACKNOWLEDGEMENTS

This study was supported by grant 76.063 from the Netherlands Heart Foundation.

REFERENCES

1. Rankin JS, McHale PA, Arentzen CE, Ling D, Greenfield JC, Anderson RW: The three-dimensional dynamic geometry of the left ventricle in the conscious dog. Circ Res 39:304–313, 1976.
2. Hugenholtz PG, Kaplan E, Hull E: Determination of left ventricular wall thickness by angiocardiography. Am Heart J 78:513–522, 1969.
3. Baan J: Model of the left ventricle based on an electromagnetic contractile analog of cardiac muscle. In: Cardiovascular System Dynamics, Baan J, Noordergraaf A, Raines J (eds), Cambridge, Mass, MIT Press, 1978, p 85–98.
4. Bann J, Hunter WC: Basic implications of a model of ventricular dynamics. Fed Proc 37:823, 1978.
5. Streeter Jr DD, Spotnitz HM, Patel DP, Ross Jr J, Sonnenblick EH: Fiber orientation in the canine left ventricle during diastole and systole. Circ Res 24:339–347, 1969.
6. Streeter Jr DD, Hanna, WT: Engineering mechanics for successive states in canine left ventricular myocardium: I: cavity and wall geometry. Circ Res 33:639–655, 1973.
7. Falsetti HL, Mates RE, Grant C, Greene DG, Bunnell IL: Left ventricular wall stress calculated from one-plane cineangiography. Circ Res 26, 71–83, 1970.
8. Yoran C, Covell JW, Ross Jr J: Structural basis for the ascending limb of left ventricular function. Circ Res 32:297–307, 1973.
9. Sasayama S, Franklin D, Ross Jr J, Kemper WS, McKown D: Dynamic changes in left ventricular wall thickness and their use in analyzing cardiac function in the conscious dog. Am J Cardiol 38:870–879, 1976.
10. Ross Jr J, Franklin D: Analysis of regional myocardial function, dimensions, and wall thickness in the characterization of myocardial ischemia and infarction. Circulation 53, 54 (suppl): I88–I92, 1976.

# 2.6. A MODEL FOR LEFT VENTRICULAR CONTRACTIONS BASED ON THE SLIDING FILAMENT THEORY

J.H.J.M. van den Broek, J.J. Denier van der Gon

## 1. INTRODUCTION

In the literature a number of studies are devoted to the simulation of ventricular stresses and pressure in thick-walled ellipsoidal models, the wall of which contains muscle fibres (1, 2). Streeter et al. (1) used force-length data from papillary muscle to calculate static fibre stress. Wong (2) used a muscle model based on Huxley's theory (3) to simulate pressure development during isovolumic contractions. In this study a model is presented which is applicable to isovolumic contractions as well as non-isovolumic contractions. The aim is to test some current theories concerning physiological and pathophysiological processes of cardiac contraction and to investigate which parameters may be estimated with reasonable accuracy from measurable quantities such as ventricular pressure and flow.

## 2. MUSCLE MODEL

The muscle model consists of a contractile element based on Huxley's sliding filament theory (3) and a series elastic element (SEE) which may also account for effects of distortion of the ventricle, inflexion of the valves, and so on. Parallel elasticity, describing the elastic behaviour of the non-activated muscle is not considered here.

Force generation by the sarcomeres in response to activation is thought to result from chemical interactions i.e. the so-called crossbridges. Crossbridge density $n$ (number of bridges per unit of bridge length) may change according to:

$$\frac{\partial n}{\partial t} + v \frac{\partial n}{\partial x} = f(N - n) - gn \qquad [1]$$

where $t$ is time, $x$ crossbridge length, $f$ and $g$ are rate functions, $v$ is sarcomere shortening velocity given by $v = dx/dt$ and $N$ is the density of myosin heads which may form crossbridges. It is supposed that:

- $N$ is a function of sarcomere length or preload, similar to the force-length relation as measured by Pollack and Krueger (4).

J. Baan, A.C. Arntzenius, E.L. Yellin (eds.), Cardiac Dynamics, 135–142.

- $g = g_1$, $x \geq 0$ and $g = 10\ g_1$, $x < 0$
- $f = 0$, $x < 0$ and $x > 10$ nm
- $f$ is time-dependent in a way suggested by Wong (2):

$$f(t) = A(e^{-b_1 t^2} - e^{-b_2 t^2}) \qquad [2]$$

where $A$, $b_1$ and $b_2$ are parameters.
- The activation function $f$ is influenced by sarcomere lengths (5), such that in particular the descending limb of $f$ is changed. This can be achieved by making $b_1$ sarcomere length-dependent and varying $A$ and $b_2$ so that, independently of $b_1$, the maximum value of $f$ and the time at which this value is reached remain constant; $b_1$ is (in first approximation) supposed to be linearly related to ventricular volume:

$$b_1 = b_0 \left( 1 - \frac{V_p - V_0}{V_0} b_p - \frac{V - V_p}{V_0} b_e \right) \qquad [3]$$

where $b_0$, $b_p$ and $b_e$ are parameters, $V_0$ is the volume at a preload of 0 mmHg, $V_p$ is the volume at a higher preload and $V = V(t)$ is the volume during ejection.
- The cross-bridges behave as linear elastic bonds with stiffness $Z$, so that the developed force equals:

$$F_s = \int_{-\infty}^{+\infty} nZx\ dx \qquad [4]$$

- The force-length relation of the SEE is given by:

$$F_e = F_0(e^{\alpha l_e / l_0} - 1) \qquad [5]$$

where $l_e$ is SEE extension, $l_0$ muscle length at zero preload, $F_0$ a constant and $\alpha$ a kind of stiffness. Equations [1] to [5] were solved numerically.

## 3. VENTRICULAR MODEL

The ventricle is approximated by a nested set of truncated ellipsoidal shells of revolution. This geometry is completely determined by two inner axes $E_i(1)$, $E_i(3)$, two outer axes $E_u(1)$, $E_u(3)$ and a factor $k$ (see Figure 1). In the reference situation (preload 0 mmHg), the nondimensional parameters $k$ and $d$, where $d = E_i(1)/E_i(3)$, where chosen from literature data on dog hearts (1). Inner volume $V_0$ and wall volume $V_w$ were determined in our experiments on rabbit hearts. Finally the ventricular parameters could be determined by using the condition that the pressure drop over the equatorial wall equals the pressure drop over the apical wall. At higher preloads and during ejection, $k$, $V_w$ and the ratio between wall thickness at the apex and the equator were kept constant; $d$ is supposed to depend on ventricular

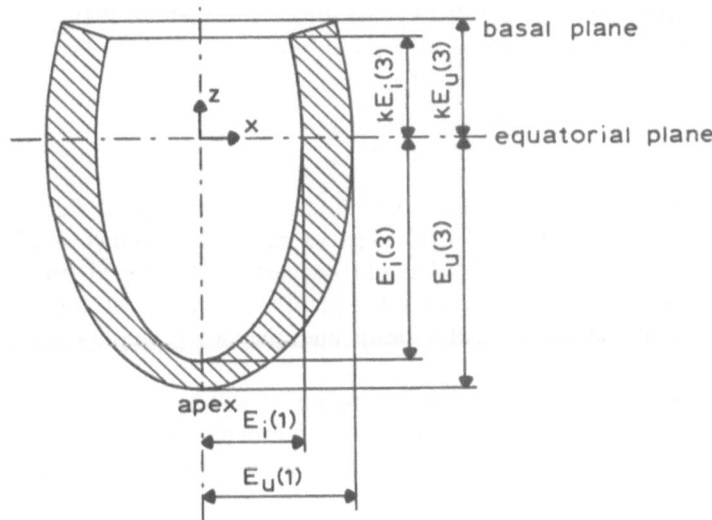

*Figure 1.* Definition of the relevant parameters of the ellipsoidal heart model.

volume. As a first approximation a linear relation is used:

$$d = d_0 \left( 1 + \frac{V_p - V_0}{V_0} d_p + \frac{V - V_p}{V_0} d_e \right) \qquad [6]$$

where $d_0$, $d_p$ and $d_e$ are parameters.

The radius of curvature in a point in the ventricular wall in a plane through the z-axis will be denoted $R$, while the radius of curvature in a plane through the normal to the ellipsoid, perpendicular to the former plane is denoted $r$. Fibre orientation in the wall is defined as the angle $\phi$ which the fibre makes with a line through that point perpendicular to $R$ and parallel to the equatorial plane. In the reference situation we will assume that $\phi$ varies linearly along a normal to the wall from $+ 60°$ (inner wall) to $- 60°$ (outer wall), and that the fibre length $l_m$ (half-sarcomere length) has a value of 0.86 $\mu$m. These values may be seen as approximations of measurements by Streeter et al. (6) and Spotnitz et al. (7). At higher preloads and during ejection new values of $\phi$ and $l_m$ can be calculated from the new geometries.

To calculate the pressure in the ventricle it is assumed that all muscle fibres are activated simultaneously and that shear stresses, influence of wall acceleration (8) and pressure gradients in the ventricle during ejection (8) may be neglected. The pressure at the inner wall is given by:

$$P = \int_{\text{wall}} \tau(u) \left( \frac{\cos^2 \phi(u)}{r(u)} + \frac{\sin^2 \phi(u)}{R(u)} \right) du \qquad [7]$$

where $\tau$ is the tension generated by the muscle fibre and $u$ is the coordinate along a normal to the inner wall.

## 4. METHODS

Experiments were carried out on isolated perfused rabbit hearts. Large sheet stimulation electrodes were used to obtain simultaneous fibre contraction. Preload and afterload could be varied. Developed pressure and flow were sampled on-line and subsequently processed. A ·more detailed description of the experimental setup and the heart preparation is given elsewhere (9).

The results of one representative experiment will be shown. All simulated pressures were calculated in the equatorial plane. Model parameters of isovolumic contractions were estimated by minimizing the sum of the

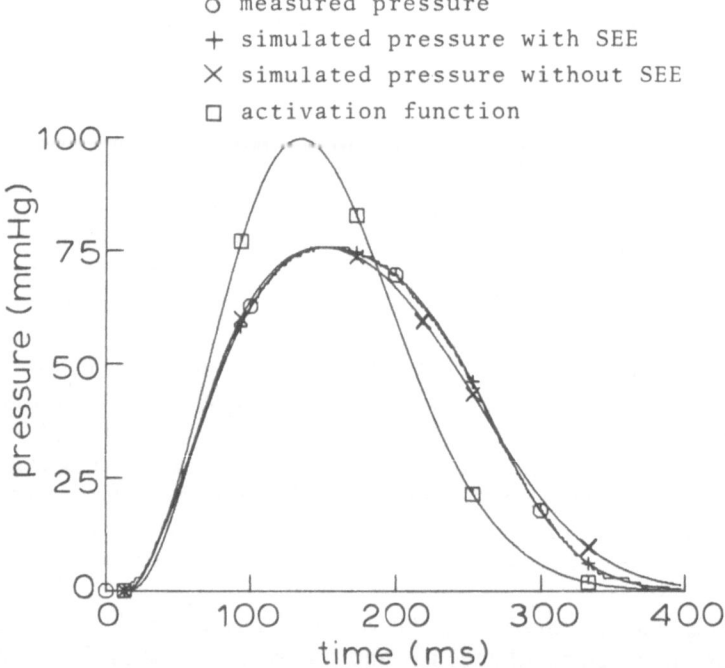

Figure 2. Isovolumic contraction in the reference situation. As a result of the A-D conversion the measured curve is not very smooth. Parameters chosen: $F_0/F_{max} = 1.0$ (where $F_{max}$ is the maximum muscle force), $V_0 = 1$ cm³, $V_w = 5$ cm³, $k = 0.5$, $d = 0.42$, $l_0 = 0.86$ μm. Calculated axes: $E_i(1) = 0.46$ cm, $E_u(1) = 1.10$ cm, $E_i(3) = 1.10$ cm, $E_u(3) = 1.40$ cm. Fitted parameters: $A = 3.44$ ms⁻¹, $b_1 = 0.62 \cdot 10^{-4}$ ms⁻², $b_2 = 0.73 \cdot 10^{-4}$ ms⁻², $g_1 = 0.184$ ms⁻¹, $\alpha = 12.56$.

squares of the deviation between measured and simulated pressure. In the reference situation $A$, $b_1$, $b_2$, $g_1$ and $\alpha[1, 2, 5]$ were fitted, together with an overall multiplicative factor in the pressure, consisting of elements such as $N$ and $Z$.

## 5. RESULTS

Figure 2 shows the result of a model without a SEE and a model with a SEE ($\alpha$ is fitted). In the latter case the (root mean square) deviation ($\Delta P$) is about equal to the experimental error ($\cong 0.5$ mmHg). Variation of $F_0$ has little effect on $\Delta P$.

At higher preloads $V_p$ and $b_p$ [3] were fitted with the use of the parameter set found in the reference situation. Figure 3 shows the results. When a preload-independent activation function was chosen ($b_p = 0$) the results became worse. Variation of $d_p$ [6] has little effect on $\Delta P$. It does, however, influence $V_p$ and $b_p$.

Pressures of non-isovolumic contractions were simulated using the parameters estimated from isovolumic contractions and the measured flow.

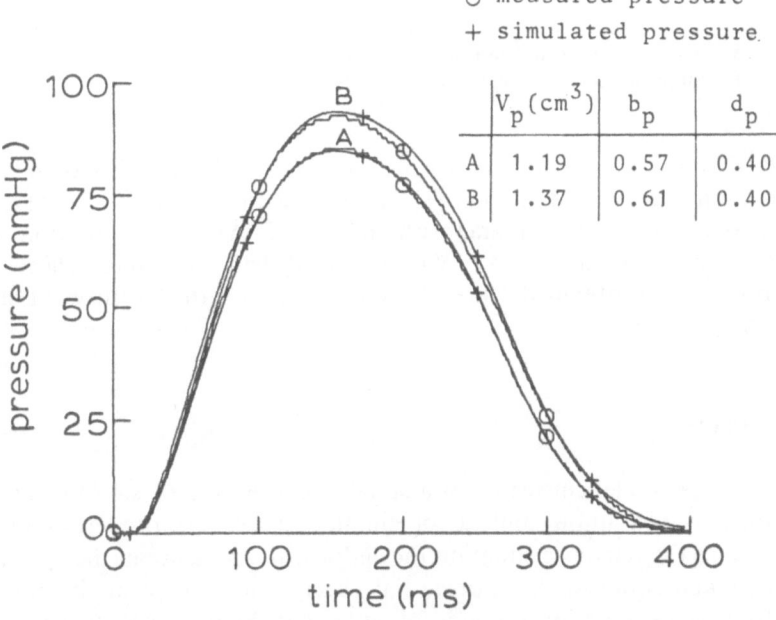

| | $V_p$ (cm$^3$) | $b_p$ | $d_p$ |
|---|---|---|---|
| A | 1.19 | 0.57 | 0.40 |
| B | 1.37 | 0.61 | 0.40 |

o measured pressure
+ simulated pressure

*Figure 3.* Isovolumic contraction at a preload of 1 mmHg (A) and at 2 mmHg (B).

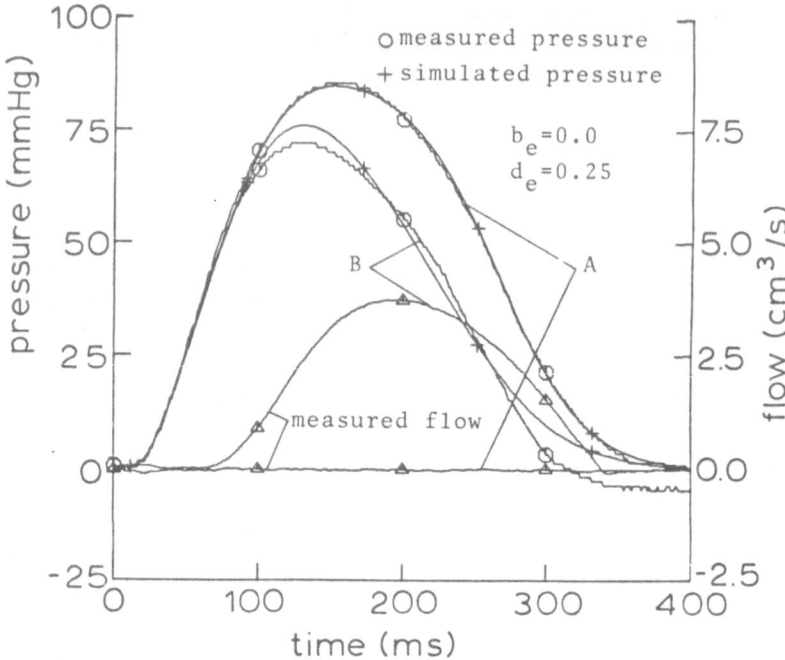

*Figure 4.* Isovolumic (A) and non-isovolumic (B) contraction at a preload of 1 mmHg. The experimental flow courses do not resemble those measured experimentally in vivo because of the use of a simple construction representing the afterload.

Figure 4 shows the results of an isovolumic (A) and a non-isovolumic (B) contraction at a preload of 1 mmHg. A model with an SEE ($\Delta P = 3.6$) again gave better results than a model without an SEE ($\Delta P = 5.8$). Variation of $b_e$ had no significant effect on $\Delta P$. Variation of $d_e$ had much more effect. The best results were obtained when the ventricular length is somewhat shortened during ejection.

6. CONCLUSIONS

A ventricular model consisting of a suitably chosen nested set of truncated ellipsoids of revolution suffices for simulating average properties of the ventricle. In the reference situation the endocardial pressure in the apex (site A) was taken equal to the endocardial pressure in a point at the equator (site B). From simulations done it followed that the pressure drop over the wall in between A and B was found to differ less than 0.15% from the equivalent endocardial pressure. So an ellipsoidal model suffices with relation to this aspect. At higher preloads and during ejection somewhat larger but still acceptable ($<5\%$) differences were found.

From curve fittings, carried out to obtain a rough estimate of the parameters, and from simulations done to test the sensitivity of some parameters it was found that:

1. In combination with the used muscle model the presence of an SEE appears to be essential to describe isovolumic as well as non-isovolumic contractions. The found values of the elasticity result in maximum sarcomere shortenings of about $6\%$ during isovolumic contractions. The elasticity may wholly or partly be due to distortion of the ventricle, inflexion of the valves and compression of the coronary arteries.

2. The chosen phenomenological activation function allows good fits. Other functions give about the same results if their shape is rather symmetrical without a plateau phase and they do not rise too abruptly at $t=0$ (horizontal derivative!). The influence of preload on activation should be taken into account.

3. Ventricular dimensions are important factors. Measurement of ventricular pressure and flow is not enough to estimate all parameters with reasonable accuracy. Simultaneous measurement of, for instance, ventricular inner and outer dimensions is necessary.

SUMMARY

A model for the left ventricle is proposed which consists of a muscle model relating contraction processes to muscle force or wall tension and a ventricular model relating wall tension to developed pressure. The muscle model is composed of a contractile element based on the sliding filament theory and a real or apparent series-elastic element. The ventricular wall is approximated by a nested set of truncated ellipsoidal shells of revolution in which the muscle fibres are located. To test the model and to fit the relevant parameters, experiments were carried out on isolated perfused rabbit hearts. It was found that non-isovolumic and particularly isovolumic contractions could be simulated rather well if rather realistic shape changes were introduced and activation was assumed to depend on preload. For accurate parameter estimation of the ventricular processes, it was found necessary to record at least pressure, flow and overall geometry.

ACKNOWLEDGEMENTS

We wish to thank Dr. A. Crowe for his criticism of the manuscript and Dr. J.H.M. Nieuwenhuijs and Drs. P. Schiereck for their cooperation with the experiments.

REFERENCES

1. Streeter Jr DD, Vaishnav RN, Patel DJ, Spotnitz JM, Ross Jr J, Sonnenblick EH: Stress distribution in the canine left ventricle during diastole and systole. *Biophys J* 10:345–363, 1970.
2. Wong AYK: Myocardial mechanics: application of the sliding-filament theory to isovolumic concentration of the left ventricle. *J Biomech* 6:565–581, 1973.
3. Huxley AF: Muscle structure and theories of contraction. In: *Progress in biophysics and biophysical chemistry* vol 7, Butler AV, Katz B (eds), Oxford, Pergamon, 1957, p 225–318.
4. Pollack GH, Krueger JW: Sarcomere dynamics in intact cardiac muscle. *Eur J Cardiol* (4) (suppl): 53–65, 1976.
5. Jewell BR: A reexamination of the influence of muscle length on myocardial performance. *Circ Res* 40:212–230, 1977.
6. Streeter Jr DD, Spotnitz HM, Patel DP, Ross Jr J, Sonnenblick EH: Fibre orientation in the canine left ventricle during diastole and systole. *Circ Res* 24:339–347, 1969.
7. Spotnitz HM, Sonnenblick EH, Spiro D: Relation of ultrastructure to function in the intact heart: sarcomere structure relative to pressure-volume curves of intact left ventricles of dog and cat. *Circ Res* 18:49–66, 1966.
8. Back LH: Left ventricular wall and fluid dynamics of cardiac contraction. *Math Biosc* 36:257–297, 1977.
9. Boom HBK, Denier van der Gon JJ, Nieuwenhuijs JHM, Schiereck P: Cardiac contractility: actin-myosin interaction as measured from the left ventricular pressure curve. *Eur J Cardiol* 1/2:217–224, 1973.

# PUMP FUNCTION AND FILLING: INTERACTION WITH THE LOW PRESSURE SYSTEM

# 3.1 DYNAMIC DETERMINANTS OF LEFT VENTRICULAR FILLING: AN OVERVIEW

EDWARD L. YELLIN, EDMUND H. SONNENBLICK,
ROBERT W.M. FRATER

## 1. INTRODUCTION

The left ventricle fills through dynamic changes in its compliance as it relaxes (by altering its wall stress), through elastic recoil from a non-equilibrium shape, and through passive acceptance of blood during diastole. The driving force necessary to accelerate the blood and to overcome dissipative energy losses is provided by the pressure in the left atrium which acts as a passively compliant reservoir (whose potential energy is provided by the right ventricular contraction), and by the active generation of force during atrial systole. The efficiency of ventricular filling, and its ability to determine the subsequent stroke volume, is in part determined by the ability of the valve to open widely and to stay open during filling, to close competently at systole, and to remain closed without leakage.

In this presentation we will provide an overview of the dynamic determinants of ventricular filling. In our laboratory we measure phasic transmitral flow along with the usual hemodynamic parameters, so that we have the unique ability to emphasize the interrelationships among these parameters and to describe their influence on filling. We will describe studies which are designed to investigate, on a beat-to-beat basis, the following determinants of left ventricular filling:

1. Phasic left ventricular relaxation rate;
2. Atrial reservoir function;
3. Contribution of atrial systole;
4. Left ventricular dynamic diastolic compliance; and
5. Mitral valve function.

The framework in which we analyze ventricular filling is based on a pressure-flow relationship between the left atrium and ventricle of the form (1),

$$\Delta p = (A)dQ/dt + (B)Q \qquad [1]$$

Thus, the driving pressure ($\Delta p$) is assumed to be proportional to an accelerative component ($dQ/dt$) and to a dissipative component linearly related to the volume flow ($Q$). We also assume that losses due to inadequate dynamic head recovery from convective acceleration across the

*J. Baan, A.C. Arntzenius, E.L. Yellin (eds.), Cardiac Dynamics, 145–158.*

valve are either insignificant, or can be lumped into the dissipative term. For purposes of this presentation we have not attempted to evaluate the coefficients ($A$, $B$) and we will focus on discussing the factors which determine the LA-LV pressure difference since this difference provides the driving force for transmitral flow.

## 2. METHODS

The animal preparation has been described previously (2) and will be summarized briefly. In the open-chest anesthetized dog, phasic mitral and aortic flows are measured electromagnetically (Carolina Medical Electronics); left ventricular and atrial pressures are measured with catheter-tip transducers (Millar); and aortic pressure is measured with a fluid-filled catheter and strain gauge (Statham). These parameters are recorded on an oscillographic recorder (Electronics for Medicine) along with the ECG and LV$dp/dt$. All pressures are at equal sensitivity and referenced to the same baseline. The records are manually digitized and analyzed with a sonic digitizer (Science Accessories) coupled to a digital computer (PDP-11).

The intact ejecting heart in the open-chest anesthetized dog is a useful analog for the study of normal and pathological filling dynamics, but it is a complex preparation because several variables may be changing at the same time. In order to minimize this problem without imposing any artificial controls on the preparation (e.g., right heart bypass with reservoir-controlled filling pressure) we have chosen to use techniques which can be classed as perturbation methods. For example, we have created the following conditions in which only a minimal number of filling parameters have changed from the control to the perturbed beat: extrasystoles, a left atrial to subclavian artery shunt which can be acutely opened or closed, and vagal stimulation. Although this approach does not solve the problem of changing only one variable at a time, it does provide significant insight into the filling dynamics of the intact ejecting heart; particularly when the instrumentation is capable of measuring instantaneous inflow, and LA-LV pressures.

## 3. RESULTS AND DISCUSSION

### 3.1. *The uniqueness of the pressure-flow relation*

Figure 1 is an oscillographic record from a dog in which an early (panel A) and a later (panel B) extrasystole were created within 10 beats of each other. Record A was duplicated on opaque paper, record B was duplicated on

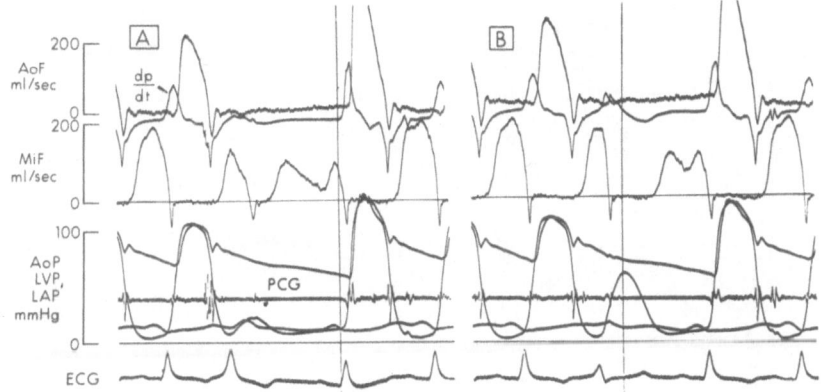

*Figure 1.* Oscillographic record from a dog with an early (panel A) and a later (panel B) extrasystole created within ten beats of each other. Note the similarity of control conditions and shape of mitral flow curves during the compensatory pause. AoF = Aortic Flow; MiF = Mitral Flow; AoP, LVP, LAP = Aortic, Left Ventricular and left Atrial Pressures; dp/dt = derivative of LVP; PCG = phonocardiogram (intracardiac); ECG = electrocardiogram.

transparent paper, and the two were superimposed as shown in Figure 2. It can be seen that for comparable patterns of atrioventricular pressure difference, there is a unique pattern of mitral flow. Two very different LVP-LAP combinations produced the same phasic difference (Figure 2: $\Delta p_A$, $\Delta p_B$), which in turn produced the same mitral flow wave-form. Only the duration of filling differed.

## 3.2. *Determinants of the pressure-flow relation*

Figure 3 shows a sequence of control (C), extrasystolic and post-extrasystolic (PES) beats which illustrates the relative importance of the atrioventricular pressure difference, particularly when compared to the diastolic filling time, and which illustrates the factors determining the pattern of the pressure difference. A comparison of the C and PES beats yields certain qualitative differences. The control LVP relaxes more rapidly and to a lower minimum than the post-estrasystolic LVP. The control LAP is slightly higher at mitral valve opening (coincident with the pressure cross-over) and decreases (i.e. unloads) at a slower rate than the post-extrasystolic LAP. The resulting pressure difference wave-forms are illustrated in the digitized data shown in A in Figure 4.

The flow patterns produced by these driving pressure differences are seen to differ in their initial rate of rise and in their peak values. As a consequence, despite the large increase in filling time for the PES beat, the C beat has a greater filling volume.

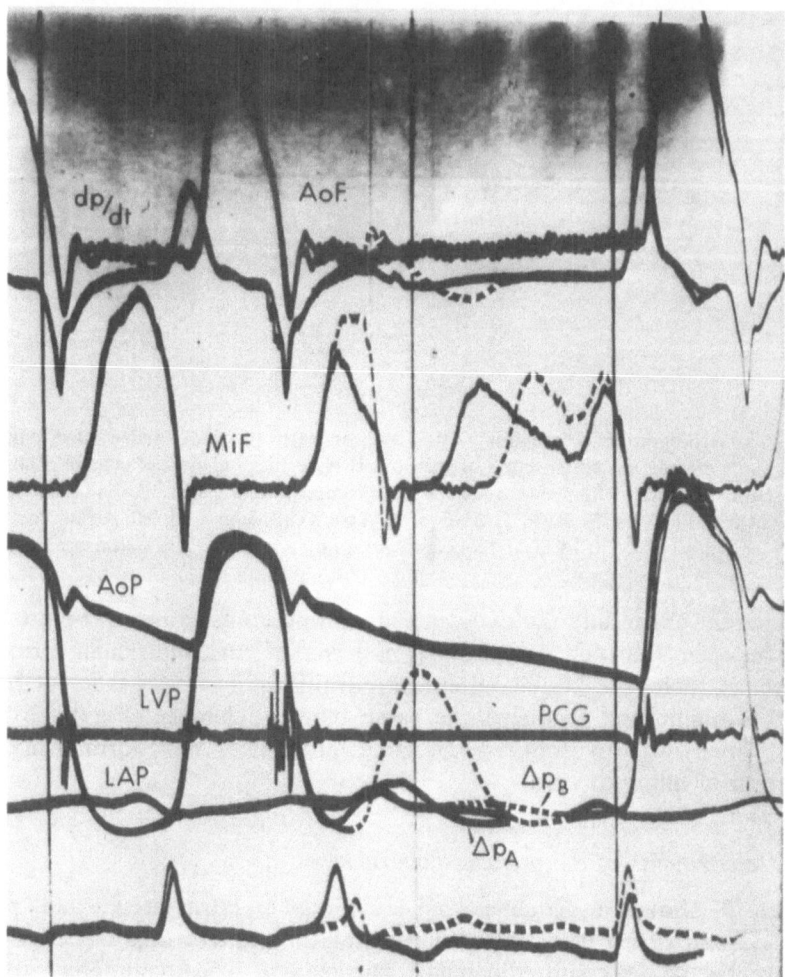

*Figure 2.* Panels A (unbroken curve) and B (broken curve) from Figure 1 overlaid to show the similarity of flow wave-forms produced by similar pressure gradients ($\Delta p_A$ and $\Delta p_B$).

3.2.1. *Left ventricular relaxation*: In order to quantify the rate of ventricular pressure fall during isovolumic relaxation as well as during early filling we have modified the method of Weiss et al. (3). An iterative procedure is used to find the best exponential fit for the data points from max-$dp/dt$ to $P_{min}$: $p = (A) \exp(t/T) + C$. The time constant ($T$) is a useful characterization of the rate of fall of LVP; B in Figure 4 shows the results of the calculations for the data from Figure 3. The time constant for the post-extrasystolic LVP is 50% greater than that for the control LVP.

The rate of ventricular relaxation influences the filling volume in many

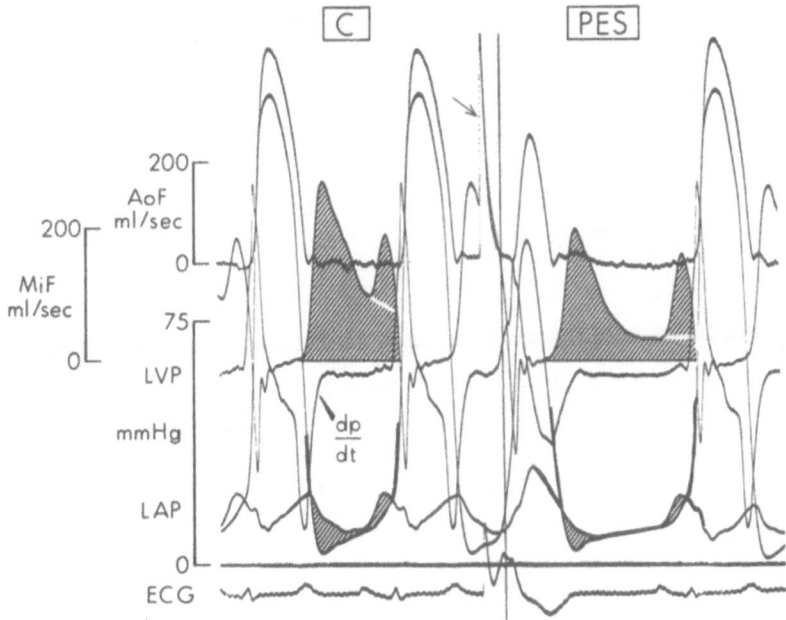

*Figure 3.* High gain oscillographic record of control (C) and post-extrasystolic (PES) beats illustrating the importance of the atrioventricular pressure difference in the generation of mitral flow (shaded areas). The break in the shading of the mitral flow curve separates the contribution of atrial systole from the inflow which would have occurred in the absence of an atrial contraction. The arrow points to the stimulus artifact.

ways. It determines the rate of development of the pressure gradient and hence the rate of early rapid filling, which, in turn, influences the amplitude of the flow curve. Since flow deceleration is accomplished by viscous dissipation in the absence of an adverse gradient during mid-diastole (which is normal), the amplitude, and hence the initial momentum, will influence the subsequent rate of flow. Finally, a rapid rate of fall of ventricular pressure increases the duration of the filling period.

*3.2.2. Left atrial reservoir function:* The level of atrial pressure at the time of mitral valve opening will clearly influence the magnitude of the developing pressure difference and hence the amplitude of early inflow. The atrial pressure also influences the rate of development of the pressure gradient in the following way: the greater the LAP at mitral valve opening, the greater the rate of pressure fall at that time, the greater the rate of gradient development, and hence the greater the filling (see above). Thus, the value of $-dp/dt$ at mitral valve opening (or pressure cross-over) is a significant determinant of filling and perhaps more important than max-$dp/dt$. These

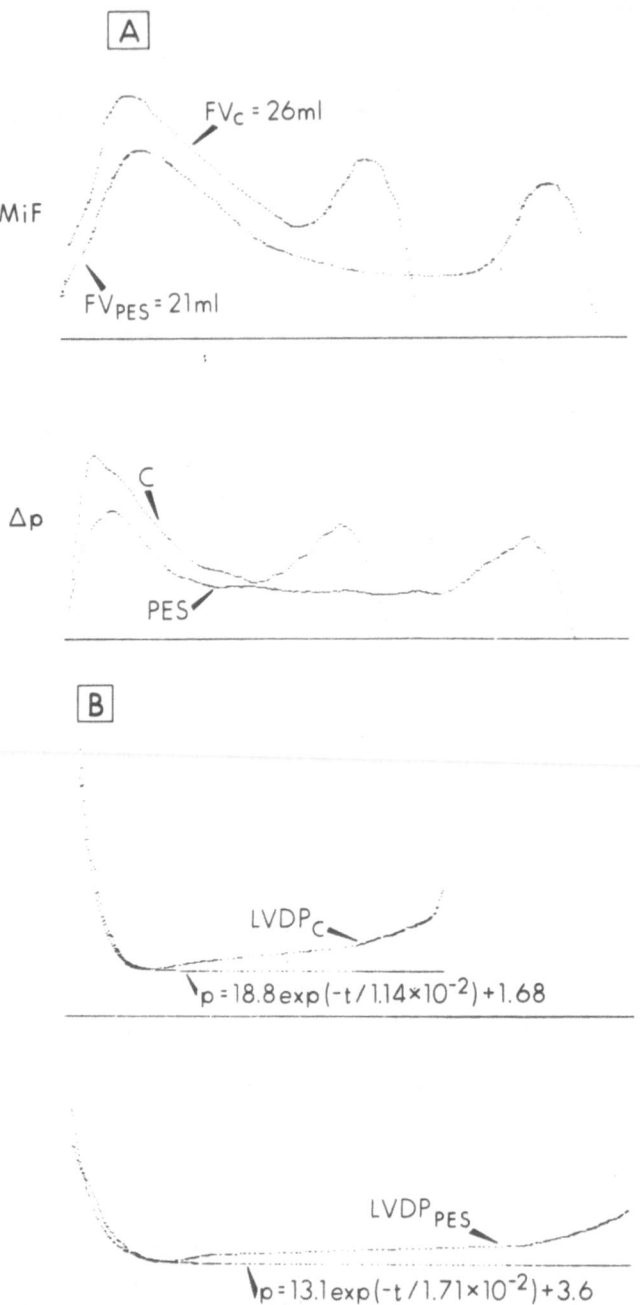

*Figure 4.* Panel A: the digitized flow and pressure difference curves obtained from Figure 3 illustrating that the duration of diastole is of secondary importance when compared to the driving pressure gradient; panel B: the digitized left ventricular diastolic pressure curve and its associated exponential fit for the C and PES beats from Figure 3. Note that the time constant, or the rate of relaxation, for the C curve is significantly greater than that for the PES curve.

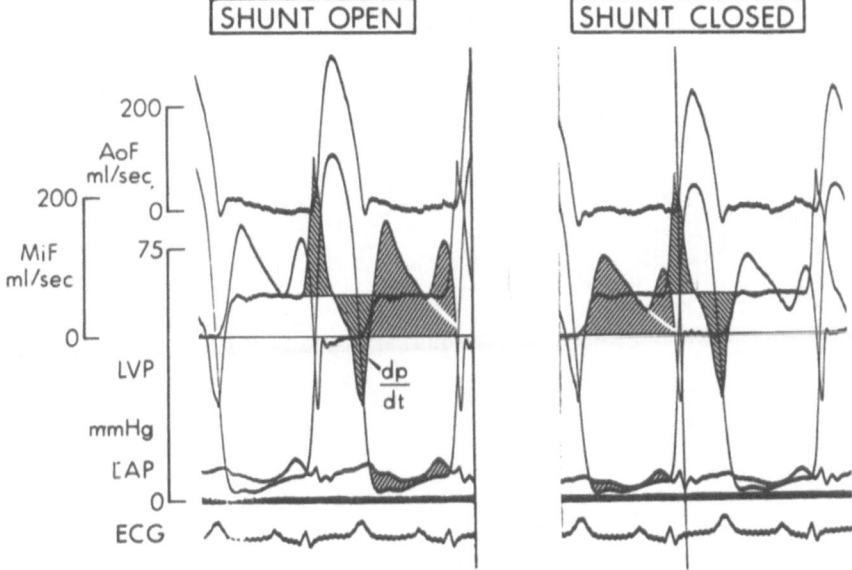

*Figure 5.* Oscillographic record illustrating the importance of the level of left atrial pressure to the mitral flow curve. In the left panel, mitral flow was enhanced by a left subclavian artery to left atrial shunt, and in the right panel the shunt was closed and left atrial pressure was reduced. Note that negative *dp/dt* maxima remained constant and that the mitral flow waveforms remained similar but were reduced in amplitude after shunt closure. The break in the shading of the mitral flow curve delineates the atrial contribution to inflow.

concepts are illustrated in Figures 5 and 6. In these records the left atrial pressure was acutely decreased by closing a subclavian artery to left atrial shunt. There was no change in either max-*dp/dt* (Figure 5) or the time constant of left ventricular pressure fall (Figure 6); as a consequence, the magnitude of the mitral flow curve changed significantly and the rate of rise changed somewhat less.

3.2.3. *Role of atrial contraction:* The quantification of the contribution to filling provided by an atrial contraction depends on the definition of the problem, which can be formulated in two ways: (1) How much volume would be lost if the diastolic filling period remained equal to control, but the atrium did not contract (e.g., atrial arrest with nodal rhythm)?; and (2) How much volume would be lost if the atrium did not contract because the diastolic period was shortened (e.g., by a ventricular premature contraction)? The answers to the questions can be determined by examining the equation of motion [1]. Under normal conditions of low to moderate HR, the LA-LV pressure difference is significant only during early diastole when

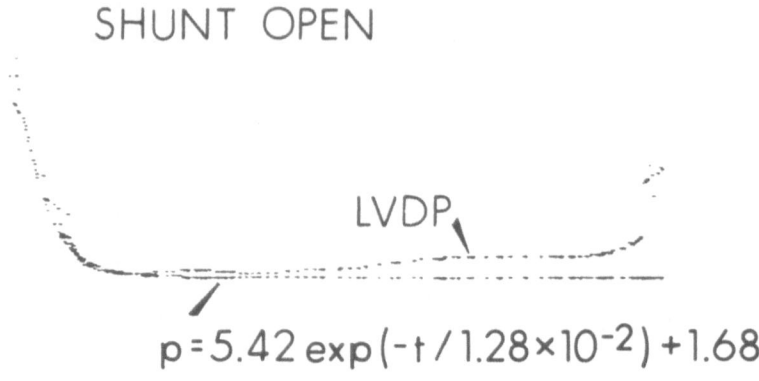

SHUNT OPEN

LVDP

$$p = 5.42 \exp(-t / 1.28 \times 10^{-2}) + 1.68$$

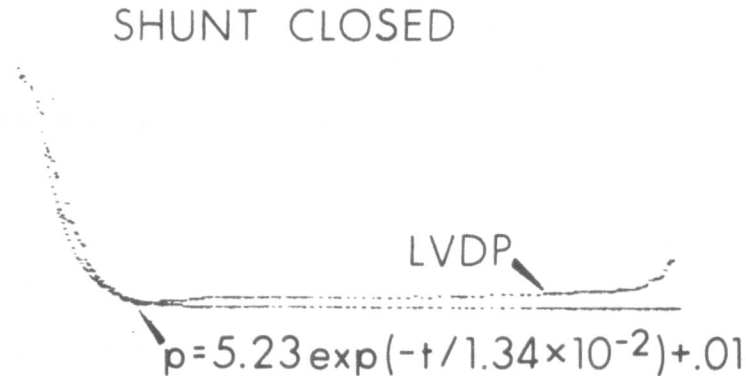

SHUNT CLOSED

LVDP

$$p = 5.23 \exp(-t / 1.34 \times 10^{-2}) + .01$$

*Figure 6.* The exponential fit to the diastolic left ventricular pressure curve from Figure 5. Note that the time constnat of exponential decay was unchanged in the two conditions. This is consistent with the similarity in negative $dp/dt$ and the rate of rise of mitral flow.

momentum is imparted to the blood for rapid early filling (Figures 3, 5). In mid-diastole, $\Delta p$ becomes zero and the solution of [1] leads to an exponential decay in flow by viscous dissipation (Figures 3, 5: break in shading). Under these conditions, the answer to the first question is that approximately 10–20% of the total filling volume is provided by the atrial contraction (the area above the broken line in Figures 3, 5). The answer to the second question is that approximately 20–30% of the total filling volume is provided by the atrial contraction (the area under the second upswing in flow, Figures 3, 5).

3.2.4. *Mitral valve function:* Mitral stenosis represents an increased imped-ance to flow with a pressure-flow relation that is best described using a square law dissipative term in the equation of motion rather than a linear term (4):

$$\Delta p = (A')dQ/dt + (B')Q^2 \qquad [2]$$

Under these conditions, the dissipative term is dominant, the LAP rises so that the gradient persists for all diastole, the flow wave-form is relatively flat, and the peak flow is diminished (Figure 7).

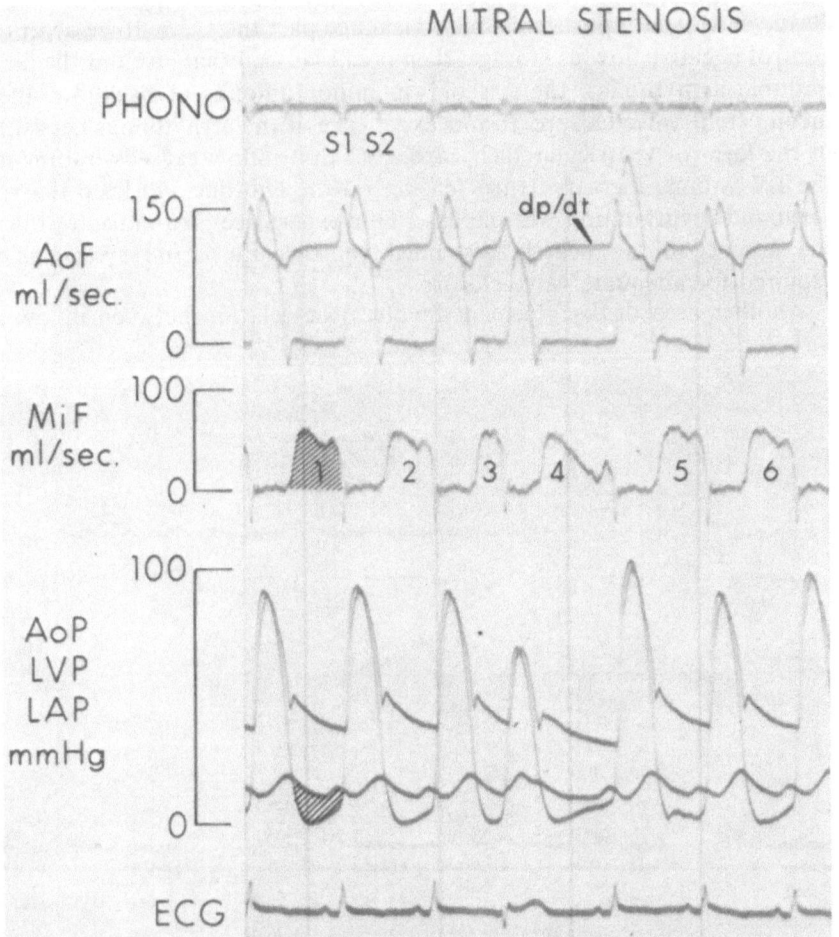

*Figure 7.* Oscillographic record from a dog with surgically created mitral stenosis. Note the decreased amplitude of mitral flow, its relatively flat wave-form, and the significant diastolic pressure gradient. The pressure-flow relations conform to [2] under the diverse conditions shown in beats 1, 3, and 4.

Mitral regurgitation may be due to an incompetent valve or incompetent closure. In the former case, if the regurgitant fraction is significant, then filling will be influenced only to the extent that it will be increased, but the dynamic relations will remain unchanged. The latter case has been the subject of some controversy and will be discussed here. Figure 8 is an oscillographic record from a dog showing a sequence of normal sinus rhythm followed by two consecutive ventricular premature contractions, a potentiated beat, and another premature contraction. The shaded areas of the flow curves represent negative flow relative to the flow probe at the annulus. Thus, a portion of the backflow is due to energy stored in the elastic valve and a portion is due to leakage past the valve. If we accept the control negative flow as storage, then it can be seen that, even in the face of multiple arrhythmias, there is only a minor amount of backflow due to incompetent valve closure. In our experience, if the arrhythmias persist, say in the form of ventricular tachycardia, so that inflow exceeds outflow and the LV volume increases, then tension on the chordae will keep the valve open and regurgitation will increase. Our experience also indicates that, in the absence of an acutely distended ventricle, an atrial systole is not required for adequate valve closure.

Another area of disagreement involves the relation between inflow and

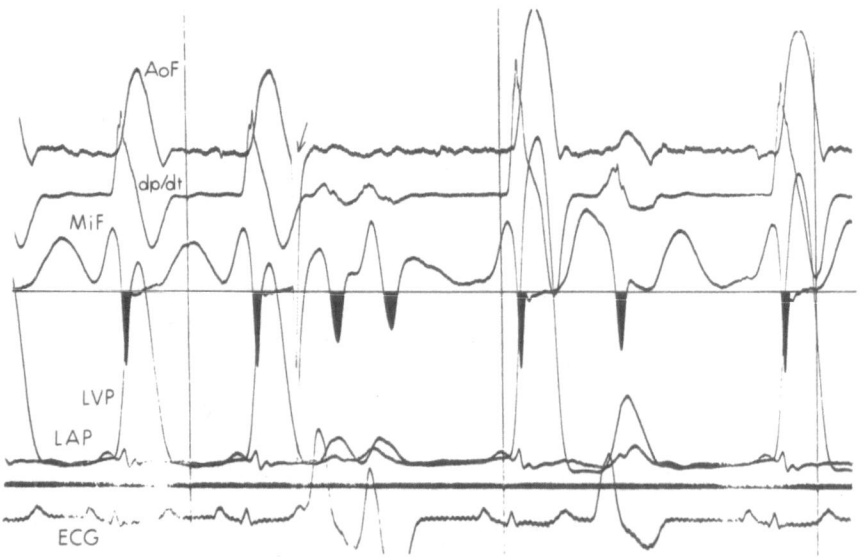

*Figure 8.* Oscillographic record showing the effect of arrhythmias on valve closure. The shaded areas of the negative portion of the mitral flow curve in the first two beats designate a valve closure artifact and is due to elastic storage, not backflow. The shaded areas in the third and fourth beats are due to storage and very small amount of backflow. The arrow points to the stimulus artifact.

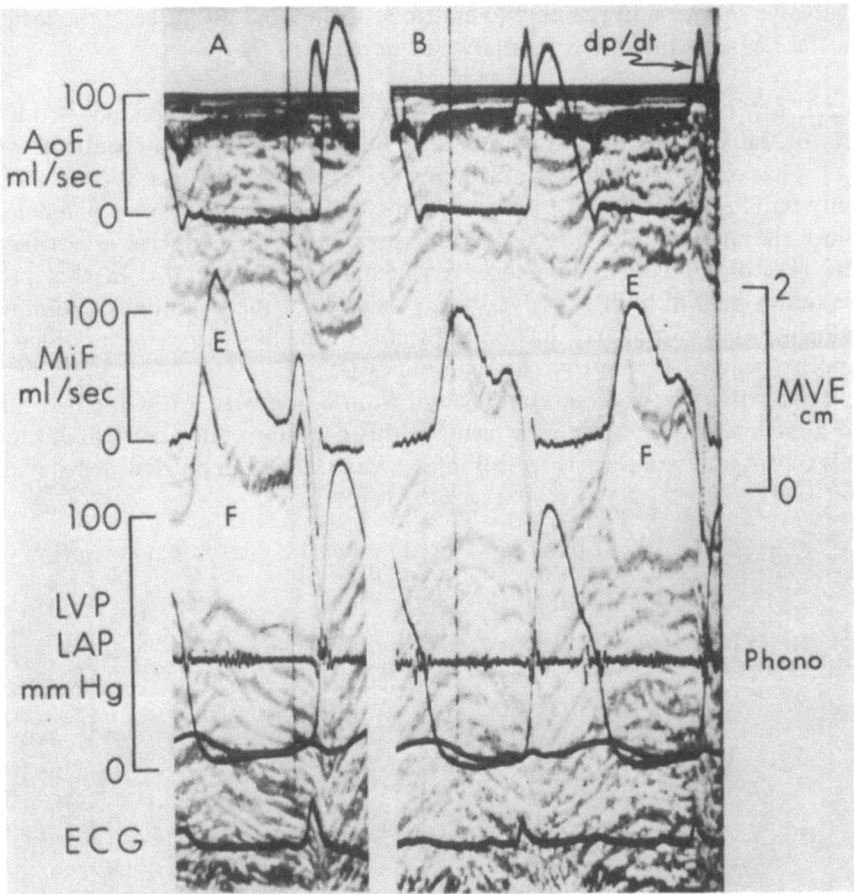

*Figure 9.* Oscillographic record from a dog with simultaneous mitral valve echo (MVE) and mitral flow. Note that the start of diastolic closure (E point) occurs while mitral flow is still accelerating. This phenomenon is independent of heart rate: Panel A is a slow rate relative to Panel B. See text for discussion.

mitral valve motion. Figure 9 shows an oscillographic record from a dog with a simultaneous measurement of mitral flow and valve motion. It can be seen that the mitral valve starts its diastolic closure motion (point E) before flow starts to decelerate. Using a probe area of 2.9 cm², a maximum volume flow of 125 cm³/sec, and a paper speed of 100 mm/sec, we calculate that the valve started to move toward closure well before a fluid particle at the leaflet edge or mitral annulus was able to reach the apex of the heart (i.e., 2 cm is the distance travelled at maximum flow and 1 cm is the distance travelled at the E point). We conclude that the size of the ventricle does not determine the ability of a vortex to move the valve toward closure (5), but rather that the vortex forms at the leaflet margin due to shearing forces at the valve surface and possibly to elastic restoring forces that keep the leaflet in the mainstream where vorticity can develop (6, 7).

3.2.5. *Left ventricular compliance:* Strictly speaking, the compliance properties of the ventricle will not exert an influence on filling independently of [1]. That is, for a given flow, changing the compliance of the ventricle will only require an increased LAP to provide the necessary pressure difference. Since the myocardium has viscoelastic properties, the converse is not true: the rate of filling will influence ventricular compliance (8). In this presentation we will limit ourselves to an example of the potentially profound influence that compliance has on the shape of the flow wave-form (which is another way of saying that $\Delta p$ determines $Q$).

Figure 10 is an oscillographic record from a dog with a low preload due to hypovolemia. Possibly as a result of this condition, the ventricle did not relax adequately and early mitral inflow was severely depressed (left panel).

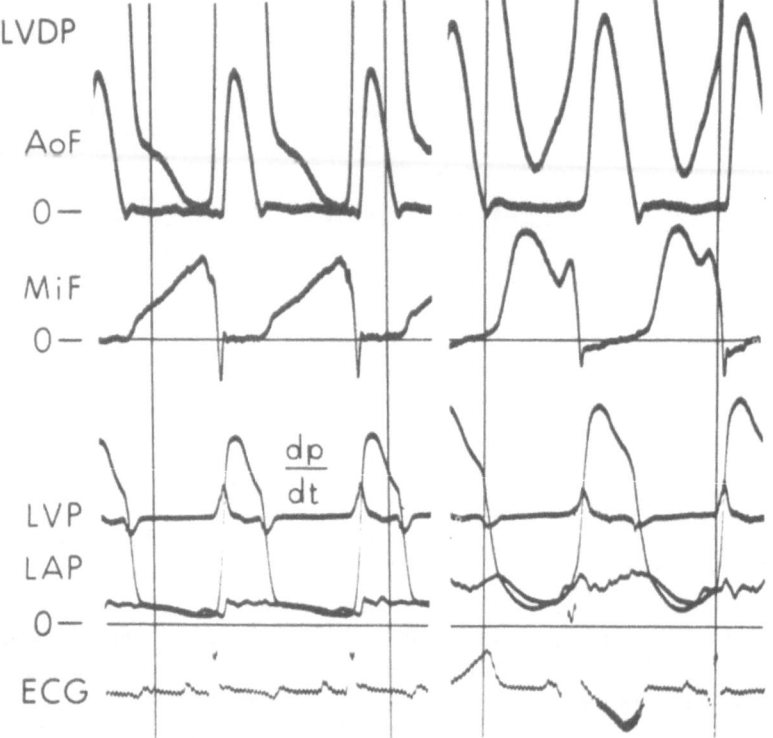

*Figure 10.* Oscillographic record showing impaired ventricular relaxation following a normal negative *dp/dt*, and its profound effect on the shape of the mitral flow curve (left panel). Restoration of normal relaxation resulted in marked improvement in mitral flow (right panel).

Volume infusion reversed the condition, adequate relaxation was achieved, and the mitral flow assumed its normal shape (right panel).

Another interesting example of the interaction between left ventricular compliance and mitral inflow is shown in Figure 11. This record illustrates the clinical entity of the "square root sign" LVP (upper trace). Under conditions of poor compliance (either because of acute volume distension or because of chronic hypertrophy) and rapid early filling, the ventricle abruptly stiffens and the pressure gradient reverses. Flow will quickly decelerate under the action of an adverse gradient (Panels A, B). Under some conditions the pressure difference will again reverse (second arrow,

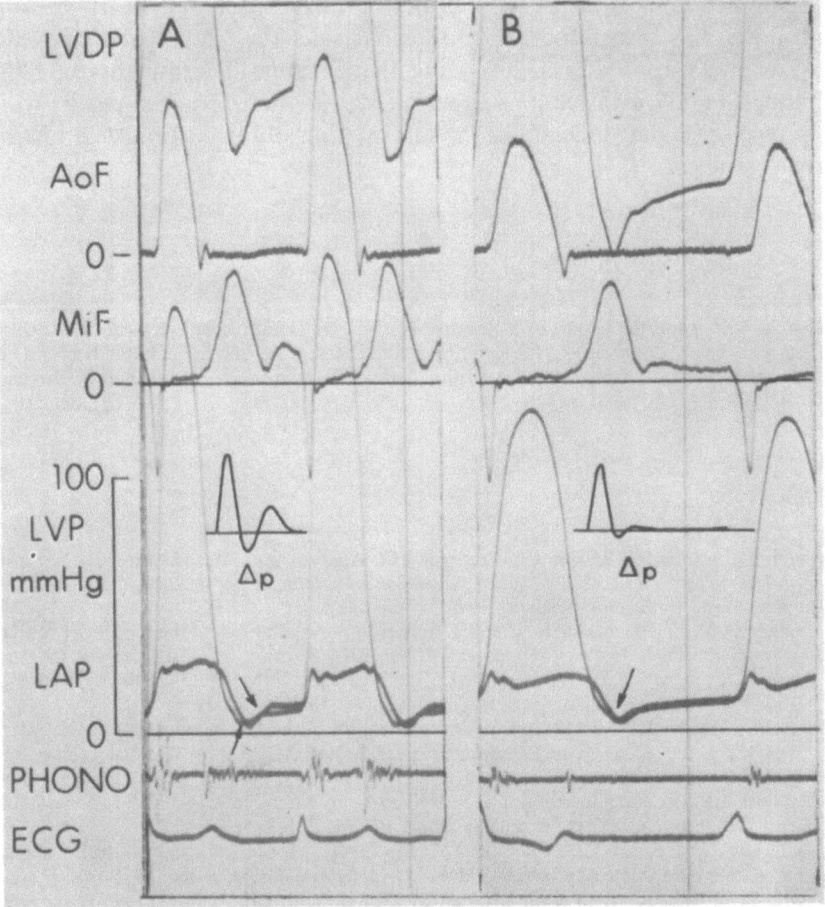

*Figure 11.* Oscillographic record illustrating the "square root sign" LVDP due to a stiff ventricle. As a result, an adverse gradient decelerates mitral flow more rapidly than normal. The arrows point to the pressure cross-over points.

Panel A) and a second phase of forward flow results (Panel A). We assume that a resonance phenomenon produces this oscillation. It is interesting to note that the pressure-flow wave-forms of Figure 11 indirectly confirm the applicability of the equation of motion [1]. Just as we predicted the diastolic exponential decay of flow when the pressure difference became zero, and stayed at that value, [1] also predicts that an adverse gradient rapidly decelerates flow.

## 4. CONCLUSION

The simultaneous measurement of phasic intracardiac left heart pressures and flows has permitted us to demonstrate the viability of a simple mathematical approach to analyzing the dynamic determinants of filling. Although highly invasive, this experimental method provides results which help us clarify and understand the information obtained from less invasive patient studies.

ACKNOWLEDGEMENTS

This work was supported in part by a National Institutes of Health Research Grant HL 19391. It could not have been done without the technical skills of Messrs. Astolfo Leon, Pablo Bon and Felix Rivera. Figure 7 was reproduced by permission of the American Society of Mechanical Engineers (Ref. 4).

REFERENCES

1. Yellin EL, Laniado S, Peskin CS, Frater RWM: Analysis and interpretation of the normal mitral valve flow curve. In *The mitral valve: a pluridisciplinary approach*, Kalmanson D (ed), Action, Mass, Publishing Sciences, 1976, p 163–172.
2. Laniado S, Yellin EL, Miller H, Frater RWM: Temporal relations of the first heart sound to closure of the mitral valve. *Circulation* 74:1006–1014, 1973.
3. Weiss JL, Frederiksen JW, Weisfeldt ML: Hemodynamic determinants of the time-course of fall in canine left ventricular pressure. *J Clin Invest* 58:751–760, 1976.
4. Yellin EL, Frater RWM, Peskin CS: The application of the Gorlin equation to the stenotic mitral valve. In: *Advances in Bioengineering, 1975*, Bell AC, Nerem RM (eds), New York, ASME, 1975, p 45–47.
5. Belhouse BJ: The fluid mechanics of heart valves. In *Cardiovascular fluid dynamics*, vol 1, Bergel DH (ed), New York, Academic Press, 1972, p 261–285.
6. Tsakiris AG, Gordon DA, Mathieu Y, Lipton 1: Motion of both mitral leaflets: a cineroentgenographic study in intact dogs. *J Appl Physiol* 39:359–366, 1975.
7. Yellin EL, Frater RWM, Peskin CS, Laniado S: Left ventricular inflow patterns and mitral valve motion: animal studies and computer analysis. In: *New England Bioengineering Conference: 4th: proceedings* Saha S. (ed), Elmsford, Pergamon, 1976, p 177–180.
8. Kennish A, Yellin E, Frater RW: Dynamic stiffness profiles in the left ventricle. *J Appl Physiol* 39:665–671, 1975.

## 3.2. EFFECTS OF THE PERICARDIUM ON LEFT VENTRICULAR PERFORMANCE

JOHN V. TYBERG, GREGORY A. MISBACH,
WILLIAM W. PARMLEY, STANTON A. GLANTZ

Several investigators have demonstrated acute, reversible shifts in the position of the diastolic, left ventricular pressure-volume curve (1, 2,3 4, 5, 6). Upward shifts tend to be associated with conditions that increase the load against which the heart ejects or conditions which decrease the capacity of the heart to meet that load. Downward shifts have followed administration of the pharmacologic vasodilators nitroglycerin or nitroprusside and are presumably associated with a more advantageous relation of the contractile capacity of the heart to the load presented by the circulation.

Sometimes these shifts appear to be critical to the heart's ability to maintain its stroke volume. For example, Figure 1 shows data from patient no. 4 from Alderman and Glantz (1), who received nitroprusside and whose diastolic pressure-volume curve shifted downward by approximately 7 mmHg. During the control condition, end-diastolic pressure was 16 mmHg, end-diastolic volume 194 ml and stroke volume 118 ml, leaving an end-systolic volume of 76 ml. After nitroprusside was given, end-diastolic volume decreased only slightly to 176 ml because of the substantial downward shift in the curve. Stroke volume was maintained at the same level (114 ml), leaving an end-systolic volume of 62 ml. Suppose, instead, that the curve had not shifted. If the reduced end-diastolic pressure of 6 mmHg (see dashed lines) corresponded to an end-diastolic volume of 100 ml, as would have been the case had the pressure-volume curve not shifted, ejection of the original stroke volume would have been impossible.

These data suggest that a shift in the pressure-volume curve is an important part of the mechanism whereby patients in cardiac failure respond to vasodilators. Without such a shift, it is difficult to imagine how stroke volume can be preserved if, at a given contractile state, systolic ejection is limited by the line describing $E_{max}$ for that contractile state (7).

In 1978 we reported the results of studies initiated by Glantz to determine the role of the pericardium on the diastolic pressure-volume relationship (8, 9). These data showed that left and right ventricular pressure-dimension relationships were remarkably different in the presence or absence of the pericardium (Figure 2). Using a stepwise multiple linear regression technique on these data, Glantz et al. (8) showed that when the pericardium was intact, right ventricular pressure actually predicted left ventricular pressure

J. Baan, A.C. Arntzenius, E.L Yellin (eds.), Cardiac Dynamics, 159–168.

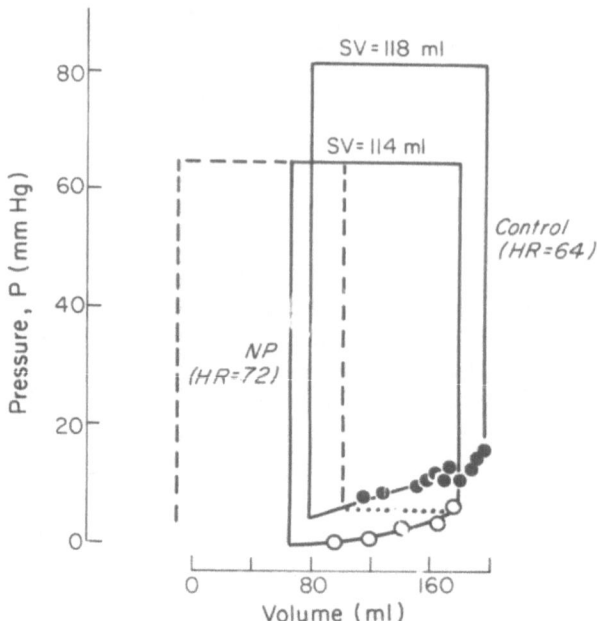

*Figure 1.* The importance of a shift in left ventricular diastolic pressure-volume curve to the maintenance of stroke volume after administration of sodium nitroprusside. Because of the shift in the curve, stroke volume was maintained despite large reductions in end-diastolic pressure. Had the control pressure-volume curve been followed, this reduction in end-diastolic pressure would have corresponded to such a small end-diastolic volume that stroke volume would have decreased greatly. Data replotted from Alderman and Glantz (1) with permission of the publisher.

better than did left ventricular dimensions. When the pericardium was open, of course, left ventricular pressure was a function of left ventricular dimensions and only minimally affected by right ventricular pressure. Furthermore, the left ventricular pressure-dimension curve could be shifted upward by constricting the pulmonary artery only if the pericardium was intact.

The statistical analysis convincingly demonstrated the association between right and left ventricular pressures and an apparent role for the pericardium. Based on the anatomy which implied that left ventricular pressure equalled the sum of the transmural myocardial pressure plus the transmural pericardial pressure (if intrathoracic pressure was zero as in our open-chest dogs), we suggested (9) that the observations could be explained by means of a simple hydraulic model (Figure 3). As long as the volume of the heart is less than the unstressed volume of the pericardium, the diastolic pressure recorded from the left ventricle will be the same whether the

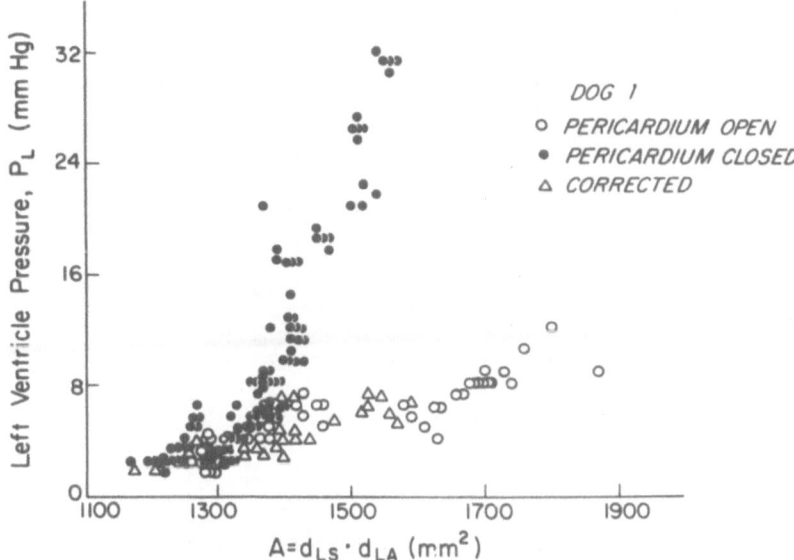

*Figure 2.* Left ventricular diastolic pressure as a function of left ventricular dimensions (*A* is the product of the two minor-axis diameters). Solid circles denote data recorded during volume loading when the pericardium was closed. Open circles denote data recorded when the pericardium was open. Open triangles indicate estimates of transmural pressure based on right ventricular pressure-diameter data. Reproduced with permission of the publisher (9).

pericardium is open or closed. However, when the volume of the heart exceeds the unstressed volume of the pericardium, the ventricular diastolic pressure equals the transmural pressure necessary to distend the ventricle plus the pericardial pressure. The importance of this model is that any condition which changes pericardial pressure (e.g., a change in volume of the right ventricle or the atria), will change the measured left ventricular diastolic pressure *in the absence of any change in the left ventricular volume.* Thus, such a mechanism can produce a shift in the pressure-volume curve.

According to this mechanism, at any instant during diastole, the pressure difference between the pericardium-closed curve and the pericardium-open curve for both the right and left ventricles must be the same, since that difference is due to the pericardial pressure. This concept is illustrated in Figure 4. Although Glantz et al. (8) did not measure pericardial pressure, we tested this hypothetical mechanism by examining the original data retrospectively (9). For each beat we measured the right ventricular end-diastolic diameter and then measured the pressure difference between the right ventricular pericardium-open and pericardium-closed curves at this diameter (Figure 4). We subtracted this pressure difference from the left

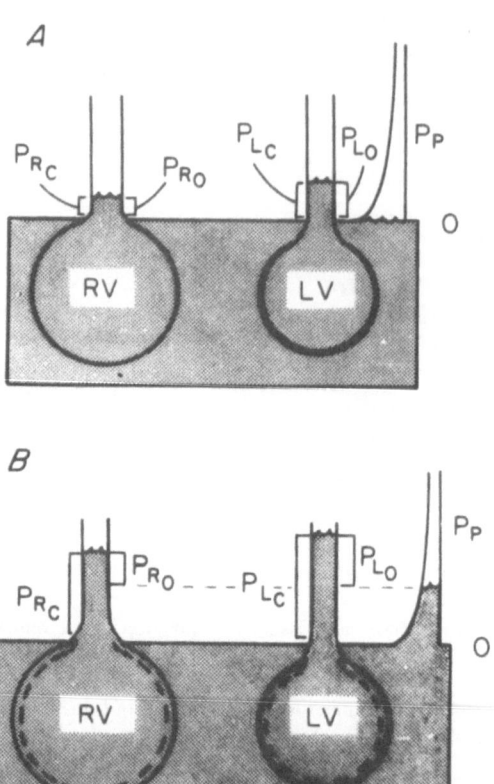

*Figure 3.* A schematic, hydraulic model for the interaction of the ventricles and the pericardium. The right and left ventricles are represented as water-filled, distensible balloons. The pressure-volume characteristics of the pericardium are modelled by a rigid, water-filled box with a narrowing vent such that successive increments in volume produce increasingly larger increments in pressure. When cardiac volume is less than the unstressed volume of the pericardium, pressure outside the ventricles is zero and ventricular diastolic pressure is the same as when the pericardium is open. When cardiac volume is greater than the unstressed volume of the pericardium, ventricular diastolic pressure equals the pressure necessary to distend the ventricle to the given volume *plus* pericardial pressure. Reproduced with permission of the publisher (9).

ventricular pericardium-closed curve at the left ventricular end-diastolic diameters recorded during that beat. Then we compared these estimates of left ventricular end-diastolic transmural pressure (diastolic pressure minus estimated pericardial pressure) and size (the product of two minor-axis left ventricular diameters) to the originally recorded curve of left ventricular diastolic pressure versus size with the pericardium open. (When the pericardium was open, diastolic pressure equalled transmural pressure.) The triangles in Figure 2 illustrate the excellent agreement which obtained.

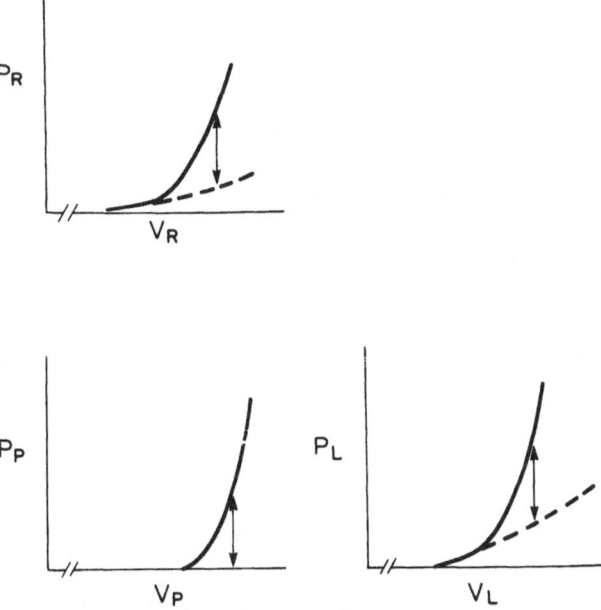

*Figure 4.* Diagrams of right (*top*) and left ventricular (*lower right*) and pericardial (*lower left*) pressure-volume relationships which show that the pericardial pressure (the length of the double-ended arrow) accounts for the pressure difference between the pericardium-open (dashed lines) and the pericardium-closed curves for each ventricle. Reproduced with permission of the publisher (9).

The role of the pericardium in the mechanism of acute shifts in the pressure-dimension curve is further illustrated in Figure 5. Assuming a spontaneous, primary increase in right ventricular volume, the pericardial volume and thus the pericardial pressure may increase by a substantial amount if the initial cardiac volume exceeds the unstressed volume of the pericardium. *With no change* in left ventricular volume, the pressure recorded in the left ventricle increases by the amount of the increase in pericardial pressure. Therefore, the magnitude of the shift is equal to the increase in pericardial pressure. (This diagram is oversimplified in that an increase in pericardial pressure would produce an equal upward shift in the right ventricular pressure-volume curve.)

This hypothesis has been supported by several observations during 1978. Shirato et al. (10) measured pericardial pressure in chronically instrumented dogs which they volume-loaded and then vasodilated with nitroprusside. Later, they repeated the measurements after removing the pericardium. When the pericardium was intact, volume loading shifted pressure-length curves upward and nitroprusside invariably lowered the curves toward control. Although they did not calculate transmural pressure, they found

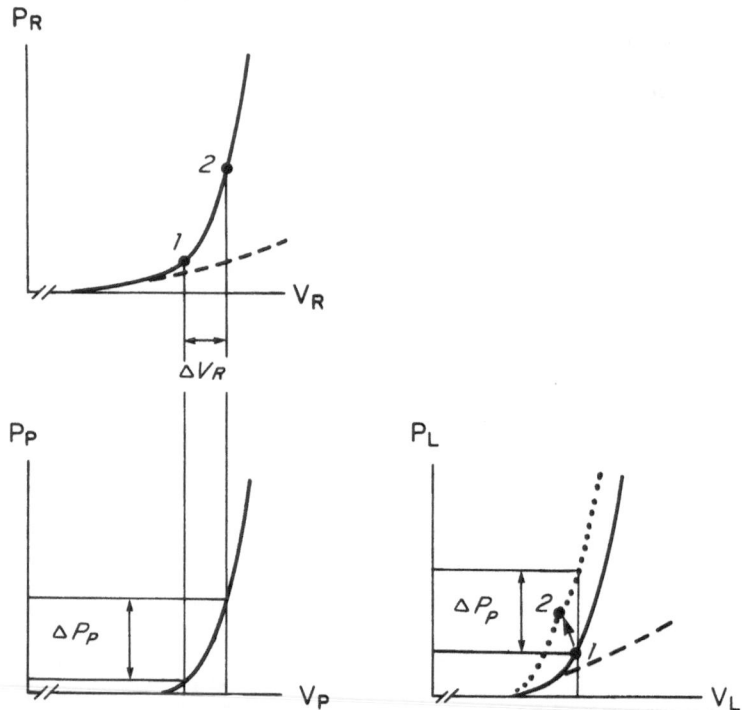

*Figure 5.* A mechanism by which an increase in right ventricular volume can shift the left ventricular pressure-volume curve upward. (Diagram is oversimplified since the right ventricular pressure-volume curve would be shifted upward also.) Reproduced with permission of the publisher (9).

that pericardial pressure increased significantly with volume loading, from $1.5 \pm 0.7$ mmHg to $8.2 \pm 0.5$ mmHg (SE). (The magnitude of this increase is similar to the displacement of the curves which they showed.) After nitroprusside, pericardial pressure decreased significantly to $4.8 \pm 0.1$ mmHg. The results of this investigation support our hypothesis, in that shifts in the curve correspond quantitatively to changes in pericardial pressure.

Padiyar et al. measured the mechanical properties of the left ventricular wall at transmural pressures up to 26 mmHg with and without the pericardium (11). The curve of transmural pressure versus volume was unchanged. Also unchanged was the relationship of myocardial stiffness to transmural pressure. This study supports the validity of our subtraction technique and the conclusion that the difference between the pericardium-closed and pericardium-open curves is the pericardial pressure.

Misbach and Glantz (12) have examined the consequences of shifts in the diastolic pressure-dimension curve on the interpretation of ventricular function curves. While measuring ventricular work, they volume-loaded the heart with the pericardium closed. Then they produced shifts in the left ventricular diastolic pressure-diameter curve by removing the pericardium and repeating the volume load. When ventricular work was plotted as a function of end-diastolic pressure, it appeared as though removing the pericardium had produced a substantial increase in contractility, because a given end-diastolic pressure corresponded to a longer fibre length which, in turn, enhanced performance via the Frank-Starling mechanism. When they plotted work against end-diastolic diameter, they found that removing the pericardium did not shift the curve. Hence, it may be quite impossible to infer the magnitude of the reduction in end-diastolic fibre length from only the observation of reduced left ventricular filling pressure. Although it is often difficult to obtain clinically, the value of direct measurements of ventricular dimensions cannot be overemphasized.

Rabson and Permutt (13) studied the interaction of the right and left ventricles and the contribution of the pericardium in an isolated dog heart preparation in which both ventricles contracted isovolumically. When right ventricular pressure was less than 5 mmHg, they found that right ventricular pressure changed left ventricular pressure to the same extent whether or not the pericardium was present. When right ventricular pressure exceeded 5 mmHg, increases in right ventricular diastolic pressure increased left ventricular pressure more when the pericardium was present. These values confirm our estimates for the point at which the effects of the pericardium become measureable.

A criticism of the work of Glantz et al. (8) was that the reconstructed pericardium was unphysiologic. Accordingly, Ringertz and Misbach have begun a series of experiments (unpublished) in closed-chest anesthetized dogs previously prepared with subendocardial tantalum screws according to Carlsson and Milne (14). They volume-loaded with dextran while recording left ventricular pressure and measuring volume by cineradiography. The experiment was repeated after the pericardium had been removed. Preliminary results confirm that the pericardium-closed curve lies substantially above the pericardium-open curve after volume-loading. Furthermore, the point at which the effect of the pericardium becomes measurable appears to be in the same range as we inferred from the earlier data and to be comparable to that found by Shirato et al. (10), i.e., a left ventricular pressure of approximately 10 mmHg.

We have also begun a series of experiments in acute, anesthetized open-chest dogs, in which we measure pericardial pressure with a Millar catheter-tip manometer enclosed in a flat, fluid-filled, unstressed balloon. Preliminary results from these experiments tend to support the hypothetical mechanism. Figure 6 shows the effect of temporary constriction of the caval veins in a previously volume-loaded animal whose pericardium had been reconstructed. Left ventricular diastolic pressure decreased by several milli-

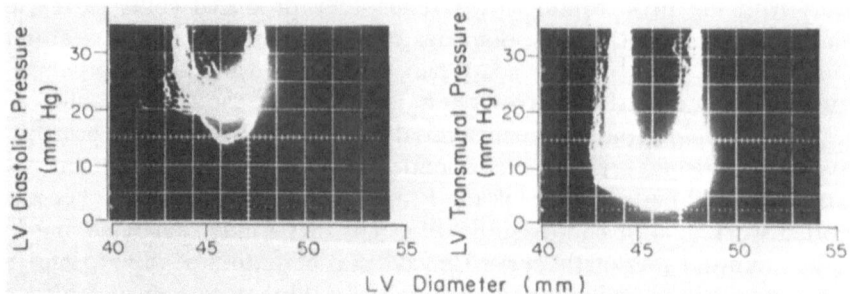

*Figure 6.* Effects of acute cardiac decompression of the left ventricular diastolic pressure-diameter relationship with closed pericardium. The experiment was performed in open-chest anesthetized dogs using manometer-tipped catheters and ultrasonic crystals to measure cardiac dimensions. The animal had been volume-loaded. When the caval veins were suddenly occluded, left ventricular diastolic pressure decreased abruptly (*left*) due to a decrease in pericardial pressure. When trans-mural pressure (left ventricular pressure minus pericardial pressure) was plotted against diameter, no displacement of the diastolic pressure-diameter relationship was seen (*right*).

meters of mercury during the initial period of cardiac decompression. However, when *transmural* (i.e., left ventricular pressure minus pericardial pressure) pressure was plotted against diameter, there was no shift. This directly supports the hypothesis that changes in the diastolic pressure-dimension are due to changes in pericardial pressure (3, 8, 9).

Recent clinical observations pertaining to the mechanism of shifts in the pressure-volume curve are less numerous. Ludbrook et al. (4) studied the effects of nitroglycerin upon left ventricular pressure-volume relations in 22 patients at the time of cardiac catheterization. Nitroglycerin produced large downward shifts in the pressure-volume curve. Most importantly, they showed that these shifts were not associated with significant changes in $T$, the time constant of ventricular relaxation shown by others to be relatively independent of peak systolic pressure and end-systolic volume (15). They concluded that the observed shifts were not due to changes in ventricular relaxation and were probably due to the effects of the pericardium.

CONCLUSIONS

We have proposed that changes in pericardial pressure are responsible for acute shifts in the left ventricular diastolic pressure-volume curve. Recent investigations support this hypothesis and show (1) that shifts in the curve correspond to changes in pericardial pressure, (2) that the transmural pressure-volume curve is not affected by the pericardium, and (3) that shifts in the curve can occur in patients without changes in ventricular relaxation.

SUMMARY

We have proposed that the pericardium has a dominant role in the mechanism of acute shifts in the left ventricular diastolic pressure-volume relationship. Relative to intrathoracic pressure, the left ventricular diastolic pressure must be the sum of the pressure differences across the left ventricular wall and across the pericardium. If pericardial pressure changes, diastolic left ventricular pressure will change even with no change in left ventricular volume. Thus, if cardiac loading or myocardial contractility changes and the heart dilates or becomes smaller, pericardial pressure changes and shifts the left ventricular diastolic pressure-volume curve, measured with respect to atmospheric pressure.

This hypothesis has been supported by a number of recent studies which show (1) that shifts in the curve correspond to changes in pericardial pressure, (2) that the transmural pressure-volume relationship is not affected by the pericardium, and (3) that shifts in the curve can occur in patients with no change in ventricular relaxation.

ACKNOWLEDGEMENTS

This work was supported in part by NHLBI Program Project Grant HL 06285. Dr. Tyberg is a recipient of an American Heart Association Grant-in-Aid 76-788 and an NIH Research Career Development Award. Dr. Misbach was supported by NIH Training Grants 05251 and GMO 1474-12. Dr. Glantz is the recipient of an NIH Research Career Development Award.

REFERENCES

1. Alderman El, Glantz SA: Acute hemodynamic interventions shift the diastolic pressure-volume curve in man. *Circulation* 54:662–671, 1976.
2. Brodie BR, Grossman W, Mann T, McLaurin L: Effects of sodium nitroprusside on left ventricular diastolic pressure-volume relations. *J Clin Invest* 59:59–68, 1977.
3. Glantz SA, Parmley WW: Factors which affect the diastolic pressure-volume curve. *Circ Res* 42:171–180, 1978.
4. Ludbrook PA, Byrne JD, Kurnik PB, McKnight RC: Influence of reduction of preload and afterload by nitroglycerin on left ventricular diastolic pressure-volume relations and relaxation in man. *Circulation* 56:937–943, 1977.
5. Mann T, Brodie BR, Grossman W, McLaurin LP: Effect of angina on the left ventricular diastolic pressure-volume relationship. *Circulation* 55:761–766, 1977.
6. Parmley WW, Chuck L, Chatterjee K, Klausner SC, Glantz SA, Ratshin RA: Acute changes in the diastolic pressure-volume relationship of the left ventricle. *Eur J Cardiol* 4 (suppl): 105–120, 1976.
7. Suga H, Sagawa K, Shoukas AA: Load independence of the instantaneous pressure-volume ratio of the canine left ventricle and effects of epinephrine and heart rate on the ratio. *Circ Res* 32:314–322, 1973.
8. Glantz SA, Misbach GA, Moores WY, Mathey DG, Lekven J, Stowe DF, Parmley WW, Tyberg JV: The pericardium substantially affects the left ventricular diastolic pressure-volume relationship in the dog. *Circ Res* 42:433–441, 1978.

9. Tyberg JV, Misbach GA, Glantz SA, Moores WY, Parmley WW: A mechanism for shifts in the diastolic, left ventricular pressure-volume curve: the role of the pericardium. *Eur J Cardiol* 7 (suppl): 163–175, 1978.
10. Shirato K, Shabetai R, Bhargava V, Franklin D, Ross Jr J: Alteration of the left ventricular diastolic pressure-segment length relation produced by the pericardium. *Ciriulation* 57:1191–1198, 1978.
11. Padiyar R, Pao YC, Ritman EL: Role of the pericardium in left ventricular stiffness: abstract. *Fed Proc* 37:920, 1978.
12. Misbach GA, Glantz SA: Changes in the diastolic pressure-volume relation produced by opening the pericardium alter the relation of systolic performance to end-diastolic pressure even at constant contractility. (Submitted.)
13. Rabson J, Permutt S: the role of the pericardium in diastolic interdependence of the right and left ventricles: abstract. *Fed Proc* 37:778, 1978.
14. Carlsson E, Milne ENC: Permanent implantation of endocardial tantalum screws: a new technique for function studies of the heart in the experimental animal. *J Assoc Can Radiol* 19:304–309, 1967.
15. Weiss JL, Frederiksen JW, Weisfeldt MC: Hemodynamic determinants of time-course of fall in left ventricular pressure. *J Clin Invest* 58:751–760, 1976.

## 3.3. BLOOD FLOW DYNAMICS DURING THE HUMAN LEFT VENTRICULAR FILLING PHASE

P. Brun, C. Oddou, P. Dantan, J.P. Laporte,
F. Laurent, P. Perrot

### 1. INTRODUCTION

Interpretation of such common phenomena as left ventricular filling and mitral valve opening or closure is still obscured by disparity between hydrodynamic models, physiological experiment and clinical investigation. Problems such as the anteriority of full mitral opening versus peak mitral flow variations, the respective role of local, viscosity-dominated, or convective vortex formation, or breaking of a jet mechanism for valve closure, remain unsolved (1, 2, 3). The multiple scanning pulsed Doppler velocimetry of the heart, an atraumatic, external, clinical investigation could open a new field of approach of the phenomena related to blood flow in the cardiac cavities in undistorted physiological conditions. This technique, in its present stage, remains semi-quantitative, and of limited applicability and performance; thus our observations concerning the left ventricular rapid filling phase do not pretend to solve any pendant problems, but to demonstrate the feasibility of the method.

### 2. MATERIALS AND METHODS

The ultrasonic velocimeter used was the D.W. Baker pulsed Doppler echocardiographic system (Advanced Technology Laboratories, Bellevue, Washington) with a 3 MHz emission frequency, emitted during very short pulses ($\cong 1$ msec), at a repetition rate of 10 KHz. After quadrature phase detection the Doppler signals were processed in order to display the frequency spectrum (zero-crossing histogram) and its mean value (unused in this work). Sampling zone depth, time-motion echogram and electrocardiographic reference were simultaneously written on a line scan recorder. (Figure 1). A real-time multiscan echocardiographic system (Organon Technika, Rotterdam, The Netherlands) with videorecorder was chosen to control the anatomical locations. Data were gathered on a young normal volunteer, a student in athletic conditions.

*J. Baan, A.C. Arntzenius, E.L. Yellin (eds.), Cardiac Dynamics, 169–181.*

## 2.1. *Data acquisition and spatial coordination*

The probe was located on the thorax on three aligned points the positions of which were previously determined by a multiscan observation giving a satisfactory long axis view of the left ventricle (LV). This observation plane was not perpendicular to the thoracic reference plane, but slightly inclined at a 12° angle. The Doppler probe was equipped with a small collimated spotlight whose beam indicated the direction of the ultrasonic beam. Therefore, the angles between probe and thoracic reference plane could be continuously determined and controlled with a reference map drawn on the laboratory ceiling (Figure 1). On each selected point, the probe was rotated successively by 1.5° steps, in order to cover corresponding sectors manually. For each of these orientations, recordings were made at various depths with steps of 0.5 or 0.25 cm between interventricular septum and posterior wall. These individual recordings included a short sequence of 3 to 10 consecutive cardiac cycles. The purpose was to cover the sector area with discrete sampling zones, taking into account their estimated size (length: 4 mm, diameter: 2 mm) related to the time gate interval and the ultrasonic beam diameter. Knowing the angles formed by the crossing beams, one could derive the respective depths to be selected in order to obtain coordinated samplings (Figure 1).

Unfortunately, a study on time-motion echograms demonstrated a sizeable gap between the two predicted locations of conspicuous anatomical points used as landmark (the junction between left auricular and LV posterior wall and posterior mitral leaflet insertion). The multiscan image

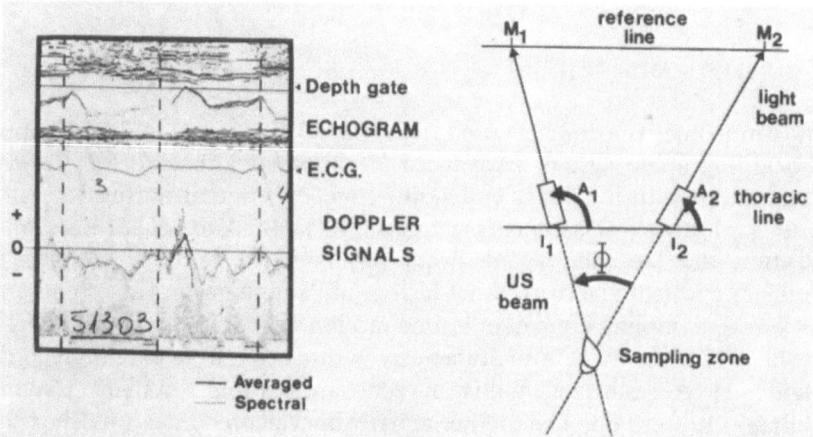

*Figure 1. Left*: simultaneous M-mode and pulsed Doppler display: line scan recorder data. *Right*: multiple beam technique: the ultrasonic probe placed on thorax on points $I_1$ $I_2$, with an orientation given by the spots $M_1$, $M_2$ (angles with the thoracic line $A_1$, $A_2$) explored the same sampling zone (angle between beams $\Phi$).

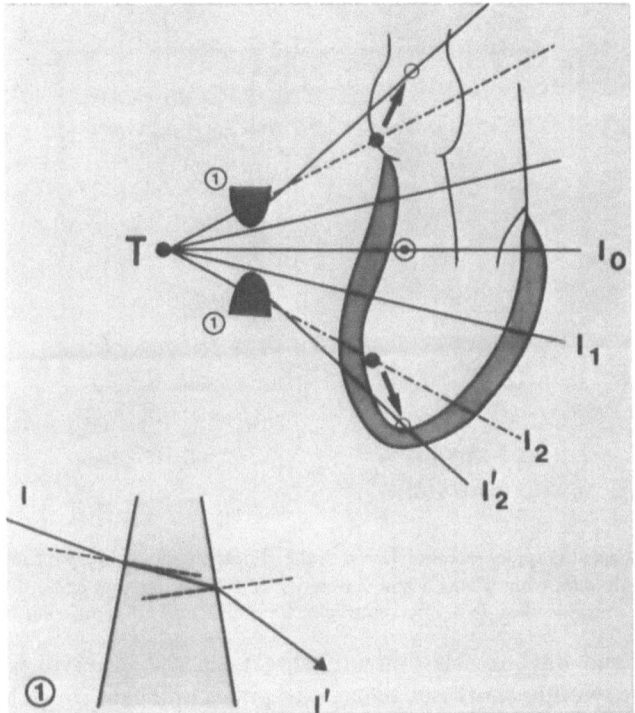

*Figure* 2. Distortion of the ultrasonic beam in the thorax. *Top*: suggested corrections for beam pathways; *bottom*: assumed pathway through a rib.

was used as reference, and it was assumed that: (1) normal or close to normal ultrasonic beams suffered no distortion; (2) oblique beam paths underwent a change in direction by refraction and the ultrasonic velocity increased while crossing the ribs (Figure 2). Doppler locations were empirically modified according to these remarks. Sampling zones from two beams were considered to be coordinated according to a sufficient proximity of their centres. In Figure 3 the overlappings between corrected sector areas can be seen. Aortic valve region and the apical zone of the L.V. remained out of the procedure.

## 2.2. *Data time corrections and post-synchronization*

Data were recorded during a six-hour session, interrupted by short breaks. Cardiac heart rate presented no drastic variations but two types of minor and similar-amplitude variations were observed: (1) variations of cycle duration in short sequences, and (2) variations of mean cycle duration between different sequences. A study on mitral echograms of the same subject demonstrated that: (1) the anterior mitral leaflet (AML.) *F* point was

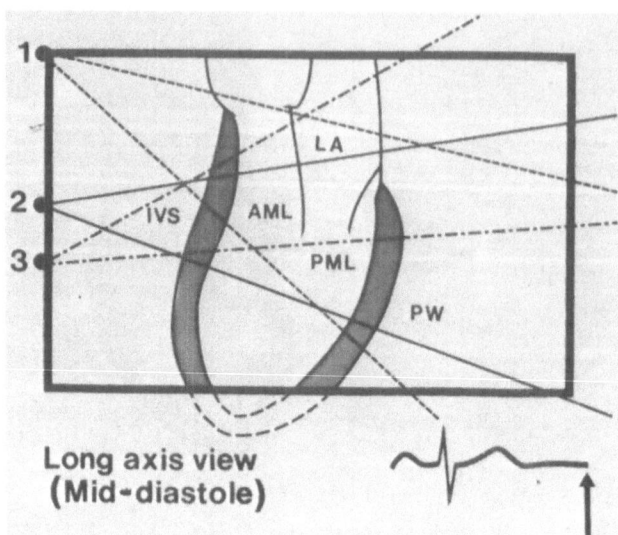

*Figure 3.* Corrected Doppler sectors referred to the multiscan image: 1, 2, 3: probe positions on the thorax (only data from points 1 and 2 were used). LA: left atrium; AML, PML: Anterior and posterior mitral leaflets; IVS: interventricular septum; PW: Left ventricular posterior wall.

constantly and unequivocally identified; (2) the *Q-F* interval was surprisingly stable within short sequences, despite significant respiratory cycle length variations; (3) in contrast, *Q-F* intervals varied if different sequences were considered. These variations measurements were correlated fairly well with the following formula:

$$(QF) = 0.7 \times (RR)^{1/3} \text{ sec}$$

where $(QF)$ is the interval between the electrocardiogram $Q$ wave and mitral $F$ point, and $(RR)$ the cardiac cycle duration; and (4) the duration of the fast-filling period (*D-F* interval on the AML echogram) demonstrated variations too small ($\cong 5$ ms) to be integrated in the computation and was assumed to be constant. In order to synchronize all Doppler recordings, even if the AML was not available on the sampling site, the following rules were applied: (1) the $F$ point was used as time reference, (2) in individual recordings the mean cycle interval was taken into account for rule 3, (3) the $F$ location on the Doppler recordings was derived from the above formula.

### 2.3. *Data processing and velocity field mapping*

The recordings issued from the forty coordinated zones retained were analysed according to the following processes: (1) on both associated sequences a cardiac cycle was randomly selected; (2) the zero-crossing histograms were redrawn according to a continuous and empirically smooth-

ed line; (3) the AML *F* point was chosen as time origin; (4) as a test for
time coherence of both data sources and first qualitative approach of the
flow orientation, the recordings were mixed, as seen in Figure 4; on the
upper base line, above the line the first beam positive values, under the line
the second beam negative values, and vice versa; (5) the documents were
then placed on a digitizing tablet and values were measured in the time
interval from −250 msec to +50 msec (*F* reference), with 10 msec steps.

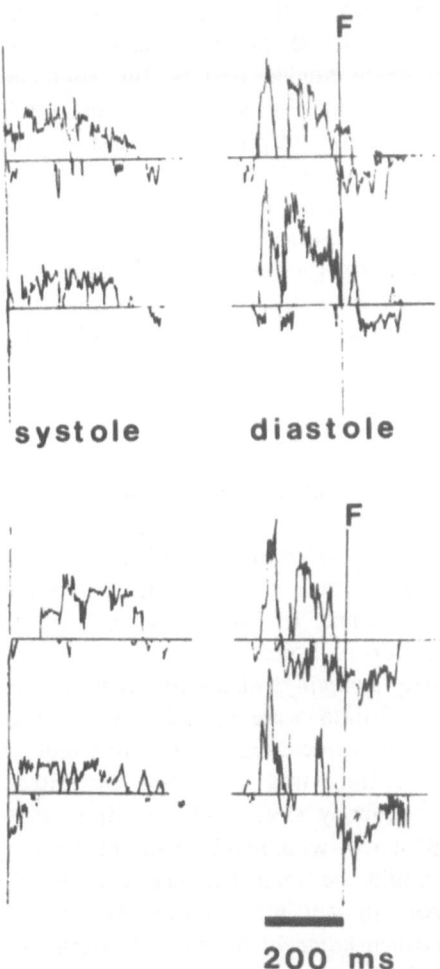

*Figure 4.* Combined frequency shift signals: data from coordinated sampling zones 11 and 22
are displayed. Time reference for systole is the electrocardiogram *Q* wave for diastole the *F*
point of the anterior mitral leaflet echogram. The negative data from beam 1 and beam 2 were
permuted to facilitate chronologic comparison.

The data inputs for a Wang-2200 desk computer were the Doppler frequency shifts, the coordinates of the sampling zones and the beam orientation parameters. All data were stored on flexible discs. Velocity computations were performed using the following algebraic formulae:

$$tg\theta_1 = \frac{1}{\sin \Phi} \frac{F_2}{F_1} - \cos \Phi \quad \text{and} \quad V = \frac{c}{2} \frac{F_1}{F_e} \frac{1}{\cos \theta_1}$$

where $V$ is the velocity component in the plane of observation, $c$ the ultrasonic velocity in blood, $F_e$ the ultrasonic emitting frequency, $F_1$ and $F_2$ the Doppler frequency shifts, $\Phi$ the angle between the beams, derived from corrected values of beam angles, and $\theta_1$ the angle between the velocity vector and one of the beams. Velocity fields were ultimately plotted, each vector being located on its sampling zone and rotated according to the beam orientation. The velocity maps thus obtained illustrated the flow structure in a fixed reference plane system, not related to the moving heart. In the figures the overall motion of the LV was taken into account. An attempt was also made to approximate the instantaneous location of the AML (a) by analysis of the velocity vectors configuration, (b) by available time-motion recordings, and (c) by continuity rules (4).

## 3. RESULTS

1. *Results concerning the similarity of data from one beam sampling zone, same angle, same depth.* If cycle per cycle frequency shifts data were compared in a sequence of consecutive beats, changes appeared, not modifying the overall pattern of the cycle, but occasionally raising or depressing part of the trace. In no case were there major objections to retaining the cycle random choice.

2. *Results concerning samplings along an ultrasonic beam, one beam, fixed angle, various depth.* If data were considered along a beam at different depths, progressive changes occured, as seen in Figure 5. Sampling 1, near the interventricular septum, was unaffected by mitral valve or chordae presence, diastolic frequency shifts were positive, as well as systolic. In sample 9, near the posterior wall, inverted signals were seen in diastole, and a transition zone could be seen between sample 5 and 6, suggesting diverging flow and/or opposite motion valve leaflets.

3. *Comparison between adjacent beams.* Comparison of samplings along different beams in a sector revealed progressive modification from zone to zone. Their significance was difficult to assess.

4. *Comparison between data in a coordinated zone.* The data display used for coordinated zones (Figure 4) facilitated the comparison between information issued from independent beams synchronized for diastolic study (F reference), and revealed apparently a fair coordination of events. For

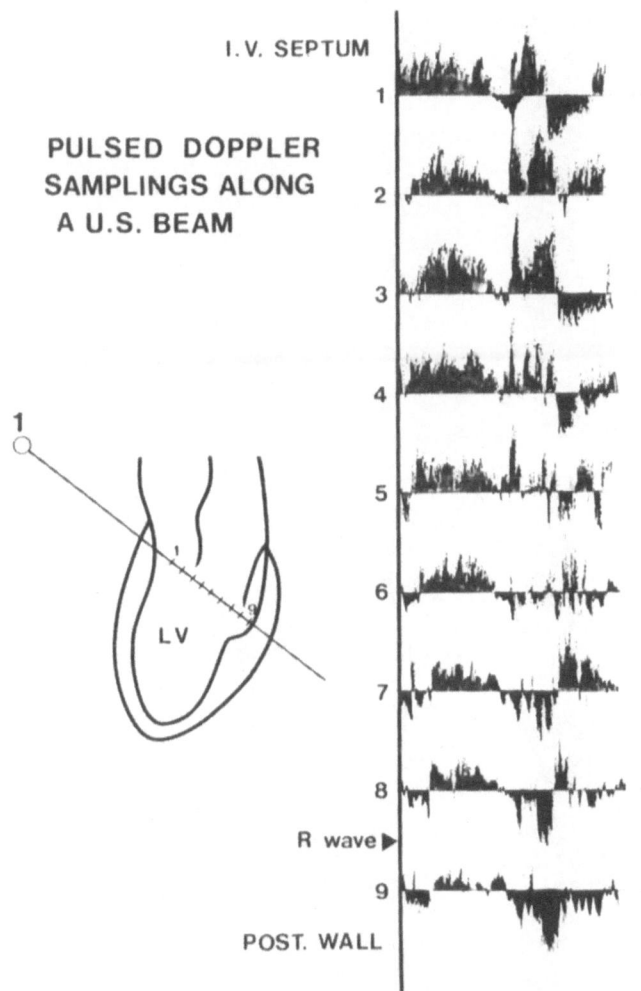

*Figure 5.* An example of Doppler shifts in different locations in the left ventricle (LV): One-beam data from interventricular septum to posterior wall. Time reference is the *R* wave of the electrocardiogram.

instance, a conspicuous phenomenon observed in one beam (an abrupt sign change, for example), would also be present, though not necessarily identically, in the adjacent beam.

### 3.1. *Velocity vector maps during diastole*

Among the instantaneous velocity field maps edited at 10 ms intervals during the fast-filling period, illustrative examples are given in Figure 6. The LV silhouettes (closed aortic cusps, interventricular septum, posterior wall)

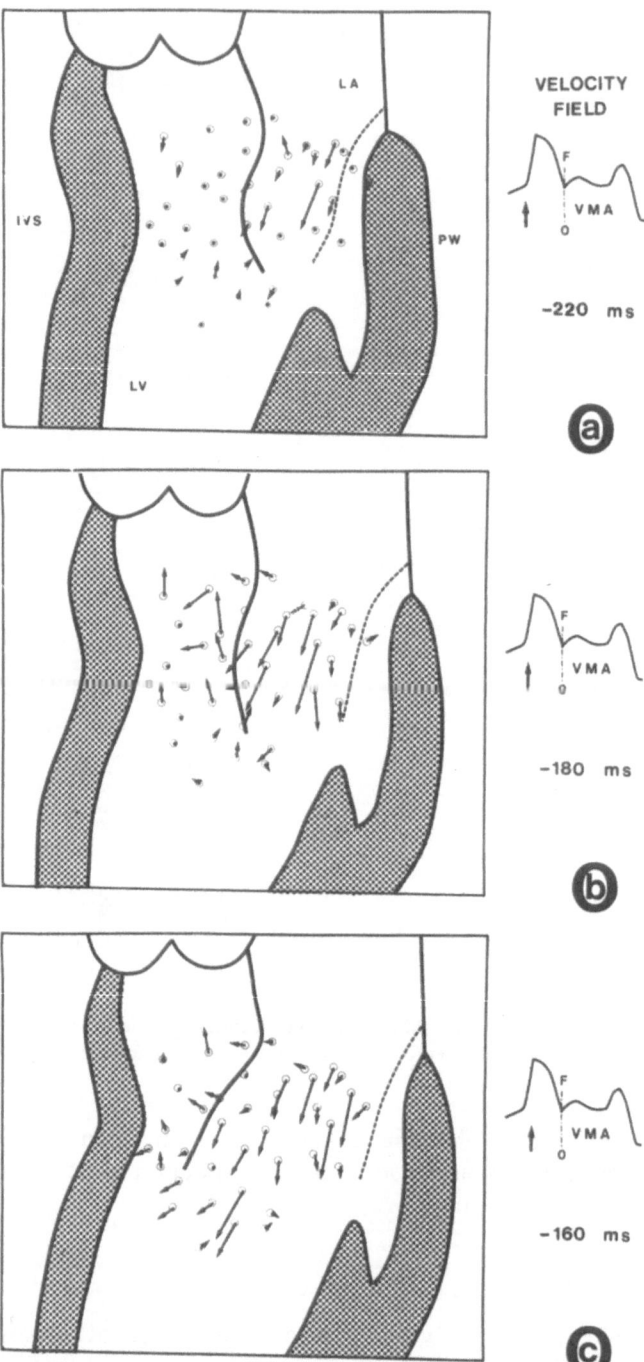

*Figure 6.* Examples of left ventricle velocity field maps: velocity fields in the ventricular cavity during the fast filling phase. Time reference is the *F* point of the anterior mitral leaflet echogram. See text for the positioning of mitral leaflets, interventricular septum (IVS) and

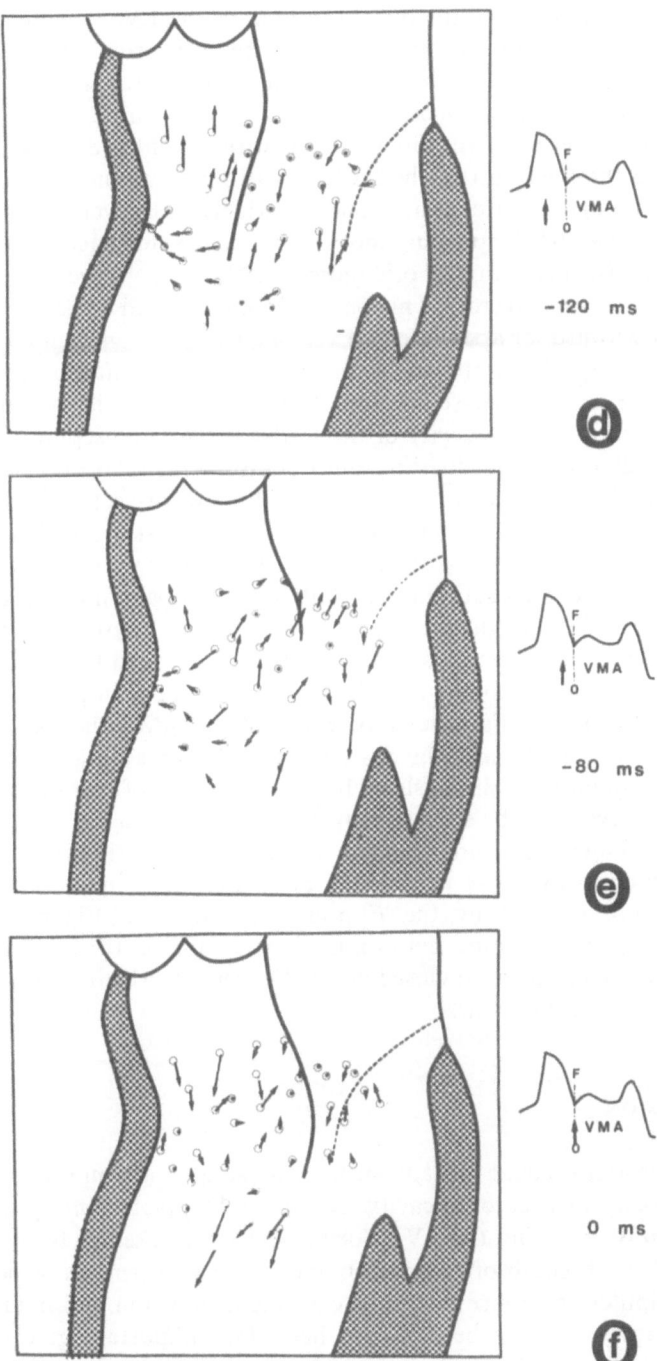

posterior wall (PW), and the velocity vector configurations. LA: left atrium LV: left ventricle, VMA.: anterior mitral leaflet echogram.

included consideration of the overall motion of the LV. The intersection of the AML with the observation plane was deduced from the velocity field analysis and corroborated by the time-motion recordings. The posterior mitral leaflet position was merely hypothetical. One can describe (Figure 6, −220 ms) the onset of the filling phase with downward velocity vectors confined to the inlet part of the LV and valve opening not extended to its tip. At −180 ms, the stream has enlarged widely in the ventricle, the whole leaflet is affected by the opening motion, but as the free edge of the AML is reached, a dispersion in the orientation of the velocity vectors occurred, including ascending vectors. This pattern, characterized by (1) an enlarging zone of downward, or apex-oriented vectors, with concomitant enlargement of the LV cavity, (2) an abrupt dispersion of vector orientation at the tip of the AML, (3) a scattered-vector zone between interventricular septum and the leaflet, and (4) a convexity of the leaflet toward the septum, started as soon as −200 ms and persisting until complete valve opening (Figure 6, −160 ms) where it seemed to vanish. The downward-vector zone extended now to the entire explored area, except the narrow triangle between valve leaflet and septum. This flow structure appeared to be particularly transient. At −120 ms, the AML, still near its fully-opened position and presenting a rectilinear profile, was surrounded by zero (or nearly zero) velocity points in a neutral sheet between an ascending stream anterior to the leaflet and the (still persisting) descending stream behind it. This pattern persisted as long as the so-called first diastolic slope event of the AML did. Afterward, as seen in Figure 6 (−80 ms), the descending-vector area became smaller and the vector amplitudes diminished. In the inlet part of the ventricle, local reversal of flow could be seen. Meanwhile, the ascending vectors in front of the AML rotated and were oriented toward the left atrium and the leaflet shape became convex toward the LV posterior wall. The end of the fast-filling period, marked by the F point, is shown in Figure 6 (0 ms). Descending vectors reappeared in a narrow channel in the inlet part of the ventricle, between the semi-closed cusps. Descending vectors were observed also in the subaortic area.

4. DISCUSSION

Many objections could be advanced against any attempt to determine blood velocity in a cardiac cavity by pulsed Doppler technique, and the present study, mapping the LV velocity field is not exempt from criticism. The problem of length of acquisition and processing periods, which would make computer assistance for both real time acquisition and data processing mandatory, will not be discussed here. Two important questions have been raised already: the need to combine signals issued from different access pathways on the thorax and from different heart beats, before the stage of velocity computation could proceed. This double uncertainty concerning the geometrical coordination of the beams and the synchronization of the heart cycles could have involved massive errors and/or an impossibility to fulfil this mapping project. Our approach was based on the choice of well-established echographic information, more thoroughly tested than pulsed Doppler data. To check the validity of the light beam technique for geometrical adjustment, we took advantage of the presence of anatomical landmarks in the field area (posterior part of the mitral annulus, inter-ventricular septum and posterior wall) but, as mentioned before, comparison led to unexpected results and required a major discussion about propagation of ultrasonic beams in body tissues. The empirical corrections we used were derived from the ultrasonic multiscan imaging method. Due to its parallel beams normal to the thorax, and its multitransducer-focused beam technique, distortion by the ribs was assumed to be negligible. The results of the study on the AML $F$ point chronology by time-motion have permitted us to find an empirical solution to the synchronization problem. However, chronological corrections could not deal with beat to beat small modifications of cardiac stroke volume, a problem which remained unsolved.

If the objects discussed above were thus at least partially resolved major problems remained in the determination of true velocity vectors, such as the complete lack of information about the velocity vector's third component. Also, the classical LV axis view we have chosen may have been only a compromise between inflow and outflow tracts, and not the ideal plane for study of ventricular filling in an assumed axisymmetric fashion. Furthermore, the frequency calibration we used was of low accuracy, the reason why no scales were given on our maps. Nevertheless, an order of magnitude for the mean value of apex-oriented vectors in Figure 6 ($-160$ ms) was 100 cm/s. The zero crossing technique is open to criticism, but the recorded signals never revealed an important range of Doppler frequency shift, which was confirmed by audio control.

A few comments about the results seem relevant:

1. In the specific area located on the proximal or medial parts of the cavity and in proximity of the AML leaflet, comparison of velocity characteristics between three aligned adjacent sampling zones allowed us to evaluate the maximal size of the pulsed Doppler device sampling zone in vivo. For instance, at $-120$ ms the point with zero velocity lying under the AML is surrounded by high amplitude velocity vectors of opposite directions. The same point at $-160$ ms or $-80$ ms contributes to entirely different vector configurations.

2. The apex-oriented vector zone clearly illustrated the course of rapid filling: small and contiguous to the annulus at $-220$ ms, increasing in

length and lateral diameter until − 160 ms and disappearing at − 80 ms. Vector orientations were in good accordance with a jet structure in the initial phase and in the subsequent maps, with the semi-parallel, slightly diverging pattern predicted from mathematical models (5, 6, 7). The vector uneven moduli was intriguing: inequality of their components, if related to geometrical or chronological discrepancies, should have randomly affected one component at a time and modified their orientation. A physiological explanation cannot be excluded: for instance its cause may lie in the uneven mixing in the atrium of the flow streams issued from left and right pulmonary veins as revealed in small atrial septal defects by selective tracer injections.

3. A striking point was a loss of jet structure at the tip of the AML (− 180 ms) appearing less than 40 ms after valve opening, suggesting the formation of small vortices. Such viscous generation could be related to the whipping motion of the leaflet.

4. At − 120 ms an important curved flow localized under the leaflet's free edge and prolonged by a large ascending stream in the entire zone between interventricular septum and AML can be observed. Later on, while the leaflet is rapidly closing, the flow takes a posterior and superior orientation, such that a recirculation process seems to have been generated.

5. Filling flow seems to stop completely during the second diastolic slope of the AML (–80 ms) which is in good agreement with the echographic left ventricular diameter rate of change and cineangiographic volume curves.

6. A stagnation zone appeared as early as − 140 ms and increased in size afterward. Later, in the same area a reversal of flow appeared, but actually no flow crossed the mitral orifice (defined as the leaflets free edge orifice) in a backward direction. The breaking of the jet mechanism could be suggested, contributing to valve closure, though it appears to be slightly preceded by a vortex closure mechanism.

SUMMARY

A first attempt was presented to derive left ventricular blood flow velocity field from ultrasonic Doppler technique in physiological conditions in man. The probe orientation was controlled by reference to a fixed coordinate system. Time motion echocardiography and real-time imaging gave additional information. A manual multiple sector scan procedure was used to create 40 sampling zones in the left ventricular cavity at the intersection of the ultrasonic beams. Problems concerning this geometrical coordination and post-synchronization of different cardiac cycles were solved empirically. Computation was restricted to the velocity component in the observation plane which was assumed to include the ventricular long axis. Estimation of velocity was considered semi-quantitatively only. Results were illustrated by instantaneous velocity maps edited at intervals during the left ventricular fast filling phase. Different flow patterns could be described: (1) a jet flow structure in the inflow tract of the ventricle with a maximal size and an acute peak velocity around the peak of the E wave; (2) various velocity orientations suggesting small and transient vortex formation at the tip of the anterior mitral leaflet, and an important recirculation of increasing magnitude between interventricular septum and anterior mitral leaflet; (3) an early appearing stagnation zone, followed by reversal of flow on the atrial side of the valve. These preliminary results, despite measurement inaccuracies and incompleteness, could lead to subtle insight into the complexity of physiological flow.

REFERENCES

1. Bellhouse BJ: Fluid mechanics of a model mitral valve and left ventricle *Cardiovasc Res* 6:199–210, 1972.
2. Taylor EEM, Wade JD: Pattern of blood flow within the heart: a stable system. *Cardiovasc Res* 7:14–21, 1973.
3. Laniado S, Yellin EL, Kotler M, Levy L, Stadler J, Terdiman R: A study of the dynamic relations between the mitral valve echogram and phasic mitral flow. *Circulation* 51:104–113, 1975.
4. Brun P, Oddou C, Kulas A, Laurent F: Small computer development of echographic information related to left ventricle and mitral valve in diastole. In: *Computers in cardiology,* IEEE catalog 77CH1254–2C, 1977 p 267–273.
5. Oddou C, Brun P, Dantan P, Beraldo E, Kulas A, De Vernejoul F: Fluid mechanics in the human left ventricle during cardiac filling phase. In: *Colloques 71 Paris INSERM,* 1977, p 321–334.
6. Yellin EL, Peskin C: A mathematical solution to mitral flow dynamics and closure of the valve (discussion). In: *The mitral valve,* Kalmanson D (Ed), Acton, Massachusetts, Publishing Sciences, 1976, p 173–181.
7. Yellin EL, Frater RM, Peskin CS, Laniado S: Left ventricular inflow patterns and mitral valve motion: animal studies and computer analysis. In: *Fourth New England bioengineering conference,* Saha S. (ed), Oxford, Pergamon, 1976, p 177–180.

# 3.4. RELAXATION OF THE LEFT VENTRICLE

J.H.M. Nieuwenhuijs, D.J. Venderink

## 1. INTRODUCTION

End-diastolic pressure (EDP) and inotropic state of the left ventricle influence the rising limb of the pressure curve (1, 2). However, little is known of the relaxation of the left ventricle as a function of EDP and inotropic state. There is some evidence that relaxation is a function of the developed force (3).

In this study isovolumically contracting rabbit hearts were used. The representation of the pressure curve of the left ventricle in a phase plot ($dP/dt$ versus $P$) was used to investigate the shape of the pressure-time curve up to maximal pressure (contraction) and the decline of this curve during relaxation. To change the inotropic state of the ventricle extrasystolic beats were generated to attain a potentiated inotropic state in the post-extrasystolic beat. The time interval between the pre-extrasystolic and extrasystolic beat was used as a parameter influencing the inotropic state. The influence of EDP and inotropic state on contraction and relaxation was investigated. The influence of maximal pressure was eliminated by normalization. In the $P - dP/dt$ plot this was achieved by normalizing along both axes. Only differences in the shape of pressure development and relaxation appear in the normalized phase plot.

## 2. METHODS

Experiments were carried out on isolated rabbit hearts perfused by an inorganic solution via an aortic cannula equipped with a countervalve. This valve prevented ejection of fluid when the ventricular pressure exceeded the perfusion pressure. Thus the heart contracted isovolumically. In some experiments this countervalve was replaced by an electric valve, which allowed coronary perfusion during a controlled period of the diastolic pause.

Another cannula, placed in the mitral orifice, connected the left ventricle via an electric valve to a fluid column. This valve was opened during every diastolic pause. The EDP was varied by changing the level of the fluid

J. Baan, A.C. Arntzenius, E.L. Yellin (eds.), Cardiac Dynamics, 183–190.

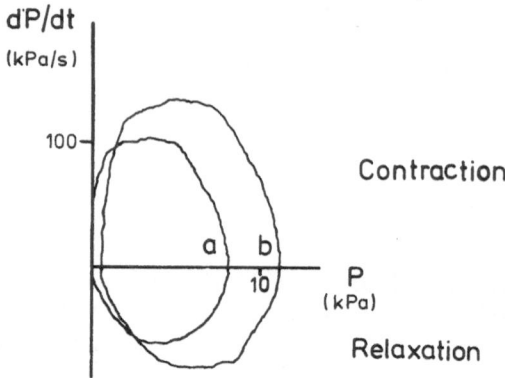

*Figure 1.* The phase plot $dP/dt$ against $P$ for two different pressure curves with EDP of a=0 and b=0.5 kPa.

column. The mitral orifice was also used as access to measure the intra-ventricular pressure with a Millar catheter-tip manometer.

After cauterizing the Hiss bundle to realize a low intrinsic heart frequency, the heart was stimulated by two plate electrodes with intervals from 500 to 1500 msec. For post-extrasystolic potentiation only the stimulation interval preceding the extrasystolic beat had a different length. The pressure and its first derivative were sampled and stored on magnetic tape.

The end-diastolic pressure, the stimulation interval and the perfusion time were varied in a series of experiments. The phase plot ($dP/dt$ versus $P$) was used to distinguish differences between the shape of different pressure curves (Figure 1). Normalizing the phase plots by dividing by $P_{max}$ eliminated its influence (Figure 2). The change in positive surface area (contraction) of this normalized phase plot and the change in the negative surface area (relaxation) were used as a figure of merit to determine differences in form of the pressure curve.

## 3. RESULTS

### 3.1. *Different end-diastolic pressures*

In the left panel of Figure 3 pressure graphs are shown for EDP 0 and 0.5 kPa; the right panel shows the time derivatives for these curves. The phase plane plots for these two EDPs are plotted in Figure 1 while Figure 2 shows the normalized phase plane plots. Both developed pressure and $dP/dt$ were multiplied with a normalization factor ($1/P_{max}$). As can be seen the normalized phase plane plots for different EDPs are equal as are the surface areas beneath the curves for the positive and negative part.

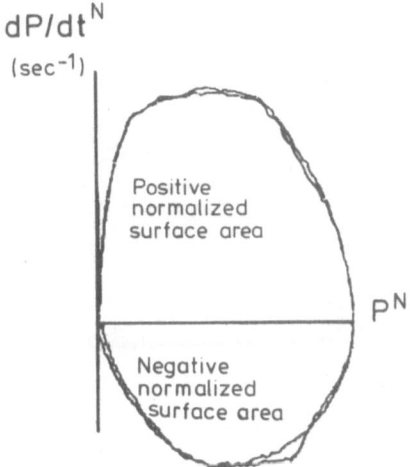

*Figure 2*. Normalized phase plots for two pressure curves with EDP $=0$ and 0.5 kPa. $P^N = P/P_{max}$; $dP/dt^N = (dP/dt)/P_{max}$.

### 3.2. *Extrasystolic potentiation*

Varying the inotropic state by means of post-extrasystolic potentiation (4, 5) resulted in pressure curves for a normal beat (a), an extrasystolic beat (b) and a post-extrasystolic beat (c) shown in Figure 4. The normalized phase plane plots (Figure 5, right) for the normal (a) and post-extrasystolic beat (c) show differences in the positive surface area only. This shows that for the

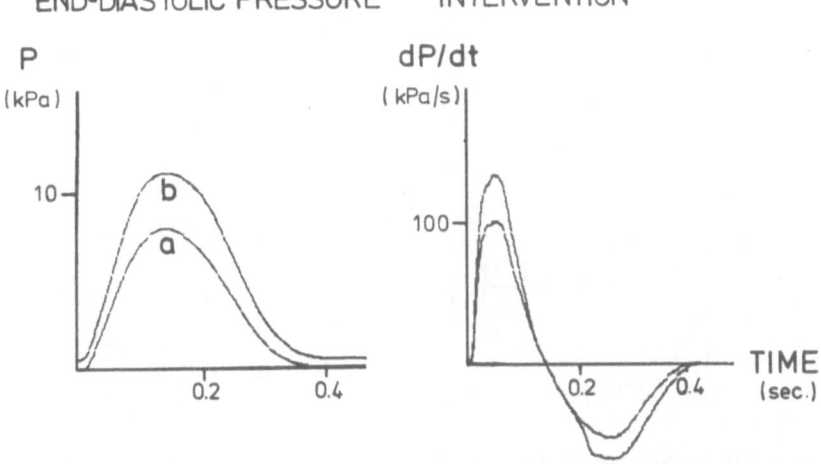

*Figure 3*. *Left*: two pressure curves with EDP of a $=0$ and b $=0.5$ kPa. *Right*: the derivatives of these curves.

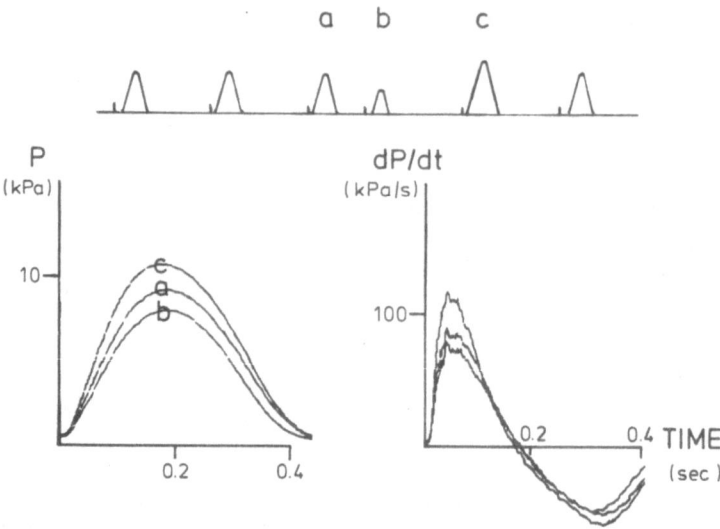

*Figure 4.* Variation in inotropic state by means of extrasystolic potentiation (*top*). *Bottom:* three pressure curves and their derivatives: normal (a), extrasystolic (b) and post-extrasystolic beat (c). Basic stimulus interval was 1200 msec and the extrasystolic interval was 700 msec.

post-extrasystolic beat the inotropic state was increased. For the extrasystolic beat (b, Figure 5, left) the negative surface area differs from the normal beat (a), while the positive surface area is equal. The influence of the extrasystolic interval on the negative surface area shows a significant change for the extrasystolic beat when compared to the post-extrasystolic beat (Figure 6).

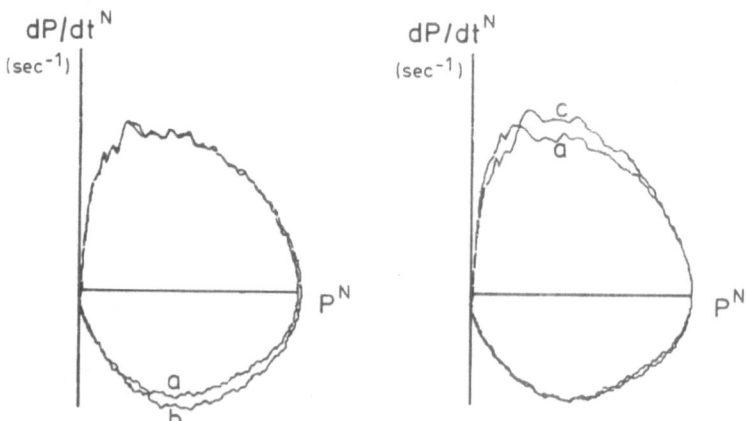

*Figure 5.* Extra systolic intervention, normalized phase plots. *Left:* normal (a) and extrasystolic beat (b). *Right:* normal (a) and post-extrasystolic (c) beat.

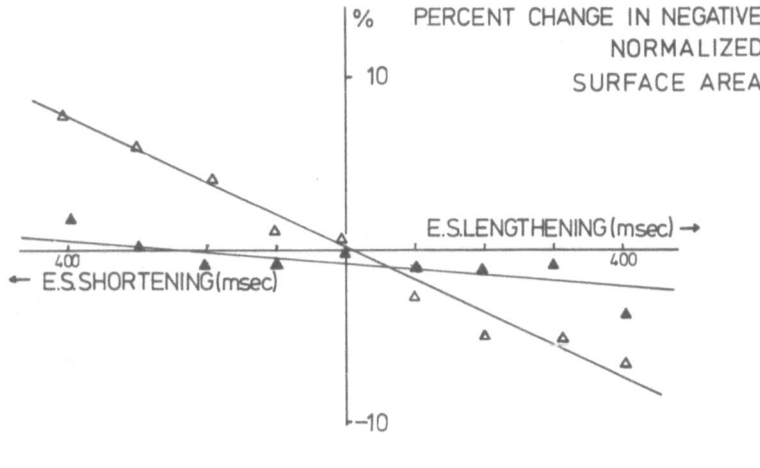

△ = EXTRA SYSTOLIC BEAT
▲ = POST - EXTRA SYSTOLIC BEAT

*Figure 6.* The proportional change in negative surface area of the phase plot for the extrasystolic and post-extrasystolic beat versus extrasystolic interval shortening and lengthening. The proportional change gives an indication for the change in the shape of the pressure curve during the relaxation period.

### 3.3. *Perfusion time variation*

Since the interval changes the shape of the pressure relaxation, we questioned if it was caused by the change in coronary perfusion (6) since the countervalve allows perfusion only during the diastolic pause, which is shortened for the extrasystolic beat. Also, the coronary flow could be affected by the pressure in the short aortic section between the aortic valve and the perfusion valve. Therefore, the influence of perfusion was investigated.

The perfusion time was varied with an electric valve in the perfusion line. In these experiments the perfusion time was shortened during a single diastolic pause. For a beat with decreased perfusion time the results are shown in Figure 7, and for a beat without perfusion in Figure 8. Apparently, there is no influence on the normalized phase plot for perfusion times of more than 100 ms. In the experiments on postextrasystolic potentiation the perfusion time always exceeded 200 ms.

### 4. DISCUSSION

In the first place the experiments show the expected influence of end-diastolic pressure on the developed pressure, both during contraction and

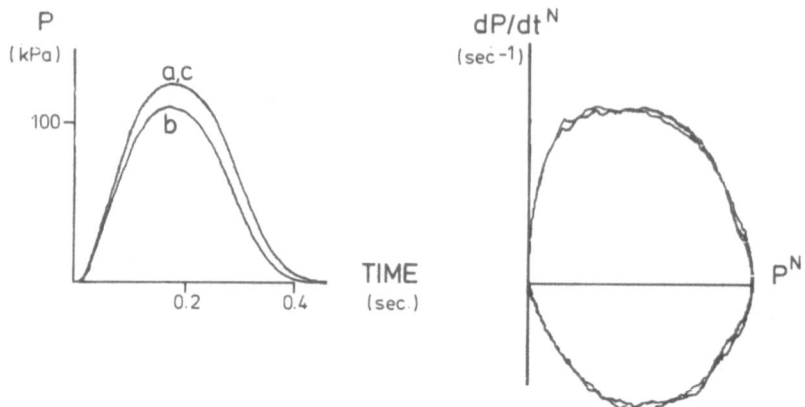

*Figure 7.* Variation in coronary perfusion time. *Left:* pressure curves for a perfusion time of 600 msec (a, c) for 100 msec (b). *Right:* the normalized phase plots for these curves.

relaxation. As in the isolated cardiac muscle preparation (3, 7) the form of relaxation of isovolumically beating hearts is not affected by EDP interventions. The higher inotropic state in post-extrasystolic beats caused no change in relaxation either. This suggests that the rate of ventricular relaxation is determined by the maximum pressure at the onset of isovolumic relaxation. In the extrasystolic beat, however, the relaxation process is affected. The dependency of the relaxation process on the interval was demonstrated (Figure 6). Under the conditions used, any influence of the coronary perfusion time on the relaxation was ruled out.

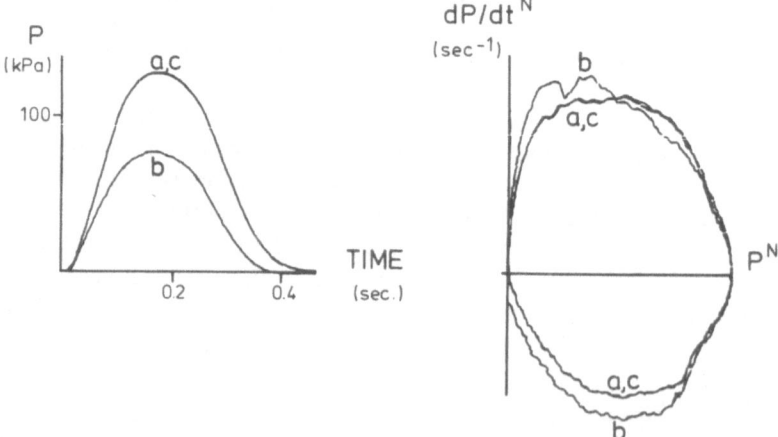

*Figure 8.* As Figure 7, but one curve (b) is without perfusion, and is the only beat with a different normalized phase plot.

It is not clear how the influence of the stimulation interval on the relaxation can be explained.

The objective of these experiments was to assess the influence of EDP and inotropic state on the process of crossbridge formation and annihilation. This influence most likely shows in those periods where the number of active crossbridges changes rapdily: therefore the phase plot was used as it emphasizes deviations in the steep parts of the pressure curve. By normalizing the phase plot the effect of maximal pressure was easily removed.

The underlying idea is that variation in EDP only changes the number of available crossbridge sites and not the process of creation and annihilation of crossbridges (1). Therefore, it should be possible to distinguish between volume dependency and dependency on inotropic state. There is much evidence now that EDP variation also changes the calcium concentration at the onset of contraction. This explains the minor change in the pressure development when varying the inotropic state or EDP, while the maximal pressure differs strongly. It is easier to understand that the relaxation process is identical for both interventions of EDP and inotropic state, because of the same low calcium concentration at that part of the pressure curve.

## SUMMARY

Left ventricular relaxation was studied in isolated rabbit hearts. In isovolumically beating hearts end-diastolic pressure (EDP), stimulation interval, and perfusion time were changed. The primary parameter determining relaxation is the maximal pressure. Minor changes in the pressure curve were investigated by normalizing the plot of $dP/dt$ versus $P$. Pressure and its derivative were divided by the maximal pressure. Variation of EDP did not change the shape of the pressure relaxation, but variation of the stimulation interval did influence this time course.

## ACKNOWLEDGEMENT

We thank P. Schiereck, E.L. de Beer and E. Lopes Cardozo for their critical remarks.

## REFERENCES

1. Boom HBK, Denier van der Gon JJ, Nieuwenhuijs JHM, Schiereck P: Cardiac contractility: actin-myosin interaction as measured from the left ventricular pressure curve. *Eur J Cardiol* 1:217–224, 1973.
2. Nieuwenhuijs JHM, Boom HBK, Denier van der Gon JJ, Schiereck P: Assessment of

myocardial contractility from intraventricular pressure recordings. *Arch Int Physiol Biochim* 82:332–337, 1974.
3. Krueger JW, Strobeck JE: Sarcomere relaxation in intact cardiac muscle. *Eur J Cardiol* 7 (suppl): 79–96, 1978.
4. Kuijer PJP, Heethaar RM, Herbschleb JN, Zimmerman ANE, Meijler FL: Postextrasystolic relaxation in the dog heart. *Eur J Cardiol* 7:133–145, 1978.
5. Werf T van der, Poelgeest van R, Herbschleb HH, Meijler FL: Postextrasystolic potentiation in main. *Eur J Cardiol* 4 (suppl):131–141, 1976.
6. Downey JM: Myocardial contractile force as a function of coronary blood flow. *Am J Physiol* 230:1–6, 1976.
7. Pollack GH, Krueger JW: Sarcomere dynamics in intact cardiac muscle. *Eur J Cardiol* 4 (suppl): 53–65, 1976.

# 3.5. INTRAMURAL STRESS AND STRAIN ANALYSIS IN THE INTACT HEART

ROBERT M. HEETHAAR, KHALED EL-SHURAYDEH, TJEERD VAN DER WERF

## 1. INTRODUCTION

To meet the demands of the body the heart needs to propel a required amount of blood. Forces generated during contraction of the individual cardiac muscle fibres result in intramural stresses and strains which lead to intraventricular pressures. Up till now indices for cardiac function, derived from pressure data, have not been satisfactory (1). This is partly due to the reflection of the contraction of all contributing wall segments; effects of regional disturbances are not clearly represented by those parameters. Therefore, especially since coronary artery disease leads to regional myocardial damage, the need for regional contractile parameters is generally felt. In this study regional parameters have been determined using overall pressure and local geometry (changes). Regional stresses and strains were derived from measurements of momentaneous cardiac geometry and transmural pressures.

## 2. METHODS

### 2.1. *Finite element analysis*

2.1.1. *Stress and strain computation from measured pressure, geometry and ventricular elasticity:* Computation of stresses and strains in any desired point of a complex elastic continuum (like the heart) cannot yet be done unless this continuum is approximated by an assemblage of subregions (or elements), each with specified elastic properties. The finer the degree of partitioning into elements the closer the solution will approximate the real situation. On the other hand, a finer partitioning implies more elements and requires larger computer facilities and longer computation times (2). In our case a partitioning of the ventricular wall is chosen so that from epicardium to endocardium three different layers of elements can be taken. This is done to be able to implement global fibre orientations in a further stage.

Cross-sections of the heart, or left ventricle (see below), were partitioned into triangular elements. Vertices (*nodes*) of triangles of adjacent cross-

J. Baan, A.C. Arntzenius, E.L. Yellin (eds.), Cardiac Dynamics, 191–196.

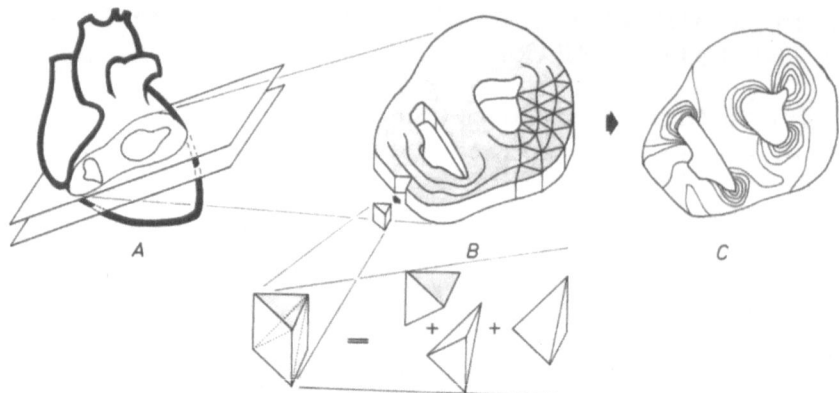

Figure 1. To apply the finite element technique cross-sections of the heart (A) from base to apex were partitioned in triangular elements (B). In (C) equi-stress lines are plotted.

sections were interconnected so that a three-dimensional structure was obtained consisting of up to 7000 tetrahedrons (Figure 1). This structure is loaded by the corresponding left ventricular pressure. If the pressure falls to zero this structure will deform ("shrink") to an assumed unstrained state. When the elastic properties of the elements, the pressure and the geometry are known the deformations of the elements to the unstrained state can be computed using the finite element theory (3). In principle this is done by solving the set of equations $[K]\{\delta\} = \{F\}$, in which $[K]$ represents the stiffness matrix of the ventricle(s); $\{F\}$ a set of forces equivalent to the transmural pressures, and acting only on the nodes; and $\{\delta\}$ a column vector of unknown nodal displacements. From the (solved) displacements the *change* of intramural stress and strain from the strained to the unstrained state can be computed. Since, in early diastole, the myocardium is assumed to be unstrained the abovementioned changes indicate also the stress and strain values in the strained state.

2.1.2. *Global elasticity determination from external work and strain energy.* By considering the ventricular myocardium during diastole as homogeneous, isotropic, and linear-elastic, the elastic modulus is constant throughout the myocardial wall. The external work $\omega$ done by the heart during the transition from phase 1 to 2 can be derived from the pressure-volume relationship:

$$\omega = \int_{1}^{2} P dV$$

At the same time the strain energy of the ventricular walls increases by an amount $U$:

$$U = \tfrac{1}{2} \sum_i \{\delta_i\}\{F_i\}$$

In this last expression the nodal displacements $\{\delta_i\}$ depend linearly on the global elastic modulus $E$. By equating both expressions the value of this modulus can be computed.

2.1.3. *Regional elasticity determination from nodal displacements*: In the basic equation of the finite element theory, $[K]\{\delta\} = \{F\}$, $\{F\}$ represents a column vector of forces acting upon the nodes and having the same effect on the structure as the transmural pressure; $[K]$ is the stiffness matrix of the object and $\{\delta\}$ the column vector of nodal displacements. The above-mentioned equation indicates a set of linear equations: $\Sigma_i k_{ji} \delta_i = F_j$, in which the coefficients $k_{ji}$ depend linearly on the elastic modulus. If subregions of the heart are assumed to have different elastic moduli $E_i$ the coefficients $k_{ji}$ will be linear functions of these moduli. Rearranging the terms in $[K]\{\delta\} = \{F\}$ will lead to $[M]\{E_i\} = \{F\}$ in which now the coefficients $m_{ij}$ of the matrix $[M]$ are linearly dependent on the displacements. When a displacement field is known the matrix $[M]$ can be constructed and the equation solved for regional elastic moduli. Analysis of regional myocardial elasticity thus requires a displacement field of nodal coordinates. Displacements of epicardial and endocardial nodes can be identified as far as they correspond to (anatomical) markers. Intramural nodes however cannot be traced yet throughout the cardiac cycle. Therefore, subregions of equal myocardial elasticity are chosen throughout the ventricular wall in a first attempt to analyse regional elasticity. By mapping two geometries, before and after a quick injection of a certain volume $\Delta V$ into the ventricle, surface displacements are found using anatomical (papillary muscle) or artificial markers (lead beads stitched on the heart).

2.2. *Isolated working left ventricle and intact heart preparation*

Experiments for the computation of stress and strain distributions in the isolated left ventricle and intact heart have been described previously (4, 5). A brief outline is given below. The isolated working left ventricle or intact heart was perfused with dextran in Ringer's solution containing 10% X-ray contrast medium at controlled filling pressure and output resistances. The ventricle was positioned in front of an X-ray imaging system and rotated 180° about the apex-to-base axis in increments of 5.4° every second heart cycle. The ventricle was electrically paced in synchrony with the 60-cycle X-ray pulses. From each angle of view X-ray silhouettes were recorded on videotape throughout the cardiac cycle. Cross-sections of the ventricle from base to apex (approximately 1 mm apart) were computed using algebraic reconstruction techniques.

## 2.3. *Patient data*

In our catheterization laboratory the geometry of the human left ventricle was obtained from cineventriculograms after contrast injection. The endocardial borders were outlined by hand using a light pen. Wall thickness was measured either echocardiographically or from the frontal X-ray projection of the free wall of the left ventricle. This value was assumed to be the same over the whole ventricular wall. The ventricular cavity was considered as a set of parallel ellipses the long and short axes of which were obtained from the X-ray projection.

## 3. PRELIMINARY RESULTS

Stress and strain computations were done in diastole assuming the myocardium to be homogeneous, isotropic and linear-elastic. In Figure 2 circumferential stress distributions are presented for cross-sections from base to apex of the isolated working left ventricle. By comparing these values for subsequent phases during the filling phase an impression of stress and strain generation in the myocardium is obtained.

Stresses and strains in the human left ventricle and intact dog heart were also computed. Similar results as for the isolated left ventricle were found: highest stresses and strains were generally computed to exist at the endocardial subregions, gradually decreasing transmurally. However in some cases, depending on the local radius of curvature and wall thickness, *local* stress and strain maxima were found intramurally.

## 4. DISCUSSION

Methods of measuring intramural stress and strain distributions in the heart do have large experimental difficulties and are only informative for the state of strain of a small part of the object under study corresponding to the site of the measuring device. A direct method to verify the computed stress and strain fields in the myocardium is not yet available. To check the developed finite element technique it was applied to thick-walled hemispheres, for which the analytic solutions are found in the classical theory of elasticity (6). For those specific cases a very close correspondence was found between the finite element and the analytical solutions. Therefore it was

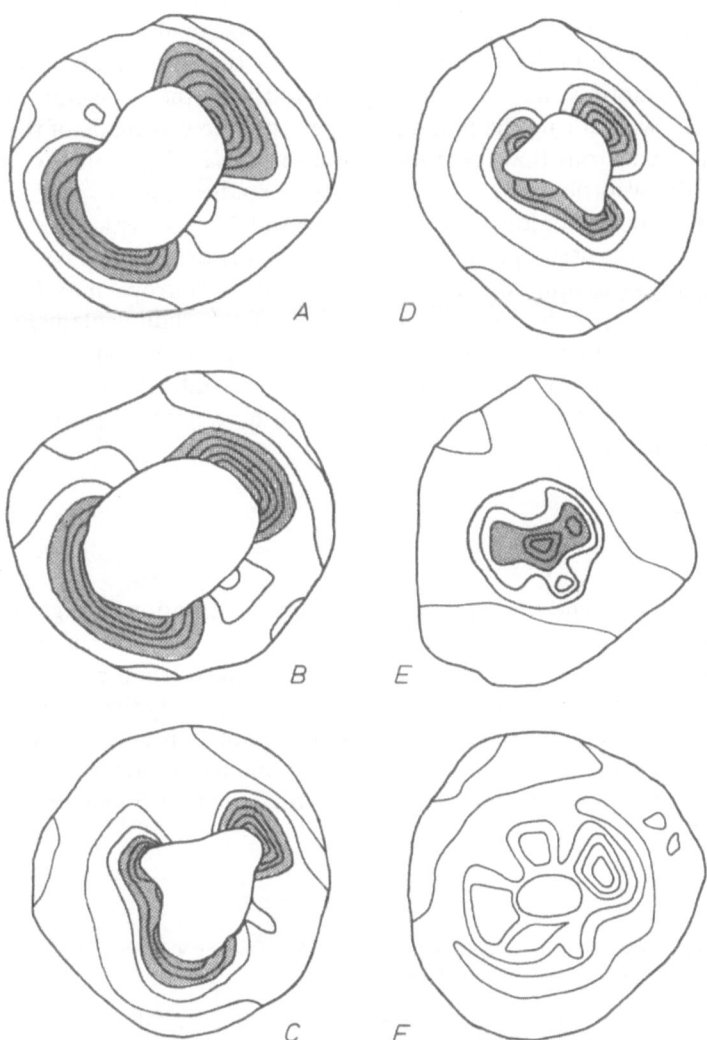

*Figure 2.* Circumferential stress distributions in cross-sections from base to apex ($A \rightarrow F$) of the isolated working dog left ventricle during diastole. Stresses are normalized on the left ventricular pressure (LVP). In the darkest areas stresses exceed LVP, in the white areas stresses are less than 0.5 LVP, in the remaining areas stresses are between LVP and 0.5 LVP. The cross-sections are scaled in $y$-direction to obtain equal-sized plots. Poisson ratio was taken 0.4, global elasticity $10^5 \mathrm{N/m^2}$.

concluded that, under the assumptions made, the stress and strain values computed in the myocardium were representative of the real values.

The method applied considers the heart at a particular moment as a non-moving structure under internal pressure. For the sake of simplicity effects of cardiac motion are being disregarded. From the acceleration of the ventricular wall during the filling phase an estimate was made of the inertial forces. It turned out that these forces were less than 5% of the nodal forces due to the ventricular pressure. In these studies the myocardium was considered to be homogeneous, isotropic and linear-elastic. For the diastolic phase these assumptions are reasonably correct. For the systolic phase however these assumptions lose their validity. Anisotropy may have to be introduced due to the intrinsic anisotropy of the sliding filaments of the sarcomere and their complex anatomical composition. The model used, however, could allow for anisotropy as well as inhomogeneity. Regional elastic moduli can be implemented as soon as reliable experimental data become available.

SUMMARY

A finite element method is presented for the computation of regional stress and strain distributions in the heart from the momentaneous cardiac geometry, transmural pressures and elasticity. This method can also be used to compute the global modulus of elasticity of the myocardium from the external work done by the heart during the transition between two phases in the cardiac cycle and the corresponding change in strain energy of the ventricular walls. Regional myocardial elasticity can also be analysed using this method.

ACKNOWLEDGEMENT

The authors wish to thank Dr. E.L. Ritman and co-workers for their willingness to provide us with the 3D canine cardiac reconstruction data.

REFERENCES

1. Bos GC van den, Elzinga G, Westerhof N, Noble MIM: Problems in the use of indices of myocardial contractility, *Cardiovasc Res* 7:834–848, 1973.
2. Heethaar RM, Pao YC, Ritman EL: Computer aspects of three-dimensional finite element analysis of stress and strain in the intact heart, *Comp Biomed Res* 10:271, 1977.
3. Zienkiewicz OC: *The finite element method in engineering science*, London, McGraw-Hill, 1978.
4. Ritman EL: Left ventricular function and myocardial contractility. *Mayo Clinic Proc* 50:147–156, 1975.
5. Heethaar RM, Robb RA, Pao YC, Ritman EL: Three-dimensional stress and strain analysis in the intact heart. *Proc San Diego Biomed Symp* 15:337–342, 1976.
6. Love AEH: *A treatise on the mathematical theory of elasticity*, New York, Dover, 1926.

## 3.6. EFFECTS OF INTRAVENOUS ISOSORBIDE DINITRATE ON FILLING PRESSURES AND PUMP FUNCTION IN PATIENTS WITH REFRACTORY PUMP FAILURE

Babeth Rabinowitz, Israel Tamari,
Henry N. Neufeld

### 1. INTRODUCTION

The role of vasodilators in the therapy of pump failure has been a subject of intensive investigation. Conflicting results have been reported about the mechanism of action of nitroglycerine and of isosorbide dinitrate. Some authors (1, 2, 3, 4) found these agents active peripherally only on the venous side of the circulation, thus merely affecting filling pressures, but others reported significant effects on the arterial side of the circulation, in particular on the so-called resistance vessels, manifested by afterload reduction and increase of cardiac output (5, 6, 7). These apparently contradictory results might be explained by the different nitrates used, by the different routes of administration, but most probably by the type of patients treated and their initial hemodynamics (8).

The present study was aimed at investigating the hemodynamic effects of isosorbide dinitrate (ISDN) administered by intravenous infusion in patients with severe refractory pump failure.

### 2. METHODS

Fifteen critically ill patients with severe pump failure, mainly on the left, were studied. The group comprised 13 men and 2 women and the age range was 48 to 77 (mean: 58.8). Twelve patients had coronary heart disease, all with a history of recurrent myocardial infarction. One patient had rheumatic aortic insufficiency (grade IV) and moderate mitral insufficiency and two had congestive cardiomyopathy. Three of the coronary patients had significant mitral regurgitation and one had a ruptured septum. The other nine coronary patients received the therapeutic trial with i.v.ISDN during an acute ischaemic episode which worsened a previously severe clinical condition. Seven of the patients (four of the coronary group, the patient with the aortic insufficiency and the two diagnosed as cardiomyopathy) had undergone cardiac catheterization and angiography, to establish their diagnosis and to evaluate their cardiac function. The patient with aortic insufficiency was the only one considered operable, although at very high risk, and was put on i.v. ISDN prior to surgery. Four coronary patients who had undergone angiography were considered inoperable on grounds of too-depressed cardiac function with low ejection fraction. The other eight coronary patients were not even considered for angiographic study, since all had extreme cardiomegaly with very poor contractions on fluoroscopic, radiographic, and echocardiographic examinations.

All patients were in severe distress, dyspneic and hypoxic and had radiographic evidence of pulmonary venous congestion prior to i.v. ISDN administration. As stated before, they were not relieved by conventional prior therapy.

## 2.1. Hemodynamic measurements

A thermodilution triple-lumen balloon-tipped catheter was introduced via an antecubital vein and right atrial (RA); pulmonary arterial (PA) and pulmonary capillary wedge (PCW) pressures were continuously monitored. Cardiac output (CO) was measured in triplicate by the thermodilution technique with a bedside computer. Arterial blood pressure (AP) was measured from cuff readings and the following quantities were calculated: mean Arterial Pressure (AP), Cardiac Index (CI), Stroke Volume Index (SVI), Stroke Work Index (SWI), Systemic Vascular Resistance (SVR), and Pulmonary Vascular Resistance. After the baseline hemodynamics were established the patients entered the study only when the measurements showed PCW pressure to be higher than 20 mmHg and systolic arterial pressure to be above 90 mmHg.

An i.v. infusion of ISDN* in glucose 5% was administered in doses of 2 to 8 mg/hour. The hemodynamic measurements were recorded 15 minutes and 1 hour after the beginning of therapy. If improvement, i.e. decrease in PCW, was slight or absent, the dose was increased. The rate at which the dose was increased varied from 1 to 3 mg/hour depending on the clinical condition of the patient and the hemodynamic parameters. The dose at which "optimal" PCW, AP and CO for the individual patient was achieved was maintained for at least 24 hours; this dosage point was considered "optimal" for each subject and the hemodynamic data, obtained at this particular dose level, are reported below.

## 3. RESULTS

### 3.1. Hemodynamic profile

The initial mean PCW pressure, which in 14 cases was not significantly different from the diastolic pulmonary artery pressures, ranged from 20 to 40 mmHg (Figure 1). Significant decreases of the mean PCW were observed

---

*Kindly supplied as Isoket ampoules by Pharma Schwarz Laboratories, Mannheim, Federal Republic of Germany.

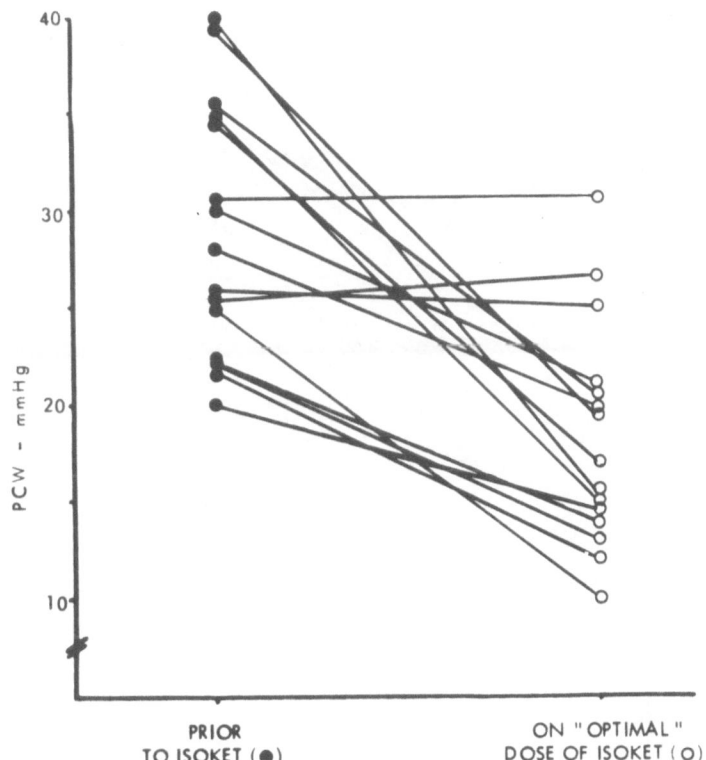

*Figure 1.* Effect of i.v. isosorbide dinitrate (Isoket) on pulmonary capillary wedge (PCW) pressure in 15 patients.

in 12 patients while 3 patients did not respond to therapy. CO was measured serially at each dose level in 12 of the patients, showing significant increases in 9 of them (Figure 2). SVR calculated in those 12 patients showed decreases in 10 patients (Figure 3). It is obvious that it did not change in patients who started at very low SVR values since probably they had already vasodilated their peripheral tree to its maximal capacitance.

Mean AP (Figure 4) was substantially and favourably decreased in those patients who had high initial arterial pressures; in the other patients it was not markedly affected.

The changes in heart rate (Figure 5) illustrated a pattern similar to that of the arterial pressure. Figure 6 illustrates the left ventricular function curves, constructed from the relation between PCW pressure, considered to reflect left ventricular filling pressure, and simultaneous measurements of CO.

The patients who had documented significant ischaemic mitral insufficiency appeared to benefit more markedly from the therapy; along with the decrease in filling pressures, the giant "V" waves on the PCW and PA

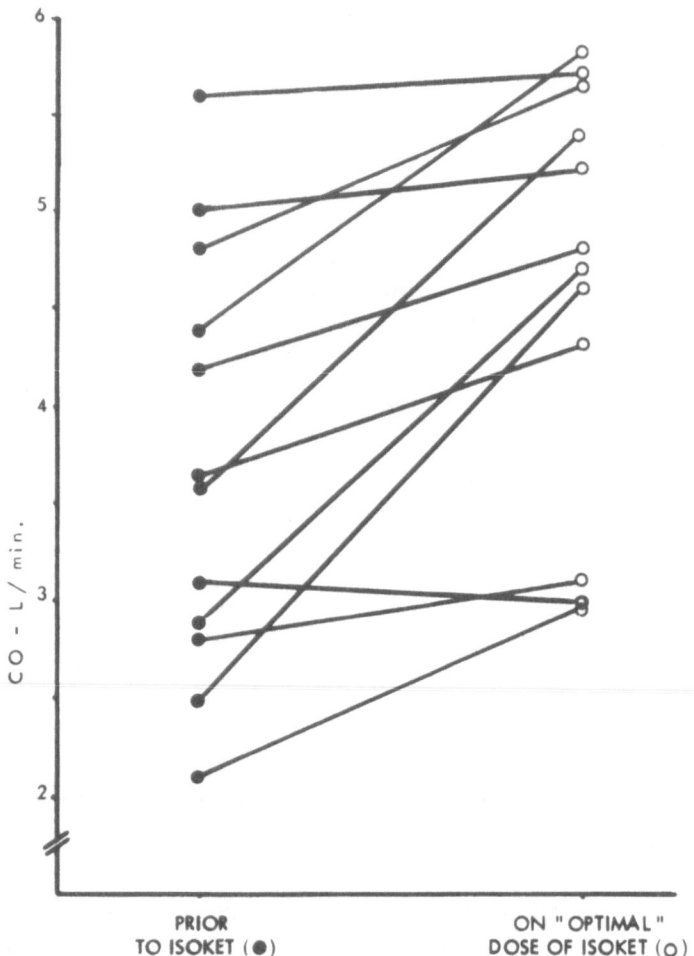

*Figure 2.* Effect of i.v. isosorbide dinitrate on cardiac output (CO) in 12 patients.

pressures and the murmur disappeared during optimal therapy (Figure 7).

A patient with rheumatic mitral insufficiency (Grade II) and aortic insufficiency (Grade IV) also benefited considerably from the treatment.

## 3.2. *Clinical results*

As described earlier, significant hemodynamic improvement was obtained in 12 cases. In each of these cases, the improvement of the hemodynamic parameters was paralleled by clinical and radiologic improvement. In 3 cases, trials to discontinue the ISDN infusion produced reappearance of

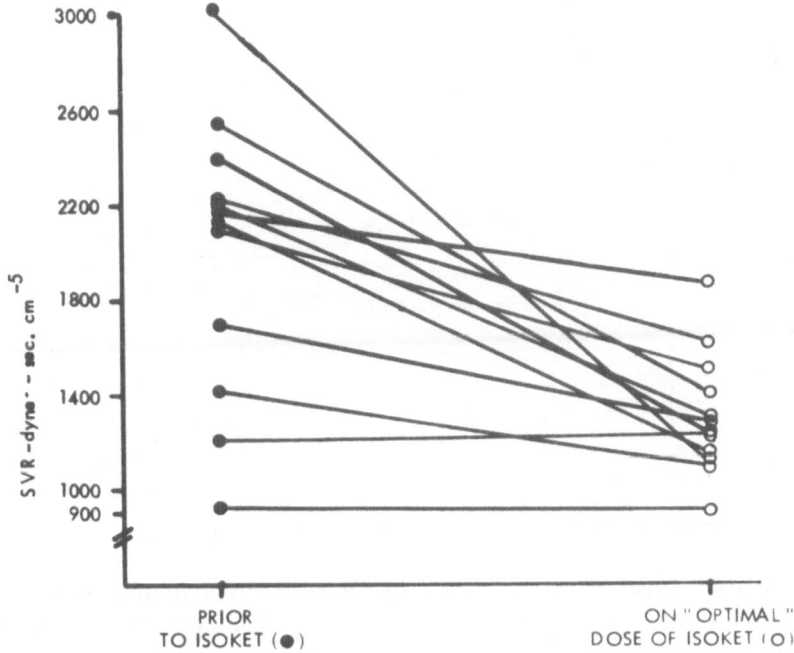

*Figure 3.* Effect of i.v. isosorbide dinitrate on systemic vascular resistance (SVR) in 12 patients.

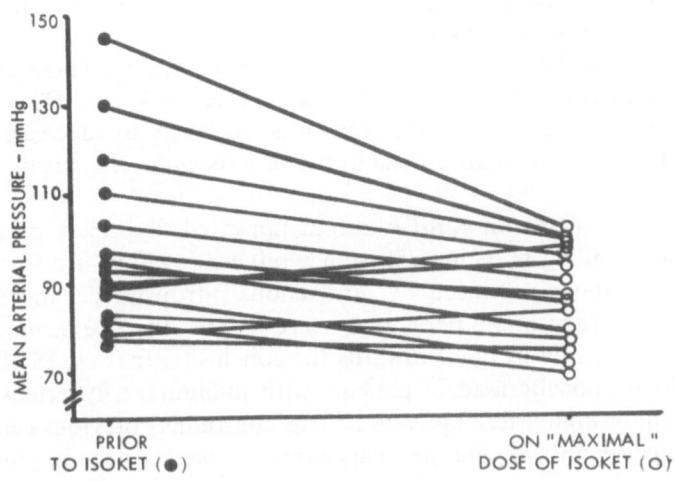

*Figure 4.* Effect of i.v. isosorbide dinitrate on mean arterial pressure in 15 patients.

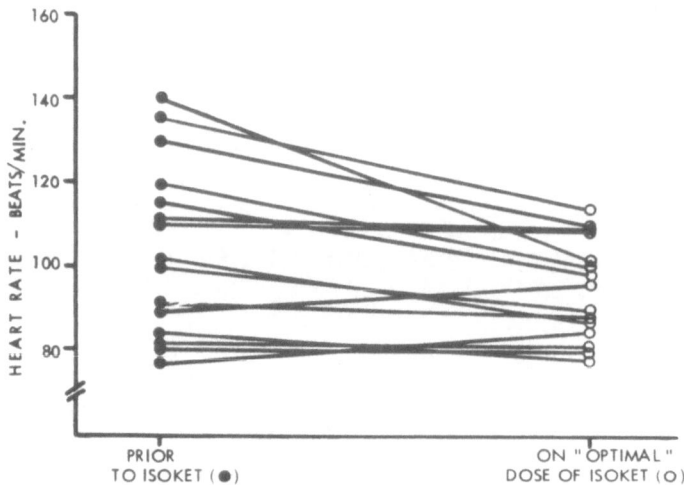

*Figure 5.* Effect of i.v. isosorbide dinitrate on heart rate in 15 patients.

pulmonary congestion and worsening of the hemodynamic profile; resumption of the treatment was followed by a marked improvement. In only 7 cases were we able to decrease the i.v. ISDN dose gradually and replace it by sublingual and oral high doses of ISDN.

4. DISCUSSION

The present study has demonstrated that ISDN administered intravenously in patients with severe pump failure, manifested clinically by left-sided failure, has remarkably favourable hemodynamic effects. These effects include substantial decreases of filling pressures, i.e. PCW and PA pressures, and increases of CO and SWI; this was achieved by decreasing total peripheral vascular resistance without deleteriously affecting aortic pressure and heart rate.

The positive effects on cardiac output appeared to be less pronounced than those on filling pressures. These hemodynamic effects are very similar in quality to those produced by intravenous nitroprusside and to those produced by prazosin in refractory heart failure (9). The hemodynamic changes observed by us point towards the conclusion that i.v. ISDN affects both preload and afterload in patients with pulmonary hypertension and with normal or high arterial pressures. This contradicts previous claims that nitrates affect mainly or only the "capacitance" vessels or the venous side of the peripheral circulation (1, 2). It appears to us from the results of the present study that ISDN also affects the arterial side of the peripheral tree,

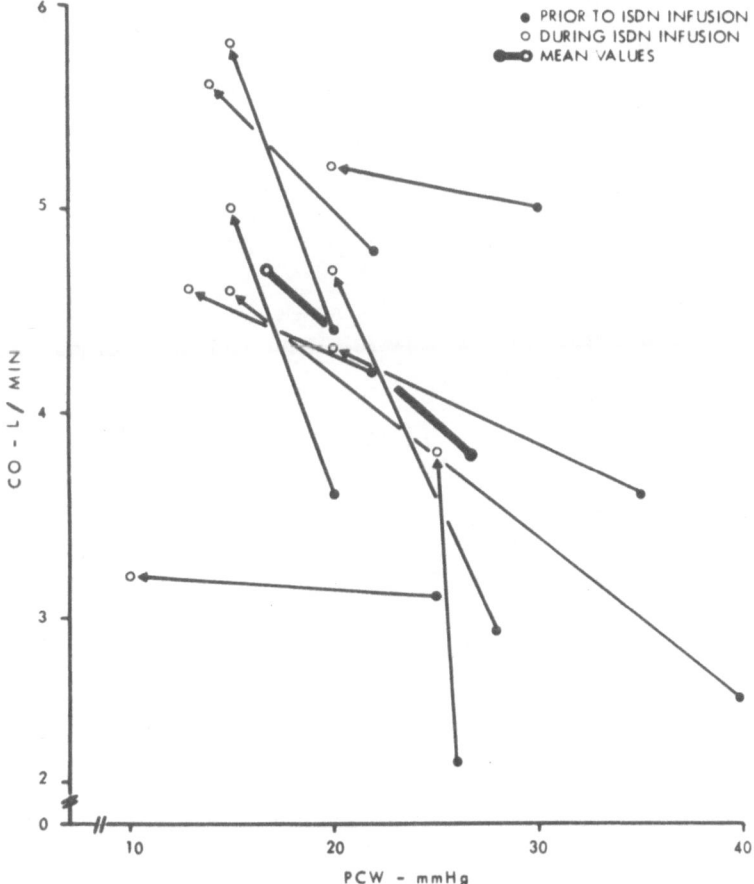

*Figure 6.* Effect of i.v. isosorbide dinitrate on left ventricular function curves in 10 patients.

the so-called "resistance" vessels. Apparently it does so more mildly than other agents such as nitroprusside or alpha-blocking agents, which are reported to produce sharp decreases in arterial pressures. These findings are in agreement with those reported by Bussman and Schupp (5) and by Baligadoo and Chiche (8). According to the findings of these authors, i.v. ISDN also appears to have an advantage over i.v. nitroglycerine by not inducing undesirable sharp decreases of AP. Reports on the effects of ISDN administered i.v. are very scarce and some of them deal with studies in acute infarction, not necessarily accompanied by pulmonary congestion. From these studies and from others dealing with orally or sublingually adminis-tered nitrates, it appears that beneficial effects on afterload with increases in cardiac output are obtained only in the presence of left ventricular failure,

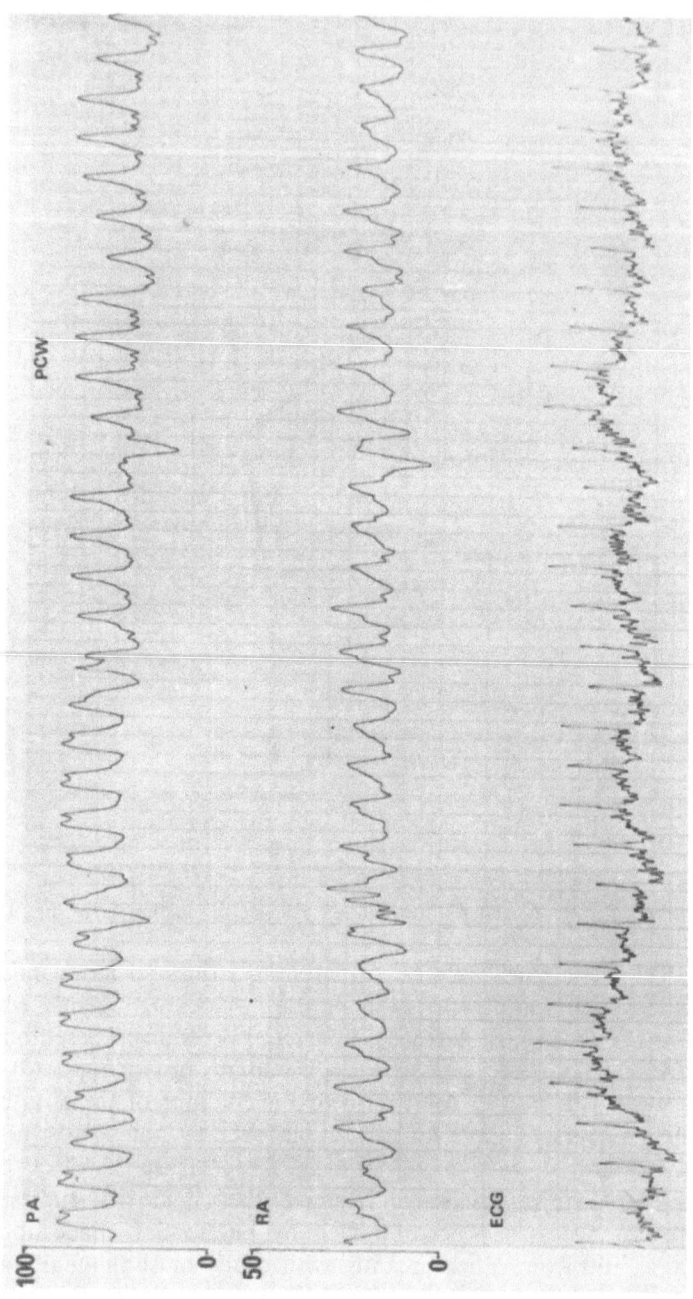

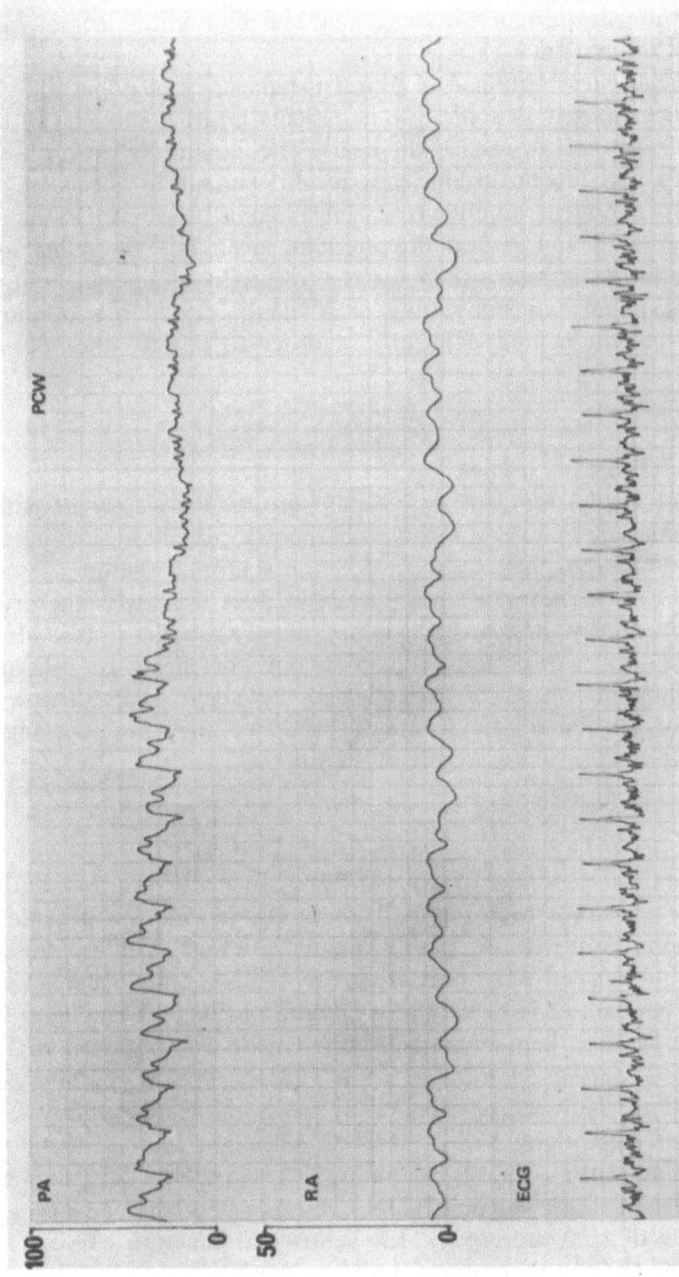

*Figure 7.* Effect of i.v. isosorbide dinitrate in a patient with mitral regurgitation before treatment; during ISDN. PA: pulmonary artery pressure; PCW: pulmonary capillary wedge pressure; RA: right atrial pressure. Scales in mmHg.

i.e. high filling pressures. Therefore, the apparently contradictory results existing in the literature on nitrates might be due to two reasons: different routes of administration of the drug, and different initial hemodynamic conditions of the patient.

The beneficial effect obtained in mitral insufficiency of ischaemic origin manifested dramatically in some of our patients is similar to that of other vasodilator drugs used to unload the heart. The favourable effect observed in the patient with aortic insufficiency is also similar to effects of other afterload reducing agents and it proves once again that i.v. ISDN acts not only at the preload, but also at the afterload level. The variability in the individual response is responsible for the variability found in "optimal" dosage. Thus, in any clinical setting, it is mandatory in our opinion to monitor the patient hemodynamically in order to achieve the "optimal" dosage and thus to avoid side effects.

### 4.1. Clinical implications

The beneficial results reported by us in a group of severely ill patients appear to encourage the use of ISDN intravenously, in left heart failure not responsive or only partially responsive to conventional therapy. It might become the i.v. vasodilator of choice, since it does not lower the arterial pressure inadvertently. Besides being a peripheral vasodilator, it is also an anti-anginotic drug with direct coronary vasodilator effects. Its role in the therapy of different subsets of patients with ischaemic heart disease and with acute myocardial infarction and its possible role in preserving the ischaemic myocardium need further evaluation.

SUMMARY

Conflicting results have been reported about the mechanism of action of nitrates in pump failure. In order to evaluate the effect on filling pressures and pump function of isosorbide dinitrate (ISDN) administered intravenously, 15 patients in refractory heart failure of different etiologies have been studied. Marked hemodynamic improvement was obtained in 12 of the 15 patients during an infusion of i.v. ISDN at 2–8 mg/hour. Left ventricular filling pressures, represented by the pulmonary capillary wedge pressures, decreased along with a marked reduction in the vascular resistance; cardiac output, stroke volume and stroke work index increased. The results demonstrate that i.v. ISDN decreases both preload and afterload, thus affecting favourably the left ventricular function curves of the failing heart by shifting them upward and to the left.

REFERENCES

1. Massie B, Chatterjee K, Werner T, Greenberg B, Hart R, Parmley WW: Hemodynamic advantage of combined administration of hydralazine orally and nitrates nonparenterally in the vasodilator therapy of chronic heart failure. *Am J Cardiol* 40:794–801, 1978.
2. Williams DO, Amsterdam EA, Mason DT: Hemodynamic effect of nitroglycerine in acute myocardial infarction: decrease in ventricular preload at the expense of cardiac output. *Circulation* 51:421–427, 1975.
3. Gray R, Chatterjee K, Vyden JK, Ganz W, Forrester JS, Swan HJC: Hemodynamic and metabolic effects of isosorbide dinitrate in chronic congestive heart failure. *Am Heart J* 90:346–352, 1975.
4. Mason DT, Braunwald E: The effects of nitroglycerine and amylnitrite in the arteriolar and venous tone in the human forearm. *Circulation* 32:755–766, 1965.
5. Bussman WD, Schupp D: Effect of sublingual nitroglycerine in emergency treatment of severe pulmonary edema. *Am J Cardiol* 41:931–936, 1978.
6. Gold HK, Leinbach RC, Sanders CA: Use of sublingual nitroglycerine in congestive heart failure following acute myocardial infarction, *Circulation* 46:839–845, 1972.
7. Bussman WD, Löhner J, Kaltenbach M: Orally administered isosorbide dinitrate in patients with and without left ventricular failure due to acute myocardial infarction. *Am J Cardiol* 39:91–96, 1977.
8. Baligadoo S, Chiche P: The influence of initial hemodynamic parameters on the hemodynamic response to isosorbide dinitrate and i.v. nitroglycerine: abstract. *Herz* 3:206, 1978.
9. Miller RR, Awan NA, Maxwell KS, Mason DT: Sustained reduction of cardiac impedance and preload in congestive heart failure with the antihypertensive vasodilator prazosin. *New Engl J Med* 297:303–308, 1977.

# 3.7. TRANSFER FUNCTION MODEL OF THE HEART

K.P. Pfeiffer, T. Kenner, J. Schaefer

## 1. introduction

The arrhythmic sequence of arterial pressure pulses in atrial fibrillation reflects the fact that any heartbeat is influenced by the properties of all preceding contractions. This viewpoint is one of the fundamental ideas in general of an autoregressive (AR) model (1).

Among the properties which especially should be described as depending on preceding contractions, diastolic filling and contractility have to be mentioned. The relatively long-lasting and exponentially declining effects of any heart beat on contractility have been examined and summarized by Koch-Weser and Blinks (2). The lasting influences of hemodynamic factors became obvious from results of a earlier study of our group (3).

We will describe in this study that the method of time series analysis (1) permits the visualization of these lasting effects by determining the model parameters of an AR model of the process which generates an arrhythmic sequence of arterial pressure pulses.

## 2. methods

For our study strip chart records of the aortic pressure, recorded by catheter-tip manometers in 12 patients with atrial fibrillation, were available. We evaluated the diastolic filling periods $d_i$, the aortic diastolic pressure $p_i$ and the aortic pressure amplitude $\Delta p_i$ of each pulse. The goal was to develop an AR model which allows the expression of the pressure amplitude of each pulse as a function of the preceding values of $d_{i-1}$ and $p_i$.

## 3. results, statistical analysis

The first part of the analysis examines the statistical properties of each variable and the relation between the variables.

The joint interval histogram of diastolic periods (Figure 1: top) does not reveal any preferential pattern of consecutive periods. As shown in Figure 1

J. Baan, A.C. Arntzenius, E.L. Yellin (eds.), Cardiac Dynamics, 209–216.

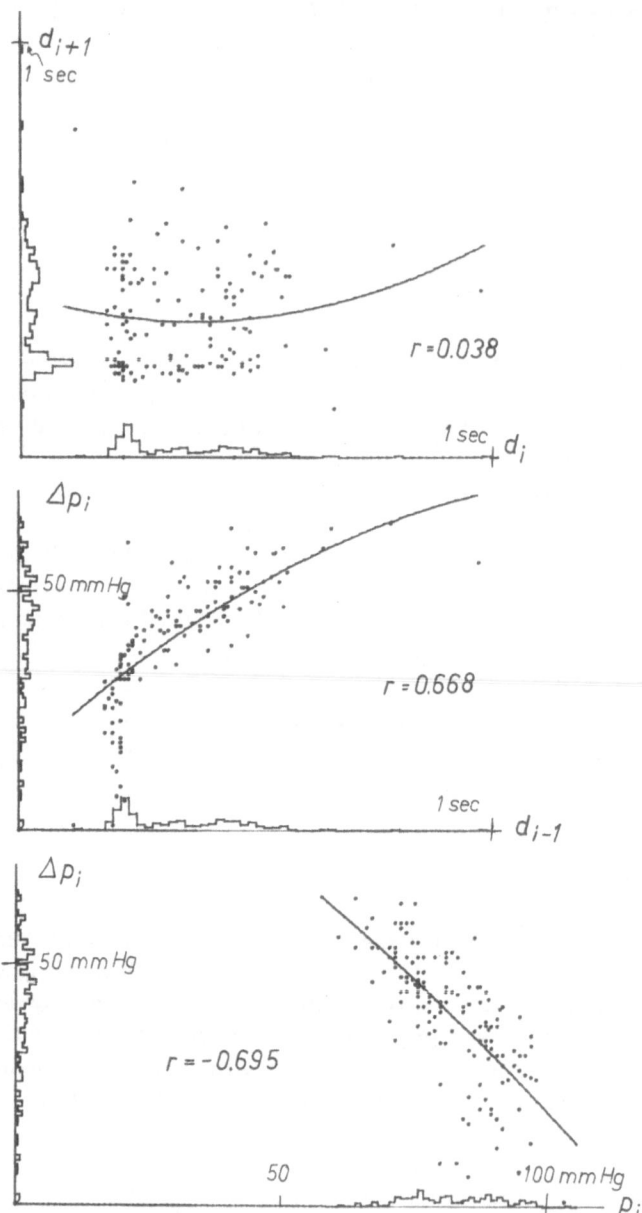

*Figure 1. Top:* joint interval histogram between one and the following diastolic period ($d_i$ and $d_{i+1}$); *middle:* relation between preceding diastolic period $d_{i-1}$ and the consecutive aortic pressure amplitude $\Delta p_i$; *bottom:* relation between diastolic pressure $p_i$ and pressure amplitude $\Delta p_i$, Data from one patient with atrial fibrillation.

(middle), the pressure amplitude rises and tends toward an asymptotic value as the filling period increases. Similar results have been reported in the literature (4, 5, 6). In the lower part of the figure the relation between diastolic pressure $p_i$ and pressure amplitude is shown. As the diastolic pressure increases the pressure amplitude decreases.

The result of a double regression allowing for quadratic and cubic terms is shown in Figure 2. The ordinates of this diagram are normalized with respect to the standard error of each variable. The diagram shows the common influence of the preceding diastolic period $d_{i-1}$ and of the diastolic pressure $p_i$ on the pressure amplitude $\Delta p_i$ of each pulse. Thus, on average, the pressure amplitude can be described as a function of the preceding diastolic period and of the diastolic pressure.

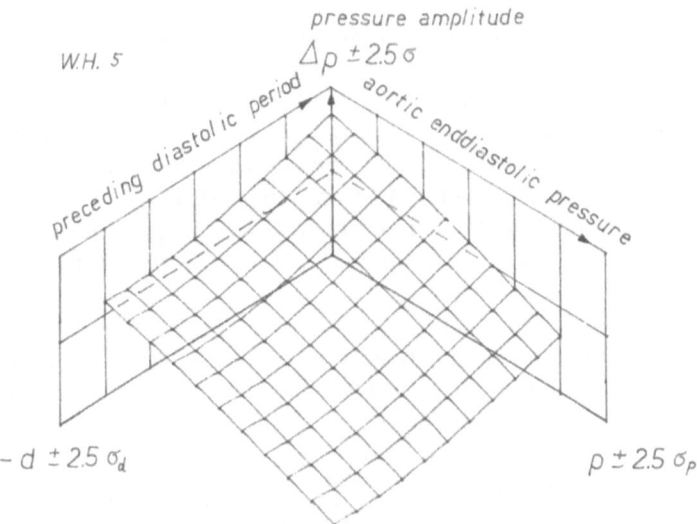

Figure 2. Three dimensional plot showing the relation between preceding diastolic period, aortic end-diastolic pressure and aortic pressure amplitude. The ordinates are normalized with respect to the standard errors ($\sigma$) of the data sets.

4. RESULTS, DYNAMIC ANALYSIS, AR MODEL

Figure 3 shows the most simple form of a so-called "moving average" type of AR model (1). In this model the number of preceding intervals $(d_{t-1}, d_{t-2} \ldots d_{t-M1})$ which have influence on each output term $\Delta p_{t-k}$ equals the model order $M1$ which can be chosen. The model of Figure 3 can be described mathematically by the following equation:

$$\Delta p_i = \sum_{k=1}^{M1} a_k \, d_{i-k} + \epsilon_i. \qquad [1]$$

The coefficients $a_k$ of the model can be calculated by the application of the criterion [2] which represents the minimization of the error term $\epsilon_i$:

$$\frac{1}{N} \sum_{i=1}^{N} \epsilon_i^2 \rightarrow Min. \tag{2}$$

$N$ is the number of analysed heart beats of the total time series which was usually chosen as 150. The application of [2] to [1] leads to a set of $M1$ equations which contain the autocorrelation coefficients of the input variable (matrix $[R_{dd}]$) and the cross-correlation coefficients between input and output (matrix $[R_{d\Delta p}]$). In matrix form the equation for the coefficient matrix is given by

$$\hat{a} = -R_{dd}^{-1} \cdot R_{d\Delta p} \tag{3}$$

The model coefficients $a_1$ to $a_{M1}$ represent the transfer characteristic of the AR model. The model order $M1$ was usually chosen to be 4 or 5.

Since the series of coefficients $a_k$ corresponds to the normalized non-dimensional impulse response of the system, any output of the model can be calculated by convolution of the coefficients with the input. As an example for such a procedure, Figure 4 shows the calculated responses of the pressure amplitudes to step changes of the diastolic period for three of the analysed patients. Thus, a comparison of the results of the analysis of arrhythmic pulses with earlier results using step changes of frequency (3) is possible.

To improve the model, the influence of the two independent variables was combined and nonlinear terms were included:

$$\Delta p_i = \sum_{k=1}^{M1} a_{1k}\, d_{i-k} + \sum_{k=0}^{M2} b_{1,k}\, p_{i-k}$$

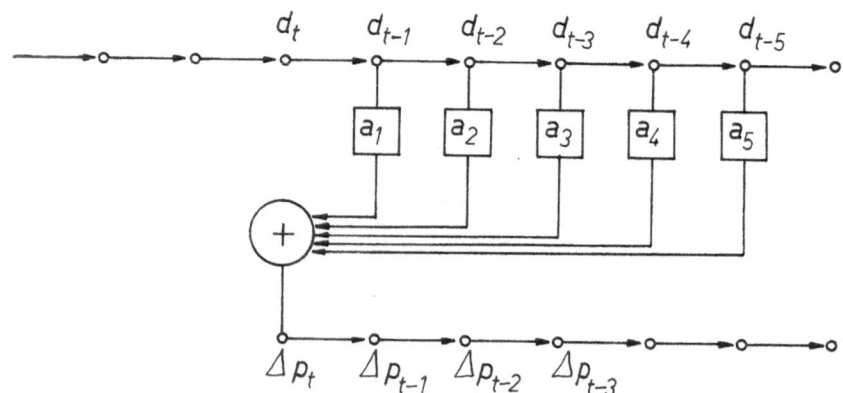

Figure 3. Schematic diagram of an autoregressive "moving average" model.

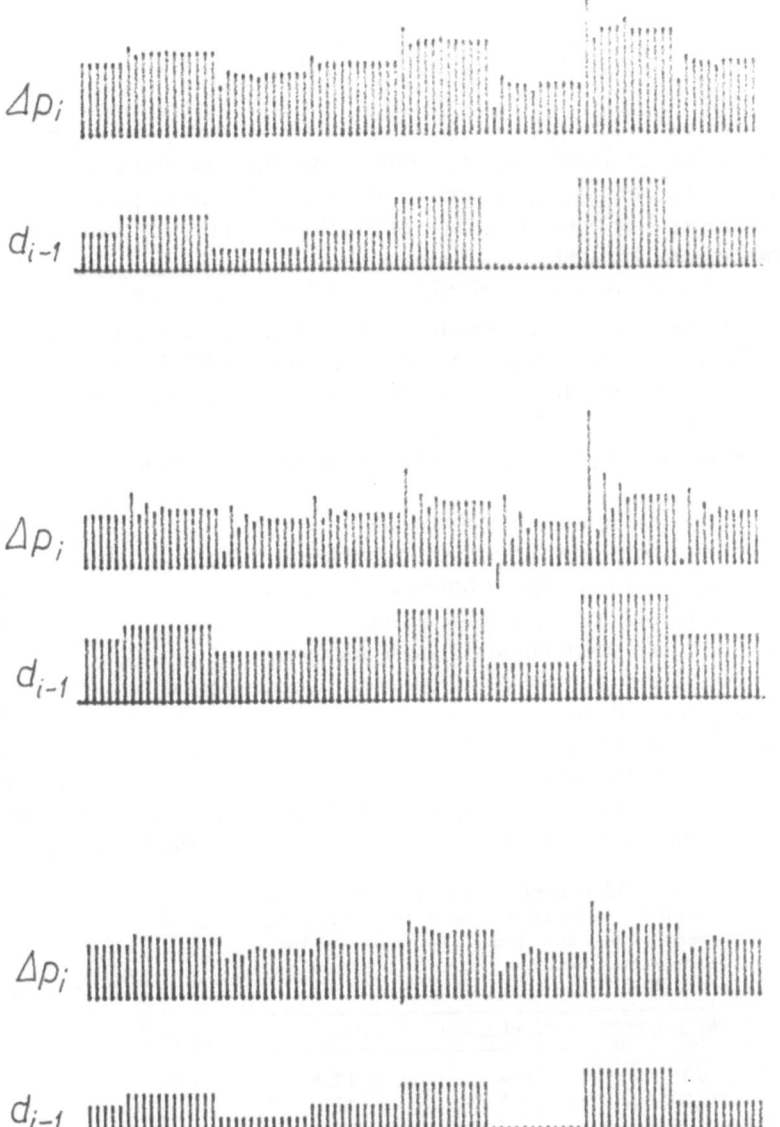

*Figure 4.* Response of the pressure amplitude ($\Delta p_i$) to step changes of the preceding diastolic period ($d_i$). Examples are taken from three patients with atrial fibrillation.

$$+ \sum_{k=1}^{M1} a_{2,k} \, d_{i-k}^2 + \sum_{k=0}^{M2} b_{2,k} \, p_{i-k}^2 \qquad\qquad [4]$$

$$+ \sum_{k=1}^{M1} a_{3,k} \, d_{i-k}^3 + \sum_{k=0}^{M2} b_{3,k} \, p_{i-k}^3 + \epsilon_i.$$

The different indexing $k=1$ or $k=0$ in the two sets of terms depends on the convenience of numbering the pulses: on the one hand the preceding diastolic period ($d_{i-1}$), on the other hand the corresponding diastolic pressures $p_i$. The basic procedure of the calculation is the same as with the simple model [1, 2, 3].

An estimate of the improvement can be given in one example if we compare the normalized mean error variance $\overline{\epsilon_i^2}$ for the nine different possible models and model combinations (patient W.H. 100 pulses, model order 5). The variance of the first model is set equal to 1.0000 for comparison.

1.  Pressure amplitude as function of diastolic duration
    only                                                                    1.0000
2.  Same, including quadratic terms                                          0.8716
3.  Same, including cubic terms in addition                                  0.8089
4.  Pressure amplitude as function of $p_i$ only                             1.6803
5.  Same, including quadratic terms                                          1.6488
6.  Same, including cubic terms in addition                                  1.6125
7.  Pressure amplitude as function of diastolic period
    and diastolic pressure                                                   0.5364
8.  Same, including quadratic terms                                          0.3378
9.  Same, including cubic terms in addition                                  0.2757

It is obvious that the complete model (no. 9) shows the most marked improvement by minimizing the error variance. As shown in Table 1 the

Table 1. An example of ten consecutive aortic pressure amplitudes (mmHg), comparing measurement and prediction with the two-dimensional nonlinear AR model, order 5, patient W.H.

| Measured | calculated | error |
|---|---|---|
| 6.250 | 3.024 | 3.226 |
| 50.000 | 52.219 | −2.219 |
| 15.000 | 13.564 | 1.436 |
| 11.250 | 8.995 | 2.255 |
| 37.500 | 36.217 | 1.283 |
| 10.000 | 12.748 | −2.748 |
| 43.750 | 41.937 | 1.813 |
| 27.500 | 24.410 | 3.090 |
| 25.000 | 24.454 | 0.546 |
| 41.250 | 43.717 | −2.467 |

pressure amplitudes can be predicted by this model with an accuracy of $\pm 3$ mmHg.

Finally it seems interesting and important to distinguish between the weights of the two influences on which the pressure amplitude depends. This is possible by analysis of the variance. The overall variance of the output variable $\Delta p$ is normalized and set equal to 1:

$$\frac{1}{N} \sum_{i=1}^{N} \Delta p_i^2 = 1. \qquad [5]$$

Then the influence of the diastolic period can be stated as

$$I_d = \frac{1}{N} \sum_{i=1}^{N} \left( \Delta p_i - \sum_{k=0}^{M2} b_k \, p_{i-k} \right)^2. \qquad [6]$$

and the influence of the diastolic pressure as

$$I_p = \frac{1}{N} \sum_{i=1}^{N} \left( \Delta p_i - \sum_{k=1}^{M1} a_k \, d_{i-k} \right)^2 \qquad [7]$$

In the examples analysed so far, the two influences turn out to be about equal (for patient W.H., $I_d = 0.4938$ and $I_p = 0.5282$).

## 5. DISCUSSION

For our study only aortic pressure pulses were available. We could therefore only examine relations between variables which could be determined from the strip chart recordings. An AR model is the discrete form of a transfer function and, in our example, provides the transfer function from diastolic filling period and diastolic pressure to the pressure amplitude. It seems tempting to try to interpret the input variables as representing influences of filling and left ventricular contractility while the output variable could represent an index of the stroke volume of the left ventricle. Such an interpretation, however, would go beyond the scope of this study.

SUMMARY

The interrelation between the diastolic filling period, the diastolic aortic pressure and the aortic pressure amplitude of arrhythmic pressure pulses from patients with atrial fibrillation was examined. A two-dimensional nonlinear AR model was developed to describe the transfer characteristics for determining the aortic pressure amplitudes from the sequence of preceding diastolic periods and diastolic pressures. It was shown that the model can predict the output with an accuracy of $\pm 3$ mmHg.

ACKNOWLEDGEMENTS

This study was supported by the Austrian research fund.

REFERENCES

1. Box GEP, and Jenkins GM: *Time series analysis*, San Francisco, Holden-Day, 1970.
2. Koch-Weser J, Blinks JR: The influence of the interval between beats on myocardial contractility. *Pharmacol. Rev* 15:601–652, 1963.
3. Schaefer J, Rumberger E, Baumann K, Schöttler M: Der systolische Spitzendruck bei sprunghafter Änderung der Stimulationsfrequenz des menschlichen Herzens. *Klin Wochenschr* 54:267–276, 1976.
4. Remington JW: Relation between length of diastole and stroke index in the intact dog. *Amer J Physiol* 162:273–279, 1950.
5. Vadot L: Mécanique du coeur et des artères. In: *L'expansion scientifique française*, Paris, 1967.
6. Pauser P, Kenner T, Bachmann, K: Beurteilung der Gleichgewichtskurven des Herzens auf Grund arterieller Druck pulse. *Zeitscher Kreislauff* 57:1049–1060 (1968).

# 3.8. DYNAMICS OF SEQUENTIAL LARGE PULMONARY EMBOLI

H.N. Mayrovitz, R. Castillo, R. Llamas, J. Raines

## 1. INTRODUCTION

The clinical importance of further clarifying the fundamental character of pulmonary embolism (PE) is amplified by recent statistics which estimate the total annual United States incidence of PE at 630,000 (1). Of the 89% of patients who survive the first hour, it is estimated that the diagnosis of PE is missed in 71% of the cases, and the total death rate sums to 200,000, almost 32% of the estimated incidence. Since early diagnosis and treatment can significantly reduce mortality (82% when diagnosed and 30% when undiagnosed), and in the light of newly available treatment modalities it is important not only to develop new and simpler methods of detecting the presence of PE, but also to provide information which will be helpful to the physician in selecting appropriate therapy (2). Since most emboli to the pulmonary vasculature originate in the leg and pelvic veins it is logical to view preventative therapy together with monitoring the development of venous thrombosis as a first line of defence in the prevention of PE in a selected class of high risk patients (3, 4, 5). Although noninvasive methods for detection of venous thrombosis are currently available, their sensitivity is limited to detecting hemodynamically significant thrombi while they are not feasible as a general screening technique (3, 6).

This state of affairs raises one of the questions which motivated the present study, namely: What is the relationship between the size of a clot and the effect it has when it embolizes to the pulmonary vasculature? Further, based on the recognition that venous thrombi may embolize, reform, and embolize again, thus producing a cardiovascular alteration attributable to multiple emboli, the second aspect of the present study was to determine the effect of sequential emboli of varying size on cardiovascular system dynamics.

## 2. METHODS

Eighteen unselected mongrel dogs (weight 11.4 to 20.5 kg) were embolized with autologous blood clots made radiopaque by mixing 6% Renographin with blood drawn 24 hours prior to each experiment. No quantitation of

*J. Baan, A.C. Arntzenius, E.L. Yellin (eds.), Cardiac Dynamics, 217–227.*

clot consistency was made. Three clot volumes (2.5, 5.0, and 10 ml) were formed in glass tubing having an inside diameter of 1.3 cm. The three clot volumes were equally divided between the total group in which, overall, 70 injections were made. In each animal the inferior vena cava (IVC) at the level of the renal vein confluence was exposed and the clots were injected via a Dacron graft sutured to the IVC. Only one clot size per animal was used. The clots were injected sequentially at times determined by stabilization of pulmonary artery pressure. Visualization of each clot was by fluoroscopy. Transit time of each clot from injection site to, and exit from the heart was observed and recorded on videotape. All animals were anesthetized using chloralose. Respiration was maintained constant and the following hemodynamic quantities were measured: pulmonary artery pressure (PAP), femoral artery pressure (FAP), left atrial pressure (LAP), right atrial pressure (RAP), and cardiac output (CO), using a thermodilution method. Arterial blood gases were measured and the electrocardiogram monitored via lead II. All data except as noted are reported as mean ± SEM; statistical significance of differences are based on students' $t$ tests with $P < .05$ taken as statistically significant.

3. RESULTS

3.1. *Typical responses associated with clot embolization*

Typical changes following clot injection are illustrated in Figure 1. Following a transit time from injection site to heart entry of $1.9 \pm 0.3$ sec the clot enters the right atrium, proceeds into the right ventricle where it

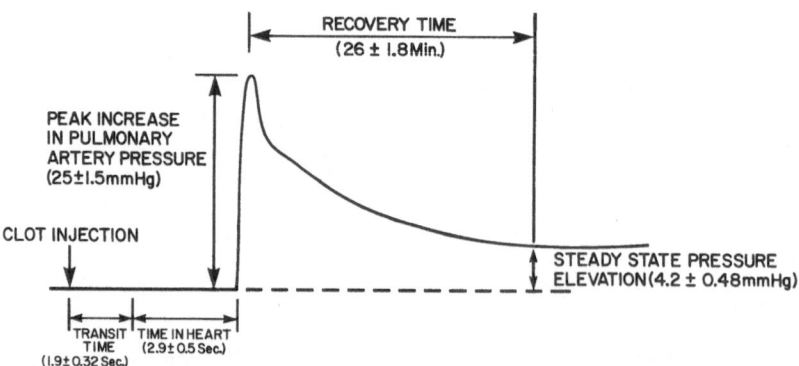

*Figure 1.* Typical response to clot injection. Data shown are mean ± SEM corresponding to all 70 clot injections. Note the rapid and gradual phase of recovery in pulmonary artery pressure.

remains on the average $2.9 \pm 0.5$ sec. Generally, the smaller the clot size, the shorter the transit time and the less time spent within the right heart. Since the mean control heart rate was 145 beats per minute the clot remained in the chamber for approximately 7 beats. Clot entry into the heart was as a single bolus in 84% of clots injected. In the remaining cases the clot was fragmented in transit and entered the heart usually in two pieces displaced in time by not more than a few seconds. Those 10 ml clots which entered the heart as a single bolus were fragmented in all but one case while in the heart. Twenty 10 ml clots entered as a single mass. Eleven were broken into two pieces, six into three pieces, and three into four pieces while in the heart. During a single injection the fragmented pieces tended to move into different pulmonary arterial vessels. The tendency for the clot to break into multiple pieces diminished as the size of the injected clot was reduced. In the case of 10 ml clots, 4% exited the heart intact, 36% in the case of 5 ml clots and 71% of the 2.5 ml clots.

Entrance of the clot into the pulmonary circulation was associated with a precipitous rise in pulmonary artery pressure (PAP). The average peak increase in pulmonary artery pressure produced by all clots was $25 \pm 2$ mmHg. In 49 of the 70 clots injected, the recovery phase of the PAP was characterized by a rapid abrupt drop, followed by a more gradual return towards the pre-injection level. The magnitude of this rapid pressure reduction was variable. The rapid phase of the recovery time never exceeded 120 sec. PAP reached a steady-state pressure level after an average time of $26 \pm 2$ min. This value was $4.2 \pm 1.8$ mmHg above control level.

In addition to the typical changes in PAP described above, several other hemodynamic changes attributable to the clot were observed. Two of these are illustrated in Figure 2. In this example the clot was seen to exit from the heart 12.8 sec after injection into the IVC. Associated with its exit was a precipitous rise in PAP and a concomitant reduction in FAP, which after a period of about 20 sec, returned to the pre-embolic value. Reductions in FAP following clot injection were noted in approximately 20% of cases and appeared to be more prevalent in larger clots. The increase in RAP concomitant with a rise in PAP may also be noted in this figure as well as the presence of two premature ventricular contractions (PVCs) denoted by the arrows in the lead II tracing of the ECG. The presence of cardiac arrythmias of this type have been quite prevalent and associated with embolus entrance into the pulmonary vasculature. The occurrence of PVCs depends on the size of the clot injected. They were observed in 80% of the 10 ml injections, 50% of the 5 ml injections and 25% of the 2.5 ml injections. In all but two experiments the effect of the emboli on cardiac output was to produce a slight transient increase (average increase 15%) followed by a return to control value; this measurement was taken approximately 2 min after the embolic event. The effect of pulmonary emboli on arterial blood

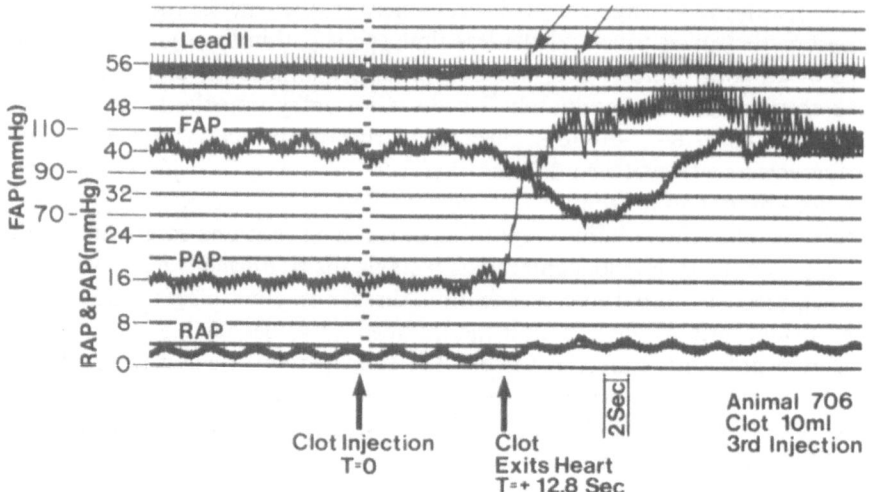

*Figure 2.* Example of response to 10 ml clot injection. Note the rapid rise in pulmonary artery pressure (PAP), transient fall in femoral arterial pressure (FAP) and occurrence of two premature ventricular contractions (denoted by arrows). RAP:right atrial pressure.

gases was rather consistent. Following each embolus there was a precipitous drop in arterial $O_2$ tension and an elevation in $CO_2$ tension. Oxygen tension tended to recover in a staircase fashion with successive injections. This staircasing effect was less evident in the smaller-sized clots.

## 3.2. *Effect of clot size and injection sequence on pulmonary pressure*

As seen in Figure 3, the transient peak increase in PAP appeared to be independent of the number of clots injected (1 to 4 injections). However, the peak increase in pressure was sensitive to the volume of clot injected. This difference showed up most dramatically between the 2.5 ml clot and the 5 or 10 ml clots. Although there was no statistically significant difference between the effect of the 5 ml as compared to the 10 ml clot, each produced a significantly greater effect than the 2.5 ml clot ($P < .05$). Comparing all data only by clot volume shows the 2.5 ml, 5 ml, and 10 ml clots produced peak PAP increases of 16, 33, and 28 mmHg ($P < .001$) respectively.

The steady-state PAP reached after each embolism was strongly dependent on the clot sequence (Figure 4). With each successive clot injection mean steady-state PAP was seen to increase with increasing clot size. This finding was statistically significant for the 5 and 10 ml clots ($P < .05$) for all injections as compared to the control PAP, but did not achieve statistical significance for the 2.5 ml clot until the third injection had been made. However, when the effects of the emboli are compared on the basis of the equivalent total blood clot volume injected (Figure 5) it is found that the

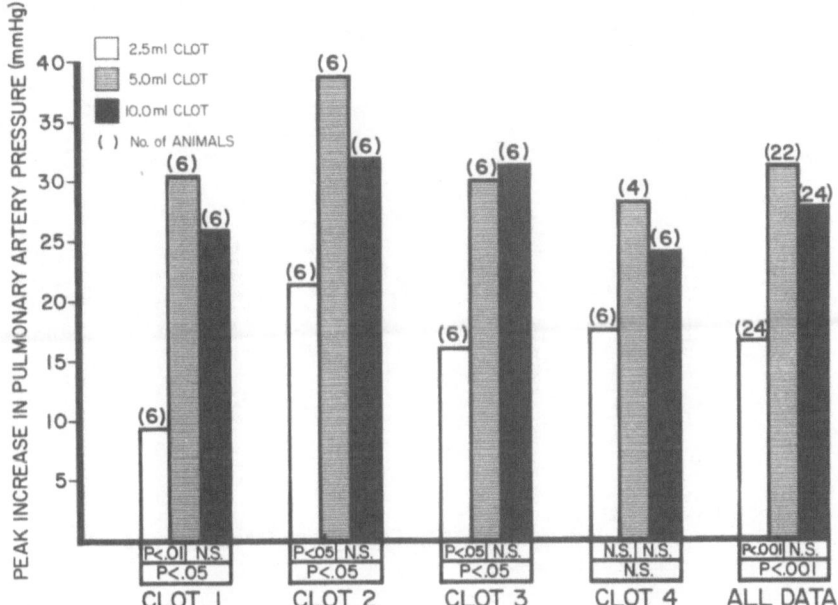

*Figure 3.* Peak increase in pulmonary artery pressure as a function of clot size and numbers of injection.

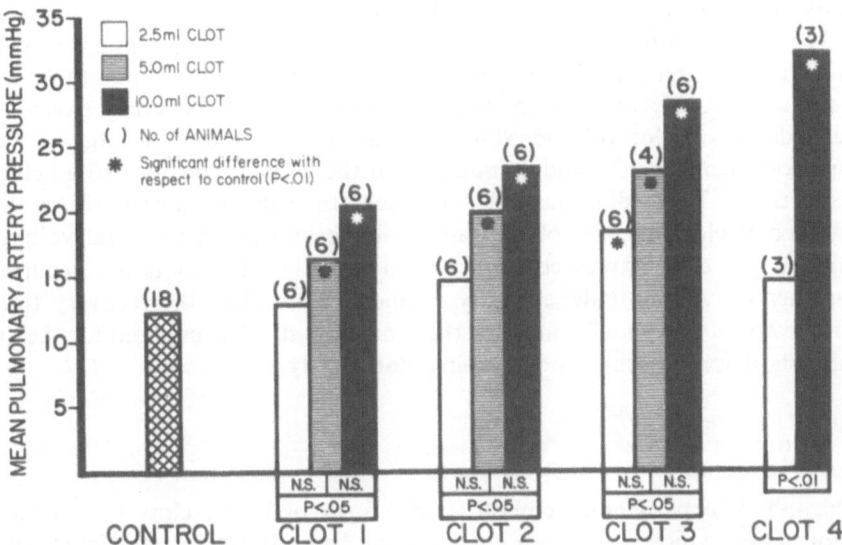

*Figure 4.* Steady-state pulmonary artery pressure after embolism (as a function of clot size and number of injection).

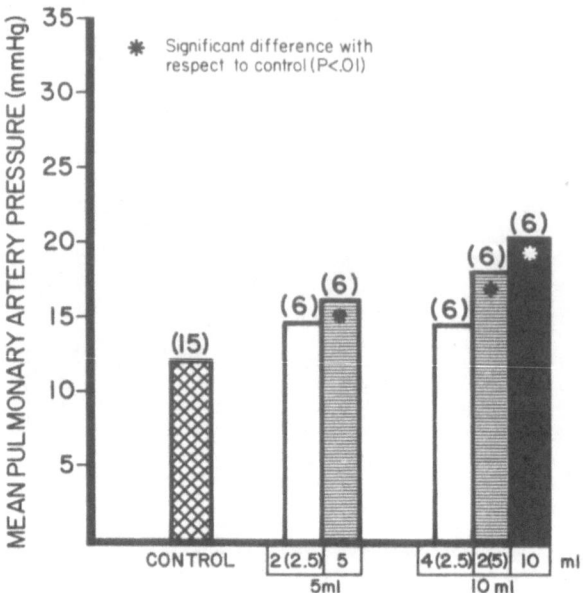

*Figure 5.* Steady-state pulmonary artery pressure after embolism with equivalent blood clot volume. Note that a single 10 ml injection results in a greater pressure than four 2.5 ml injections.

difference between the 2.5 ml, 5 ml, and 10 ml clots becomes smaller and non-significant although the trend suggests greater effects for larger-size individual clots as well as greater effects for the larger total volume.

The recovery time dependence on clot sequence and clot volume is shown in Figure 6. First injection recovery times for the 2.5 ml, 5 ml, and 10 ml clots were 9, 23, and 38 minutes respectively, demonstrating a strong dependence on clot volume. Similar results were obtained for the second injections, being 19, 25, and 40 minutes for the 2.5 ml, 5 ml, and 10 ml clots respectively. These data suggest a recovery time dependence both on the number of clots injected of the same volume as well as the total volume injected per clot. Expressed somewhat differently when clots are grouped together by volume independently of injection number, the recovery time with a 2.5 ml clots is 17.2 min, for the 5 ml clots it is 24 min, and for the 10 ml clots it is 31.5 min, all data being statistically significant.

## 4. DISCUSSION

The use of experimental emboli in the form of blood clots has yielded information which has helped elucidate the hemodynamics associated with pulmonary emboli. Just-Viera and Yeager, using barium-loaded blood clots,

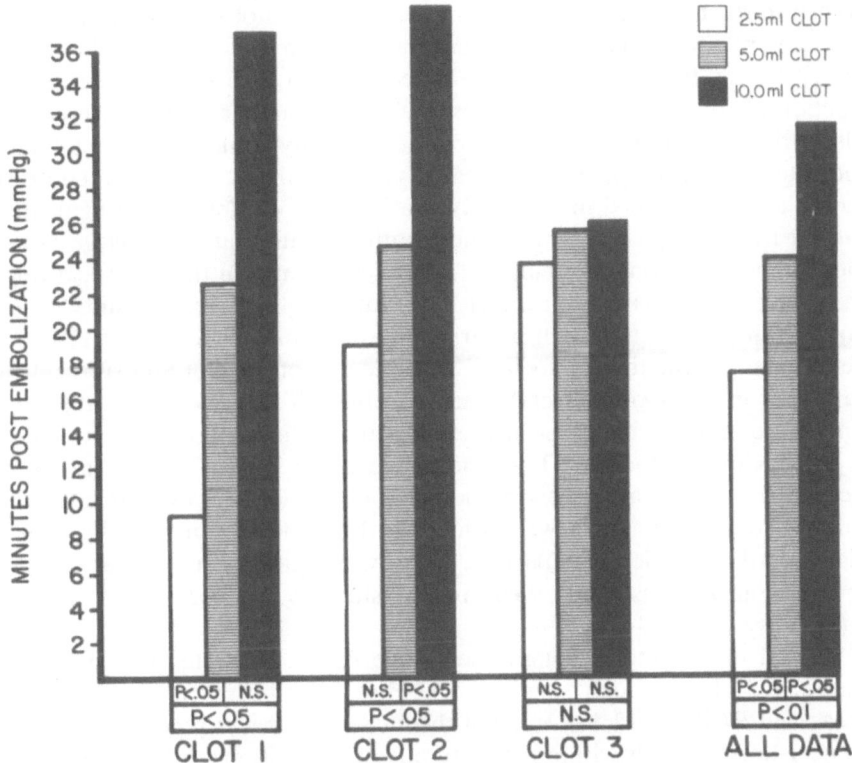

*Figure 6.* Recovery time required for pulmonary artery pressure to reach new steady state (as a function of clot size and number of injections).

determined that the single dose of embolus injected through the external jugular vein required to cause death in 50% of canines studied, was 0.81 ml/kg (7). In unanesthetized dogs a value of 0.86 ml/kg was found (8). If blood clots without barium were used these values were 1.5 ml/kg in anesthetized dogs and 2.86 ml/kg in unanesthetized animals. In the present study no single dose exceeded 0.18 ml/kg. However, the toal cumulative dosage per animal varied from 0.58 to 2.94 ml/kg. Since only 2 of 18 animals used in our study succumbed to the effects of the emboli (cumulative doses for these animals were 2.84 and 2.94 ml/kg) it may be that the use of Renographin as the radiopaque substance renders the consistency of the clot more physiological. Allison et al. used Dionicil to produce radiopaque clots approximately 5.5 ml in volume; these were injected into the left jugular vein and/or the inferior vena cava (9). Using cineradiography they reported that the time required for the clot to transmit from the systemic vein to the pulmonary artery was about 6 seconds. Distinction between transit to the heart and time spent in the heart was not made. The results of the present study clarify this issue and confirm the vein-to-pulmonary-artery transit time to be less than 6 seconds but also show that a larger fraction of that time is spent within the heart chamber itself. Allison et al. also briefly described the action of the heart dynamics on the clot and indicate that most clots exit the heart as a single piece, which is in contrast to the results obtained in this study: we found most clots were fragmented into at least two pieces. Finally, these authors state that the passage of the clot into the pulmonary circulation caused no change in the electrocardiogram. This finding is also in direct opposition to the present results which confirm the presence of multiple arrythmias often in the form of premature ventricular contractions associated with the exit of the clot and subsequent rapid rise in pulmonary artery pressure. Although Just-Viera et al. reported on severe abnormalities of the electrocardiogram subsequent to lethal injected clots including ST segment depression and T wave inversion occurring as early as 5 seconds post embolus (10), it is evident from the present results that clots well below the lethal level can and do induce electrocardiographic irregularities. The consequences of these emboli-induced arrythmias and their relationship to sudden death remain speculative.

Several investigators, using either single bolus injections or injection of masticated clot through small-bore needles have observed immediate increases in PAP (11, 12, 13). In all of these cases PAP was reported to return to near-normal levels within hours. In one of the most careful hemodynamic studies related to the effects of emboli on PAP, Dalen et al. showed a correlation between the changes in PAP and the diameter change of the main pulmonary artery (11). In their study, as well as most other related studies, pulmonary hemodynamic data is not systematically reported for times less than three minutes after embolus injection. As a consequence, the initial instantaneous pressure transient discovered in the present study has not been previously included as a component in the PAP response to PE. For a complete characterization two separate aspects of the transient hypertension produced by pulmonary emboli must be dealt with. The first is to account for the initial rise and rapid fall of the pulmonary artery pressure and the second is to account for the more gradual reduction in pulmonary artery pressure toward pre-embolic levels.

To address the first aspect it is useful to examine two working hypotheses as to the cause of the initial elevation. Two possibilities are: mechanical blockage superimposed upon arteriolar vasoconstriction or mechanical blockage alone. The vasoactive aspect of pulmonary hypertension associated with pulmonary emboli is quite controversial, however, the temporal character of the rapid phase of PAP recovery is consistent with a neural or vasoactive component. On the other hand, if the vasoactive component is small or nonexistent and the response is due solely to mechanical blockage then there are three principal mechanisms whereby one could account for the rapid recovery phase (14). These are (1) passive recruitment of pulmonary arterial vessels, (2) passive dilation of already patent pulmonary vessels, and (3) movement of the clot. Both vessel recruitment and vessel dilation are known to be pressure-dependent. Therefore it could be argued that the observed initial peak pressure rise caused by emboli lodging in pulmonary vessels will be the stimulus to dilate or recruit additional vessels. This would cause the initially elevated vascular resistance to fall from its peak value until a quasi-steady state is achieved. Data from our present experiments do not support these possibilities for the following reasons. If either mechanism were at work one would predict that the rapid phase of recovery should diminish with increasing clot injection. This follows because with each injection, both distension and recruitment reserve should become diminished. However, the data show no reduction in the presence or magnitude of the rapid recovery phase. Therefore, the above passive methods are probably not responsible for rapid recovery. The third mentioned mechanism, slight movement of the clot, may account for this phenomena. If for example the clot is initially lodged in one or more labar arteries at a point near a first order branch the resultant elevated PAP would have the tendency to push the clot distally. If conditions were favourable it may be pushed into one or more of the first order branches. The hemodynamic effect would be to reduce abruptly the magnitude of the initially elevated vascular resistance and subsequently reduce PAP. The phenomena would not be dependent upon the number of clots injected in the same manner as would passive dilation or recruitment. Further, there is additional evidence to support this conclusion. Lockhead et al., using angiography, noted that many vessels initially occluded by emboli were only partially occluded seconds or minutes later (15); similar observations were made by Dalen et al (11). If this is the mechanism of PAP recovery from severe hypertensive states subsequent to PE, it implies that the propensity of clot deformation, as well as its size, can play an important role in the ability of the pulmonary vasculature to accommodate.

The slower phase of PAP recovery can be related to both clot movement and dissolution. As shown, steady-state pressure after embolization increases both with number of clots injected and with the volume of the clot injected. Further it was shown that the time to reach this new steady-state pressure increased with clot size. Data on the dissolution rate of pulmonary emboli in the form of blood clots over the small time spans measured in these experiments could not be found in the literature. However, other investigators using angiography have shown that after embolization gradual reduction in PAP was accompanied by a reduction in the number of first-order arteries that were initially occluded (11). Although the angiographic data was inconclusive concerning mechanism it was noted that small changes in the position of radiopaque blood clots often resulted in a change from complete to partial obstruction of embolized pulmonary vessels. Further, Moser et al, showed that 3 hours after injection of 4 ml clots at autopsy only half the injected clot volume could be recovered (16). This suggests a rather high clot dissolution rate. These investigators felt fibrinolysis was primarily responsible. Based on observations of the present study it is clear that at least in part the slow phase of the recovery is due to a reduction in the embolic material in previously occluded vessels. We observed that, when a clot fragments within the heart, the fragments embolize to different pulmonary vessels. However, once pressure reaches its new equilibrium level and a second injection is made, clot fragments frequently are seen to propagate in the same vessel which had been previously embolized. Extrapolated to the clinical setting the present findings indicate that the ultimate effect of pulmonary embolism depends not just on the size of the embolus but on the time interval between successive emboli.

SUMMARY

Radiopaque autologous blood clots (2.5, 5.0, and 10 ml) have been used to study the dependence of cardiovascular dynamics on pulmonary emboli size and embolization sequence. Each embolus caused an initial peak increase in pulmonary artery pressure which after partial recovery resulted in a sustained pulmonary hypertension. The magnitude of the hypertension was greater for larger individual clots and increased with the number of clots injected. For equal total injected volumes the sustained hypertension was less when produced with multiple 2.5 ml clots as compared to the larger-size clots. The initial peak increase in PAP and subsequent recovery time increased by an amount dependent on the volume of each clot injected and not on the number. Further it was discovered that the recovery of PAP occurred in two phases characterized by an initial rapid reduction in PAP explainable on the basis of emboli movement, followed by a more gradual reduction attributable to additional effects. The data suggest that individual clots of larger volume produce greater functional derangements but that factors other than size, such as clot consistency, may be of fundamental as well as clinical importance.

ACKNOWLEDGEMENTS

The research for the work is supported by grant HL-19427 from the National Heart, Lung and Blood Institute.

REFERENCES

1. Dalen JE, Alpert JS: Natural hisotry of pulmonary embolism. In: *Pulmonary embolism*, Sasahara AA (ed), New York, Grune and Stratton, 1975, p 77–88.
2. Sasahara AA, Hyers ThM: The urokinase pulmonary trial. *Circulation* 47 (suppl 2):1–108, 1973.
3. Wheeler HB, O'Donnel JA, Anderson FA, Benedict K: Occlusive impedance phlebography: a diagnostic procedure for venous thrombosis and pulmonary embolism. In: *Pulmonary embolism*, Sasahara AA (ed), New York, Grune and Stratton, 1975, p 37–43.
4. Clagett GP, Salzman EW: Prevention of venous thromboembolism. In: *Pulmonary embolism*, Sasahara AA (ed), New York, Grune and Stratton, 1975, p 117–129.
5. Kakkar VV, Corrigan TP: Efficacy of low dose heparin prophylaxis. In: *Pulmonary embolism*, Sasahara AA (ed), New York, Grune and Stratton 1975, p 139–141.
6. Kakkar VV, Corrigan TP: Detection of deep vein thrombosis: survey and current status. In: *Pulmonary embolism*, Sasahara AA (ed), New York, Grune and Stratton, 1975, p 45–55.
7. Just-Viera JO, Yeager GH: Massive pulmonary embolism II: predictable mortality and cardiopulmonary changes in dogs breathing room air. *Ann Surg* 154:636–644, 1964.
8. Just-Viera JO, Yeager GH: Pulmonary embolism in unanesthetized dogs. *Surg Gynec Obstet* 27:19–26, 1967.
9. Allison PR, Dunhill MS, Marshall R: Pulmonary embolism. *Thorax* 15:272 283, 1960.
10. Just-Viera JO, Gonzalez LF, Yeager GH: Massive pulmonary embolism III: immediate electrocardiographic changes. *Ann Surg* 161:201–208, 1965.
11. Dalen JE. Matnur VS. Evans H, Haynes FW, Pur-Shahirari AA, Stein PD, Dexter L: Pulmonary angiography in experimental pulmonary embolism. *Am Heart J* 72:509–520, 1966.
12. Dalen ME, Haynes FW, Hoppin FG, Evans GL, Bhardwaj P, Dexter L: Cardiovascular responses to experimental pulmonary embolism. *Am J Cardiol* 20:3–9, 1964.
13. Jacques WE, Hyman AL: Experimental pulmonary embolism in dogs. *Arch Path* 64:487–492, 1957.
14. Kinsely WH, Wallace JM, Mahaley BS, Scatterwhite WM: Evidence, including in vivo observations, suggesting mechanical blockage rather than reflex vasospasm as the cause of death in pulmonary embolization. *Am Heart J* 54:483–497, 1957.
15. Lockhead RP, Roberts DJ, Dotter CT: Pulmonary embolism, experimental angiographic study. *Am J Roentgenol* 68:625–635, 1952.
16. Moser KN, Guisan M, Bartimmo EE, Longo AM, Harsanyi PG, Choriazzi N: In vivo and post morten dissolution rates of pulmonary emboli and venous thrombi in the dog. *Circulation* 48:170–178, 1973.

SECTION 4

# PUMP FUNCTION AND EJECTION: INTERACTION WITH SYSTEMIC LOAD AND CORONARY PERFUSION

## 4.1. PUMP FUNCTION AND ITS INTERACTION WITH THE SYSTEMIC LOAD

D.L. SCHULTZ, L.B. TAN, G. DE J. LEE,
B. RAJAGOPALAN, G.W. CHERRY, W.D. GUNDEL,
J.J. SCHIPPERHEYN, P. HUISMAN

### 1. INTRODUCTION

Many parameters have been used to categorize the mechanical function of the myocardium, such as the rate of rise of ventricular pressure $(dP/dt)$ and the velocity of fibre shortening $(dV/dt)$. Such factors attempt to relate the performance of the intact ventricle to that of isolated muscle strips and while a deeper understanding of ventricular function will eventually come from such isolated muscle studies there are still many unresolved difficulties in the way. An alternative approach is to investigate the function of the intact ventricle through measurements of pressure and flow which are the integrated external effects of tension and shortening velocity in the individual muscle segments. If the ventricle is regarded as a source of mechanical power coupled to the circulatory system which has as its chief characteristic an input impedance it is apparent that the simultaneous measurement of the aortic pressure and flow enables two further functions to be derived. Firstly, the product terms (pressure × flow) at each harmonic yield the power transferred into the circulation, and secondly, the quotient terms (pressure/flow), again at each harmonic and making due allowance for phase angle, give the input impedance.

It can be argued that the power flow from the ventricle to the aorta is an important feature of myocardial function in that it combines the two separate parameters of pressure and flow and its variation during the cardiac cycle may be useful in distinguishing normal and abnormal behaviour. The measurement of power flow alone, however, would be incomplete since, with a ventricle delivering constant power, there is an infinite range of pressures and flows which would satisfy the criterion $P \times Q = $ constant. When coupled to the systemic load, however, there is only one condition which will simultaneously satisfy $P \times Q = $ constant and $P/Q = Z$, the input impedance of the circulation; the calculations being done at each harmonic in the Fourier series expressing the individual wave forms with the phase angle considered in each case. This approach to the assessment of cardiac function is particularly valuable when inotropic interventions, such as isoprenaline, are used to apply graded stress to the ventricle. This technique has been used during routine catheterization to

*J. Baan, A.C. Arntzenius, E.L. Yellin (eds.); Cardiac Dynamics, 231–247.*

estimate cardiac response to exercise but in both cases two effects occur simultaneously. Firstly, there is a change in the inotropic state of the ventricle, and secondly, there is usually a change in the impedance of the circulatory system. It will be shown that it is possible to state whether there has been, as a result of inotropic intervention, an unambiguous change in myocardial function as determined by measurements of the power output or whether such changes could have been due to changes in impedance. It is particularly important to be able to draw such distinctions when a product term such as power is used to define the state of the ventricle. In all these arguments it is assumed that the system is linear in order that the wave forms of flow and pressure may be analysed in terms of the Fourier components. The range of validity of this assumption has been examined by Van der Werff et al. (1) for aortic flow and pressure wave forms and it was concluded that the hypothesis is reasonable.

## 2. Power transfer to aorta and input impedance

If the aortic flow and pressure wave forms are expressed in the form:

$$q(t) = q_0 + \sum_{m=1}^{\infty} q_m \cos(m\omega t - \theta_m)$$

$$p(t) = p_0 + \sum_{n=1}^{\infty} p_n \cos(n\omega t - \phi_n),$$

the cycle average power may be expressed as

$$\overline{W} = \frac{1}{T} \int_0^T \dot{w}(t)\, dt = \frac{\omega}{2\pi} \int_0^{\frac{2\pi}{\omega}} p(t)\, q(t)\, dt$$

$$= \frac{\omega}{2\pi} \int_0^{\frac{2\pi}{\omega}} \left\{ \left[ \sum_{n=0}^{\infty} p_n \cos(n\omega t - \phi_n) \right] \left[ \sum_{m=0}^{\infty} q_m \cos(m\omega t - \theta_m) \right] \right\} dt$$

Each term in the integral may be expressed as

$$w_{mn} = \frac{p_n q_m}{2T} \int_0^T \left\{ \cos\left[ (m+n)\,\omega t - (\theta_m + \phi_n) \right] \right.$$

$$\left. + \cos\left[ (m+n)\,\omega t - (\theta_m - \phi_n) \right] \right\} dt.$$

For $m \neq n$, the cross products

$$\int_0^T \cos\left[ (m \pm n)\,\omega t - (\theta_m \pm \phi_n) \right] dt$$

$$= \left[ \frac{1}{(m \pm n)\, \omega}\, \sin\left\{ (m \pm n)\, \omega t - (\theta_m \pm \phi_n) \right\} \right]_0^{\frac{2\pi}{\omega}}$$

$$= \frac{1}{(m \pm n)\, \omega} \left[ \sin\left\{ (m \pm n)\, 2\pi - (\theta_m \pm \phi_n) \right\} - \sin\left\{ -(\theta_m \pm \phi_n) \right\} \right]$$

$$= 0.$$

For $m = n$, however,

$$w_{mn} = \frac{p_n q_n}{2T} \int_0^T \left[ \cos\left\{ 2n\omega t - (\theta_n - \phi_n) \right\} + \cos\left\{ -(\theta_n - \phi_n) \right\} \right] dt$$

and since $\displaystyle\int_0^T \cos\left[ 2n\omega t - (\theta_n - \phi_n) \right] dt \cong 0$

and $\displaystyle\int_0^T \cos(\phi_n - \theta_n)\, dt = \frac{2\pi}{\omega}\, \sin(\phi_n - \theta_n)$

the cycle-average power becomes

$$\overline{W} = p_0 q_0 + \tfrac{1}{2} \sum_{n=1}^{\infty} p_n q_n \, \sin(\phi_n - \theta_n)$$

It is therefore seen that by calculating the cycle average power only the mean term $p_0 q_0$, the product of mean pressure and mean flow, and the power at each discrete harmonic appear. The same measurements of aortic flow and pressure used in the manner outlined above to calculate the cycle averaged power are used to determine the impedance spectrum:

$$Z(j\omega) = \left| \frac{P_m}{Q_m} \right| \frac{|\phi - \theta}{},$$

the real part of the complex impedance being

$$R(j\omega) = \frac{P_m}{Q_m} \cos\ (\phi - \theta).$$

The average power may be calculated either from the product terms of pressure and flow or from the expression

$$\overline{W} = |Q(\omega)|^2\ R(j\omega) = |P(\omega)|^2 / R(j\omega).$$

Having calculated the cycle average power at each harmonic and the corresponding arterial impedance it is now necessary to establish a technique for distinguishing the effect of inotropic changes from those of arterial impedance changes on power output.

This may be done by considering the nomogram in Figure 1. In this figure the three vertical axes represent the root-mean-square flow

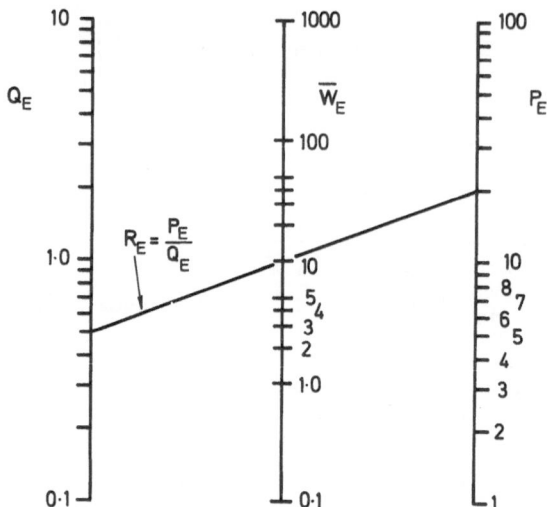

*Figure 1.* Nomogram illustrating relationship between effective flow $Q_E$, pressure $P_E$ and power $W_E$ for one harmonic.

$Q_E = Q_m/\sqrt{2}$, the cycle average power $\overline{W}_E = P_E Q_E \sin(\phi - \theta)$ and the root-mean-square pressure $P_E = P_m/\sqrt{2}$, respectively, for each harmonic term. For the zeroth harmonic, the average pressure flow and pressure give average power $P_0 Q_0$ directly. For simplicity in graphical analysis the cosine term may be incorporated into $P_E$ so that $P_E$ is now defined as $P_m \cos(\phi - \theta)/\sqrt{2}$.

The scales are shown logarithmically for convenience so that of the centre axis is the square of the outer two which are equidistant from it. For a given

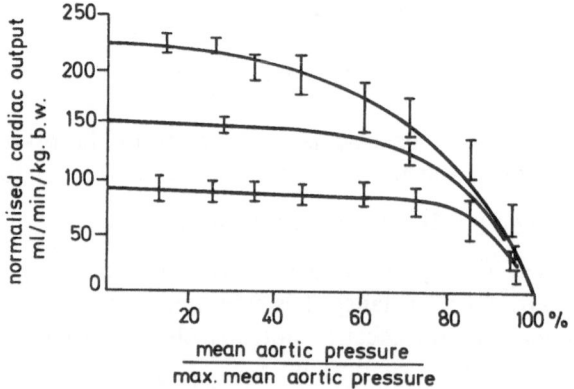

*Figure 2.* Cardiac output as a function of aortic pressure. Top curve: high LAP; middle curve: medium LAP; lower curve: low LAP. Redrawn from Sagawa (2).

operating point on the $Q_E$ and $P_E$ axes a line joining them intersects the central axis at the value $\overline{W}_E = Q_E P_E$ and the slope of the line may be labelled $R_E = P_E/Q_E$ although because of the logarithmic scales the normal geometric relationship does not hold. In order to make further use of this presentation of cardiac function it is necessary to assume the limiting behaviour of the ventricle as at one extreme a constant flow source or at the other a constant pressure source. This limiting performance has been illustrated by, for example, Sagawa (2) and Figure 2 illustrates the measured dependence of normalized left ventricular output on both aortic pressure and left atrial pressure. It will be seen that the curves may be bounded by two limits of constant flow and constant pressure and that at constant left atrial pressure the LV output must decrease monotonically as the mean aortic pressure is increased. At low mean aortic pressures the LV is seen to behave as a constant flow generator while at higher mean aortic pressures the LV tends towards a constant pressure generator. The sensitivity of the actual curve to mean left atrial pressure should, however, be noted.

Referring to Figure 3 and assuming for example that the ventricle is operating against an arterial pressure $P_0$, producing a flow $Q_0$ and thus operating at a power level of $W_0$ with an arterial impedance of $R_0$, if an inotropic agent such as isoprenaline, which changes both the impedance and the power output, is administered, a line may be drawn from the original value of $P_0$ to intersect the $Q$ axis ordinate at $Q_P$, the increased flow

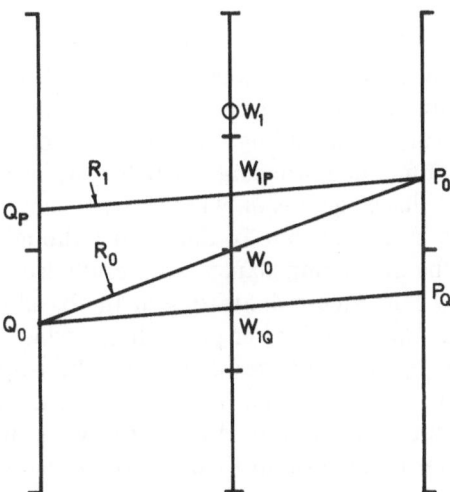

*Figure 3.* Nomogram illustrating effect of altered aortic impedance on power flow. $R_0$ initial resistance, $R_1$: reduced resistance.

to which would result from a constant pressure source when faced with a reduced impedance. The power at 1 under these conditions would be $W_{1P}$. Alternatively, if the LV had been functioning as a constant flow source at a level $Q_0$ and the impedance had been lowered the pressure would have fallen to $P_Q$ and the power reduced to $W_{1Q}$. Thus, if the ventricle was originally operating at a power level $W_0$ into a load impedance $R_0$ and the impedance was changed to $R_1$, then power levels between $W_{1P}$ and $W_{1Q}$ could be ascribed solely to changes in impedance and no inotropic alterations may have taken place. If, however, the observed power in this condition is $W_1$, say, above $W_{1P}$ in Figure 3, then it would be possible to state that there had been an unambiguous change, in this case an improvement, in the inotropic state of the LV. If the new measured operating power level is within the limits $W_{1P}$ and $W_{1Q}$ then counteracting changes in inotropic state and impedance may have taken place and no firm conclusions may be drawn from the measurement.


3. ANIMAL EXPERIMENTS

In order to test this method of myocardial assessment trials were carried out on a series of five dogs in which aortic flow was determined by a cuff electromagnetic flow meter and aortic pressure by an external transducer coupled to the aorta with a short stiff cannula. Graded doses of isoprenaline from 0.5 to 2 micrograms per minute were administered and after a settling period of about 5 minutes a series of aortic pressure, aortic flow, ECG and left ventricular pressure signals was recorded on magnetic tape for subsequent analysis on a digital computer. At each infusion level a run of 10 to 20 beats of aortic flow and pressure were averaged. The averaged wave form was then used to obtain, after Fourier analysis, the aortic impedance and power at each harmonic including the mean term. The basis for the selection of isoprenaline as a stressing agent for the heart is dealt with in more detail later. At this stage it is only necessary to employ some stimulant which will alter the inotropic state of the heart although it may well, and indeed does, alter the aortic impedance. The results from one such animal experiment are shown in Figure 4. Starting at the basal level two lines are drawn indicating the upper and lower power limits which could be ascribed to the measured impedance changes caused by the isoprenaline infusion. These two limits are labelled $p$ and $q$, representing the constant pressure and constant flow source assumptions respectively, as outlined above and illustrated for one harmonic term in Figure 3. It will be noted that with the exception of the 1.5 microgram/minute infusion the slightly increased mean power levels $W_0$ are explicable simply in terms of resistance changes. At the heart rate, the first harmonic, however, there is at every infusion level a

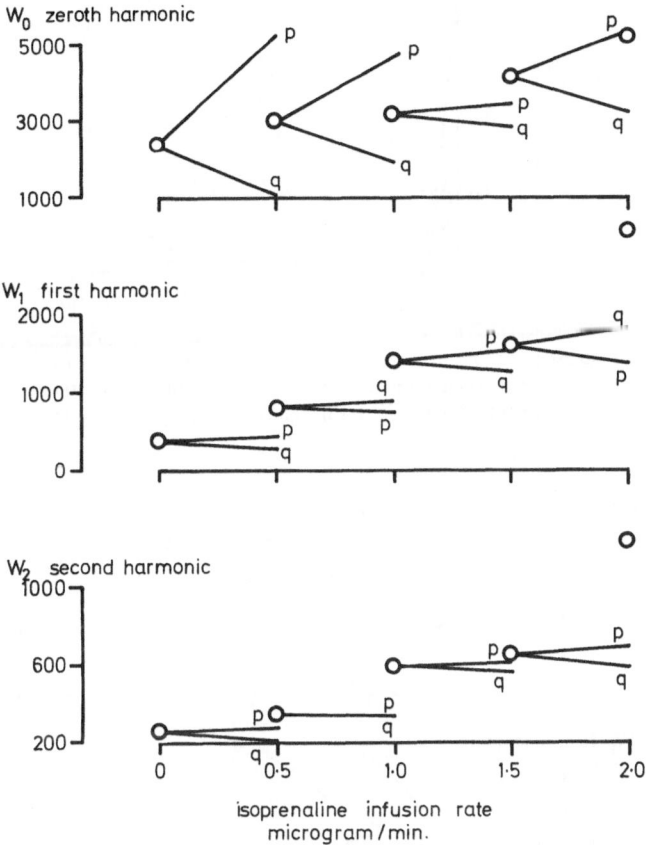

*Figure 4.* Effect of isoprenaline infusion on mean (zeroth harmonic) power flow and power at first harmonic (heart rate) and second harmonic of dog LV. Units are mmHg × ml/sec which can be converted to watts by multiplying by $1.33 \times 10^{-4}$.

substantial increase in power which is greater than that which could be due to changes in peripheral impedance. The 1.5 microgram/minute power level is not so far outside the *pq* limits as at the other infusion levels but the overall trend is clear at both the heart rate and its harmonic. The aortic impedance spectra for this particular experimental preparation is shown in Figure 5. It is apparent that there is a marked reduction in peripheral resistance as the isoprenaline dosage is increased from 0 to 2 microgram/ minute. This is consistent with the wide angle subtended by the *p* and *q* generator limits illustrated in Figure 4. Small changes in the impedance result in smaller subtended angles and this is seen to be the case in the power terms at the heart rate and twice the heart rate, $W_1$ and $W_2$ respectively in Figure 4.

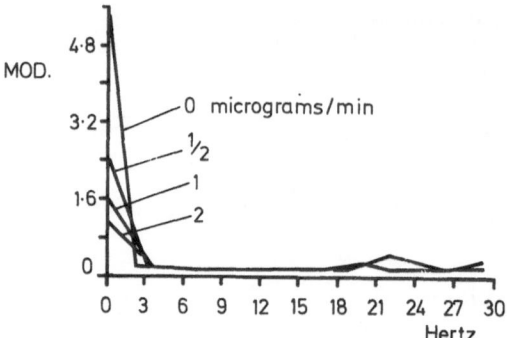

*Figure 5.* Superposed aortic input impedance spectra showing effect of isoprenaline on load impedance of dog. Note marked reduction in systemic peripheral resistance as isoprenaline dosage is increased from 0 to 2 μg/min and insignificant change in characteristic impedance.

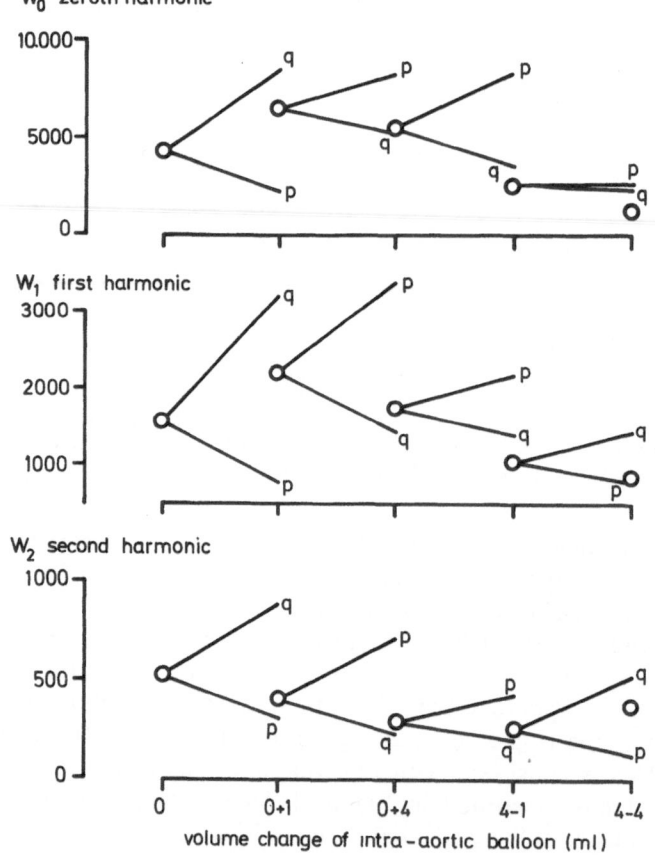

*Figure 6.* Effect of intra-aortic balloon inflation on power flow in dog. Units are mmHg × ml/sec.

A further indirect test of the method in the intact animal was obtained by gradually inflating an intra-aortic balloon catheter located at the mid-thoracic level in a dog in which aortic flow was measured by the same means, that is to say a cuff electromagnetic flow meter and external aortic pressure transducer. The mean power and that at the heart rate and harmonic are shown in Figure 6. As would be expected the first balloon inflation of 1 ml results in an increase in power output. The increased aortic pressure leads to an increase in coronary flow but with a further balloon inflation of 4 ml the mean power output and that at the heart rate fall as venous return is reduced and permanent myocardial damage is caused. Deflation of the balloon confirms this hypothesis and although the test cannot be regarded as conclusive the results are in accordance with previous experience, the peripheral resistance reflecting the incremental changes in balloon volume.

## 4. CLINICAL INVESTIGATIONS

Clinical studies have been carried out on a series of 51 patients admitted for routine catheterization. All patients in the series were shown to have angiographic evidence of disease of the coronary arteries compatible with atherosclerosis, but without significant dysrhythmias or valvular disorders. The highest level of isoprenaline infusion for each patient was determined on the day prior to catheterization by continuous infusion via a superficial vein accompanied by electrocardiographic monitoring and heart rate measurement. Infusion was commenced at 1 $\mu$g/min and continued for 6 to 7 minutes. The procedure was continued with step increments in infusion rate until the heart rate had increased by 30 to 40 per beats/min or until the patient experienced chest pain, shortness of breath or until marked ST depression on the ECG was observed. Tests on three patients showed that the increase in total circulating catecholamines was directly proportional to the infusion rate of isoprenaline after about 4 minutes, the assay used being unable to distinguish noradrenaline and isoprenaline. A specially built catheter incorporating an electromagnetic velometer (3) approximately 10 cm from the tip, a left ventricular pressure lumen at the tip and an aortic pressure lumen 1.1 cm distal from the flow meter electrodes was inserted via a femoral artery. The introduction of the catheter was aided by the use of a sleeve previously manoeuvred into the left ventricle over an 8F pigtail catheter. Retraction of the pigtail enabled the velometer catheter to be inserted such that this tip was in the LV and the aortic lumen and electrodes of the velometer were 3 to 4 cm distal from the aortic valve. The aortic diameter at the location of the velometer electrodes was determined from calibrated angiographic records and from comparison of mean cardiac outputs from catheter and indicator dye results. Mean cardiac output was also determined using standard dye output techniques. The calibration of the velometer was done in normal saline and found to be relatively insensitive to flow alignment, a 30° angulation causing only a 3% reduction in sensitivity. If, however, one electrode touched the arterial wall the signal could be grossly distorted without any warning change in baseline so that care had to be taken to ensure that the velometer electrodes were approximately central in the aorta with the tip of the catheter in the LV cavity. The frequency response of the catheter was checked using an electrical method reported by Gessner and Bergel (4) when operated with the commercially available control unit (EMI Flowmeter SEM 275). The amplitude and phase errors were automatically corrected in the data analysis program and were found to have a minimal effect on wave shape, causing a slight forward timeshift of the entire wave form. Left ventricular and aortic pressures were determined by external pressure transducers (S.E. 4–82) attached directly to the catheter end connections. This method, although having a limited frequency response of approximately 50 Hz natural resonant frequency, had the advantage of direct calibration and zero setting which is essential for accurate power measurement. The wave form of the measured ventricular and aortic pressures may be corrected in the same program used to calculate the power flow. As in the case of the animal experiments a run of 10 to 15 cardiac cycles was recorded on magnetic tape in analog form for subsequent analysis.

The selection of an inotropic stimulant to stress the heart was narrowed to a choice between calcium gluconate and isoprenaline. Some preliminary studies in human subjects indicated that calcium gluconate caused profound bradycardia or paraesthesia and lightheadedness. In addition, the infusion rate required to elicit an adequate inotropic response exceeded the recommended safety limits. Isoprenaline has the additional advantages that its action is rapid and found to reach a stable level after approximately 5 minutes of steady infusion. The effect can be quickly reversed by β-adrenergic blocking agents. The most common adverse effects on patients with ischaemic heart disease were ectopic beats which caused difficulties in data analysis, occasional chest pain, or shortness of breath. Cessation of the infusion caused these adverse effects to disappear in 1 to 4 minutes. Isoprenaline does not act by releasing endogenous catecholamines, nor is it taken up by the autonomic nerve endings so the conclusion is that the level of circulating isoprenaline is unaffected by the state of the autonomic nerve endings in the myocardium, *and* that the myocardial response to isoprenaline is not modified by changes in the autonomic nerve endings (e.g. increased, sympathetic efferent stimulation and noradrenaline vesicle depletion in congestive heart failure). The hemodynamic effects of isoprenaline in human subjects have been well documented and its use as a stressing agent suggested by other workers (5, 6) although the use of graded increments in the rate of steady infusion has not been reported elsewhere.

The ability of the patient to exercise is greatly reduced during cardiac catheterization but it is important to establish that graded doses of isoprenaline reproduce the main features of exercise in a repeatable manner. Isoprenaline reproduces *some* of the effects of exercise, principally the increased heart rate. Mean vascular resistance, for example, may not be as affected by exercise, the vasodilatation in skeletal muscle being offset by reflex vasoconstrictions in the splanchnic circulation. Rushmer (7, 8) noted that a major difference was that isoprenaline produced a greater ventricular "impulse", the duration of systole being reduced and the stroke volume diminished. The conclusions of the present study support these findings. In addition it should be noted that the positive chronotropic influence of isoprenaline is generally more pronounced than that caused by exercise. In the absence of a systematic study, which would of necessity involve an assessment of total energy consumption, it is not possible to state whether exercise or the infusion of isoprenaline exerts more demand on the myocardial energy supply. It is sufficient at this stage to note that both exercise and isoprenaline infusion stress the heart into response patterns which are not dissimilar.

Between 10 and 15 cardiac cycles were analysed at each infusion level to obtain an average beat for LV pressure, aortic velocity and pressure. Digital filtering techniques were used to smooth the data points obtained after digitization, the smoothed wave forms analysed into Fourier components and the impedance and power computed. The analysis was repeated at each isoprenaline infusion level. A typical result from a patient with a moderately responsive ventricle is shown in Figure 7. In this patient the ECG was normal at rest but showed ST depression after short exercise, heart sounds were normal, the LV angiogram indicated a normal-sized ventricle with good contraction. Selective coronary arteriography revealed an irregular left anterior descending artery, narrowed proximally, and a small circumflex artery with severe local narrowing at the equator. From Figure 7 it will be seen that isoprenaline infusion up to 3 $\mu$g/min results in a steady increase in left ventricular output power in the mean, heart rate and all harmonic terms. The mean power increase is, however, within the limits which are defined by the changes of resistance or impedance as described earlier in this paper and illustrated in Figure 3. At the heart rate and its harmonics the increase in power is unambiguous and outside any limits set by the measured changes in peripheral impedance. An example of a patient with a poorly responsive ventricle is illustrated in Figure 8. In this patient the ECG revealed evidence of old antero-inferior MI and ischaemia. The heart

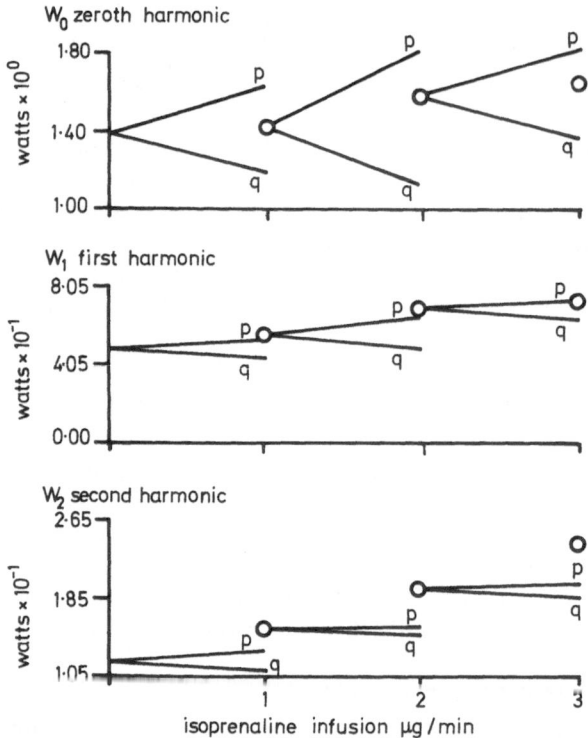

*Figure 7.* Isoprenaline infusion in human subject showing effect on mean power flow and power at heart rate and 2 × heart rate. Patient with normally responsive LV.

sounds were normal and the LV angiogram showed that although wall movements were good the apex was akinetic. Coronary arteriography showed severe proximal narrowing of the LAD, a beaded and circuitous circumflex artery. It will be seen from Figure 8 that both the mean power and the power supplied at the heart rate fall with increasing isoprenaline infusion but this decrease could be due in most cases to a change in peripheral resistance or impedance. The results at harmonics of the heart rate show marked changes in impedance and no improvement in inotropic state with increasing isoprenaline infusion. In this patient the stroke volume varied from a resting value of 94.7 cm$^3$ to 86.2 cm$^3$ at the 2 $\mu$g/min infusion level. Other indices of cardiac performance in this case, such as $dP/dt$, showed reasonable improvement from 1482 mmHg/sec at rest to 2433 at 2 $\mu$g/min isoprenaline infusion, although the peak power rose from 7.35 watts to only 8.19 watts at 2 $\mu$g/min.

A further clinical assessment of the technique may be obtained by the

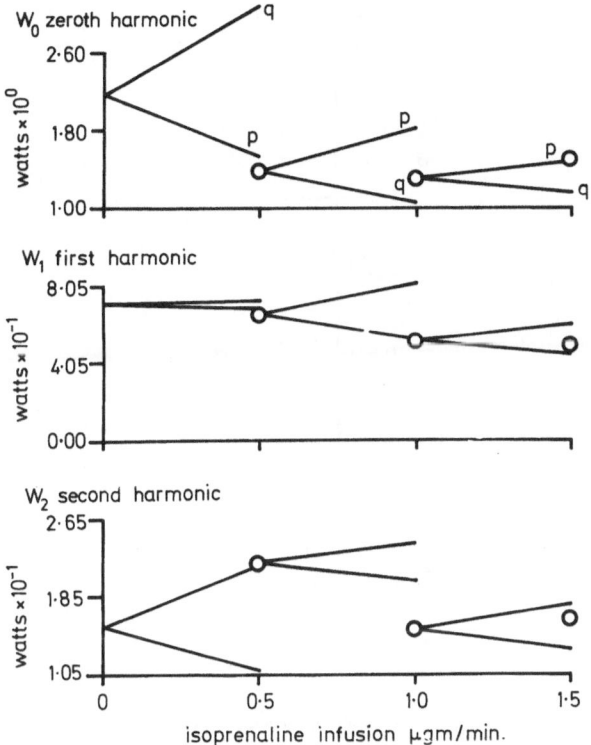

*Figure 8.* Effect of isoprenaline infusion in patient with poorly responsive LV.

measurement of power output when the circulatory bed is vasodilated with nitroprusside. Following a period of baseline hemodynamic measurements, nitroprusside was administered by calibrated Watson-Marlow "sigma" pump in a concentration of 7.5 $\mu$g/cm$^3$. Infusion was begun at a rate of 15 $\mu$g/min and the dose was increased in increments of 10 to 20 $\mu$g/min every 2 minutes until the mean aortic blood pressure had fallen by 20 to 30 mmHg or until the systolic pressure had dropped to 90 mmHg. Nitroprusside has no *direct* effects on the inotropic state of the myocardium (9, 10) and is a pure vasodilator, exerting a potent effect upon both the venous (capacitive-preload) and arterial (resistance-afterload) vascular beds. However, nitroprusside has been demonstrated (11) to affect adversely regional myocardial bloodflow to marginally perfused vascular beds distal to coronary occlusive disease in *some* patients, an effect independent of changes it may induce in aortic perfusion pressure. Thus, by reducing bloodflow to underperfused areas of myocardium, nitroprusside could induce an indirect depression of

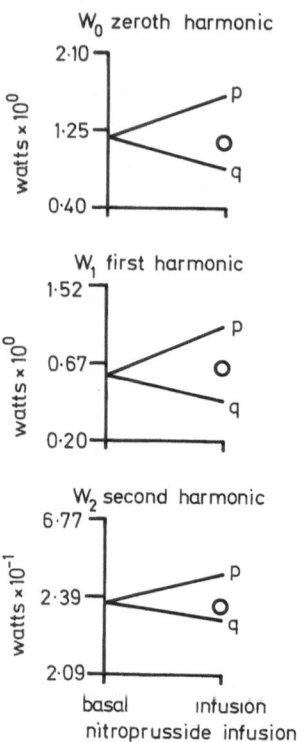

*Figure 9.* Effect of nitroprusside infusion on LV power requirement in human subject.

regional myocardial function by augmenting ischaemia. It would be expected that the measured power changes at mean, heart rate and harmonics would be explicable predominantly in terms of a pure impedance change and, as will be seen from the example in Figure 9, this is the case. The power levels with the nitroprusside infusion are seen to be almost constant and within the limits set by the change of impedance. The mean power level is slightly reduced from its resting level of 0.77 watts and the power at the heart rate increased slightly from a resting level of 0.41 watts but both power measurements move to values within the constant pressure and constant flow limits. The same patient, when infused with isoprenaline, was able to increase the power output at all harmonics and in this trial also the changes were ambiguous, the increased power levels being within the constant pressure and constant flow source limits. Of equal interest were the changes in cardiac output and aortic pressure. The cardiac output increased from 5 litres/min to 6 litres/min, the aortic pressure fell from 157/74 mmHg to 126/57 and the average power rose only slightly from 1.38 watts to 1.48 watts.

A further series of clinical trials to assess the usefulness of power measurements has been conducted and compared with the conventional indices of cardiac performance. Catheter studies have been made as part of a routine screening for possible coronary artery surgery and compared with similar studies made where applicable six months after surgery. Patients were again infused with graded doses of isoprenaline and measurements of cardiac output power and aortic input impedance made at each infusion level. An example of pre- and post-operative cardiac function in a patient whose myocardium was improved by this surgery is shown in Figures 10 and 11. It will be seen that output power at the heart rate has been increased and that the increase for 1 and 2 μg/min is outside the limits due to the changed impedance. Cineangiography pre-operatively revealed anterior wall akinesis which had disappeared by the post-operative study. At the heart rate the power at 3 μg/min is seen to have improved from just over 0.3 watts to about 0.8 watts and there has also been an increase at the second harmonic from just over 0.1 watts to over 0.2 watts.

This technique of pre- and post-operative cardiac assessment has been

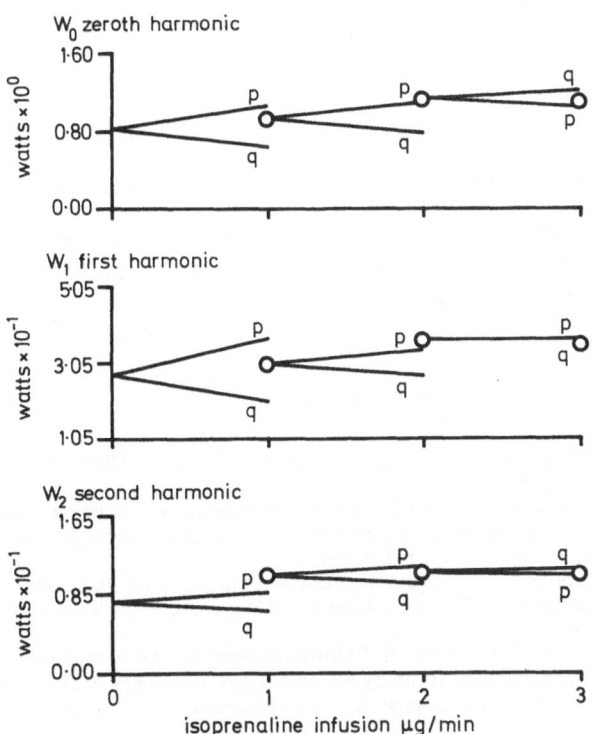

*Figure 10.* Power flow in human subject prior to coronary artery bypass surgery.

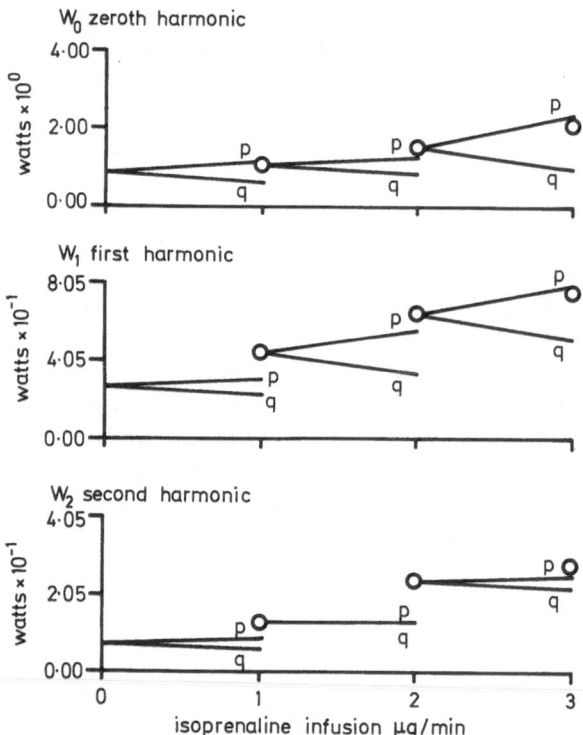

*Figure 11.* Power flow in human subject after coronary artery bypass surgery.

applied systematically to a series of 15 patients and may now be considered a valuable method for the measurement of improvements, if any, which are effected by coronary artery bypass surgery.

REFERENCES

1. Van der Werff TJ: Studies in cardiovascular fluid dynamics. Thesis, D Phil, University of Oxford, Oxford, 1971.
2. Sagawa K: Analysis of the ventricular pumping capacity as a function of input and output pressure loads. In: *Physical basis of circulatory transport*, Reeve EB, Guyton AC (eds), Philadelphia, Saunders, 1967, p 141–149.
3. Mills CJ: A catheter-tip electromagnetic velocity probe. *Phys Med Biol* 11:323, 1966.
4. Gessner U, Bergel DH: Frequency response of electromagnetic flowmeters. *J Appl Physiol* 19:1209, 1964.
5. Wexler H, Kuaity J, Simonson E: Electrocardiographic effects of isoprenaline in normal subjects and patients with coronary atherosclerosis. *Brit Heart J* 33:759, 1971.
6. Combs DT, Martin CM: Evaluation of isoproterenol as a method of stress testing. *Am Heart J* 87:711, 1974.
7. Rushmer RF: Initial ventricular impulse: a potential key to cardiac evaluation. *Circulation* 29:268, 1964.

8. Rushmer RF: *Cardiovascular dynamics*, Philadelphia, Saunders, 1970.
9. Adams AP, Clarke TNS, Edmond-Seal D, Foëx P, Prys-Roberts C, Roberts DG: The effects of sodium nitroprusside on myocardial contractility and haemodynamics. *Brit J Anaesthesia* 46:897, 1974.
10. Ross G, Cole PV: Cardiovascular actions of sodium nitroprusside in dogs. *Anaesthesia* 28:400, 1973.
11. Mann T, Cohn PF, Holman BL, Green LH, Markis JE, Phillips DA: Effect of nitroprusside on regional myocardial blood flow in coronary artery disease. *Circulation* 57:4, 1978.

## 4.2. QUANTIFICATION OF EXTRAVASCULAR CORONARY RESISTANCE

BERND WÜSTEN, WOLFGANG SCHAPER

### 1. INTRODUCTION

Myocardial perfusion depends upon the pressure and is a function of the resistance of the coronary vessels. The resistance changes with the diameter of the vessels and with the number of flow-limiting vascular structures. A restriction of coronary flow may be caused by "autoregulation" which causes changes in the width of the resistance vessels, controlled by a feedback mechanism, according to the metabolic demand of the myocardium. In addition myocardial contraction causes a decrease of flow within the intramural coronary branches during systole by extravascular compression. Such an increase and decrease of coronary arterial and also coronary venous flow during the cardiac cycle has been experimentally confirmed by previous investigations (1, 2, 3, 4). With these observations evidence was brought forward that coronary resistance is composed of a vascular and an extravascular component.

Coronary resistance can be calculated from coronary flow and the pressure difference between perfusion pressure and post-capillary pressure. This approach, however, does not identify the vascular and extravascular components that contribute to the total coronary resistance. To determine the extravascular resistance by itself Standfuss (5) and Bretschneider (6) suggested the measurement of flow and pressure during maximal vasodilation in order to exclude vascular regulation of resistance or measurement at a constant minimal vascular resistance respectively. The obvious advantage of this approach is a direct determination of the extravascular resistance, as it is transmitted to the coronary vessels during the cardiac cycle. This approach led to a number of observations showing an increase of coronary extravascular resistance with increasing heart rate, left ventricular pressure, and contractility (7, 8, 9, 10). In addition, further observations led to the assumption that the intracavitary left ventricular pressure may be the primary determinant of the extravascular coronary resistance, therewith assuming a passive role during diastole, and an active role during systole (11, 12).

Intramyocardial pressure can be described as a passive transmission of the intraventricular pressure across the ventricular wall and hence will

J. Baan, A.C. Arntzenius, E.L. Yellin (eds.), Cardiac Dynamics, 249–259.

generate extravascular compressive forces. This postulation implies that passive elastic wall stress, i.e. the radial component of wall stress, may account for the extravascular coronary resistance under the assumption that intramyocardial pressure acts on the coronary circulation as a Starling resistor (13,14,15); this mechanism was compared to so-called "vascular waterfalls" which model has been favoured by Permutt (16) and applied to the pulmonary circulation. His theory implies that the arterial driving pressure equals the difference between arterial pressure and intramyocardial pressure. The hypothesis that such a mechanism may be responsible for the extravascular resistance in the coronary circulation was the subject of our own experimental work. The feasibility of quantifying extravascular flow impedance has been investigated with respect to overall ventricular flow and regional coronary blood supply, since regional coronary flow, i.e. transmural flow distribution, might be of major importance for the pathogenesis of the increased vulnerability of the subendocardium.

For this purpose any investigation should be based on a determination of

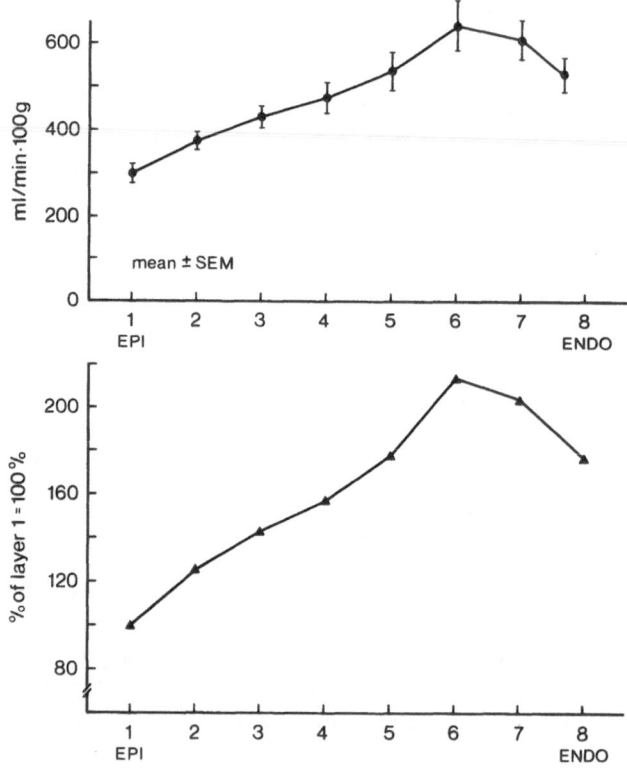

*Figure 1.* Maximal coronary flow values in 8 different wall layers of the diastolic arrested left ventricle at a perfusion pressure of 76 mmHg.

the vascular dilatory capacity of the coronary resistance vessels, since the actual coronary flow is influenced by both vascular and extravascular coronary resistance.

Therefore the functional capacity of the regional vasculature in the left ventricular wall was measured at maximal vasodilation on the isolated unloaded canine heart. In isolated hearts which were perfused under constant pressure with arterial blood from a support dog, maximal vasodilation was achieved by adenosine infusion and the hearts were arrested by procainamide infusion. Coronary flow was measured by the injection of radioactive labelled tracer microsphere (TM). Regional coronary flow was determined in eight different transmural wall layers from the prevailing tissue radioactivity. Results from nine experiments obtained at a perfusion pressure of 76 mmHg (mean) are shown in Figure 1.

Mean left ventricular coronary resistance at maximal vasodilation amounted to 0.157 mmHg·min·100 g·ml$^{-1}$ in absence of any extravascular compression of the coronary arteries. The ratio of subendocardial over subepicardial flow was $1.62 \pm 0.28$ (mean $\pm$ SD). The transmural flow distribution evaluated in eight different layers revealed a progressive increase of flow from the most superficial layer towards the subendocardium with a maximum in layer 6. A slight decrease in the deepest layers (7 and 8) was noted. When maximal coronary flow was measured in the unloaded diastolic arrested left ventricle the dilatory capacity of the supplying vessels could be demonstrated to increase with ventricular wall depth which suggested a better vascularization of the subendocardium.

## 2. INFLUENCE OF VENTRICULAR FIBRILLATION AND CONTRACTION ON CORONARY FLOW

There is little information in the literature whether ventricular contraction or fibrillation per se affect coronary blood supply. Contradictory data have been reported (11, 17, 18, 19). Therefore in isolated heart experiments the transmural flow distribution was measured in the unloaded left ventricle, during adenosine-induced vasodilation, by TM injections in hearts beating at 100 beats/min and in addition in hearts during electrically induced ventricular fibrillation. Our results are shown in Figure 2. In both groups the ratio of subendocardial versus subepicardial left ventricular flow (ENDO/EPI) was only slightly different from 1.0 at a perfusion pressure of 70 mmHg. The mean values were 1.1 and 0.95 in empty beating and in fibrillating hearts respectively. These data show that the increased subendocardial dilatory capacity that is demonstrable in diastolic arrested hearts is reduced during unloaded cardiac contraction and completely abolished during ventricular fibrillation. In previous experiments we found that at a

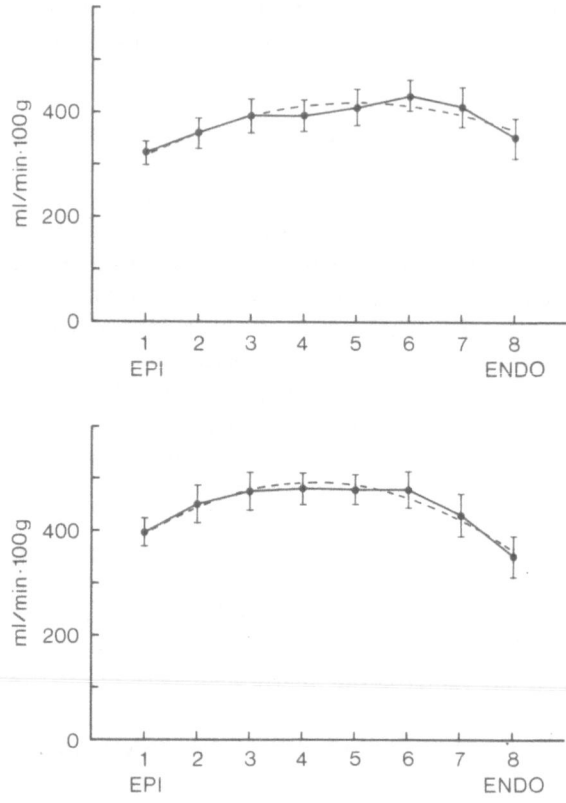

*Figure 2.* Transmural distribution of maximal coronary flow at a perfusion pressure of 70 mmHg demonstrated for the unloaded left ventricle of (*top*) hearts beating at a pacing rate of 100 beats/min and (*bottom*) fibrillating hearts.

low heart rate of 35–40 beats/min (complete atrioventricular block) under comparable experimental conditions the ENDO/EPI ratio was 1.30 which suggests a frequency dependence of the extravascular component of resistance during ventricular contraction.

## 3. EXTRAVASCULAR CORONARY RESISTANCE DUE TO INTRAVENTRICULAR LOAD

We chose to perform these investigations in isolated hearts also because of numerous advantages to this approach: above all a rigid control of ventricular load, coronary perfusion pressure and coronary vasomotor tone. In order to control ventricular volume and pressure loads a thin latex balloon with an unstressed volume of about 80 ml was placed into the left ventricle via the mitral annulus.

In one group (A) experiments were performed at cardiac arrest during maximal vasodilation. Coronary flow was measured at volume loads corresponding to intraventricular pressure values of zero and at four to five different intraventricular pressures between zero and a maximum value close to the coronary perfusion pressure. In a second group (B) identical experiments were carried out during electrically induced ventricular fibrillation. In a third group (C) of experiments isovolumetrically beating hearts were studied at various diastolic and systolic loads, due to alterations in heart rate, diastolic pressure and volume load, systolic isometric peak pressure, and contractility.

Total coronary resistance (CRT) of the entire left ventricle and regional resistances of the different layers of the left ventricular wall were calculated for each experimental condition. Since CRT equals the sum of vascular (CRV) and extravascular (CRE) components of resistance: CRT = CRE + CRV, and all measurements were performed at maximal coronary dilation, CRV can be assumed to be constant for each individual heart, and CRT in the unloaded ventricle represents CRV: CRT = CRV, when CRE is zero.

However such an assumption is only valid for diastolic arrested hearts, since extravascular influences must be considered in beating and fibrillating hearts. Therefore CRV needs to be defined for each experimental condition. At an intraventricular pressure of zero this represents the minimal possible coronary resistance. Total coronary resistance and the ENDO/EPI ratio of flow were expressed as a function of intraventricular pressure load in all groups. CRT at maximal vasodilation showed a linear increase with the augmentation of intraventricular pressure, while the ENDO/EPI ratio was found to decrease continuously. Accordingly it could be concluded that changes of coronary resistance at maximal vasodilation can be mainly attributed to the state of subendocardial flow. This finding is supported strongly by the determination of extravascular coronary resistance for the different wall layers as a function of intraventricular pressure. In Figure 3 data from isovolumetrically beating hearts are shown. The results obtained in group A and B were comparable.

4. DETERMINANTS OF THE EXTRAVASCULAR CORONARY RESISTANCE

Intraventricular pressure has been assumed to be the major determinant of extravascular coronary compression. The theoretically well-founded theory suggests that intraventricular pressure forces, acting perpendicularly on the inner surface of the ventricular wall are transmitted through the wall and

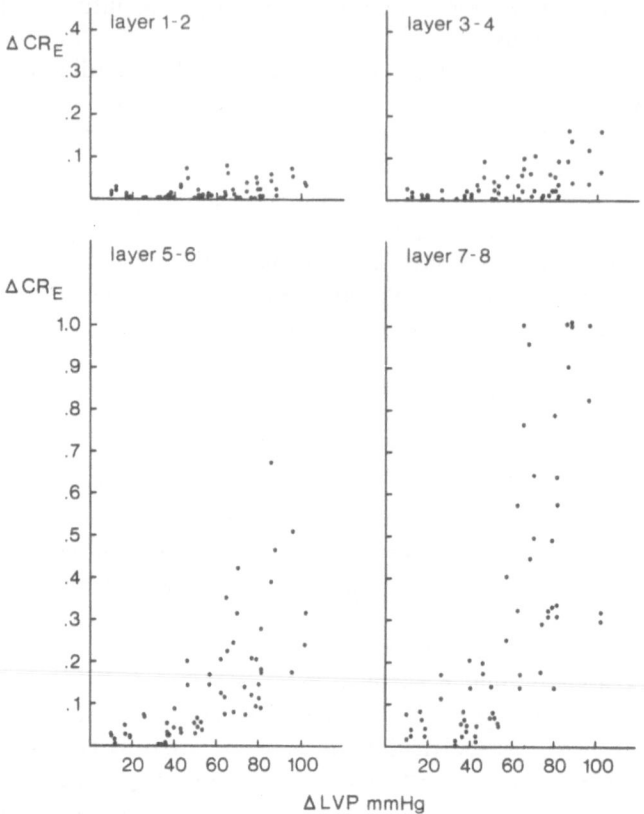

*Figure 3.* The extravascular coronary resistance (CR$_E$) in mmHg·min·100g·ml$^{-1}$ in iso-volumetric beating hearts plotted against left ventricular mean pressure (LVP) for different layers of the ventricular wall.

generate radial and circumferential wall stress forces. Radial wall stress is the compressive force which supposedly equals intraventricular cavity pressure in the subendocardial layer, decreasing towards the epicardium and approaching zero at the outer surface (20). The radial component of wall stress has been favoured as the major determinant of intramyocardial tissue pressure (IMP). Based on the relationship between CRT, perfusion pressure (CP), and coronary flow (CBF): CRT = CP/CBF, and on the waterfall theory which implies that local coronary driving pressure (CPL) equals the difference between CP and IMP: CPL = CP − IMP, vascular coronary resistance at abolished autoregulation can be given as a quotient of CPL and CBF: CRV = CPL/CBF. At the same time the equation can be converted to: IMP = CP − CRV · CBF.

Hence IMP can be determined from coronary flow measurements as

long as vascular coronary resistance is known. The concept that intramyocardial pressure can be determined indirectly from measurements of
coronary flow in the maximally dilated coronary bed was applied to the
heart in order to overcome methodological difficulties of direct measurements of intramyocardial tissue pressure. Controversial results with respect
to absolute values of intramyocardial pressure measured directly by various
methods, can be considered to result from local trauma caused by placement of the measuring devices that have been used. Previous work from
others has pointed out that all direct measurements of tissue pressure are
questionable (13).

Calculations of IMP in eight different wall layers were performed in
diastolic arrested, fibrillating and beating hearts for all given values of
intraventricular pressure load. In Figure 4 regional IMP for the different
wall layers are shown as a function of intraventricular pressure in isovolumetrically beating hearts. In this group as well as in groups A and B an
increasing slope of the regression lines with increasing wall depth has been
demonstrated, suggesting a progressive increase of IMP towards the subendocardium. The regression coefficient near 1.0 in the subendocardial layers
7 and 8 proves that IMP in these layers is comparable to the intraventricular cavity pressure. The data support the hypothesis that the radial

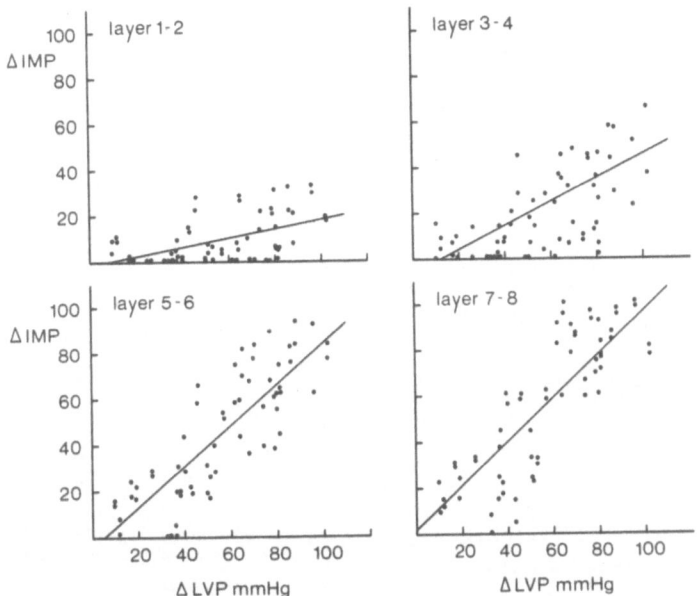

*Figure 4.* The behaviour of regional intramyocardial pressure (IMP) in different wall layers with
increasing mean left ventricular pressure (LVP) in isovolumetric beating hearts.

component of wall stress may account for the dominant determinant of the extravascular coronary resistance.

In order to support this finding further, wall stress forces due to the passive elastic conductance of intraventricular cavity pressure were calculated and compared to IMP values measured from changes of regional coronary flow. In order to calculate wall stress within the thick wall, the left ventricle was considered to be a thick-walled sphere and the myocardium was assumed to consist of an elastic homogeneous and isotropic material.

The wall stress values calculated for diastolic arrested and fibrillating hearts were compared to the respective values of IMP calculated from changes in coronary flow ($IMP_Q$) for all wall layers and intraventricular pressure levels (see Figure 5). The relationship between $\sigma R$ and $IMP_Q$ in both groups is described as a linear function. The regression equation and the correlation coefficients are:

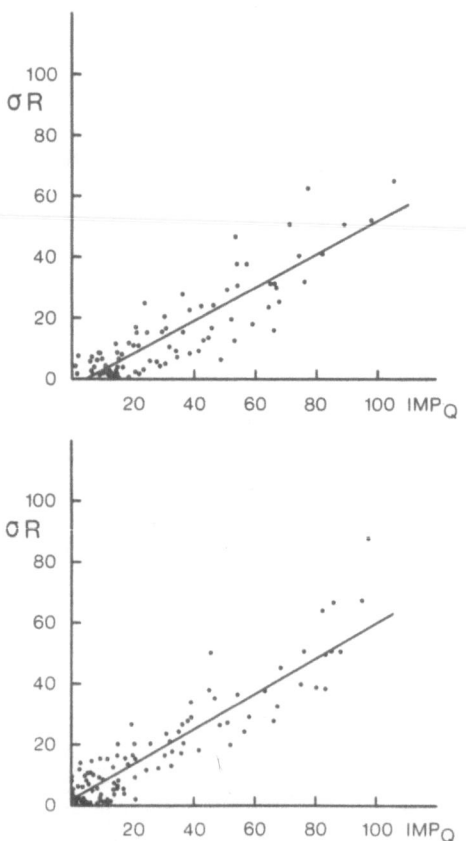

*Figure 5.* The correlation between radial wall stess ($\sigma R$) and intramyocardial pressure (IMP) in the pressure-loaded diastolic arrested (*top*) and fibrillating (*bottom*) left ventricle.

group A: $\sigma R = 0.54 \ IMP_Q - 2.4 \ (r = 0.88)$;

group B: $\sigma \ R = 0.59 \ IMP_Q + 2.7 \ (r = 0.92)$.

A regression coefficient of 0.54 in group A and 0.59 in group B reveals, obviously, that neither in diastolic arrested hearts nor in fibrillating hearts can intramyocardial pressure be explained by the radial component of wall stress alone. Since wall stress cannot be caused by ventricular contraction in diastolic arrested hearts and has already been considered in fibrillating hearts, the hypothesis has been brought forward that in addition to radial compressive forces tangential wall stresses might be responsible for the extravascular compression of the coronary supply vessels.

From our data on diastolic arrested and fibrillating hearts the fractional contribution of tangential wall stress in the different wall layers has been calculated in order to describe $IMP_Q$ by wall stress forces. Correlation of the individual data points between IMP measured from regional coronary flow changes ($IMP_Q$) and IMP calculated from wall stresses ($IMP_\sigma$) revealed regression coefficients of 0.99 for group A and 0.91 for group B. Since it is possible to explain extravascular compression of the coronaries in terms of wall stresses in diastolic arrested and fibrillating hearts by the described method the same should be equally applicable to the beating heart. In the case of the beating heart it has to be considered that during intraventricular pressure increases, and during systol, IMP in the subendocardium may reach values above coronary perfusion pressure, with the consequence that flow ceases completely, and values of IMP greater than CP at further increase of intraventricular pressure consequently will be ineffective since flow has reached zero already. For each experimental hemodynamic condition and for each wall layer this so-called critical intraventricular pressure was determined. Intraventricular pressures above this level were not taken into account for the calculation of extravascular compressive forces. The effective mean IMP over the entire cardiac cycle was calculated from diastolic and systolic IMP values. When, for all layers and each evaluated left ventricular load, i.e. altered heart rate, diastolic and systolic intraventricular pressure, and contractile state, was calculated from both changes of maximal coronary flow ($\Delta IMP_Q$) and wall stresses ($\Delta IMP_\sigma$) a correlation near the line of identity was obtained: $IMP_Q = 0.90 IMP_\sigma + 1.31$, $r = 0.91$ (see also Figure 6).

SUMMARY

Our experiments demonstrate that the left ventricular extravascular compression of the coronary arteries correlates with intraventricular cavity pressure.

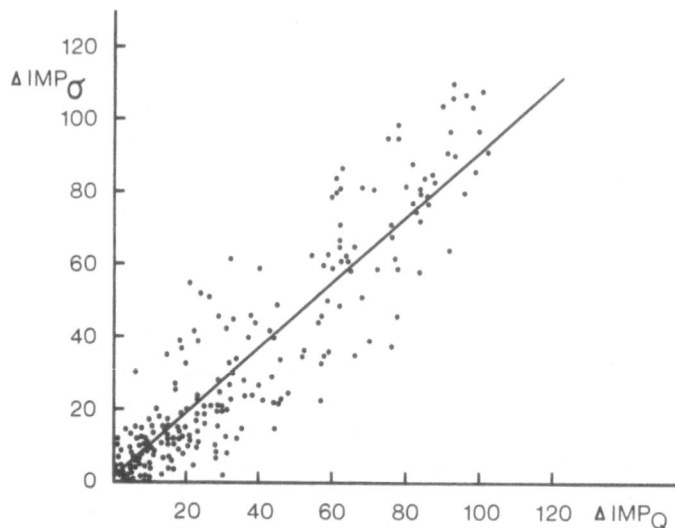

*Figure 6.* The correlation between both values of intramyocardial pressure (IMP$_Q$ and IMP$_\sigma$) for isovolumetrically beating hearts.

Measurements of regional coronary perfusion revealed a redistribution of coronary flow away from the subendocardium with increase of extravascular coronary resistance. Augmented left ventricular loading caused an elevation of extravascular resistance in the subendocardial wall layers to reach 1.0 mmHg·min·100g·ml$^{-1}$, which led to a restriction of flow in the concerned myocardium amounting to 10 to 15% of the normal dilatory capacity. This reduction of subendocardial perfusion represents subendocardial ischaemia, at normal anatomy of the coronary arteries. Elastic conductance of intraventricular cavity pressure causes a local extravascular compression of the coronaries which is negligible in the superficial wall layers and increases towards the subendocardium.

The values of intramyocardial pressure in any location within the ventricular wall and at any ventricular loading condition correlate with the radial component of wall stress.

The actual values of IMP, however, cannot be accounted for entirely by radial wall stresses alone; therefore, it has been suggested that extravascular resistance is partially due to circumferential wall stress forces. The validity of this hypothesis could be established in isovolumetrically beating hearts with alterations of ventricular load over a wide range.

A decreased subendocardial vascular resistance due to a better vascularization which could be demonstrated in the unloaded diastolic arrested heart is proposed as an important mechanism to compensate for extravascular compression during normal cardiac contraction. This finding contradicts the commonly acknowledged hypothesis of a diminished vascular tone in the subendocardium as a single mechanism to provide for a homogeneous distribution of flow in the normal beating heart.

REFERENCES

1. Anrep GVon, Cruickshank EWH, Downing AC Subba Rau A: Coronary circulation in relation to the cardiac cycle. *Heart* 14:11, 1927.
2. Gregg DE, Fisher LC: Blood supply to the heart. In: *Handbook of physiology*, Washington DC, American Physiological Society, 1963.
3. Sabiston DC, Gregg DE: Effect of cardiac contraction on coronary flow. *Circulation* 15:14–20, 1957.
4. Wiggers CJ: The interplay of coronary vascular resistance and myocardial compression in regulation coronary flow. *Circ Res* 2:271–279, 1954.
5. Standfuss K: Die mechanische Wirkung der Herzkontraktion auf die Coronardurchblutung. Inaugural dissertation, Cologne, 1963.
6. Bretschneider HJ: Aktuelle Probleme der Coronardurchblutung und des Myokardstoffwechsels. *Regensb Jb Ärztl Fortb* 15:1–27, 1967.
7. Raff WK, Kosche F, Lochner W: Extravasale Komponente des Coronarwiderstandes und Coronardurchblutung bei steigendem enddiastolischen Druck. *Pflügers Arch* 327:225–233, 1971.
8. Raff WK, Kosche F, Lochner W: Herzfrequenz und extravasale Komponente des Coronarwiderstandes. *Pflügers Arch* 323:241–249, 1971.
9. Raff WK. Kosche F. Lochner W: Die extravasale Komponente des Coronarwiderstandes bei Steigerung der linksventrikulären Druckanstiegsgeschwindigkeit durch Isoproterenol. *Pflügers Arch* 325:323–333, 1971.
10. Raff WK, Kosche F, Lochner W: Extravascular coronary resistance and its relation to microcirculation. *Am J Cardiol* 29:598–603, 1972.
11. Downey JM, Downey HF, Kirk ES: Effects of myocardial strains on coronary blood flow. *Circ Res* 34:286–292, 1974.
12. Snyder R, Downey JM, Kirk ES: The active and passive components of extravascular coronary resistance. *Cardiovasc Res* 9:161–166, 1975.
13. Archie JP: Intramyocardial pressure: effect of preload on transmural distribution of systolic coronary blood flow. *Am J Cardiol* 35:904–911, 1975.
14. Downey JM, Kirk ES: The distribution of coronary blood flow across the canine heart wall during systole. *Circ Res* 34:251–257, 1974.
15. Downey JM, Kirk ES: Inhibition of coronary blood flow by a vascular waterfall mechanism. *Circ Res* 36:753–760, 1975.
16. Permutt S. Bromberger-Barnea B, Bane HN: Alveolar pressure, pulmonary venous pressure, and vascular waterfall. *Med Thorac* 19:239–260, 1962.
17. Baird RJ, Dudka F, Okumori M, De La Roche A, Goldbrock MM, Hill W, MacGregor DC: Surgical aspects of regional myocardial blood flow and myocardial pressure. *J Thorac Cardiovasc Surg* 69:17–29, 1975.
18. Hottenrott CE, Maloney Jr JV, Buckberg GD: Studies on the effects of ventricular fibrillation on the adequacy of regional myocardial blood flow: electrical *vs* spontaneous fibrillation. *J Thorac Cardiovasc Surg* 68:615–625, 1974.
19. Reis RL, Cohn LH, Morrow AG: Effects of induced ventricular fibrillation on myocardial performance and cardiac metabolism. *Circulation* 36 (suppl 1):234–243, 1967.
20. Wong AYK, Rautaharju PM: Stress distribution within the left ventricular wall approximated as a thick ellipsoidal shell. *Am Heart J* 75:649–662, 1968.

# 4.3. STUDIES ON THE OPTIMAL MATCHING BETWEEN HEART AND ARTERIAL SYSTEM

T. KENNER, K.P. PFEIFFER

## 1. INTRODUCTION

A large number of parameters and variables contribute to the control of heart and circulation. It has been argued since about half a century ago that some kind of optimal relationship contributes to the design as well as to the regulation of some of these magnitudes (1). Broemser (2) in 1935 was the first to propose that some optimal relationship exists between heart rate and stroke volume. One special aspect of optimal control in the circulation was found to be the time course of the ejection of blood from the left ventricle. The hypothesis that the ejection pattern follows such a function that the external energy loss per stroke is minimized is part of Broemser's original problem. A solution of this problem was first given by Yamashiro et al. (3) and has been further developed by Kenner and Estelberger (4) and by Pfeiffer and Kenner (5). At the same time, Noldus (6) developed similar methods. In this study we will discuss a further improvement of the method of calculus of variations which appears important for any practical application of the method, such as comparison between model and measurement for the purpose of parameter estimation.

One of the main problems in uncovering presumably optimal control mechanisms is the unsolved question of biological optimization criteria. Usually the optimal condition consists of a compromise between different parameters and functions, minimizing a certain loss which, from a practical point of view, is mostly assumed as energy loss.

Another problem which will be discussed in the study is the magnitude of the economic or energetic advantage of certain optimal adjustments. We will show that even in the apparently optimal relationship between heart and circulation the energetic advantage of optimization is surprisingly small. Furthermore, we will discuss additional factors which, besides optimization, influence the time course of central aortic flow and pressure.

## 2. CALCULATION OF OPTIMAL PULSES

The characteristics of the central aortic flow pulse contour are its steep ascent, which leads to a peak flow early in systole, and a slow descent which, together, give the pulse a more or less triangular shape. During the.

J. Baan, A.C. Arntzenius, E.L. Yellin (eds.), Cardiac Dynamics, 261–270.

descent of the flow a "shoulder" or "nose" can usually be found, as shown in
the typical pulse in Figure 1.

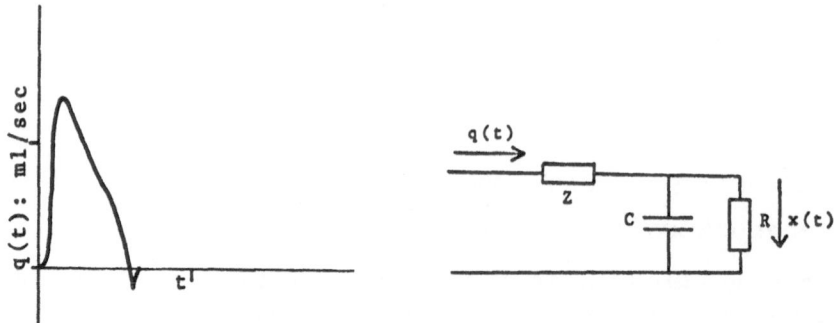

*Figure 1. Left*: characteristic human aortic flow pulse as used by Anliker et al. as standard
input for their model (11); *right*: model of the arterial system.

Following first the method described by Yamashiro et al. (3) we use as
model of the arterial system a windkessel model with a resistance $Z$ which
simulates the characteristic impedance of the aorta, a peripheral resistance
$R$, and a capacitance $C$. The model is shown in Figure 1.

During systole $[0, S]$ the arterial or ventricular pressure $p(t)$, the central
aortic flow $q(t)$ and the peripheral flow $x(t)$ through the resistance $R$ can be
described by the following equations:

$$q(t) = x(t) + RC \; \dot{x}(t),$$
$$p(t) = Z \; q(t) + R \; x(t). \qquad\qquad 0 \le t \le S \qquad\qquad [1]$$

We assume as optimization criterion that the ejection pattern of the
ventricle takes place in such a time course that the total external stroke
work is minimized:

$$W = \int_0^S p(t)q(t)dt \to \min. \qquad\qquad [2]$$

Furthermore, we assume that the pulses are periodic with period $T$ such
that

$$x(0) = x(T) = x_0. \qquad\qquad [3]$$

During systole a given stroke volume $V_s$ is being ejected

$$\int_0^S q(t)dt = V_s. \qquad\qquad [4]$$

During diastole

$$q(t) = 0$$
$$x(t) = x_0 \exp((T-t)/RC) \qquad\qquad S \le t \le T \qquad\qquad [5]$$

Besides that, the following boundary condition is given for the central aortic flow:

$$q(0) = q(S) = 0 \tag{6}$$

By considering the [1] for $q(t)$ and $p(t)$ the condition for optimization can be written as a function of $x(t)$, $\dot{x}(t)$ and $t$:

$$\int_0^S F(x, \dot{x}, t)dt \to \min, \tag{7}$$

with

$$F(x, \dot{x}, t) = x^3(R + Z) + x\dot{x}\ RC(2Z + R) + \dot{x}^2(R^2C^2Z). \tag{8}$$

A function $x(t)$ which makes this functional to an extremum has to be a solution of the Euler-Lagrange equation:

$$\frac{\delta F}{\delta x} - \frac{d}{dt}\frac{\delta F}{\delta \dot{x}} = 0. \tag{9}$$

A necessary condition for this extremum to be a minimum is the fulfilment of the Legendre inequality

$$\frac{\delta^2 F}{\delta \dot{x}^2} > 0. \tag{10}$$

The flow pulses computed according to these assumptions have a strange appearance insofar as the steepness of the ascent of the flow pulse is infinite as can be seen in Figure 2. (The computations described in this paper were performed on a Hewlett-Packard 2100A digital computer.) Pulses of the kind shown in Figure 2 have been presented by Yamashiro et al. (3) and by Kenner and Estelberger (4). With respect to the steep ascent these pulses do not agree sufficiently with physiological pulses.

### 3. CALCULATION OF OPTIMAL PULSES WITH FINITE STEEPNESS

In order to improve these results and to reach conditions which are compatible with the biological properties of the system involved, we considered also the condition

$$\dot{q}(0) = 0 \tag{11}$$

in our computations.

A new extended functional allows us to calculate flow pulse contours by iteration in order to satisfy the condition of periodicity $x(0) = x(T)$. As can be seen in Figure 3 the flow contours according to the extended conditions agree much better with the characteristic physiological shapes.

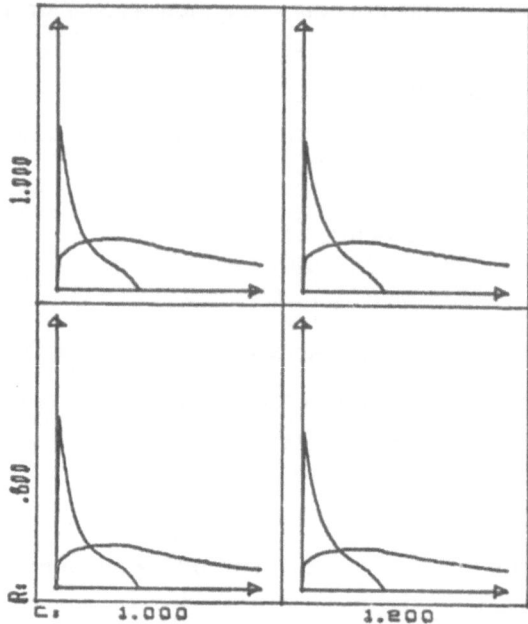

*Figure 2.* Optimal contours of flow (peaked pulse) and pressure with infinite ascending slope of the flow pulse for two different values of the peripheral resistance $R$ (mmHg·sec/ml) and for compliance $C$ (ml/mmHg). $T$ is pulse period (1.000 sec), $S$ is duration of systole (0.400 sec), $VS$ is stroke volume (75.000 ml), $Z = 0.006$ mmHg·sec/ml.

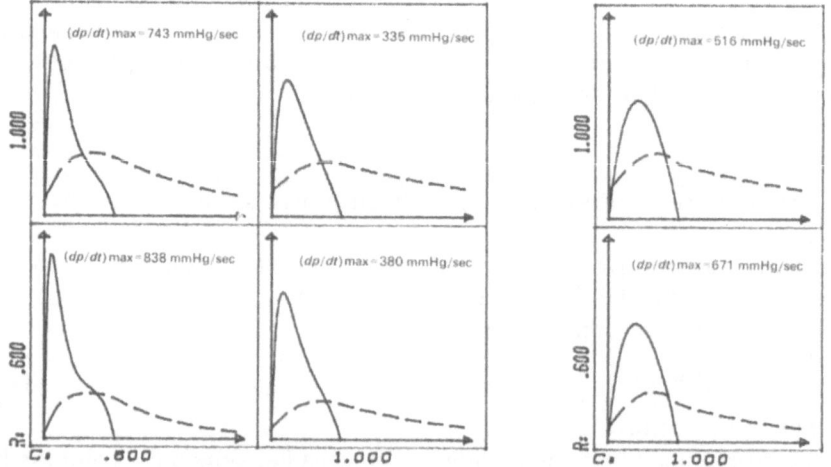

*Figure 3.* Optimal flow and pressure pulses calculated under the additional constraint $\dot{q}(0) = 0$. $T = 1.000$; $S = 0.350$; $VS = 80.000$; $Z = 0.010$.

In a series of flow and pressure pulses Figure 3 shows the influence of the variation of peripheral resistance $R$ (normal value 1.0 mmHg·sec/ml), capacitance $C$ (normal value 1.0 ml/mmHg) and of the characteristic impedance $Z$ (normal value 0.1 mmHg·sec/ml) of the windkessel. The following parameters were kept constant: pulse period $T=1$ sec, duration of systole $S=0.35$ sec, stroke volume $VS=80$ ml.

It is interesting that the shoulder in the downslope of the flow pulses can only be seen at low values of the characteristic impedance $Z$. This fact, apparently, does not agree completely with physiological conditions since the shoulder can be seen in vivo at higher (normal) values of the characteristic impedance. At $Z=0.1$ mmHg·sec/ml in our model the shoulder is absent in all pulses.

Nevertheless, the improvement of the pulse contours is sufficient to expect further clarification of these open questions. The new results allow us to examine additional parameters with respect to optimal conditions. From the pressure pulses shown in Figure 3 the values of the maximal pressure slope $(dp/dt)_{max}$ were measured. Since the magnitude of this slope depends on the parameter values of the model, a comparison with in vivo measurements seems possible. It can be seen that the slope of optimal pulses increases with reduction of peripheral resistance and of capacitance. The less distensible the aortic windkessel, the steeper the slope of the pulse pressure was found. At high values of the resistance $Z$ an increase of the maximal slope of optimal pressure pulses was found in such a way that doubling $Z$ would increase $(dp/dt)_{max}$ by about 20%. A similar behaviour of the parameter $(dp/dt)_{max}$ can be found in physiological pulses (7).

## 4. EFFECTIVENESS OF OPTIMIZATION

In the preceding calculations of optimal pressure and flow contours we have assumed that the optimization in this system consists in the minimization of the external work of the heart. The fundamental shape of the central flow pulse can be described as triangular. For this reason we have attempted to determine the effectiveness of the optimization by comparing optimal to triangular pulses. The triangular pulses with different time position of the systolic peak of the triangle and with the same given stroke volume are considered as suboptimal pulses. The energy loss was compared with that of optimal pulses. It was found that the external stroke work for generating suboptimal triangular pulses is only slightly higher than the energy necessary to generate optimal pulses. As is shown in Figure 4, some effect can be observed if the influence of the peripheral resistance $R$ is examined. In the left ordinate of Figure 4, the external work of optimal pulses is set at 100%. The three lines designated curve 1 represent the relative energy loss

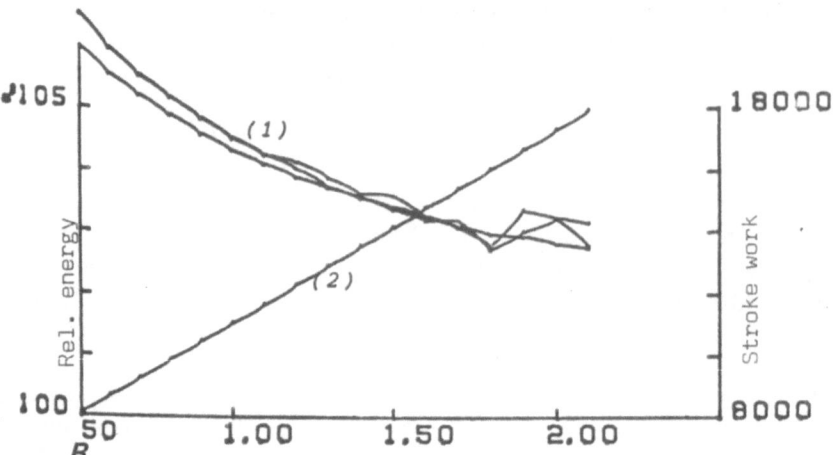

*Figure 4.* Influence of the peripheral resistance $R$ on the effectiveness of optimization. Curve 1 shows the relative energy loss for the generation of triangular flow pulses with three different positions of the peak of the flow pulse. Curve 2 shows the increase of stroke work with rising peripheral resistance $R$. $VS = 80.000$; $T = 1.000$; $C = 1.000$; $S = 0.350$; $Z = 0.200$.

for the generation of triangular flow pulses. Three different positions of the peak were considered, which apparently made no difference in the result (beginning, middle, and end of systole). The right ordinate represents the absolute value of stroke work. The trend of curve 2 shows, that stroke work increases with rising peripheral resistance. An increase of $Z$ would raise absolute stroke work as well as the relative energy loss of suboptimal pulses. The influence of the capacity $C$ is small.

It may be concluded that the gain or saving of energy due to optimization of the cardiac ejection pattern is rather small and may not exceed 5% under physiological conditions.

## 5. DETERMINATION OF THE DURATION OF SYSTOLE

The relative duration of systole was a possibility of adjustment which Broemser (2) had taken into account for the maximization of stroke volume. It can easily be shown that an increase of the systolic duration leads to a steady decrease of the energy expenditure of the ventricle (Figure 5). The way the ventricle would save the most energy may be achieved by pumping a steady flow, i.e.: $S = T$.

Mathematically, the final pulse shapes were calculated by iteration. The solution of the corresponding Euler-Lagrange equation [9] was repeated with ever-improving choice of the parameters until the condition $p(0) = p(T)$, which is the same as $x(0) = x(T)$, was met. In our examples the

duration of systole was kept fixed at a given value while the initial values of
$x(0)$ and $p(0)$ were varied. Another possibility would be to assume a fixed
given value for the diastolic pressure $p(0)$ and try to satisfy the condition of
periodicity by variation of the duration of the systole. A priori it can be
stated that in this case, under the prerequisite that the value of $p(0)$ lies
within realistic boundaries, the solution will find the longest possible
systolic duration which just satisfies the condition. Thus we are faced with
the problem that in the assumption of this model so far, the duration of
systole cannot be determined exactly by using an optimization criterion
because the solution would possibly be physiologically unrealistic if no
additional constraints are given.

One of the constraints which may be assumed for such a calculation is
that the energy supply to the heart is provided solely by coronary flow
which is proportional to the aortic blood pressure $p(t)$ and takes place only
during diastole $(S-T)$. Obviously more sophisticated criteria might be
introduced as well. If we simply assume that the energy supply to the heart
is proportional to the area under the diastolic part of aortic pressure this
implies that it decreases linearly with the duration of systole (Figure 5).
Thus the two curves for energy expenditure and supply tend to diverge as
the duration of systole increases.

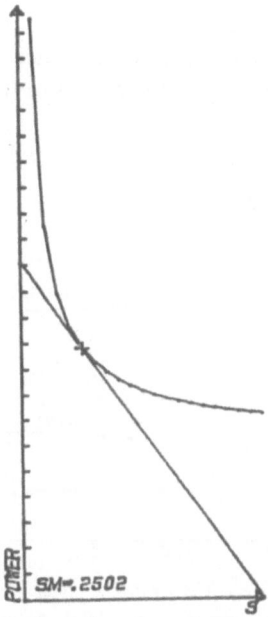

Figure 5. External work (curved line) and energy supply (straight line) by coronary flow
depending on the duration of the systole S. An optimal duration of the systole (SM) may be
determined by the limiting case in which both curves just touch. $R = 1.000$; $C = 1.000$; $VS =$
80.000; $Z = 0.100$; $T = 1.000$.

As Kenner (8) discussed recently, any condition in which the two curves either intersect and cross each other or in which they just touch is physically and biologically imaginable. It can be assumed that the first case usually prevails because the supply exceeds the expenditure of energy by a certain margin. A more detailed discussion has to take into account the fact that the effective supply is less than the actual supply since, due to the limited thermodynamic efficiency of the heart, a large part of the supply is wasted as heat. The limiting condition of both curves just touching each other is shown in Figure 5. A further decrease of the supply would be equivalent to apparent coronary insufficiency.

6. DETERMINATION OF THE HEART RATE

The adjustment of frequency played the most important role in Broemser's (2) argumentation. His model of the arterial system had a very marked minimum of the input impedance at a certain "optimal" frequency. In the arterial system such a minimum is hardly observable, if at all present (1, 9).

If we examine the influence of increasing frequency under the condition of constant $S/T$ ratio in our model we find that pressure amplitude as well as external power for a given cardiac output decreases with increasing frequency. Thus, if no other constraint were present, the heart should increase its frequency in order to minimize external power expenditure. One possible actual constraint may be deduced from Figure 6. It consists in the marked

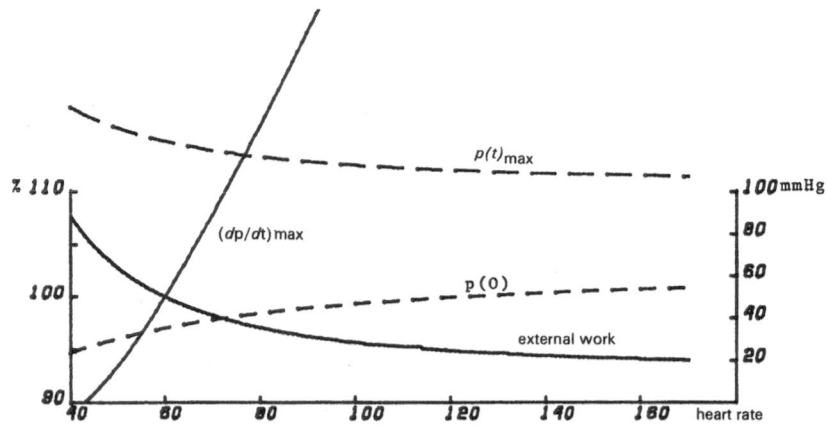

*Figure 6.* Relative decrease of external work for a given cardiac output (5000 ml/min) with increasing heart rate. Relative increase of the maximal ascending slope of pressure $(dp/dt)_{max}$, with increasing frequency. Also shown are systolic, $p(t)_{max}$ and diastolic, $p(0)$ aortic pressures (dashed lines). $PP(0) = 687$; work/min (Hz) $= 519071$; $VS/min = 5000$; $C = 0.800$; $T/TS = 3.000$; $Z = 0.100$; $R = 0.800$.

increase of the ascending slope $dp/dt$ in optimal pressure pulses with increasing frequency, indicating a considerable rise in internal energy demand and in total energy expenditure of the heart.

## 7. DISCUSSION

Optimization of the relation between heart and arterial system by adjustment of the properties of the heart is just one part of a more general problem. Properties of the arterial system also play a role, including the possible optimization of the characteristic impedance with respect to arterial pressure and the more or less optimal matching between characteristic impedance and peripheral resistance by tapering of the arterial system found by Taylor (9) and Kenner (1).

Our presentation has shown that the criteria of minimization of the external energy expenditure leads to a surprisingly small economic advantage for the pump compared with suboptimal ways of pumping. Other criteria may be examined, including one recently described by Noldus (6):

$$\int_0^S (p^2(t) + p(t)q(t))dt \to \min, \tag{12}$$

which apparently attempts to include elastic properties of the ventricle. This criterion, however, leads to pulse contours which have finite but surprisingly slow ascending slope not in agreement with physiological pulses and thus does not seem to improve the results.

It appears that inclusion of a more detailed description of the geometric properties of the ventricle mechanics into our criteria will be needed to improve the results. Such an attempt will also be necessary for further development of the interpretation of parameters which can now be calculated with our method and are related to ventricular contractility, such as $(dp/dt)_{max}$. So far our results can only be interpreted as arising from the requirement of optimality. Yet proceeding further along this road may well lead to deeper insights.

Finally it should be mentioned that the procedure of optimization could be used for purposes of parameter estimation. Estelberger (10) has attempted to use the criterion of optimality for a noninvasive calculation of stroke volume from pulse contours by parameter adjustment. At this stage of development, however, such detailed computations may lead to erroneous results at large computational expense. We rather envision a comparison between experimentally obtained and calculated optimal pulses using a model the parameters of which have been derived from physiological measurements.

SUMMARY

We have described the calculation of optimal pulse contours of central aortic flow and pressure pulses using a procedure which was described first by Yamashiro et al. (3) and was developed further in our laboratory. The improved method allowed us to calculate flow pulses with finite ascending slope and characteristic shapes. In addition to earlier results we could calculate values for the parameter $(dp/dt)_{max}$ of optimal pressure pulses. A condition was discussed which permits the calculation of optimal values for the duration of systole. Furthermore it was found that the energy saving by optimization is surprisingly small. This indicated that, under physiological conditions, additional constraints are of equal importance for the purpose of circulatory control.

REFERENCES

1. Kenner T: Beziehung zwischen Dynamik und Regulation des Arteriensystems. *Verhandl Deut Ges Kreislaufforsch* 40:41–60, 1974.
2. Broemser P: Über die optimale Beziehung zwischen Herztätigkeit und physikalischen Konstanten des Gefässystems. *Zeitschr Biologie* 96:1–10, 1935.
3. Yamashiro SM, Daubenspeck JA, Bennett FM, Edelmann SK, Grodins FS. Optimal control analysis of left ventricular ejection. In: *Cardiovascular system dynamics*, Baan J, Noordergraaf A, Raines J (eds), Cambridge, MIT Press, 1978, p 427–431.
4. Kenner T, Estelberger W: Zur Frage der optimalen Abstimmung der Herzkontraktion an die Eigenschaften des Arteriensystems. *Verhandl Deut Ges Kreislaufforschg* 42:1976, 132–135.
5. Pfeiffer KP, Kenner T: Minimization of the external work of the left ventricle and optimization of flow and pressure pulses. In: *The arterial system*, Bauer RD, Busse R (eds), Berlin, Springer, 1978, p 216–223.
6. Noldus EJ: Optimal control aspects of left ventricular ejection dynamics. *J Theor Biol* 63:275–309, 1976.
7. Elzinga G, Westerhof N: Pressure and flow generated by the left ventricle against different impedances. *Circ Res* 32:178–186, 1973.
8. Kenner T: Zur Frage der Optimierung in der Abstimmung zwischen Herztätigkeit und Kreislauf. In: *Wechselwirkung zwischen Herztätigkeit und Kreislauf*, Hamburg, 1976.
9. Taylor MG: The elastic properties of arteries in relation to the physiological functions of the arterial system. *Gastroenterology* 52:358–363, 1967.
10. Estelberger W: Eine neue nichtinvasive Pulskontur-Schlagvolumsbestimmungsmethode aufgrund eines Optimierungsmodells der Herzarbeit. *Biomed Technik* 22:212–217, 1977.
11. Anliker, M, Stettler JC, Niederer P, Holenstein R: Prediction of shape changes of propagating flow and pressure pulses in human arteries. In: *The arterial system*, Bauer RD, Busse R (eds), Berlin Springer, 1978.

# 4.4. END-SYSTOLIC PRESSURE AS DIRECT DETERMINANT OF STROKE VOLUME FROM FIXED END-DIASTOLIC VOLUME IN ISOLATED CANINE LEFT VENTRICLE

Hiroyuki Suga, Kiichi Sagawa

## 1. INTRODUCTION

Ventricular systolic pressure as a whole has been considered the determinant of stroke volume of the ventricle which is contracting from a given end-diastolic (preload) volume under a given contractile state. However, the relative importance of the instantaneous ventricular pressure at different instants of systole remains unknown. In the present study, we investigated the effect of changing the magnitude of systolic ventricular pressure at the onset, middle, or end of ejection on stroke volume of isolated left ventricles, which contracted from a fixed end-diastolic volume. The results indicate that end-systolic pressure, rather than early or mid-systolic pressure, is the direct determinant of stroke volume in the ventricle contracting from a given end-diastolic volume under a given contractile state.

## 2. METHODS

The details of the surgical preparation were described elsewhere (1). Briefly, in each experiment, a pair of mongrel dogs (9–19 kg) were anesthetized with sodium pentobarbital (30 mg/kg, i.v.), an excised cross-circulated heart preparation was instituted, and a thin latex balloon was fitted in the left ventricle. Left ventricular thebesian flow was drained out. The heart preparation was perfused at a constant pressure between 75 and 125 mmHg (mean = 88 mmHg) at 35–37°C. The heart beat at a regular sinus rhythm between 75 and 130 beats/min (mean = 102) for 4–6 hours.

The balloon placed in the left ventricle was connected via the mitral annulus to the volume servo pump (Figure 1). The balloon and the water housing of the pump were primed with tap water without leaving any air bubbles. The water was reciprocated between the ventricle and the pump in synchrony with ventricular contraction in a programmed manner by the volume command signal which was generated by a specially designed signal generator. End-diastolic and end-systolic volumes were fixed at desired values by electrically clamping the corresponding voltages of the volume

J. Baan, A.C. Arntzenius, E.L. Yellin (eds.), Cardiac Dynamics, 271–278.

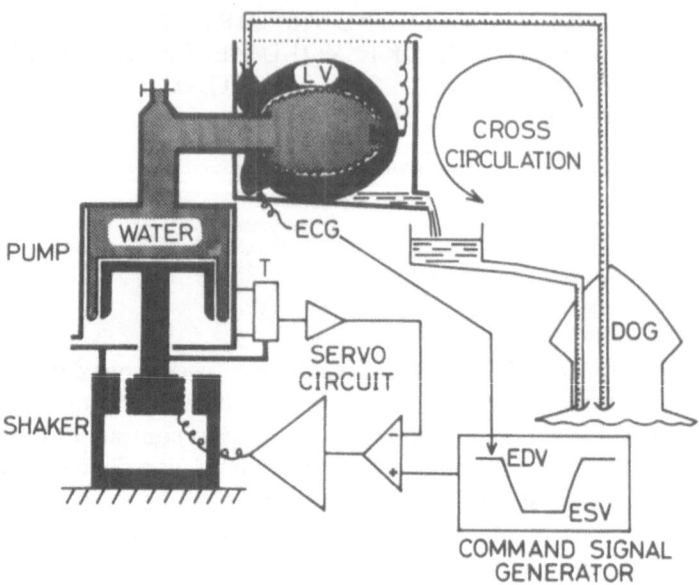

*Figure 1.* Schematic diagram of the volume servo pump. EDV and ESV = volume reference voltages corresponding to the desired end-diastolic and end-systolic volumes, respectively. LV = left ventricle. The servo circuit compares the volume signal from the linear displacement transducer T and the volume reference signal to produce the control signal.

command signal. Left atrial ECG signal was used to trigger the command signal generator. The servo pump enabled us to vary the onset and velocity of ventricular ejection while clamping the end-diastolic and end-systolic volumes at desired values and producing a flow pattern resembling the natural flow pattern observed in vivo. Intraventricular pressure was measured with a miniature pressure gauge placed inside the apical end of the balloon.

Since the end of ejection does not necessarily coincide with the end of systole when the ventricle is connected to an artificial afterload system without any valve between them (2), we attempted to simulate the natural type of ejection as much as possible by making end of ejection coincide with the end of ventricle's own systole as in a natural type of contraction (3).

Consequently the end of systole could be identified as the end of ejection in the pressure and volume tracings and also as the left upper corner of the pressure-volume loop trajectory in the pressure-volume plane, as indicated at the tip of the solid triangles in Figures 2, 3 and 4.

The inotropic background of the preparation without any intentional inotropic intervention was considered to be the control contractile state in this study. End-diastolic volume of the ventricle was set at a value within the range of 10 to 45 ml, which was accompanied by peak isovolumic pressure of 50 to 250 mmHg. In the first protocol, the time of the onset of ejection was varied so that the pressure at which ejection begins would be varied (Figure 2). In the second protocol the velocity of ejection was varied appropriately, while fixing the time and pressure of the onset of ejection constant (Figure 3).

In the two series end-systolic (residual) volume as well as end-diastolic volume of the ventricle was maintained constant to determine end-systolic pressure necessary for generating a constant stroke volume. In the third protocol the end-systolic volume was varied appropriately to determine end-systolic pressure for generating varied stroke volumes from a constant end-diastolic volume (Figure 4).

Ventricular pressure, volume, and velocity of ejection (i.e., $-d$ [volume]$/dt$) were traced on a strip chart as a function of time (panel A in Figures 2, 3, 4). The same pressure and volume signals were recorded on a storage oscilloscope as the pressure-volume loop trajectory (panel B). All data were taken only from steady-state contractions. The steady state was reached in 2–3 min after changes in loading conditions.

## 3. RESULTS

Figure 2 shows a representative set of left ventricular pressure ($P$), volume ($V$) and flow ($-dV/dt$) tracings and pressure-volume loops in one heart. End-diastolic volume, end-systolic volume, and therefore stroke volume were fixed. The flow pattern was also fixed. The onset of ejection was widely varied, which resulted in extensive changes in the ventricular pressure at the onset of ejection as shown at the tip of the open triangles in panels A and B. Marked differences in the ventricular pressure were seen during most of the ejection period. However, the end-systolic pressures were very close to each other, as shown at the tip of the solid triangles. This suggests that the end-systolic pressure did not have to be changed to maintain the same stroke volume regardless of the marked differences in the time course of systolic pressure.

The larger solid circles in panel C are plots of the end-systolic pressures against the ventricular pressures at the onset of ejection in those contractions shown in panels A and B. Evidently, the relationship curve is almost flat, indicating that little change in end-systolic pressure was required to maintain the same stroke volume. All of the other ten ventricles showed similar lack of effect of early ejection pressure. Small solid circles exemplify some of the data. Statistically, increases in the pressure at the onset of ejection by $114 \pm 10$ (SE) mmHg, $N = 11$, from $22 \pm 4$ to $136 \pm 9$ mmHg were accompanied by decreases in the end-systolic pressure of as

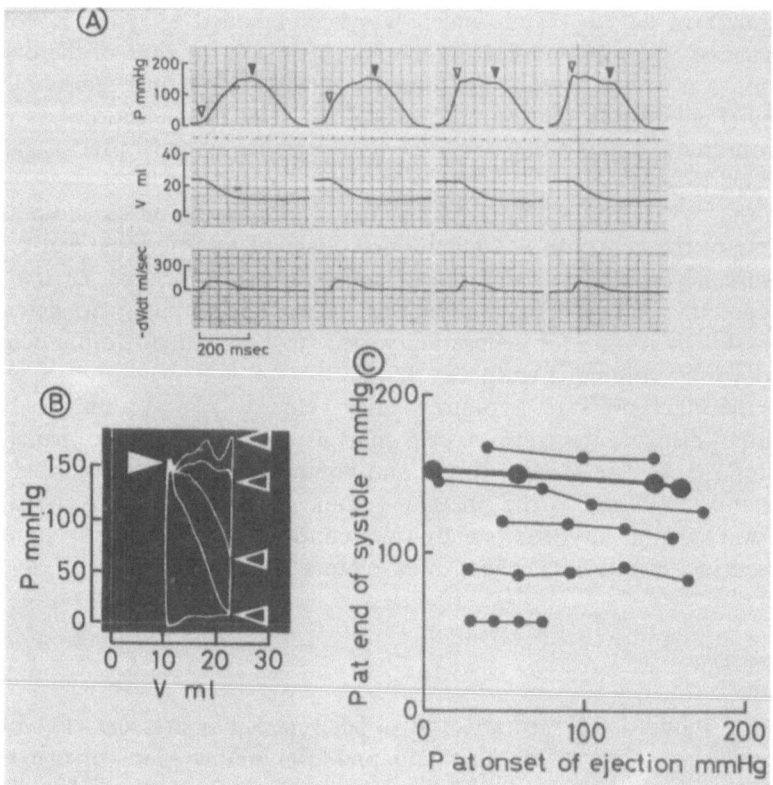

*Figure 2.* Effect of the primary changes in ventricular pressure at the onset of ejection on end-systolic pressure required for a constant stroke volume. Panel A shows simultaneous tracings of ventricular pressure (P), volume (V) and velocity of ejection (−dV/dt) in four steady-state contractions in which the onset of ejection was gradually delayed. Panel B is a picture of superimposed pressure-volume loop trajectories obtained from the same contractions shown above. The open triangles in panels A and B indicate the onset of ejection and the solid triangles the end of systole. In panel C, the four larger solid circles are the plots of the end-systolic pressures against the pressures at the onset of ejection in the example shown in panels A and B. The other smaller circles show similar data in 5 other ventricles. Although not shown, 5 other ventricles also showed similar relationships.

small as $11 \pm 2$ mmHg ($p < 0.001$) from $117 \pm 11$ mmHg with the same stroke volumes of $14 \pm 2$ ml. (1 mmHg = 133.3 Pa in SI units.)

Figure 3 shows a representative set of left ventricular pressure, volume and flow tracings and pressure-volume loops in one heart. End-diastolic volume was fixed at a constant value. Stroke volume was maintained to be constant. The velocity of ejection was primarily changed over a wide range so that ventricular pressure at the middle of ejection would be vastly different. Despite these markedly different mid-ejection pressures, the end-

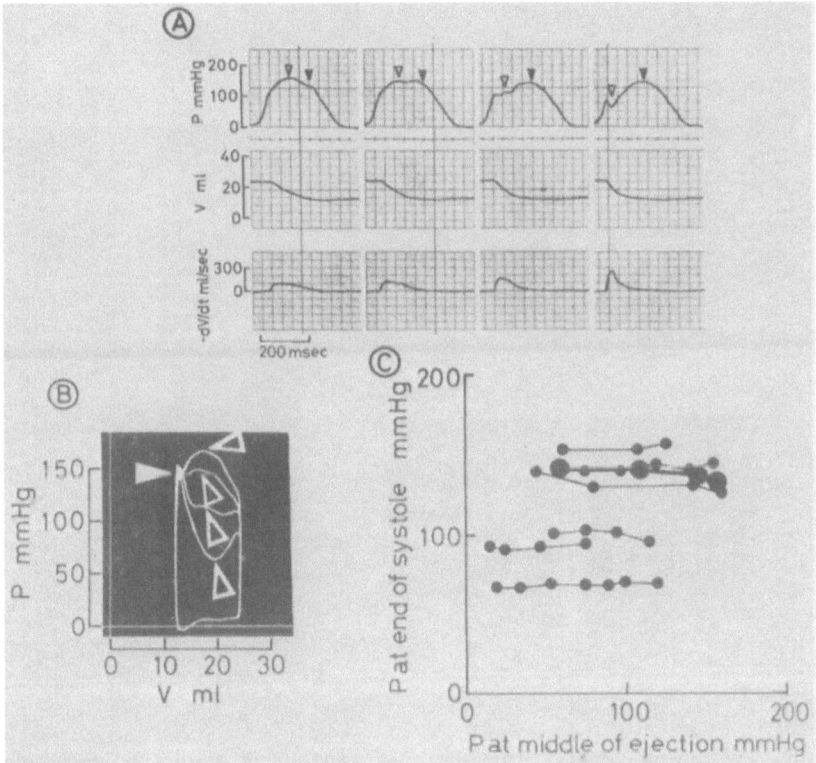

*Figure 3.* Effect of the primary changes in ventricular pressure at the middle of ejection on end-systolic pressure required for a constant stroke volume. Panel A shows simultaneous tracings of ventricular pressure, volume and velocity of ejection in four steady-state contractions in which the velocity of ejection was gradually increased. Panel B is a picture of superimposed pressure-volume loop trajectories obtained from the same contractions shown above. The open triangles in panels A and B indicate the mid-ejection time at which ventricular pressures were read for analysis. The solid triangles indicate the end of systole. In panel C, the four larger solid circles are the plots of the end-systolic pressures against the mid-ejection pressures in the example shown in panels A and B. The other small circles show similar data in 6 other ventricles. Although not shown, 5 other ventricles also showed similar relationships.

systolic pressures (at the tip of the solid triangles in panel A) with which the ventricle achieved the same stroke volume from the fixed end-diastolic volume were not significantly different from each other. The insensitivity of the end-systolic pressure is shown by the large solid circles plotted in panel C. Eleven other ventricles also yielded similar results. Small solid circles exemplify some of the data. Statistically, decreases in ventricular pressure at the middle of ejection by $71 \pm 6$ (SE) mmHg, $N = 12$, from $118 \pm 9$ to $44 \pm 6$ mmHg were accompanied by insignificant ($p > 0.1$) increases in end-systolic pressure of $4 \pm 2$ mmHg from $110 \pm 7$ mmHg with the same stroke volumes

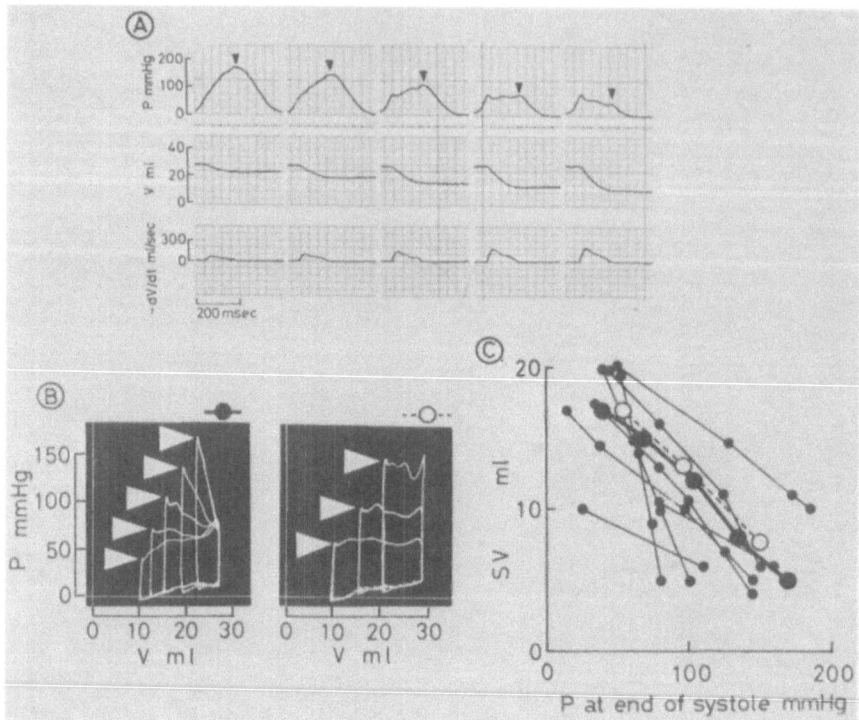

*Figure 4.* Inversely proportional relationship between end-systolic pressure and stroke volume from a fixed end-diastolic volume. Panel A shows simultaneous tracings of ventricular pressure, volume and velocity of ejection in five steady-state contractions in which the end-systolic pressure was gradually decreased and thereby stroke volume was increased. The left picture in panel B superimposes the five pressure-volume loops from those contractions shown above. The right picture in panel B superimposes three other loops from the same heart but under different load conditions as explained in the text. The solid triangles indicate the end of systole. In panel C, the five large solid circles are the plots of the stroke volumes against the end-systolic pressures in the left-side picture of panel B. The open circles are the plots of the stroke volumes against the end-systolic pressures in the right-side picture of panel B. The small solid circles are similar plots of the data in 8 other cases in 5 ventricles. Although not shown, 7 other cases in 4 other ventricles showed similar relationships.

of $14 \pm 1$ ml. These results suggest that as long as end-systolic pressure remains unchanged stroke volume is little affected by the ventricular pressure during the mid-ejection period.

Figure 4 shows the relationship between changes in the end-systolic pressure and stroke volume from a fixed end-diastolic volume. Decreases in end-systolic pressure (indicated at the tips of the solid triangles in panels A and B) were accompanied by reciprocal increases in stroke volume regardless of how the systolic pressures at the onset and middle of ejection changed during ejection. The large solid and open circles in panel C represent the relationship of stroke volume to the end-systolic pressure measured in those two ventricles shown in panel B. Similar inverse relationships were obtained in 12 other ventricles, as exemplified by 8 curves in panel C (small circles and thin lines). Statistically, the correlation coefficients were $-0.992 \pm .003$ (SE), $N = 13$, and the slopes of the relationship lines ranged from $-0.047$ to $-0.407$ ml/mmHg with a mean of $-0.137 \pm 0.026$ (SE) ml/mmHg, $N = 16$.

From all the present results, we conclude that it is the end-systolic pressure, not the early or mid-systolic pressure, which directly determines stroke volume from a fixed end-diastolic volume under a given inotropic background.

4. DISCUSSION

The conclusion stated above seems to be consistent with known physiological properties of the ventricle and heart muscle. First, the end-systolic pressure (or force) and volume (or length) relationship has been shown to be largely independent of the end-diastolic volume and the mode of contraction (2, 3, 4, 5). This load insensitivity suggests that the end-systolic volume is almost uniquely determined by end-systolic pressure. Thus, when an ejection ends at the end of systole as under natural loading conditions, the stroke volume is expected to be determined by the end-systolic pressure, with little influence of the pressure prior to the end of systole. This expectation was directly confirmed by the present results. Secondly, in cardiac muscle contracting from a fixed initial length, the amount of shortening of excised cardiac muscle was shown to be unaffected by the time course of afterloaded force if the afterload force at the end of shortening was maintained constant in contractions from a fixed initial length (6). This property of cardiac muscle seems to be the basis of the present observations in the ventricle. Thirdly, the deactivation effect of shortening on the force that heart muscle eventually attains at a prespecified length seems insensitive to the velocity of shortening. Rather the amount of shortening has a greater effect (7, 8). This velocity insensitivity seems to be another property of cardiac muscle which is underlying the present observations.

Because of the interaction between the ventricle and the afterload system, end-systolic pressure cannot be independent of the preceding course of systolic pressure in the in vivo ventricle. Therefore, it will be difficult to confirm the validity of the present findings in the in situ heart. Nevertheless, we consider, based on the present study, that even in the in vivo ventricles its stroke volume is determined directly by the end-systolic pressure if the ventricle contracts from a fixed end-diastolic volume under a given contractile state.

SUMMARY

Systolic courses of left ventricular pressure and volume of the isolated cross-circulated canine heart were varied by a servo pump under a given inotropic background. Maintenance of a desired constant stroke volume from a given end-diastolic volume required almost constant end-systolic pressure regardless of the marked changes in ventricular pressures at the onset and middle of ejection. Changes in stroke volume from a given end-diastolic volume required inversely proportional changes in end-systolic pressure. These results indicate that end-systolic pressure, not the entire time course of systolic pressure, is the direct determinant of stroke volume from a fixed end-diastolic volume of the left ventricle under a given contractile state.

ACKNOWLEDGEMENT

This study was partly supported by U.S. Public Health Service Grant HL14903.

REFERENCES

1. Suga H, Sagawa K: End-diastolic and end-systolic ventricular volume clamper for isolated canine heart. *Am J Physiol* 233:H718–H722, 1977.
2. Suga H, Sagawa K: Instantaneous pressure-volume relationship and their ratio in the excised, supported canine left ventricle. *Circ Res* 35:117–126, 1974.
3. Suga H, Sagawa K, Shoukas AA: Load independence of the instantaneous pressure-volume ratio of the canine left ventricle and effects of epinephrine and heart rate on the ratio. *Circ Res* 32:314–322, 1973.
4. Downing SE, Sonnenblick EH: Cardiac muscle mechanics and ventricular performance: force and time parameters. *Am J Physiol* 207:705–715, 1964.
5. Weber KT, Janicki JS, Hefner LL: Left ventricular force-length relations of isovolumic and ejecting contractions. *Am J Physiol* 231:337–343, 1976.
6. Paulus WJ, Claes VA, Brutsaert DL: Physiological loading of isolated mammalian cardiac muscle. *Circ Res* 39:42–53, 1976.
7. Brutsaert DL, Claes VA, Donders JJH: Effects of controlling the velocity of shortening of force-velocity-length and time relations in cat papillary muscle velocity clamping. *Circ Res* 30:310–315, 1972.
8. Méiss RA, Sonnenblick EH: Controlled shortening in heart muscles: velocity-force and active state properties. *Am J Physiol* 222:630–639, 1972.

# 4.5. PUMP FUNCTION OF THE LEFT VENTRICLE EVALUATED FROM PRESSURE-VOLUME LOOPS

PETER L.M. KERKHOF, ARJAN D. VAN DIJK,
TJONG AOUW JONG, JAN KOOPS, RUDOLF J. MOENE, JAN BAAN

## 1. INTRODUCTION

Evaluating the performance of the left ventricle and assessing contractility in a quantitative manner in the normal and failing heart constitute major problems in cardiology. The classical viewpoint has been to characterize the contractile behaviour of the heart in terms of quantities derived from cardiac muscle mechanics, i.e. force-velocity-length relations. Yet the application of these basic muscle concepts to the intact heart remains controversial (1).

Another approach is based on the pumping aspect of the heart and its determinants are governed by dynamic pressure-volume-flow relations during the cardiac cycle. Employing this concept requires faithful techniques to measure instantaneous pressure and volume of the left ventricle, especially when diagnostic interpretations are to be ascribed to properties of individual pressure-volume (P-V) loops (2, 3).

Although the method to analyse P-V loops has new elements, there is nevertheless a close relationship with formerly described LV function curves. We deduced some immediate implications of the linear end-systolic P-V relations which have been proposed by other investigators (3, 4). These theoretical digressions are compared with our experimental results in order to verify the range and conditions for which the linear model is valid.

We developed an isolated ejecting heart preparation and applied a new method for determining ventricular cavity volume in order to investigate preload and afterload dependence of P-V loops. Additional experiments were conducted in open-chest dogs employing essentially the same volume measurement technique.

## 2. THEORETICAL CONSIDERATIONS

Recently, many investigators (3, 5, 6) have introduced the concept of "elastance" as an approach to the problem of identifying the mechanical properties of the ventricle. Such a functional model regards the left ventricle as a compliant, volume-storing structure whose elastance varies during the

J. Baan, A.C. Arntzenius, E.L. Yellin (eds.), Cardiac Dynamics, 279–291.

cardiac cycle and depends on inotropic state. Its presumed independence of loading conditions is still a matter of discussion (5, 6). Time-varying elastance $E(t)$ is defined as the instantaneous ratio of pressure over volume as indicated in the so-called Katz-Wiggers plot illustrated in graph A of Figure 1. Incorporating such factors as extrapolated volume $V_0$ at zero pressure, energy losses, and so on, these authors arrive at mathematical expressions for $E(t)$ which display unique characteristics as a function of time. The interpretations of these findings are obviously based upon underlying assumptions, while experimental observations may be limited by technical imperfections. Supposing a linear relation between end-systolic pressure-volume points when loading conditions are varied under constant inotropic state, one can deduce immediate implications for the derived quantities stroke volume (SV) and ejection fraction (EF).

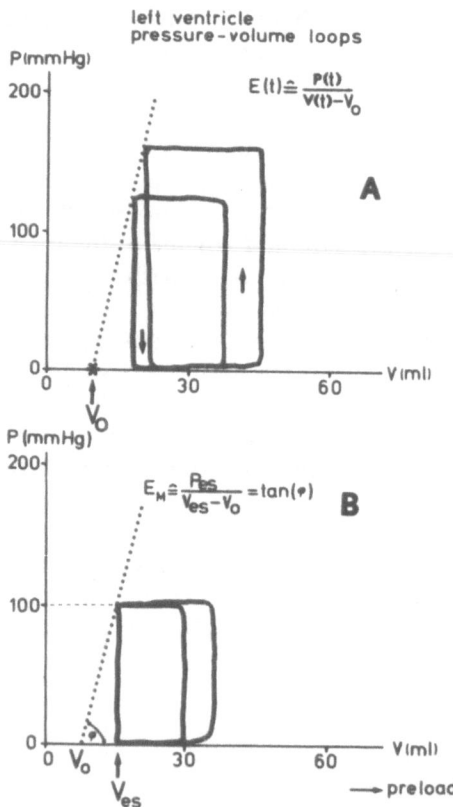

*Figure 1.* A: pressure-volume loops for different preloads and afterloads, while end-systolic points form a linear relationship, modified after Sagawa et al. (4); B: P-V loops converging to the same end-systolic volume when preload is elevated while end-systolic pressure is kept constant, modified after Sagawa et al. (4); C: applying the properties indicated in A and B the

Applying these linearity concepts rigorously leads to absolutely straight LV function curves always crossing the abscissa at an angle of 45 degrees (Figure 1: graph C). Changes in inotropic state merely shift the line in a parallel fashion, as do alterations in afterload. In fact, the position of each function curve is solely determined by the end-systolic volume $V_{es}$ which in turn depends on the particular combination of the maximal $E(t)$ value (i.e. $E_M$), $V_0$, and end-systolic pressure $P_{es}$ in the following way:

$$V_{es} = \{P_{es}/E_M\} + V_0 \qquad\qquad [1]$$

Consequently, common function curves will be found for a multitude of contractile levels and afterloads as long as the ratio of $P_{es}$ over $E_M$ remains constant.

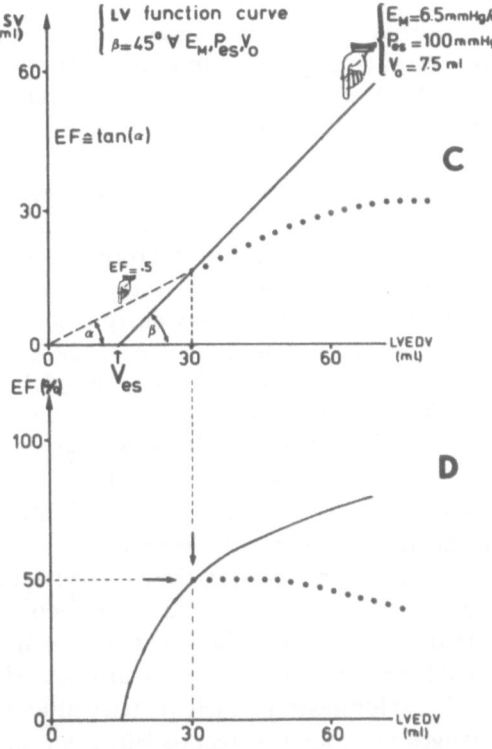

LV function curve results in a straight line. The dotted curve indicates possibly nonlinear behaviour; D: ejection fraction as a function of preload as derived from the linear as well as the nonlinear (dotted curve) function curves.

Another implication is that EF can only increase with preload $V_{ed}$ (graph D), because of the relation:

$$EF = 1 - \{V_{es}/V_{ed}\} \tag{2}$$

$E_M$ (graph B) has been claimed as an unambiguous index of contractility, being independent of preload and afterload by virtue of the linear behaviour of the maximal elastance (2, 3), while $V_0$ is supposedly independent of inotropic state.

Facing these striking consequences and the importance of the "elastance issue," we felt it desirable to test the linearity concept and to verify its implications as mentioned above.

3. METHODS AND MATERIALS

Mongrel dogs (18–30 kg body mass) were premedicated with 5 ml Hypnorm and 0.5 ml atropine i.m. and anesthetized using 6 mg/kg Nembutal and 0.1 ml/kg Methadon i.v. The animals were ventilated with a 2:1 mixture of oxygen and nitrogen. After midsternal thoracotomy the heart and major vessels were exposed. In the open-chest dog, a Millar 8F catheter-tip manometer with fluid channel was inserted into the carotid artery and advanced to the center of the ventricular cavity. A perivascular flow probe was snugly fitted around the aortic root and a solenoidal sensing coil was placed around the entire heart for the purpose of left ventricular volume measurements using a method previously described (7).

Similarly prepared dogs were utilized for isolated heart experiments. The thoracic aorta was cannulated so that the heart could fill the hydraulic circuit replacing the systemic circulation with the dog's own blood. The heart together with the lungs were then rapidly excised and transferred to the experimental setup. Appropriate hydraulic conditions were created for the isolated ejecting heart while many hemodynamic variables could be controlled independently. The details of this preparation are documented elsewhere (8) and the hydraulic pathways are schematically shown in Figure 2. The coronary and systemic circulation were functionally decoupled by supplying oxygenated blood to the entire myocardium via two special cannulas inserted into the orifices of the right and left coronary arteries. Millar catheter-tip manometers were utilized for measuring left ventricular and aortic pressures. Statham P23Db gauges were used to record left atrial and both coronary inflow pressures. Three cannulating flow probes (Skalar, Delft, Netherlands) were included in the fluid pathways for the purpose of measuring aortic and both coronary perfusion flows.

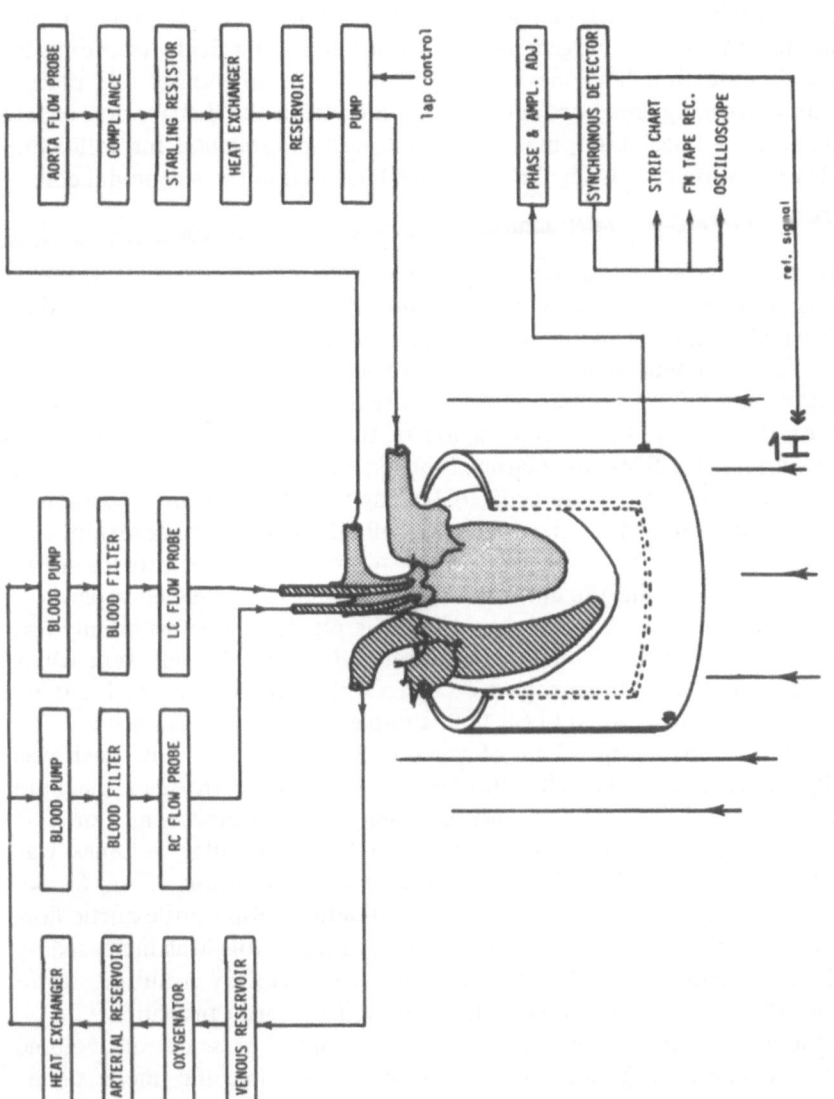

*Figure 2.* Schematic representation of isolated heart preparation showing separate coronary and systemic circulations along with the method used for measuring left ventricular volume.

The method for determining left ventricular volume in the open-chest dog as well as in the isolated heart is based upon the principle of electromagnetic induction. After being slightly diluted with a ferromagnetic tracer fluid (Ferrofluid®, Ferrofluidics Co., Burlington, Mass.), the ventricular contents act as a variable-size core of a sensing coil positioned around the heart and within an originally homogeneous alternating magnetic field. According to Faraday's induction law, the voltage induced in a solenoidal coil placed around a ferromagnetic core can be calculated from the distribution of the magnetic field lines. Lumping together several parameters, the following simple expression results for the voltage $e(t)$ induced in the solenoidal coil:

$$e(t) = C\{1 + m(t)\} \sin \omega_0 t, \qquad\qquad [3]$$

where $t$ denotes time, $\omega_0$ the angular frequency of the external magnetic field, $C$ summarizes several constants and $m(t)$ represents the modulation index which is related to the instantaneous volume of the core constituted by the ferromagnetic fluid (7). The use of an equivalent coil in the same magnetic field allows for balanced measurements applying a synchronous detector (Figure 2). The output signal of this device has been shown to provide a sensitive linear estimator of the ferromagnetic core size and hence of left ventricular cavity volume (7, 9). During the isolated heart experiment, systemic blood uniformly mixed with Ferrofluid entered the left atrium and was ejected by the left ventricle during each cardiac cycle into the aorta without contaminating the coronary blood which was provided separately to the myocardium. The left atrium itself was placed in a substantially less sensitive region of the coil so that essentially only the left ventricular contents served as a ferromagnetic core. Calibration was carried out by measuring the output signal of a fluid sample of known volume.

In the open-chest dog 0.3 ml of Ferrofluid followed by saline flush was rapidly injected into the left ventricle during diastole through the fluid channel of the Millar pressure catheter using a Cordis power injector. The time-varying pattern of successive residual left ventricular volumes was recorded and essentially reflected an instantaneous dilution curve. Stroke volume was calibrated by the simultaneous readings of pulsatile aortic flow integrated over each ejection period. Preload in these dogs was increased by rapid infusion of up to 500 ml Macrodex intravenously, resulting in an increase of ventricular diastolic volume as well as aortic pressure.

In the isolated heart preparation the behaviour of pressure and volume during elevation of preload were observed while keeping mean aortic pressure constant and omitting inotropic interventions. A possible deterioration of the preparation and a concomitant decline in contractility were monitored by comparing the initial and final values of relevant hemodynamic parameters (cardiac output, maximal $dp/dt$) during every series of experiments which took about 30 minutes each. Data from series in which these values differed considerably were discarded.

The following parameters were recorded on strip-chart and FM tape recorders during each experiment: ECG, aortic and left ventricular pressure, ventricular volume, ventricular *dp/dt*, and aortic flow. Mean left atrial and both coronary pressures and flows from the isolated heart were also registered. Instantaneous P-V loops were generated using an X-Y oscilloscope.

Dynamic P-V loops, stroke volume, cardiac output and ejection fraction were plotted as functions of end-diastolic volume which was varied over a large range by increasing mean left atrial pressure from 0 to about 6 mmHg.

## 4. RESULTS

Representative tracings of left ventricular pressure and volume in an isolated heart are shown in Figure 3 (top) Figure 3 (bottom) shows P-V loops in the same heart for various preloads with constant mean aortic pressure. It is evident that P-V loops do not have a common end-systolic

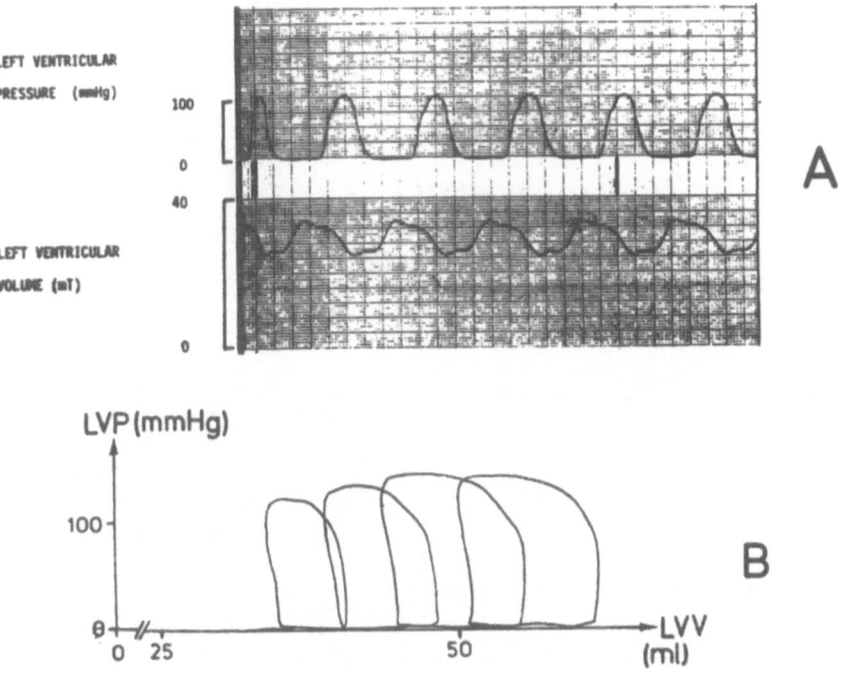

*Figure 3.* A: left ventricular pressure and volume tracings obtained from an isolated heart preparation (18 kg dog, mean aortic pressure: 80 mmHg, CO: 1.3 1/min); B; several P-V loops obtained from the same isolated heart for increasing preloads while mean aortic pressure was kept constant at 80 mmHg. Diastolic volume was varied by controlling mean left atrial pressure.

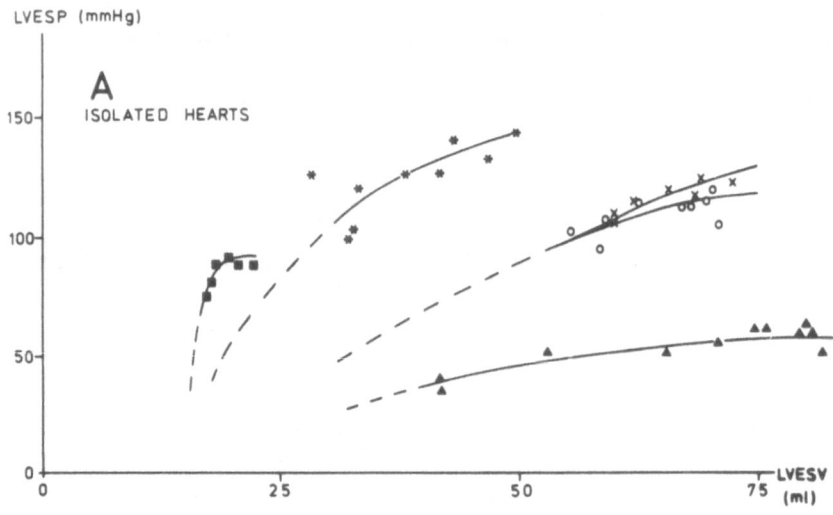

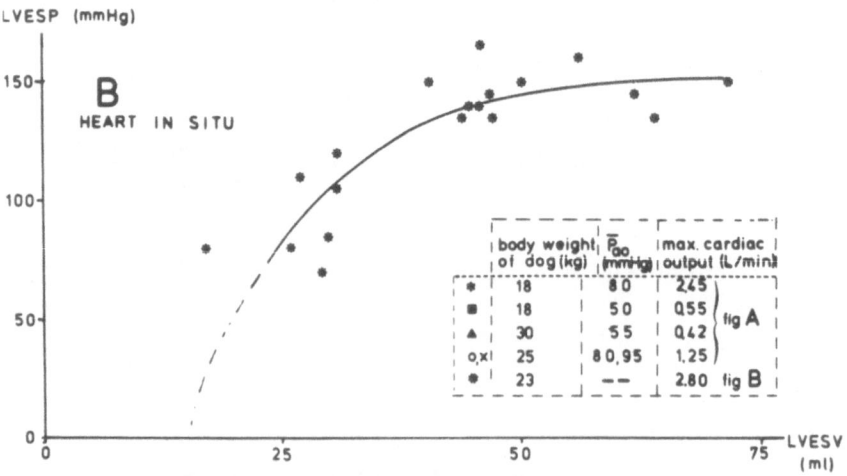

*Figure 4.* End-systolic pressure as a function of end-systolic volume A: in isolated hearts from four dogs – preload (EDV) was increased by raising left atrial pressure while mean aortic pressure was kept constant at the levels indicated in the table; B: for a dog heart in situ – preload was increased by volume loading, resulting in concomitant increase of aortic pressure.

point when preload was increased under otherwise unchanged conditions. End-systolic P-V points collected from four isolated hearts are shown in Figure 4 (top). At elevated filling pressures maximal COs between 0.42 and 2.45 l/min were produced by the various hearts while mean aortic pressure remained constant at the levels indicated in the table.

None of the series of data resulted in an unambiguously straight line connecting end-systolic points. In contrast to the alleged linearity, a best-fitting curve was drawn for each series. The reasons for doing so will be elaborated upon in the discussion. The continuation of the curves by broken lines indicates their hypothetical behaviour if all hearts could be assumed to converge to a positive intercept on the volume axis which would be the volume $V_0$ at zero pressure (3).

Figure 5 (top) shows an LV function curve in which SV is plotted against end-diastolic volume in an isolated heart. EF is identified by the slope of the line connecting the origin with each point on the LV function curve (C in Figure 1) and its dependence on preload is given in Figure 5 (bottom). In all experiments it was consistently found that SV (or alternatively CO) tends to level off at elevated filling volumes. This observation implies that EF first increases with preload, then reaches a plateau, while at even higher volumes EF tends to be depressed as demonstrated in Figure 5.

Results of experiments performed in the open-chest dog are shown in Figure 4 (bottom) summarizing a collection of end-systolic points obtained from a 23 kg dog. In this heart, CO increased from 1.2 to 2.8 l/min while both preload (EDV) and afterload (aortic pressure) increased substantially. Again a nonlinear relation is strongly evident.

The finding of curvilinear relationships between systolic pressure and volume is supported by theoretical considerations (Hunter and Baan, this volume), in which systolic P-V relations of the left ventricle were predicted based upon realistic force-length relations of sarcomeres.

## 5. DISCUSSION

If $V_0$ is defined as left ventricular cavity volume at zero pressure, then this point must be located somewhere between 0 and 20 ml, the exact number most likely being related to body surface area. Sagawa et al. (3) reported a value of 4 to 6 ml for 20 kg dogs. This suggestion would require our curves to converge to a narrow region around the 8 ml point (Figure 4) if indeed their model is applicable to our experimental conditions. However, starting from such a positive intercept the end-systolic P-V coordinates clearly cannot constitute a straight line, neither in the isolated nor in the in situ heart. The distribution of the measuring points on the other hand does not preclude a linear relationship between end-systolic P-V points in most

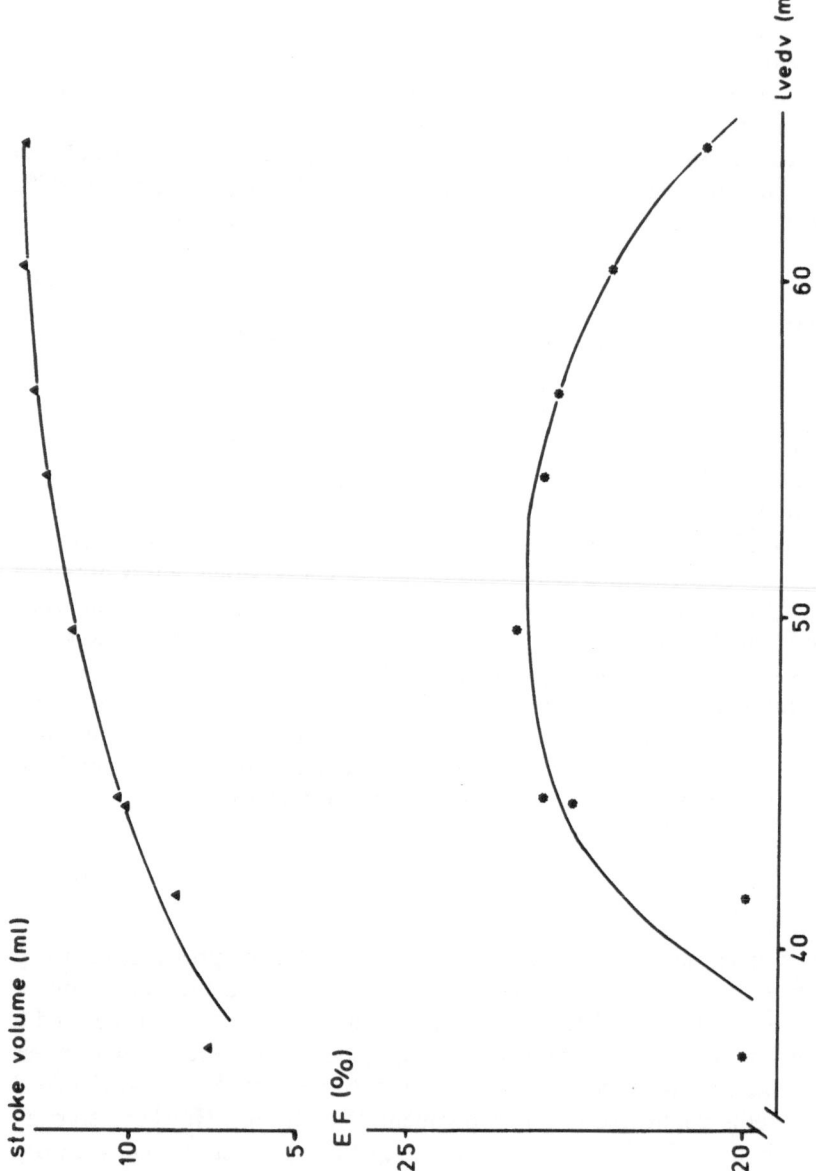

*Figure 5. Top:* stroke volume as a function of preload in an isolated heart preparation (18 kg dog); *bottom:* the increasing, plateau, and declining phases of the ejection fraction from the same heart when preload is increasing while mean aortic pressure remains constant.

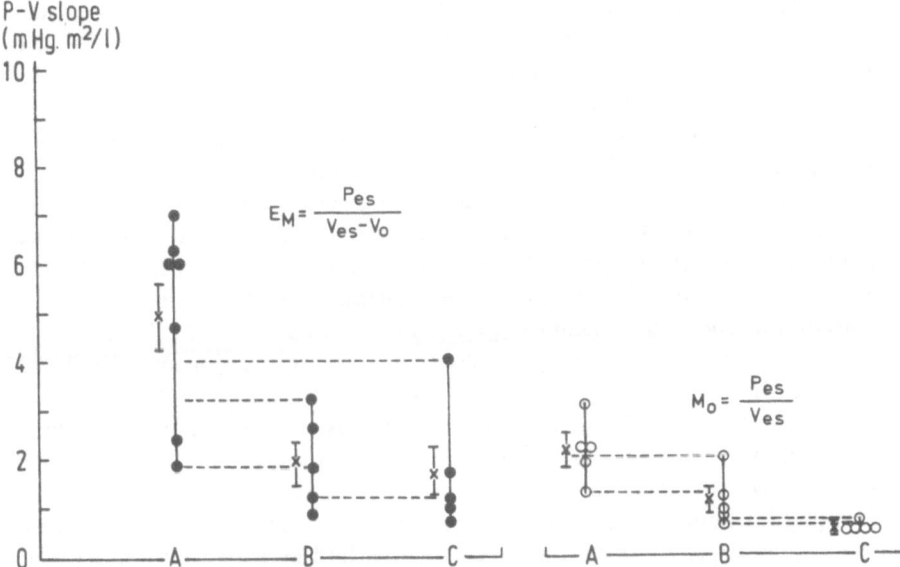

*Figure 6.* Comparison of two end-systolic P-V indexes to evaluate cardiac performance in three groups of patients indicated as A, B and C, exhibiting mean EFs of 69, 52 and 25% respectively. Closed circles refer to index $E_M$ and open circles to Mo. For explanation see text. Note the difference in overlap for both parameters. Data collected from Grossman et al (2).

hearts if the requirement of a certain positive $V_0$ value is abandoned. In fact, in the majority of the isolated hearts studied, a straight line fit through the data points would extrapolate into a negative intercept on the volume axis. Such a point obviously has no physical meaning, but retains its mathematical relevance as an extrapolation. In man, Grossman et al. (2) found negative values for $V_0$ in 5 out of 19 patients when employing peak systolic pressure in relation to ventricular end-systolic volume. These authors evaluated both $E_M$ and $V_0$ (corrected for body surface area) as indices of contractile state while the patients were categorized into three groups according to their ejection fraction having mean values of 69, 52 and 25% for the respective groups. Judging from their observations, the effectiveness of the parameters $E_M$ and $V_0$ to discriminate different groups of patients was not nearly as good as that of the parameter EF. The same is true for the use of the single parameter $V_{es}$. Thus, if only $V_{es}$ had been measured, a very significant difference between the groups would have been found. Interestingly, some of the same conclusions could have been reached without invoking any elements of the linear elastance theory (Figure 6).

The complicating problem of nonlinearity obviously may be overcome in good approximation by considering only a small portion of the nonlinear end-systolic P-V curve, as essentially also done by Grossman et al. (2). Two points then suffice to determine the linearized small trajectory under investigation. Our data show that the slope $E_M$ and the volume intercept $V_0$ of these trajectories are quite dependent on preload and afterload. Also, these parameters are subject to large experimental error caused by relatively small inaccuracies in $P_{es}$ en $V_{es}$. Thus, the power and effectiveness of these parameters to assess contractility remains to be proven. A better choice might be to use the slope of the line connecting the origin with each end-systolic P-V point. In terms of the elastance theory, this means the computation of total elastance ([1], with $V_0 = 0$), rather than "differential elastance" which is defined by the slope of a line connecting two points on the curve in close proximity.

Indeed, analysing Grossman's data (2) in this manner leads to excellent discrimination between the groups of patients. Additionally, this approach possesses the distinct advantage of not having to stress the patient by changing his hemodynamic state, since only one point would be required to obtain this slope. By the same token, the method considerably reduces the experimental error (associated with volume measurements in man) inherent to the differential elastance calculation.

SUMMARY

A theory based on linear elastance of end-systolic pressure-volume points proposed by others was shown to lead to unrealistic behaviour of left ventricular function curves and ejection fraction. To test these implications, left ventricular performance was studied in the isolated heart as well as in the open-chest dog analysing P-V relations under different loading conditions. For this purpose a new technique to measure ventricular volume was developed featuring minimal interference with hemodynamics. The results show a pronounced nonlinear behaviour of the end-systolic P-V relation in both experimental situations. Possible implications of these findings for assessing LV function were discussed, especially with respect to application in patients.

ACKNOWLEDGEMENTS

The authors gratefully acknowledge the help during various stages of the experiment by Drs. N.J. Elzenga, and W.C. Hunter and Messrs. P. Lems, C.M. van Wel, M.G. Hazekamp and E.T. van der Velde. This study was supported by the Foundation for Medical Research (FUNGO), the Netherlands Organization for the Advancement of Pure Research (ZWO), and by grant 76-063 from the Netherlands Heart Foundation.

REFERENCES

1. Brutsaert DL, Paulus WJ: Loading and performance of the heart as muscle and pump. *Cardiovasc Res* 11:1–16, 1977.
2. Grossman W, Braunwald E, Mann T, McLaurin LP, Green LH: Contractile state of the left ventricle in man as evaluated from end-systolic pressure-volume relations. *Circulation* 56:845–852, 1977.
3. Sagawa K, Suga H, Shoukas AA, Bakalar KM: End-systolic pressure/volume ratio: a new index of ventricular contractility. *Am J Cardiol* 40:748–755, 1977.
4. Sagawa K, Suga H, Nakayama K: Instantaneous pressure-volume ratio of the ventricle versus instantaneous force-length relation of papillary muscle. In: *Cardiovascular system dynamics*, Baan J, Noordergraaf A, Raines J (eds), Cambridge, MIT Press, 1978, p 99–105.
5. Demoment G: Application de la méthode du modèle à l'étude d'un système biologique complexe: le ventricule gauche. *Automatisme* 19:591–600, 1974.
6. Greene ME, Clark Jr JW, Mohr DN, Bourland HM: A mathematical model of left ventricular function. *Med Biol Eng* 11.126–134, 1973.
7. Silage DA, Stewart S, Baan J, Noordergraaf A: Phasic left ventricular volume of the canine heart in situ. *Bibl Cardiol* 35:56–63, 1976.
8. Baan J, Kerkhof PLM, Elzenga NJ, Moene RJ: Isolated ejecting canine heart with controlled coronary perfusion. (Submitted.)
9. Baan J, Elzenga NJ, Kerkhof PLM, Moene RJ: Phasic left ventricular volume in the isolated heart. *Fed Proc* 36:935, 1977.

## 4.6. SIMULATION STUDY OF FLOW DISTRIBUTION ACROSS MYOCARDIUM

FUMIHIKO KAJIYA, NORITAKE HOKI,
MICHITOSHI INOUE

### 1. INTRODUCTION

The distribution of intramyocardial blood flow is influenced by several flow determinants such as perfusion pressure, vascular active tension, intramyocardial pressure and heart rate. Among these factors, the contribution of vascular active tension and intramyocardial pressure to flow distribution within myocardium is not clarified, explicitly due to a difficulty in measuring these factors directly.

In this study, we developed a theoretical coronary circulation model (1, 2) in order to analyse, first, individual effects of the gradients of intramyocardial pressure and vascular active tension across the myocardium on flow distribution (endomyocardial/epimyocardial, i.e., endo/epi, flow ratio), and, second, the relationship between the endo/epi flow ratio and the diastolic/systolic pressure time index (DPTI/SPTI ratio) introduced by Buckberg et al. (3). The result of model predictions was also compared with that of animal experiments.

### 2. CORONARY CIRCULATION MODEL

Figure 1 shows a schematic representation of the coronary circulation model used in this study. The intramyocardial vessels, which are composed of arterioles, capillaries and venules, are disposed at one fourth and three fourths the depth from the endocardial site in order to evaluate the endo/epi flow ratio.

The intramyocardial flow is affected by the phasic change in vascular resistance and vascular volume throughout the cardiac cycle, as known by the "throttling mechanism." It is necessary to calculate the phasic change in variable resistances and volume in each vascular segment for simulating intramyocardial flows. These variables were calculated by estimating the change in vascular radii under the assumption that the quasi-static treatments were applicable during each calculation period (2 msec).

The vascular radii were estimated by the "thick wall theory" of tension-pressure-radius relationship proposed by Fung (4) and Azuma and Oka (5).

J. Baan, A.C. Arntzenius, E.L. Yellin (eds.), Cardiac Dynamics, 293–299.

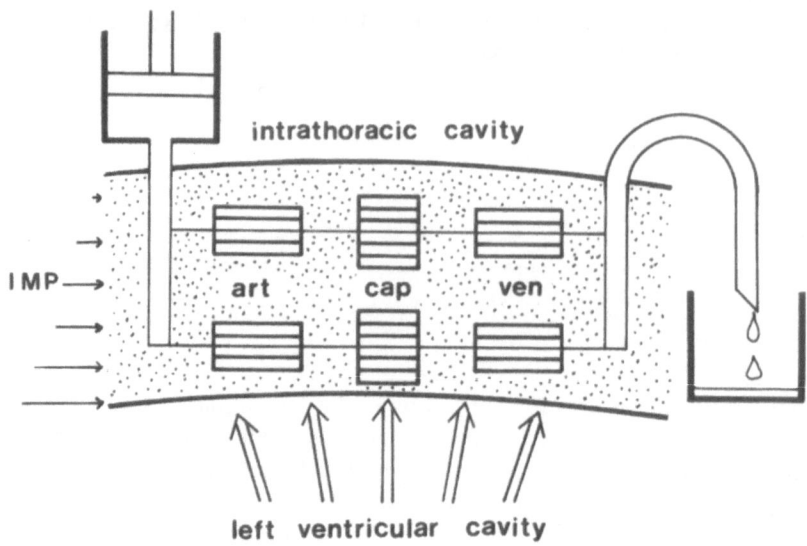

*Figure 1.* Schematic representation of coronary circulation model: *art, cap* and *ven* represent arteriole, capillary and venule, respectively.

The tension, $T$, of vascular wall in "physical" equilibrium can be expressed by

$$T = P \cdot r_i - P_t \cdot r_0, \tag{1}$$

where $P$, $P_t$, $r_i$ and $r_0$ are intravascular pressure, extravascular pressure ($\equiv$ intramyocardial pressure), inner and outer radius of a vessel, respectively. In physiological equilibrium, the tension, pressure and radius relationship can be approximated by the following equation

$$T = a \cdot r_i + b + T_a \tag{2}$$

where $a$ and $b$ are parameters representing the nature of the vascular wall in the state of complete dilatation and $T_a$ is the active tension developed by vascular smooth muscle. The inner radius $r_i$ has a limiting value, $r_c$, beyond which the vessel cannot practically dilate. Then we can calculate $r_i$ from [1] and [2] in each quasi-static calculation period through the cardiac cycle.

The intramyocardial pressure, $P_t$, was assumed to decrease linearly from the endocardial to the epicardial site as in the model proposed by Downey and Kirk (6).

On the boundary of epimyocardium and endomyocardium, the pressure at the epimyocardial site was chosen as 0 mmHg and that at the endomyocardial site was expressed by $k \cdot P_o$, where $P_o$ is the ventricular pressure and $k$ a parameter. In the present study, the value of $\dot{K}$ was chosen as 0.8 to 1.6 so as to cover the values of intramyocardial pressure reported by Armour and Randall (7) and Brandi and McGregor (8).

Concerning the values of vascular active tension developed in the vascular wall, Gould et al. (9) showed that vasodilatation causes a roughly threefold increase in coronary flow. Since this flow change corresponds to a change in active tension from 0 to 600 dyn/cm in our model, we considered that the vascular active tension varied between 0 and 600 dyn/cm according to the active state of the vascular wall.

The intramyocardial flow and endo/epi flow ratio were calculated by giving various perfusion pressures to the input of the present model.

3. RESULTS AND DISCUSSION

In order to investigate the effect of an intramyocardial pressure gradient on intramyocardial flow and endo/epi flow ratio, the parameter $k$ was varied from 0.8 to 1.6, while the active tension was kept constant at 200 dyn/cm through the myocardium.

The endomyocardial flow and the endo/epi flow ratio decreased with an increase in the intramyocardial pressure gradient, especially in the systolic phase. The values of the endo/epi flow ratios, however, were lower than those reported by Downey and Kirk (5)–0.52 during systole – and by Hess and Bache (11) – 0.38 during systole and 1.24 during diastole – even when the value of $k$ was taken as 0.8 to reduce the resistance to endomyocardial flow, i.e., the ratios were 0.17 during systole, 0.77 during diastole and 0.51 through the cardiac cycle (Figure 2).

To study the effect of vascular active tension on the intramyocardial flow distribution, the value of active tension of endo- and epimyocardial vessels was altered from 0 to 600 dyn/cm simultaneously. The endo/epi flow ratios for these simultaneous changes in active tension of the myocardial vessels varied from 0.82 to 0.71 during diastole and from 0.30 to 0.15 during systole. Then the vascular active tension in the endomyocardium was changed from 600 to 0 dyn/cm, while that in the epimyocardium was kept constant at 600 dyn/cm. In this case, the endomyocardial flow increased significantly with the decrease in the endomyocardial vascular active tension, e.g. the endo/epi flow ratio with 400 dyn/cm of the vascular active tension was 0.48 during systole and 1.06 during diastole (Figure 2).

These results indicate that the intramyocardial gradient of the vascular active tension plays an important part in controlling the intramyocardial flow distribution both in diastolic and in systolic phase.

Subsequently we analysed the relation between the DPTI/SPTI and endo/epi flow ratios. A simulation study was made in the following ways: the parameter, $k$ was varied from 1.6 to 0.8, while (A) the vascular active

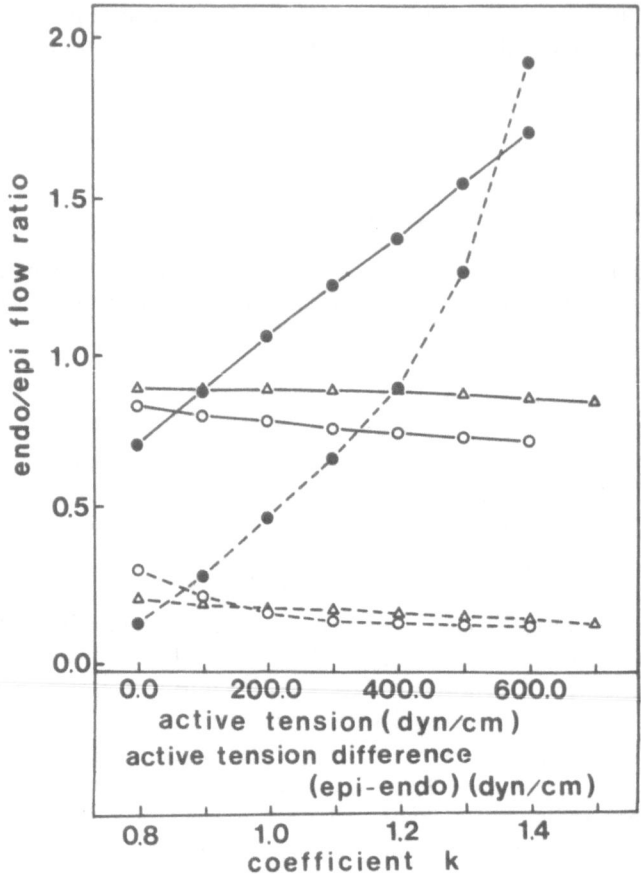

*Figure 2.* The effects of intramyocardial pressure, vascular active tension and vascular active tension gradient on the flow distribution within the myocardium. Solid lines represent the relations in diastole and dotted lines in systole. Triangles represent the change in parameter $k$, open circles the simultaneous change in the vascular active tension within the myocardium, and closed circles the change in the difference between the epi- and the endomyocardial vascular active tension.

tension was kept constant and distributed uniformly across the myocardium: and (B) the intramyocardial gradient of vascular active tension was introduced by 500 dyn/cm.

In both A and B, the endo/epi flow ratio increased linearly with the DPTI/SPTI ratio and it converged to a certain level with a break point (Figure 3). This tendency was in good agreement qualitatively with the data reported by Buckberg et al. (3). The converged value of the endo/epi flow ratio in their data is almost unity. In simulation A, the endo/epi flow ratio varied slightly from 0.4 to 0.61 with the change in $k$, while in B the ratio reached roughly unity with introduction of the vascular active tension gradient

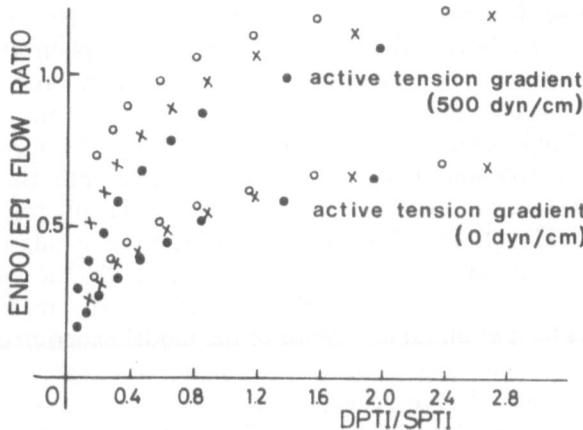

*Figure 3.* The model prediction of the relationship between the DPTI/SPTI and the endo/epi flow ratio. Note that the converged value of endo/epi flow ratio is lower than unity, if the vascular active tension gradient is taken at zero. Open circles indicate the results with $k = 0.8$, crosses with $k = 1.1$ and closed circles with $k = 1.4$.

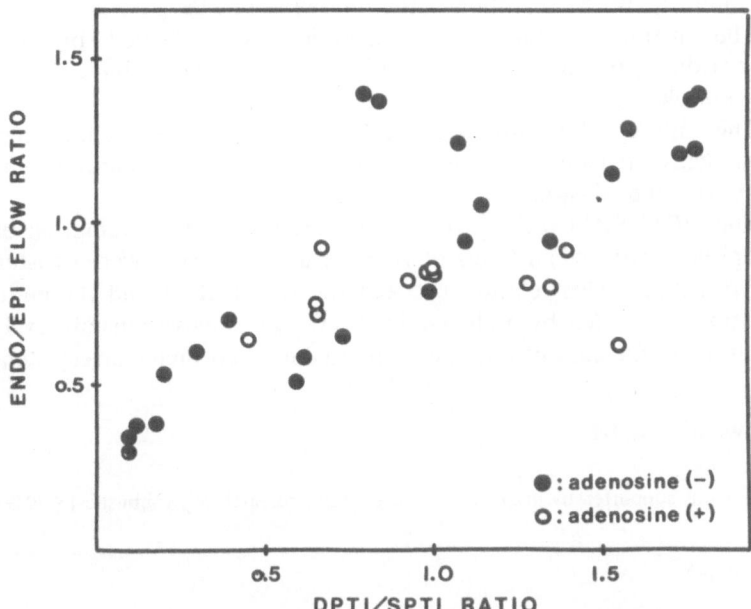

*Figure 4.* The relationship between the DPTI/SPTI and the endo/epi flow ratio. Open circles show the cases with the infusion of adenosine and closed circles the ones without adenosine.

across the myocardium. These results indicate that the vascular active tension should be introduced to some extent to explain the measured relation between the DPTI/SPTI and the endo/epi flow ratio.

In order to evaluate the results from the model predictions, we have also performed animal experiments with 5 mongrel dogs. Two platinum microelectrodes of 100 $\mu$m in diameter were inserted into the endo- and epimyocardial portion to measure the flows by the hydrogen gas clearance method. The DPTI/SPTI ratio was varied by changing the proximal and/or distal aortic constriction variously (Figure 4). The endo/epi flow ratios obtained in the control experiments were in good agreement with the results of Buckberg et al. (3) and those of the model experiment (B) with a certain degree of vascular tension gradient across the myocardium.

To examine the effect of changes in active tension, the relationship between the DPTI/SPTI and endo/epi flow ratios was studied with the same dogs by using the infusion of adenosine at a rate of 0.75–3 mg/min, which was sufficient to abolish the reactive hyperemic response to a 10-second coronary occlusion. The converged value of the endo/epi flow ratios in adenosine treatments was less than unity. These results coincided well with those in the model experiment (A) in which the gradient of vascular active tension was zero (or small). This implies that decrements in vascular active tension and small gradients of the tension produce low endo/epi flow ratios.

In summary, we have obtained the following results:

1. The intramyocardial flow distribution was affected by the intramyocardial pressure and its gradient across myocardium, especially during systole.

2. The endo/epi flow ratio was increased markedly by the increment in vascular active tension gradient from epicardium to endocardium, during both systole and diastole.

3. The DPTI/SPTI ratio gave a good measure for the estimation of the endo/epi flow ratio when levels of vascular active tension were constant in the myocardium. This relation between the DPTI/SPTI and the endo/epi flow ratio was altered by a change in the vascular active tension level and gradient, as in the case of adenosine treatment or coronary artery stenosis.

ACKNOWLEDGEMENTS

This study was supported by grants in aid for scientific research of Monbusho (337049).

REFERENCES

1. Hoki N: Simulation study of coronary circulation system. *Jap Circ* 41:409–420, 1977.
2. Kajiya F, Inada H, Hoki N, Furukawa T: A simulation study of coronary circulation. *Tech Rep Osaka Univ* 25:91–100, 1975.

3. Buckberg GD, Fixler DE, Archie JP, Hoffman JIE: Experimental subendocardiac ischaemia in dogs with normal coronary arteries. *Circ Res* 30:67–81, 1972.
4. Fung YC: Biomechanics. *Appl Mech Rev* 21:1, 1968.
5. Azuma T, Oka S: Mechanical equilibrium of blood vessel walls. *Am J Physiol* 221:1310–1318, 1971.
6. Downey JM, Kirk ES: Inhibition of coronary blood flow by a vascular waterfall mechanism. *Circ Res* 36:753–760, 1975.
7. Armour JA, Randall WC: Canine left ventricular intramyocardial pressures. *Am J Physiol* 220:1833–1839, 1971.
8. Brandi G, McGregor M: Intramural pressure in the left ventricle of the dog. *Cardiovasc Res* 3:472–475, 1969.
9. Gould KL, Lipscomb K, Hamilton GW: Physiologic basis for assessing critical coronary stenosis. *Am J Cardiol* 33:87–94, 1974.
10. Downey J, Kirk ES: Distribution of the coronary blood flow across the canine heart wall during systole. *Circ Res* 34:251–257, 1974.
11. Hess DS, Bache RJ: Transmural distribution of myocardial blood flow during systole in the awake dog. *Circ Res* 38:5–15, 1975.

## 4.7. EXPERIMENTAL STUDIES: THE APPEARANCE OF LARGE CORONARY ARTERIES DURING ARTERIOGRAPHY

ANDREW P. SELWYN, TIM CLAY, KIM M. FOX

### 1. INTRODUCTION

The clinical approach to angina pectoris is based mainly on the belief that rigid stenosis of a coronary artery limits changes in regional perfusion needed to meet myocardial metabolism (1). Fleckenstein has shown some of the biochemical pathways and responses that influence the tone of coronary arteries in vitro (2). Spasm of the coronary arteries in man has been proposed as an alternative mechanism in a proportion of patients with angina pectoris. This hypothesis is supported by the finding that a large coronary artery may transiently fail to opacify when selective arteriography is repeated during an episode of spontaneous angina or during an episode induced with ergonovine maleate (3,4).

The purpose of this work is to investigate the opacification of large coronary arteries during arteriography. The experiments test the hypothesis that mechanical and hemodynamic factors that are associated with acute regional myocardial ischaemia could cause this angiographic finding.

### 2. METHODS

Fifteen dogs (weighing between 20 and 35 kg) were anaesthetized with sodium thiopentone (16 mg/kg Pentothal). Ventilation was maintained with a cuffed endotracheal tube and a mechanical ventilator. Intravenous (i.v.) sodium pentobarbitone (2 mg/kg Sagatal) was used intermittently to continue the anaesthesia. A left thoracotomy was performed and the heart was supported in a pericardial cradle. An eight-French cardiac catheter was introduced via a left femoral arteriotomy and positioned in the mid-cavity of the left ventricle (LV). Left ventricular pressure was measured by connecting the catheter to a P23dB Statham transducer and a Hewlett-Packard 7788A multichannel recorder. A curved end was moulded on a seven-French cardiac catheter. This was introduced via a right femoral arteriotomy and positioned in the left aortic sinus. This catheter was shaped and positioned to allow quick positioning and selective injection of 5 ml of Urografin 370 (76%) into the left coronary artery (Figure 1).

Epicardial electrocardiograms (ECGs) were recorded from regions of the

*J. Baan, A.C. Arntzenius, E.L. Yellin (eds.), Cardiac Dynamics, 301–309.*

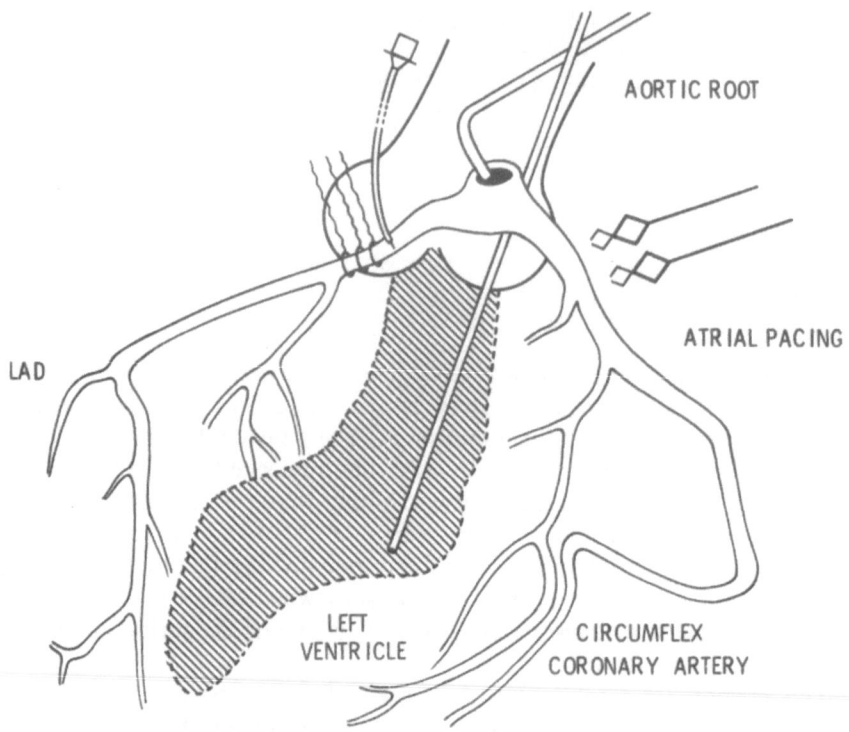

*Figure 1.* An outline' of the experimental model used to investigate the effects of regional ischaemia on the angiographic appearance of coronary arteries.

myocardium supplied by the left anterior descending coronary artery (LAD) and the left circumflex using a cotton wick electrode. This was connected to a Hewlett-Packard 7788A multichannel recorder (input impendence 50MOhm) with the calibration set at 1 mv = 1mm. The methods of Maroko et al. (5) were used to record and analyse ST segment changes. Pacing wires were stitched to the left atrium in the 5 dogs of group A. Cineangiograms were recorded using Ilford Pan-F 35 mm film recording 48 frames per second with Siemens (Pantoskop 2) equipment. Fifteen dogs were divided equally into three groups.

*Group A.* LV angiocardiograms and left coronary arteriograms were recorded with the chest open in 3 dogs and closed in 2. A reversible snare was positioned around the proximal 4 cm of the LAD. This was tightened sufficiently to reduce the diameter of that vessel by at least 60%. Care was taken not to produce significant epicardial ST segment changes. The LV angiogram and coronary arteriograms were repeated. Left atrial pacing was then used to increase the heart rate by 10 beats/min every 2 minutes until the epicardial ECG showed significant ST segment depression ($\geqq$ 2 mm) or elevation ($\geq 2$ mm) at positions within the distribution of the LAD. The LV angiogram and coronary arteriogram were then repeated. Nitroglycerine was then given as an i.v. infusion (10 $\mu$g/ml/min) that was sufficient to reduce the LV end-diastolic (LVEDP) and LV systolic pressure (LVSP) by at least 15% each. The LV angiogram and left coronary arteriogram was then repeated.

*Group B.* LV angiograms and left coronary arteriograms were performed. A reversible snare was positioned on the LAD and tightened as described for group A. No ST segment changes were noted in the epicardial ECG. The LV angiograms and coronary arteriograms were repeated and then 0.4 mg of ergonovine maleate were given by i.v. injection. Significant ST segment changes were noted between 4 and 7 minutes and the LV angiograms and coronary arteriograms were repeated before and 5 minutes after the administration of nitroglycerine i.v. as described for group A.

*Group C.* LV angiograms and left coronary arteriograms were performed in 5 dogs. A 28-gauge needle was introduced into the LAD 1 cm beyond the position where this vessel emerges from under the LA. The angiograms were repeated and then 1.0 ml/min of a 5% dextrose solution containing barium sulphate microspheres (particle size, 15–100 $\mu$g) was injected into the LAD. As soon as the LVEDP increased by 20% and the epicardial ECG showed significant changes in the ST segments the LV angiogram and left coronary arteriogram were repeated. Intravenous nitroglycerine was administered and the angiograms were repeated as described for group A.

## 3. RESULTS

Figure 2 (A, B) shows typical examples of the LV angiograms and left coronary arteriograms before and after stenosis of the LAD in group A. No regional myocardial dyskinesia or significant changes in epicardial ST segments were noted and the LAD distal to the stenosis is clearly shown. LA pacing increased the heart rate from 128 to 180 beats/min (mean for 5 dogs). This was accompanied by a rise in the LVEDP (from 4 to 24 mmHg, mean), and significant ST segment changes. The LV angiograms showed regional dyskinesia and the segment of the LAD associated with the dyskinetic segment failed to opacify during the coronary arteriogram (C). Intravenous nitroglycerine was followed by a 26% fall in LVEDP (mean) and a 17% fall in LVSP. The LV angiograms showed a reduction in LV cavity size and the LAD opacified throughout its length showing an angiographic appearance identical to B of Figure 2.

In group B, LV angiograms and left coronary arteriograms were performed before and after stenosis of the LAD. Synergic contractions of the LV and both coronary arteries were shown. Intravenous ergonovine caused a 14% increase (mean) in heart rate and an 8 to 10% increase in LVSP. There

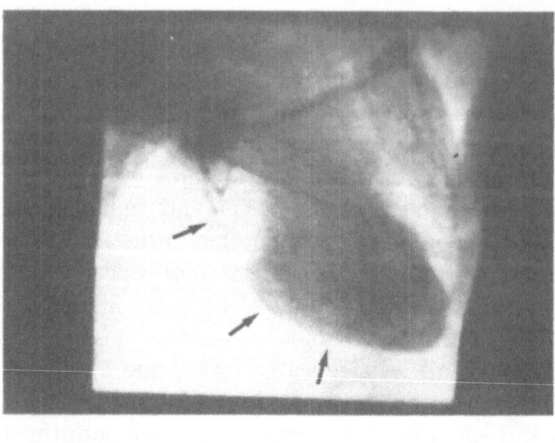

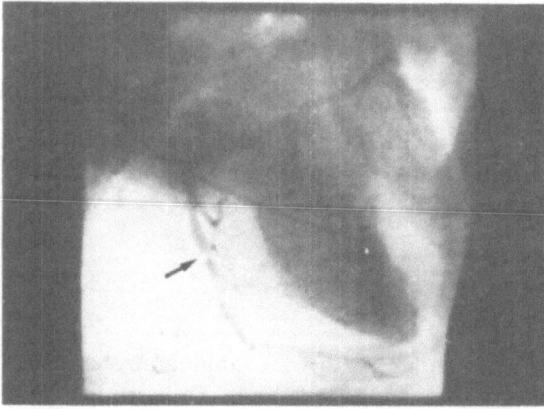

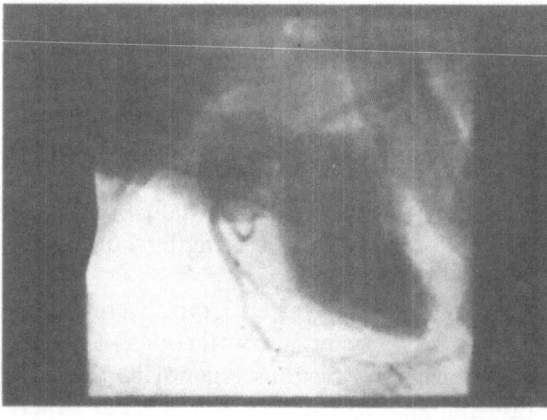

*Figure 2.* A: the left ventricular cavity shape at end-systole and the left coronary arteriogram before any interventions; B: the left coronary arteriogram shows stenosis of the left anterior descending coronary artery (LAD) – the entire vessel was opacified when the ECG and the LV angiogram showed no ischaemia or dyskinesia: C: regional myocardial ischaemia and dyskinesia produced with left atrial pacing – the length of LAD associated with the ischaemic segment failed to opacify.

was also a progressive rise in the LVEDP from 6 to 18 mmHg (mean) accompanied by significant changes in ST segments in the epicardial ECG (Figure 3). Repeat angiocardiograms at this stage showed regional myocardial dyskinesia and failure to opacify the LAD associated with the dyskinetic segment. This was reversed within 4 minutes with i.v. nitroglycerine. These changes occurred in the 5 dogs and were identical to those seen in group A.

In group C, LV angiograms and left coronary arteriograms were performed before the intervention with the microspheres (A in Figure 4). Five minutes after administration of this agent all 5 dogs showed a rise in LVEDP from 5 to 23 mmHg (mean) and significant abnormal ST segment changes. The angiography was repeated and this showed regional myocardial dyskinesia. The LAD associated with this segment appeared narrowed and abnormal during coronary arteriography (B).

Following the administration of nitroglycerine the LV cavity size was diminished and the LAD was visualized. The appearance of the LAD appeared to return towards that seen before the injection of the microspheres (C).

## 4. DISCUSSION

The simultaneous opacification of the left ventricle and coronary arteries in these experiments showed the relationships between stenosis of a coronary artery, acute regional myocardial ischaemia, and the appearance of that length of a coronary artery associated with the dyskinetic segment of the LV. The angiograms showed that when acute regional myocardial ischaemia produced distortion of the LV cavity shape with dyskinesia, the coronary artery associated with that segment failed to opacify during arteriography. It is unlikely that the variety of interventions used could all have caused coronary spasm and direct inspection in those experiments performed with the chest open supports this view.

Acute regional myocardial ischaemia is associated with regional ventricular dyskinesia, increased wall tension and impaired myocardial perfusion with failure of normal systolic and diastolic coronary flow (6, 7, 8). It seems possible that the vessel could be under increased tension from the dyskinetic segment and that the runoff of blood flow from this vessel into the ischaemic myocardium is severely reduced. These mechanisms may account for the failure to opacify a coronary artery associated with acute regional myocardial ischaemia.

Clinical work has shown that a large coronary artery may transiently fail to opacify during arteriography in patients with spontaneous angina or angina associated with the administration of ergonovine maleate (10). This

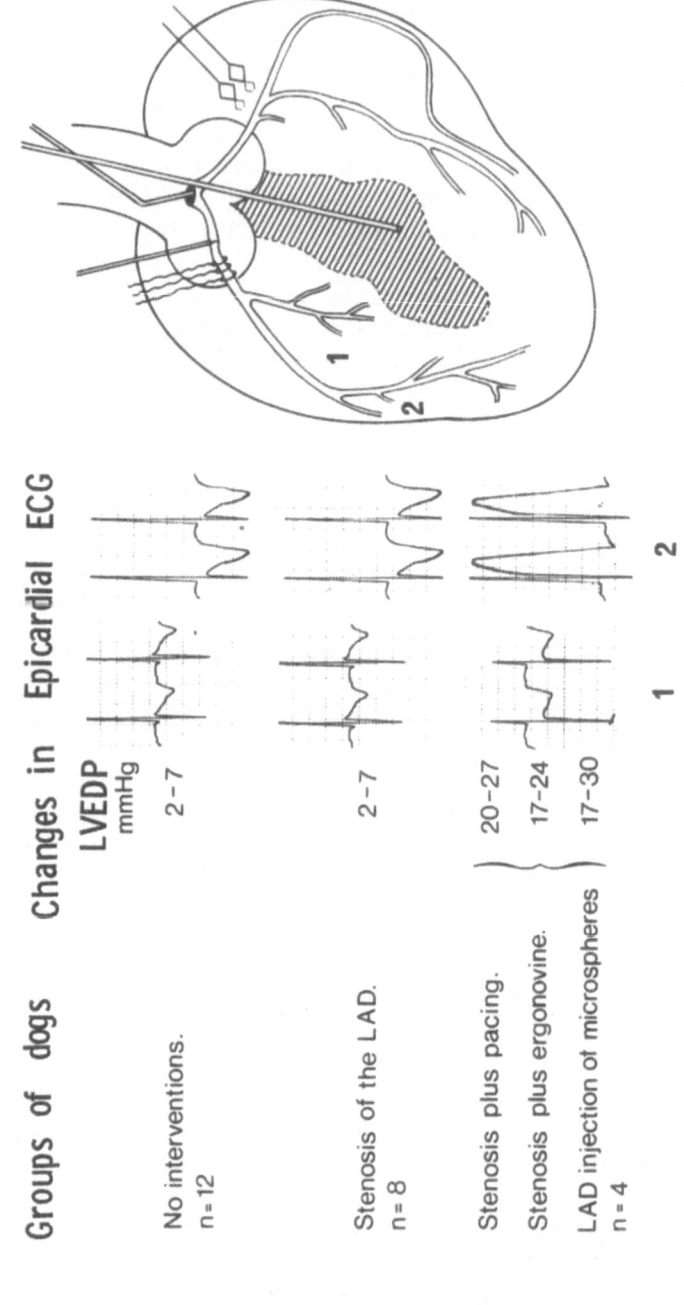

*Figure 3.* The groups of dogs studied, the changes in LVEDP caused by each intervention, and examples of the epicardial ECG recorded with each angiogram.

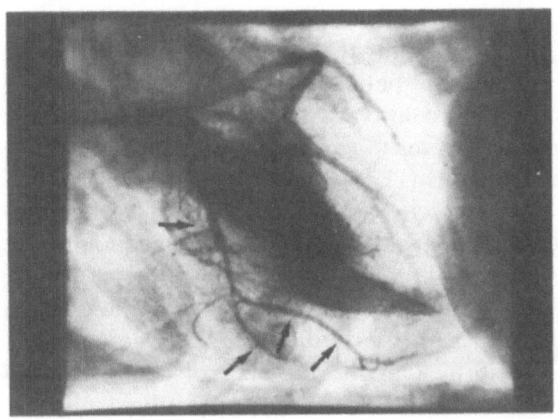

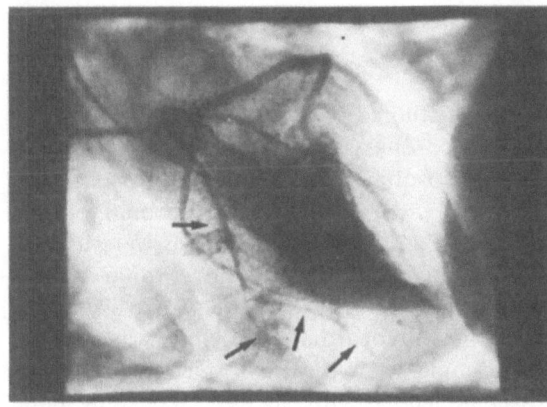

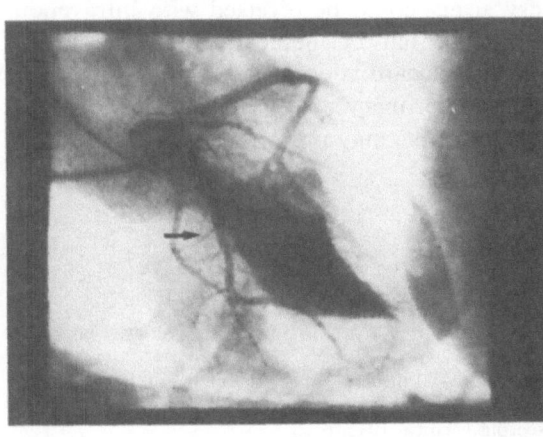

*Figure 4.* A: the LV angiogram and left coronary arteriogram before the injection of microspheres into the LAD – the 27 gauge needle in the LAD can be seen; B: regional myocardial ischaemia and dyskinesia followed the injection of microspheres into the LAD – the length of the LAD associated with the ischaemic segment failed to opacify; C: following i.v. nitroglycerine the LV cavity size was diminished and the LAD with no stenosis was opacified and shown throughout its length.

drug causes an increase in heart rate and aortic blood pressure and this affects myocardial contractility. It might therefore precipitate regional myocardial ischaemia and angina in patients with critically balanced myocardial perfusion and metabolic requirements in the presence of stenosed coronary arteries. In addition, this agent causes an 18 to 21% reduction in the diameter of all coronary vessels (11, 12, 13).

These experiments have also shown that acute regional myocardial ischaemia without coronary artery stenosis may impair opacification of the coronary artery associated with that lesion. This study does not preclude the possibility of coronary spasm in man. A number of hypotheses have been tested to investigate the transient disappearance of a large coronary artery when angiography is performed in the presence of acute regional myocardial ischaemia. The results suggest that this angiographic finding in patients may not necessarily be due to coronary spasm.

SUMMARY

Fifteen anaesthetized dogs have been studied to investigate the factors that cause transient failure to opacify a coronary artery during arteriography. Left ventricular angiograms and left coronary arteriograms were performed before and after stenosis of the left anterior descending coronary artery (LAD), with no regional ischaemia. In addition, microspheres were used to produce regional myocardial ischaemia in dogs with no coronary artery stenosis. The entire LAD was opacified before and after stenosis of that vessel. However when acute regional myocardial ischaemia was induced with left atrial pacing, ergonovine maleate or the LAD injection of microspheres, the portion of that vessel associated with the dyskinetic ventricular segment failed to opacify during arteriography. This transient disappearance of a large coronary artery could be reversed with intravenous nitroglycerine. These results suggest that mechanical and hemodynamic factors related to acute regional myocardial ischaemia may explain the transient failure to opacify a large coronary artery during arteriography. This angiographic finding, in patients, may not necessarily be due to coronary spasm.

REFERENCES

1. Epstein SE, Redwood DR, Goldstein RE: Angina pectoris: pathophysiology, evaluation, and a treatment. *Ann Intern Med* 75:263–296, 1971.
2. Fleckenstein A: On the basic pharmacological mechanism of nifedipine and its relation to therapeutic efficacy. In: *Third international adalat symposium*, Domengos A, Jatene Lichtlen P (eds), Amsterdam, Excerpta Medica, 1975, p 1ff.

3. Maseri A, Mimmo R, Chierchia S, Marchesi C, Pesola A, l'Abbate A: Coronary artery spasm as a cause of acute myocardial ischaemia in man. *Chest* 68:625–630, 1975.
4. Curry RC, Pepine CJ, Sabom MB, Feldman RL, Christie LG, Conti CR: Effects of ergonovine in patients with and without coronary artery disease. *Circulation* 56:803–809, 1977.
5. Maroko PR, Kjekshus JK, Sobel BE, Watanabe T, Covell JW, Ross Jr J, Braunwald E: Factors influencing infarct size following experimental coronary artery occlusion. *Circulation* 43:67–80, 1971.
6. Tyberg JV, Yeatman, LA, Parmley WW, Urschel CW, Sonnenblick EH: Effects of hypoxia on the mechanics of cardiac contraction. *Am J Physiol* 218:1780–1791, 1970.
7. Tyberg JV, Forrester JS, Parmley WW: Altered segmental function and compliance in acute myocardial ischaemia. *Eur J Cardiol* 1:307–312, 1974.
8. Rivas F, Cobb FR, Bache RJ, Greenfield Jr JC: Realtionship between blood flow in ischemic regions and extent of myocardial infarction: serial measurements of blood flow. *Circ Res* 38:439–450, 1976.
9. Maseri A, Pesola A, Mimmo R, Chierchia S, l'Abbate A: Pathogenetic mechanisms of angina at rest. *Circulation* 51–52 (suppl 2): 11–89, 1975.
10. Weiner L, Kasparian H, Duca PHR, Walinski P, Gottlieb RS, Hanckel F, Brest AN: Spectrum of coronary artery spasm: clinical, angiographic and myocardial metabolic experience in 29 cases. *Am J Cardiol* 38:945–953, 1976.
11. Heupler F, Proudfit W, Siegel W, Shirey E, Razair M, Sones FM: The ergonovine maleate test for the diagnosis of coronary artery spasm. *Circulation* 51–52 (suppl II): II-11, 1975.
12. Wassef MR, Pleuvry BJ: The cardiovascular effects of ergonnetrine in the experimental animal in vivo and in vitro. *Brit J Anaesthesia* 46:473–480, 1974.
13. Orlick AE, Ricci DR, Cipriano PR, Guthaner DF, Harrison DC: Coronary hemodynamic effects of ergonovine maleate in man: abstract. *Circulation* 55–56 (suppl III): III-130, 1977.

## 4.8. HEMODYNAMIC EFFECTS OF REDUCTIONS IN CORONARY BLOOD FLOW CAUSED BY MECHANICAL STENOSIS AND PLATELET AGGREGATES FORMING IN DOG CORONARY ARTERIES

JOHN D. FOLTS

### 1. INTRODUCTION

Coronary blood flow has been measured by a variety of techniques in normal vessels for over sixty years. It is only recently that attempts have been made to measure coronary blood flow in vessels which have been given mechanical stenosis. Ameroid constrictors have been used to produce gradual, but uncontrollable narrowing of coronary arteries (1). Gould et al., in open-chest dogs, developed a snare device which could be placed around the coronary artery and attached to a machinists micrometer (2). Khouri and Gregg developed a mercury-filled pneumatic device which could produce graded amounts of coronary artery stenosis in chronically instrumented dogs (3). The partial obstruction produced with these devices has been evaluated in physiologic terms by measuring the reactive hyperemic response to temporary complete occlusion, the pressure gradient across the stenosis, and the decrease in the resting coronary blood flow. These devices do not allow for fine control of the amount of stenosis or small reductions in the coronary blood flow, such as 5–10 ml/min increments. Therefore a technique is described here which produces known controlled amounts of coronary or other arterial stenosis, which can be easily altered to produce more or less stenosis, and allows for small controlled changes in coronary blood flow.

### 2. METHODS

Twenty-six open-chest anesthetized dogs were prepared as shown in Figure 1. Electromagnetic flow probes were placed on the circumflex coronary artery and the ascending aorta. Coronary artery stenosis was produced with the plastic cylinder shown in the upper right-hand corner. The technique for constructing and using these cylinders has been previously described (4). To obtain finer control over the amount of stenosis, a smooth tapered nylon fishing leader is placed in the lumen of the plastic cylinder, between the outside of the vessel wall and the inside of the cylinder. When this leader is pulled to the left a larger diameter of the leader enters the lumen and

J. Baan, A.C. Arntzenius, E.L. Yellin (eds.), Cardiac Dynamics, 311–319.

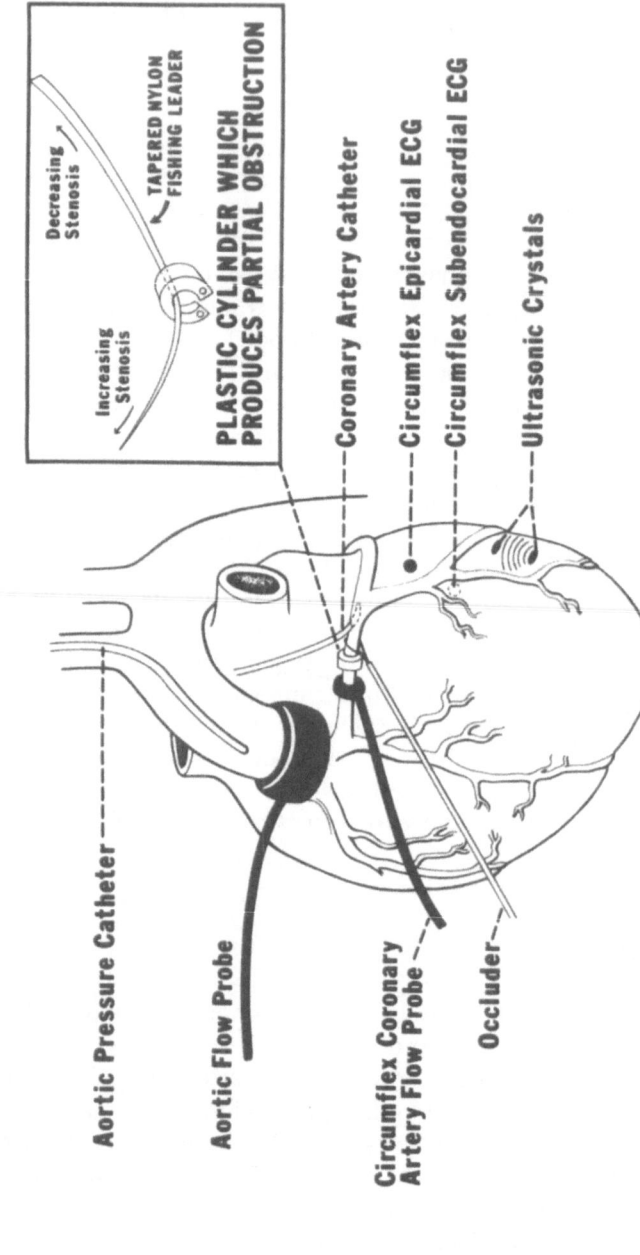

*Figure 1.* Technique for producing fixed partial obstruction in a branch of the left coronary artery. A plastic cylinder of appropriate internal diameter 3 mm in length is placed on the coronary artery. Then the tapered fishing leader is placed in the lumen of the cylinder. This leader is pulled in either direction to increase or decrease the stenosis.

produces more stenosis. This in turn reduces the coronary flow. If the leader is pulled to the right less stenosis is produced and coronary flow will increase. Pairs of ultrasonic crystals are placed in the mid-myocardium in the distal circumflex and left anterior descending (LAD) beds for measuring myocardial cord length and regional contractility. A Millar catheter-tip pressure transducer is placed in the left ventricle for left ventricular pressure and LV $dp/dt$ measurements. Epicardial ECG leads were placed in the areas supplied by the circumflex and LAD coronary arteries respectively.

An initial amount of coronary artery stenosis was chosen which just eliminates the reactive hyperemic response to a temporary 20-second complete occlusion using the occluding snare shown in Figure 1. We have previously shown that this requires about a 72% coronary diameter reduction and this was confirmed by microscopic examination of silastic rubber casts made of the stenosed artery (5). Then, using the tapered fishing leader the amount of stenosis can be increased, to reduce coronary flow. Three levels of stenosis were obtained, $S_1 = 72 \pm 8\%$, $S_2 = 80 \pm 5\%$, and $S_3 = 90 \pm 4\%$, with appropriate decreases in coronary flow, and each level of stenosis was maintained for ten minutes to allow for hemodynamic stabilization.

## 3. RESULTS

A representative record from one of the experiments in which the coronary artery was given several levels of stenosis is shown in Figure 2. There were no significant changes from control in cardiac output, aortic or left ventricular pressure, LV $dp/dt$ or ECG with the first level of stenosis which averaged 78% (panel B). Contractility, however, was impaired, as measured by increasing myocardial length, and a decrease in the myocardial shortening length. When the stenosis was increased to 86% and the coronary flow decreased 40% from control, there were now slight decreases in peak LV pressure, LV $dp/dt$ and ST segment deviation suggestive of ischemia (panel C). The last panel shows significant changes in all parameters with a 92% stenosis.

The results of the 26 dogs are summarized in Table 1. An 80% stenosis in this group of experiments reduced coronary blood flow by 26% from control. This produced a 34% decrease in maximum shortening length, but did not produce any other hemodynamic abnormality. The severe 90% stenosis produced a 62% reduction in coronary blood flow, and further impairment of contractility, with a 59% reduction in maximum shortening length. There were also significant reductions in cardiac output, LV $dp/dt$, and a 3.1 mv rise in ST segment deviation on the epicardial ECG.

In 19 of the 26 dogs there were periodic cyclical reductions in coronary

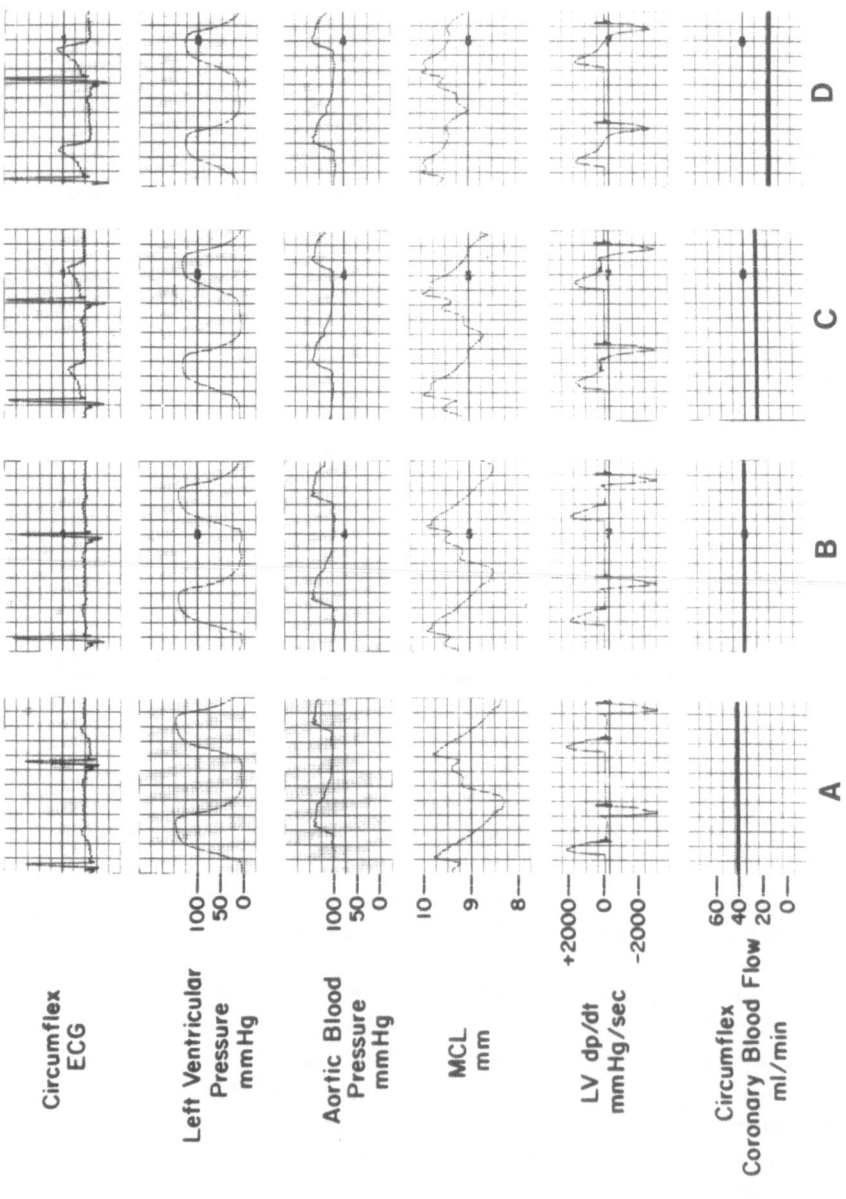

*Figure 2.* Coronary and hemodynamic effects of three levels of coronary artery stenosis. Panel A shows the effects of a 68% stenosis in the circumflex coronary artery with coronary flow at control levels. In panel B there is a 78% stenosis in the circumflex coronary artery, and myocardial cord length (MCL) is decreased. In panel C the stenosis was increased to 86%, and in panel D the stenosis was increased to 90%.

Circumflex
ECG

Left Ventricular
Pressure
mmHg
100 — 50 — 0 —

Aortic Blood
Pressure
mmHg
100 — 50 — 0 —

MCL
mm
10 — 9 — 8 —

LV dp/dt
mmHg/sec
+2000 — 0 — -2000 —

Circumflex
Coronary Blood Flow
ml/min
60 — 40 — 20 — 0 —

A          B          C          D

*Table 1.* Percent changes in hemodynamic parameters with three levels of coronary arterial stenosis.*

| Level of stenosis | $S_1 = 72\%$ | $S_2 = 80\%$ | $S_3 = 90\%$ |
|---|---|---|---|
| Coronary blood flow | $-6 \pm 9\%$ | $-26 \pm 9\%$ | $-62 \pm 15\%$ |
| Maximum shortening length | 0 | $-34 \pm 11\%$ | $-59 \pm 10\%$ |
| Arterial blood pressure | 0 | $-2 \pm 1\%$ | $-19 \pm 9\%$ |
| Cardiac output | 0 | 0 | $-15 \pm 6\%$ |
| LV $dp/dt$ | 0 | $-4 \pm 1\%$ | $-21 \pm 9\%$ |
| ECG (mv) | 0 | $0.3 \pm 0.1$ | $3.1 \pm 0.6$ |

*The data for all parameters, except ECG ST segment deviation, were normalized by expressing changes as a percentage change from control measurements.

blood flow followed by a spontaneous return to control levels as shown in Figure 3. This occurred in spite of the fact that the amount of fixed mechanical stenosis was not altered. We have previously shown that these flow reductions are caused by blood platelets periodically aggregating in the narrowed arterial lumen (6, 7). This platelet plugging produces a gradual decline in coronary flow and associated hemodynamic changes. There is a decrease in peak aortic ejection velocity, and LV $dp/dt$ due to this decline in coronary blood flow. Figure 4 shows that a 40% decline in coronary flow, from 40 ml/min to 24 ml/min produces a significant change in myocardial cord length but only a small change in blood pressure and LV $dp/dt$.

## 4. DISCUSSION

This technique, using the tapered fishing leader, produces much more stable changes in coronary flow than we could achieve using a micrometer snare (8) or a balloon, pneumatic occluder (9). It appears from these studies that the earliest measurable physiologic change due to ischaemia is a loss of regional contractility. Significant ECG or LV $dp/dt$ changes did not occur until coronary flow was decreased by more than 40% from control. This may be due in part to the collateral flow known to develop rapidly in the dog. We have previously shown that with more than 80% stenosis or when coronary blood flow is reduced to 40% of control there is a relative under-perfusion of the endocardium with respect to the epicardium and endocardial ischaemia occurs (10). This may well not be detected with epicardial ECG leads or with a measurement of global function such as LV $dp/dt$, although this level of ischaemia would be expected to affect mid-myocardial contractility as measured with the ultrasonic crystals.

The cyclical reductions in flow caused by platelet plugging can be very bothersome in studies of coronary artery stenosis. This phenomenon can be

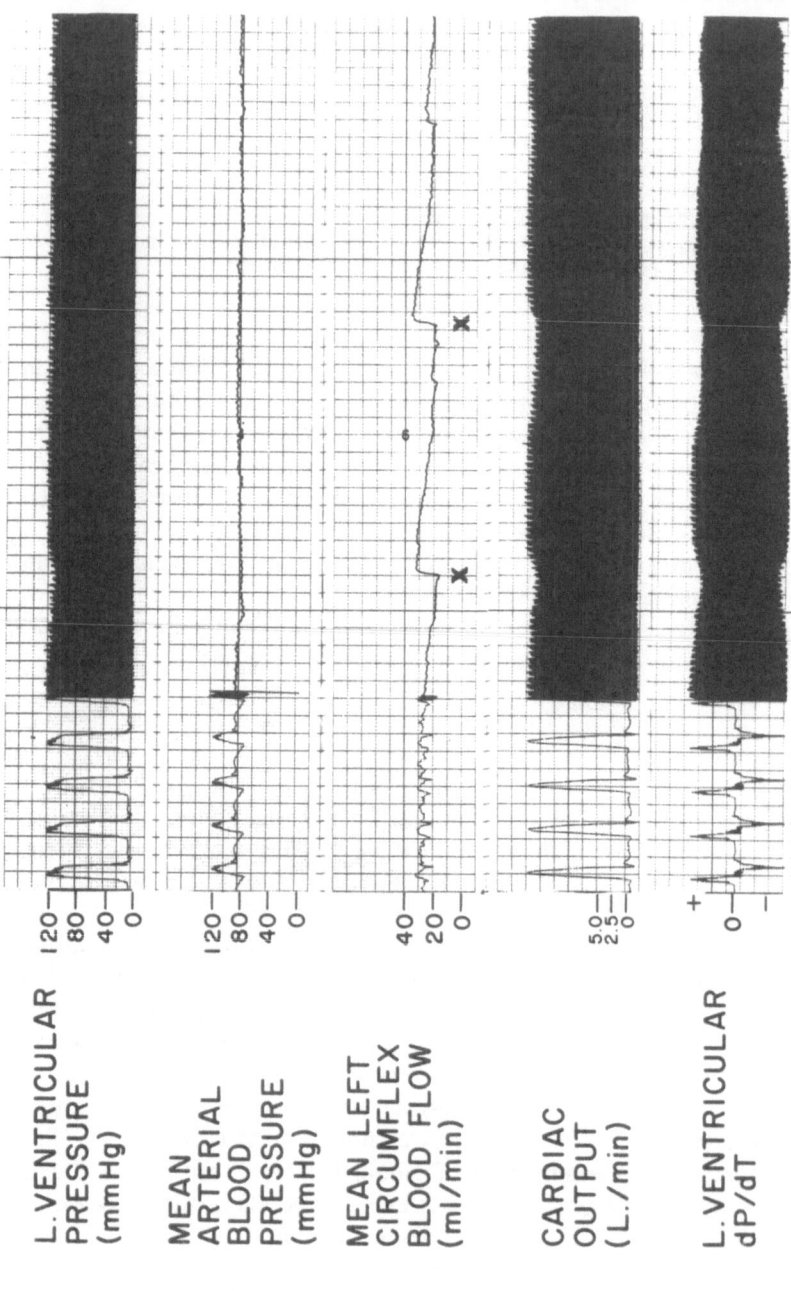

*Figure 3.* Mean coronary and aortic flows, left ventricular and aortic pressure and LV *dp/dt* recorded at fast and slow (0.25 mm/sec) paper speed. The coronary artery has a fixed 80% stenosis, and the coronary flow gradually declines, due to platelet aggregates collecting in the narrowed lumen. At the points marked with crosses the flow suddenly increases, when the platelet plug breaks loose.

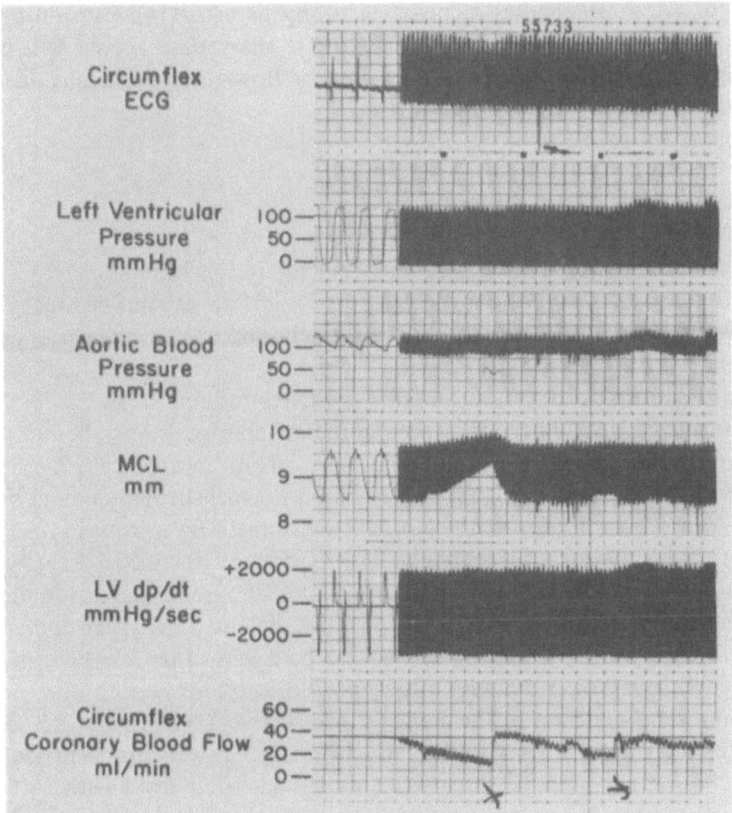

*Figure 4.* Mean coronary flow, in an artery stenosed 85%, aortic and left ventricular pressure and myocardial cord length, as measured with ultrasonic crystals, are shown along with circumflex ECG. As the coronary flow declines, due to platelet plugging in the area of stenosis, the myocardial cord length increases and myocardial shortening length decreases.

partially eliminated by pretreating the dog with 35 mg/kg of aspirin i.v. (7). However if the dog releases endogenous catecholamines this platelet plugging may still occur (11). These cyclical reductions in coronary flow in stenosed arteries have been shown to be exacerbated by i.v. infusions of oleic acid 75 mg/kg and epinephrine 2 $\mu$g/kg and can be inhibited by agents such as indomethacin 15 mg/kg, propranolol 4 mg/kg, or caffeine 25 mg/kg (12).

We postulate that patients with a 70–90% arterial stenosis may form platelet plugs in the areas of stenosis, which could further reduce the blood flow through the stenosed artery. If this were to occur in a human coronary artery reducing flow to 40% of control this could lead to pump failure or a fatal arrhythmia (13). This is the rationale for placing patients with covonary or cerebral arterial stenosis on daily aspirin (14), or sulfinpyrzone (15), known platelet inhibitors. The hope is that these agents will prevent the platelet plugging, thereby preventing the flow reductions and protecting them against heart attacks and stroke.

5. SUMMARY

In 26 acute open-chest dogs, cardiac output (CO), blood pressure (ABP), epicardial ECG, regional contractility (RC), LV $dp/dt$, and coronary blood flow (CBF) were measured, with electromagnetic flow meters, pressure transducers, and ultrasonic crystals. Three levels of controlled coronary stenosis ($S$) were produced, producing diameter reductions of $72\% = S_1$, $80\% = S_2$ and $90\% = S_3$. There was no significant change in any hemodynamic parameter with $S_1$. CBF decreased $26 \pm 9\%$ from control with $S_2$, and RC was diminished $34 \pm 11\%$ from control with no measurable change in ABP, CO, LV $dp/dt$ or ECG. With $S_3$ CBF, RC and ABP decreased $62 \pm 15\%$, $59 \pm 11\%$ and $19 \pm 6\%$ respectively. LV $dp/dt$ was decreased $21 \pm 9\%$ from control levels. ECG showed $3.1 \pm 0.6$ mv of ST segment deviation, and CO was decreased $15 \pm 9\%$. The first sign and the most sensitive indicator of regional myocardial ischaemia appears to be a loss of regional contractility. With each level of $S$ platelet plugs periodically formed in the stenosed coronary artery adding to the stenosis and further decreasing CBF, causing impaired contractility and pump function, and producing ventricular arrhythmias. These platelet plugs were abolished in all cases with i.v. aspirin (ASA) 30 mg/kg. However, 2 $\mu$g/kg of epinephrine i.v., in 12 of the 26 dogs still provokes acute platelet plugging in spite of pretreatment with ASA. Thus platelet plugging can occur after pretreatment with ASA, leading to death of the dog. We postulate that platelet plugging may occur in the stenosed coronary arteries of man acutely reducing coronary flow, leading to impaired contractility and decreased ventricular function and sudden death by ventricular fibrillation.

REFERENCES

1. Elliot EC, Jones EL, Bloor CM, Leon AS, Gregg DE: Day-to-day changes in coronary hemodynamics secondary to constriction of the circumflex branch of the left coronary artery in conscious dogs. Circ Res 22:237, 1968.
2. Gould KL, Lipscomb K, Calvert C: Compensatory changes of the distal coronary vascular bed during progressive coronary constriction. Circulation 51:1085, 1975.
3. Khouri E, Gregg DE: Flow in the major branches of the left coronary artery during experimental coronary insufficiency in the unanesthetized dog. Circ Res 23:99, 1968.
4. Folts JD, Gallagher K, Rowe GG: Hemodynamic effects of controlled amounts of coronary artery stenosis in acute open chest and chronically instrumented dogs. J Thor Cardiovasc Surg 73:722–727, 1977.

5. Gallagher KP, Folts JD, Rowe GG: Comparison of coronary arteriograms with direct measurements of stenosed coronary arteries in dogs. *Am Heart J* 95:338–347, 1978.
6. Folts JD, Rowe GG: Cyclical reductions in coronary blood flow in coronary arteries with fixed partial obstruction and their inhibition with aspirin. *Fed Proc* 33:413, 1974.
7. Folts JD, Crowell EB, Rowe GG: Platelet aggregation in partially obstructed vessels and their elimination with aspirin. *Circulation* 54:365–370, 1976.
8. Folts JD, Shug AL, Koke JR, Bittar N: Protection of the ischemic dog myocardium with l-carnitine. *Am J Cardiol* 41:1209–1214, 1978.
9. Folts JD, Rowe GG: Coronary and hemodynamic effects of temporary acute aortic insufficiency in intact anesthetized dogs. *Circ Res* 35:238–246, 1974.
10. Gallagher KP, Folts JD, Rankin JHG, Shebuski RJ, Rowe GG: Myocardial blood flow with four degrees of coronary stenosis. *Fed Proc* 37:468, 1978.
11. Folts JD, Gallagher KP: Epinephrine-induced platelet aggregation in mechanically stenosed dog coronary arteries occurring after aspirin administration. *Clin Res* 26:231A, 1978.
12. Folts JD: Platelet aggregation in stenosed coronary or cerebral arteries: a possible explanation for sudden coronary death or stroke. Submitted to *Science*.
13. Folts JD, Rowe GG: Platelet plugging or aggregation in stenosed coronary arteries as a cause of sudden death. Presented at International symposium on atherosclerosis, Milan, November, 1977 (in press).
14. Coronary Drug Project Research Group: Aspirin in coronary heart disease. *J Chron Dis* 29:625–642, 1976.
15. Anturane Reinfarction Trial Research Group: Sulfinpyrazone in the prevention of cardiac death after myocardial infarction. *New Engl J Med* 298:289–295, 1978.

SECTION 5


MEASURING CARDIAC PERFORMANCE:
AIMS AND VALIDITY OF INVASIVE
AND NONINVASIVE MEASUREMENT

# 5.1. ISAAC STARR LECTURE: INVASIVE AND NON-INVASIVE MONITORING OF CARDIOVASCULAR DYNAMICS IN CLINICAL PRACTICE

H.J.C. SWAN

## 1. INTRODUCTION

One of the striking features of cardiology in the 1970s has been a decisive alteration of practice to substitute quantitative measurement for clinical impression regarding cardiovascular function. This is a consequence of the recognition of the limitations of clinical findings as accurate indicators of the state of cardiovascular function or of its change in relation to the natural history of a disease process or resulting from a therapeutic intervention. Essentially, this has resulted from the application of knowledge defined initially in experimental laboratories and subsequently adapted in specialized cardiac catheterization laboratories to effective use in the setting of acute clinical care – at the bedside, in the operating room, the intensive care unit and the outpatient clinic. Measurement of cardiovascular dynamics in these settings has required re-evaluation of the practical utility of such measurements to clinical decision making. The purpose of this paper is to review the impact of currently available methods for quantitative measurement of cardiovascular dynamics in acute clinical care.

The term *cardiovascular dynamics* is inclusive and encompasses control of the peripheral blood vessels, the function of veins and regional circulations as well as the functions of the atria and ventricles. However, current considerations will be confined to the global and regional function of the left ventricle. While the principal attention of basic and clinical investigators has been directed, heretofore, to the contraction phase of the cardiac cycle, greater attention is now being properly placed to those factors which influence filling, namely, diastolic compliance.

Although the measurement of *global* (or total) function of the right and left ventricle has markedly increased out of understanding of the circulation in health and disease, *segmental* or *regional* disorders of function in both the left and the right ventricle are common findings associated with many circulatory disorders since they characterize the most frequent cause of heart disease, namely, coronary atherosclerosis with resultant ischaemia, infarction, or scar. Hence, description of global function alone may be insufficient in many instances and the regional contractile and compliant characteristics of segments of the ventricles become highly relevant. This lecture will consider several separate approaches to the measurement of cardiovascular dynamics, discuss the advantages and disadvantages of each in a clinical setting, and identify broad areas of application. The potential of such measurements to define responses to stress are currently attracting considerable investigator interest. Both invasive and noninvasive techniques can, and probably should, be employed, depending upon the particular circumstances. Methodology which is noninvasive is undoubtedly desirable, but imprecision, technological complexity, equipment size and cost frequently limit its usefulness. Policies, equipment and procedures must be compatible with the environment if specific procedures are to be generally useful in a clinical care setting. The equipment must be convenient and of a size not to interfere with necessary medical or surgical care. The size and mobility of a device or rack is importantly relevant to the crowded environment of an intensive care facility. In highly specialized units, effective mounting design and miniaturization of equipment with multiple functions is essential. Equipment used in a clinical setting must be highly reliable and instruments subject to even infrequent breakdowns are not acceptable. Medical and nursing staff members will dispense with such devices and rely on other guidance. Equipment must be simple and the principles of operation must be readily understandable by personnel with different backgrounds and levels of competence who change shifts of responsibility several times each day. Its function cannot be dependent upon a resident engineer for effective utilization. Preferably, data output should be automatic and the procedures to obtain relevant information readily defined and simple to follow. Likewise, the technical procedures to obtain the measurements desired preferably should be noninvasive and/or minimally hazardous. They should be reasonably comprehended by and acceptable to the patient and not significantly increase either his apprehension or discomfort. Those technical skills to perform necessary invasive procedures should be achieved and competence maintained by qualified health care personnel by participation on a frequent basis. Above all, the information obtained by such means should be relevant to the clinical situation in providing information for diagnosis or treatment not obtainable by conventional clinical evaluation. This should facilitate the establishment of a *complete diagnosis*, a *more accurate* prognosis and identify that *form of therapy* most likely to cause improvement. In addition, it should detect promptly therapeutic interventions which result in no improvement or deterioration. The information should be available immediately so as to facilitate the above objectives. The data must be obtained with a sufficient degree of *precision and accuracy* so as to provide relevant and important assistance in the decision-making process to the health care personnel involved.

The procedures used in critical care practice must demonstrate a high "benefit-risk" ratio. Even noninvasive techniques which require maintenance of fatiguing positions by the patient, frequent interventions or movement, or the close proximity of a large and threatening device such as a gamma camera, are likely to become procedures of non-acceptance by personnel in clinical care units unless they clearly contribute to a more favourable therapeutic outcome. Careful discussion of the benefits of such information with all patient care related personnel is essential.

In regard to patient benefit from rapid assessment of cardiovascular function and effective therapeutic decision making, regrettably there is no data to allow one to quantify the efficacy or lack of benefit in clinical practice. In general, the standards of practice seem to have improved as knowledge of the disease entities and the short-term effects of therapeutic interventions have been clarified. As in the case of cardiac catheterization, it may be possible to decide when certain measurements are no longer necessary for a sufficient diagnosis, and the therapeutic responses can be monitored by suitable clinical guides. This will be possible when the various and relevant sub-elements of disease states are defined with sufficient clarity and responses to differing therapies are sufficiently uniform. However, this is not the case today and appears unlikely for several years to come.


## 2. HEMODYNAMIC MONITORING

It is in the last five to ten years that the principles of hemodynamic monitoring have allowed basic physiologic measurements to be applied in a consistent manner in the management of cardiovascular aspects of critical illnesses. In this regard, hemodynamic monitoring is fundamentally an extension of the basic physiologic concepts developed in the early part of this century by Otto Frank, Ernest Starling and their contemporaries. The demonstration of the relationship of fibre stretch to velocity and force of fibre shortening has been translated into more practical terms relative to cardiovascular dynamics. Changes in left ventricular filling pressure may be considered both as a determinant of cardiac performance and, when left ventricular filling pressure is importantly elevated (in excess of 20 mmHg), a direct reflection of the competence of ventricular emptying in relation to a given afterload.

Such concepts were slow in their application to disease states in that the techniques for the accurate measurement of flow and pressure were constrained to the experimental animal laboratory. However, these matters were translated into practical terms with the introduction of diagnostic cardiac catheterization between 1942 and 1950 by Cournand and Richards, McMichael and Schaffer, Dexter and others. This procedure allowed the passage of a fluid-filled catheter into the right atrium and right ventricle of the heart with measurement of pressure by appropriate manometer systems. Cardiac output could also be measured by application of Fick's principle. In this manner, measurement of the intravascular pressures and cardiac output could be generated.

However, these techniques, useful in the definition of cardiac performance, found their primary utilization in the *diagnosis* of various diseases of the heart. In the early 1950s, the developing discipline of cardiac surgery strongly influenced diagnostic catheterization in the field of congenital heart disease. Later, the adverse effects of abnormalities of cardiac valve function were studied. In this application, knowledge of the pulmonary capillary wedge pressure did give considerable insight into the behaviour of the left ventricle and of mitral valve abnormalities. The pulmonary capillary wedge pressure is a phase-delayed and amplitude-damped version of the pressure in the next active segment of the circulation – the pulmonary capillaries and pulmonary veins downstream to the obstructed segment. Because of the need for physical manipulation of the semi-rigid catheters used for these purposes, these techniques found their application only in specialized catheterization laboratories which provided fluoroscopic facilities for deliberate guidance of the catheter into the right heart and pulmonary arteries. The semi-rigid nature of such catheters usually resulted in atrial or ventricular extrasystoles at the time when the catheter tip impacted forcibly on the endocardium of these chambers. A small but significant incidence of atrial fibrillation and ventricular fibrillation could be caused particularly in patients with moderate or severe degrees of circulatory insufficiency.

3. FLOTATION CATHETERS

In 1970, Swan, Ganz and colleagues introduced the balloon flotation catheter, which permitted the techniques of cardiac catheterization to be transferred to the clinical setting. The principles of flotation catheterization specified a high degree of flexibility of the tip of the catheter and the proximal shaft so that it might be flow-guided into appropriate locations in the circulation. As recognized earlier, such a catheter, when provided with an inflatable balloon at its tip, readily passes with the blood-stream into the right ventricle and is then propelled into the pulmonary artery to impact in a distal pulmonary vessel of moderate or even large calibre. In addition, appropriate placement of the balloon close to the tip of the catheter prevents the catheter tip from impinging upon ventricular or atrial endocardium, thus reducing the complication of serious cardiac arrhythmias from a frequent to an unusual event. Thus, the particular value of these catheters included a high frequency of automatic and uncomplicated flotation into the pulmonary artery without the use of fluoroscopy and, therefore, greatly broadened the locations in which catheterization of the right heart could be employed.

Balloon flotation catheter techniques are now generally accepted in the disciplines of anaesthesia, cardiology and critical care. Monitoring of pulmonary arterial and pulmonary capillary pressures, as well as right atrial pressure, allows for the prompt recognition of unsuspected alteration in right and left-sided cardiac dynamics.

Such catheters have similar dynamic characteristics to conventional woven catheters and a frequency response adequate to obtain systolic mean and diastolic pulmonary arterial pressure. Phasic wedge pressures, right atrial and right ventricular pressure are readily obtained.

The commonest single complication of this technique is the development of small pulmonary infarcts which, in the great majority of instances, do not result in symptoms. Inflation of the tip-balloon can result in rupture of a pulmonary artery branch. This complication is one which has proven to be fatal in several reported instances.

4. MEASUREMENT OF CARDIAC OUTPUT

Use of the Cournand catheter allowed for the measurement of cardiac output as a function of total oxygen consumption and the arterial-venous oxygen difference. This application of Fick's principle has been extended to include the dilution of an indicator on its first passage through the circulation. For many years, a variety of dyes detectable by appropriate optical devices in the arterial system or in pulmonary arterial blood were used. Of these, Indocyanine (Cardiogreen) was the most widely used. Usually, these procedures required withdrawal of blood (approx. 30 ml) from the circulation through an appropriate sensing device. Principally because of the latter equipment, the dye dilution method was never generally accepted into routine clinical practice. The need for spirometers or similar devices as well as systemic and pulmonary arterial blood sampling obviate the use of the oxygen Fick method.

The *thermal dilution technique* possesses the practical characteristics necessary for clinical application. A thermistor located 4 cm from the tip of the balloon flotation catheter acts as an accurate and effective sensor for alteration in blood temperature in the pulmonary artery occasioned by injection of bolus of cold solution in the region of the superior cava – right atrium. Adequate mixing is achieved between the chamber of the right atrium, the tricuspid valve, the chamber of the right ventricle and the pulmonary valve. Recirculation of "heat" through the systemic capillaries is small and the first passage curve in the pulmonary artery can be readily reduced and analysed by automated techniques. The precision (reproducibility) of the measurement is high. Agreement between successive (triplicate) determinations in a patient in a steady state is approximately $\pm 4\%$ (variance). The accuracy is also high in most instances, with comparisons between other (e.g., flow meters) or similar (e.g., Indocyanine green) methods shown to lie within approximately $\pm 3$–$10\%$. Occasionally, comparisons have shown a greater systematic deviation in regard to absolute agreement (coefficients of regression: $+10\%$ to $-5\%$) but retain a high correlation coefficient (0.95). Although accuracy is a highly desirable characteristic in cardiac output measurement, precision is more important in clinical applications. Decisions as to prognosis and therapy are defined initially from rather broad absolute ranges (i.e., $>1.8>2.2>L/min/m^2$). However, prognosis is more importantly affected by subsequent, relatively modest changes in response to therapy ($\pm 0.1\ l/min/m^2$). Cardiac output is now routinely measured by the thermodilution method in the operating room and recovery areas and in the medical, cardiologic and respiratory critical care units. The thermodilution technique is practicably suited to such units since blood is not withdrawn from the patient and the procedure is rapidly and readily carried out without the use of large pieces of equipment or the need to alter other important evaluation of therapeutic procedures. In this regard, nuclear scintigraphic techniques will allow measurement of cardiac output with a relatively high degree of accuracy within the immediate future. However, the expense and, at this time, the difficulties of frequent application of such procedures to more than a few patients will probably necessitate that measurement of cardiac output be based on the thermodilution technique for a considerable time to come.

## 5. MEASUREMENT OF LEFT-SIDE DYNAMICS

While left ventricular filling pressure can be estimated from the pulmonary capillary wedge pressure or from the pulmonary artery diastolic pressure when the pulmonary vascular resistance is not increased, nevertheless, important differences between pulmonary capillary wedge pressure and end-diastolic ventricular pressure may exist. In the absence of mitral valve disease, mean pulmonary capillary wedge pressure correlates closely with mean diastolic ventricular pressure. When ventricular compliance decreases and end-diastolic ventricular pressure rises, a major discrepancy develops between the mean pulmonary capillary wedge pressure and the end-diastolic ventricular pressure.

Transaortic catheterization of the left ventricle allows for the direct measurement of diastolic and systolic left ventricular pressures and with suitable dynamic response determination of positive and negative $dP/dT$. However, transaortic catheterization is associated with a significant incidence of ventricular ectopic rhythms as well as damage or injury in the arterial system. This procedure is not widely practiced, although a high-fidelity recording of diastolic ventricular pressure and of left ventricular $dP/dT$ and the left ventricular electrogram could prove most useful.

## 6. LEFT VENTRICULAR GEOMETRY

Conventionally, left ventricular volumes and changes in volume are measured in man by contrast ventriculography obtained by high-speed single or biplane cine filming of the passage of radiopaque material injected in the pulmonary artery or left ventricle to the aorta. Apart from research studies, contrast ventriculography is impractical in a critical care setting. Hence, heretofore, contrast ventriculography with determination of ejection fraction and regional wall motion has been rarely employed in the evaluation of acute illnesses or in the care of the critically ill.

## 7. NONINVASIVE DETERMINATION OF EJECTION FRACTION

Scintigraphy allows for a highly precise determination of ejection fraction by first pass or equilibrium techniques. Using the continuous circulation of Tc99m in vitro labelled red blood cells, the ejection fraction of the right or the left ventricle can be calculated from the sum of counts over a defined region of interest. The ejection fraction is the ratio of the difference between the detected counts at end-diastole minus the counts detected at end-systole divided by the counts detected at end diastole, or $EF = (CED-CES)/CED$. The precision of such measurements appears to be high within and between observers since the calculation is carried out by automated means. The correlation with single plane left ventriculography is also high; ejection fraction determined by contrast angiography from the left anterior oblique projection is systematically greater as compared to scintigraphy.

Segmental motion can be derived by means of a computerized edge-detection system using multiple frame "regions of interest." The inter- and intra-observer variability is acceptable. This may also be translated into a global definition of ventricular function in which the sum of the function of predefined regions is accumulated in an average wall motion score. Scintigraphic ejection fraction and regional wall motion score correlate satisfactorily.

Nuclear scintigraphy has the important advantage of being noninvasive and, in the case of Tc99m labelled red blood cells, the measurements are repeatable for several hours. In its current application, the limitations include not only the size of equipment but the high unit cost for data acquisition and computer data reduction devices. The approach has unique capabilities concerning abnormalities of regional wall motion, including the magnitude and rates of contraction and relaxation. The advent of the smaller "nuclear stethoscope" which will define ejection fraction alone may be a valuable and widely used tool.

## 8. CROSS-SECTIONAL ECHOCARDIOGRAPHY

This technique possesses many of the advantages of the nuclear scinti-graphy but at present lacks the degree of quantitative reliability which characterizes the scintigraphic technique. The variability in the echo image is occasioned by instrumentation resolution, the availability of a satis-factory intercostal "window" and the variability of the position of the heart with relation to specific chest wall position within and between individuals. Also, the patient has to be positioned so as to allow for minimal lung tissue to intervene between the transducer and the cardiac chambers. In addition, the recognition of epi- and endocardial surfaces does not appear to be satisfactory in approximately 20% of subjects. However, application of computer smoothing techniques may allow an improved quality of image comparable to nuclear scintigraphy in the future. Further, echocardio-graphy is continuously applicable within and between cardiac cycles since the frequency response of the total system identifies the particular events of an individual heart cycle. This is not possible with current scintigraphic techniques.

## 9. APPLICATIONS

The introduction of elementary hemodynamic measurements of intracardiac pressures and flow, described by the giants of cardiovascular physiology of the first part of this century, has been broadened to clinical practice from the specialized cardiac catheterization laboratory. Relatively safe invasive measurements can provide intracardiac and intravascular pressures, cardiac output and derived parameters of cardiac function with a high degree of practicality and minimal hazard. Baseline values, spontaneous trends and direct responses to interventions can be used to define the global cardio-vascular status. In the setting of critical illness, these values are of sufficient precision to indicate clearly effective treatment forms with a minimum of delay. Applications of such measurements, which were developed prin-cipally in the cardiac intensive unit, are now undergoing most rapid acceptance in the discipline of anaesthesia. Particular utilization is reported in patients undergoing cardiac and aortic and vascular surgical procedures such as aneurysmectomy and endarterectomy as well as general surgical procedures in the older high-risk patient with a greater likelihood of concurrent coronary artery disease. Respiratory intensive care units and general medical intensive care units experience more frequent use of invasive monitoring than cardiac intensive care units. Although a minority of cardiac patients are subjected to bedside catheterization, it has a prime and, probably, increasing application in the young patient with early and possibly large acute infarction who may be a candidate for prompt intervention, including early revascularization, or use of an intra-aortic balloon assist device. Cardiac patients with recurrent chest pain, perforated ventricular septum or acute mitral regurgitation as well as those requiring acute impedance reduction should also be treated with mandatory monitoring of hemodynamic parameters.

Techniques for detection of regional dysfunction, although noninvasive, are less readily applicable in the critical care setting by reason of size of equipment and complexity of technique. At present, these applications are confined to research settings or special laboratories in a manner very similar to the restrictions associated with formal diagnostic cardiac catheterization. Refinements in noninvasive techniques should allow a wider application of these procedures which currently complement invasive (global) measurements. It is to be hoped that in the future noninvasive procedures will largely supersede the invasive ones.

REFERENCES

1. Borer JS, Bachrach SL, Green MV, Redwood DR, Epstein SE: Real-time radionuclide cineangiography in the noninvasive evaluation of global and regional left ventricular function at rest and during exercise in patients with coronary artery disease. *New Engl J Med* 296:838–844, 1977.
2. Chatterjee K, Swan HJG, Ganz W, Gray R, Lobel H, Forrester JS, Chonette D: Use of balloon-tipped flotation electrode catheter for cardiac monitoring. *Am J Cardiol* 36:56, 1970.
3. Cournand A, Riley RL, Reed ES, Baldwin WF, Richards Jr DW: Measurement of cardiac output in man using the technique of catheterization of the right auricle or ventricle. *J Clin Invest* 25:106, 1946.
4. Forrest JS, Ganz W, Diamond G, McHugh T, Chonette D, Swan HJC: Thermodilution of cardiac output determinations with a single flow-directed catheter. *Am Heart J* 83:306, 1972.
5. Guyton AC: *Circulatory physiology, cardiac output and its reservation*, Philadelphia, Saunders, 1963.
6. Kisslo J, Von Ramm OT, Thurstone FL: Cardiac imaging using phased array ultrasound system: clinical technique and application. *Circulation* 53:262, 1976.
7. Reduto LA, Berger HJ, Cohen LD, Gottschalk A, Zaret BL: Sequential radionuclide

assessment of left and right ventricular performance after acute transmural myocardial infarction. *Annals Int Med* 89:441, 1978.

8. Russell RO, Rackley CE: *Hemodynamic monitoring in a coronary intensive care unit*, New York, Futura, 1974.

9. Swan HJC: The role of hemodynamic monitoring in the management of the critically ill. *Crit Care Med* 383, 1975.

10. Swan HJC, Ganz W, Forrester JS, Marcus HS, Diamond G, Chonette D: Catheterization of the right heart by means of balloon-tipped flotation catheters. *New Engl J Med* 283:447, 1970.

## 5.2. MEASURING CARDIAC PERFORMANCE: AIMS AND VALIDITY OF INVASIVE AND NONINVASIVE ASSESSMENT

PAUL H. HEINTZEN

In the collection on *Cardiac mechanics*, edited by Mirsky, Ghista and Sandler (1) it is stated that *contractility* is a loosely worded term, often used to describe the *performance* of the heart muscle. One could continue in saying that *cardiac performance* is a loosely worded term often used to describe pump function, dynamic geometry of the ventricles, the overall mechanical behaviour of the heart or, still more extensive, the complex mechanisms which enable the heart to fulfill its pump function, including the underlying electrical and biochemical processes.

This presentation will not deal with all these different aspects of cardiac performance but will be confined to some general aspects, recent trends in technology and a brief report on some work from our own group, related to quantitative and noninvasive angiocardiography.

With respect to the aims of noninvasive and invasive assessment of cardiac performance I would like to stress the point that the aims of assessing cardiac performance may be considerably different from the point of view of a basic scientist and from that of a clinical cardiologist, and may also be different even for a general cardiologist who wants to apply (only) the best available method, developed elsewhere, and those cardiologists who feel responsible for the development of new methods and concepts and who therefore have to study today's patients more extensively in order to have the chance to improve patients' care in the future.

For the clinical cardiologist the main goal is to arrive at a correct diagnosis, quantitatively or qualitatively, and to do this at the lowest risk and discomfort for the patient and with the minimum expenditure and cost for the community. Naturally we would only try to arrive at a correct diagnosis and a degree of accuracy which is relevant. But what is relevant? In clinical cardiology it means that the result of the investigation, the diagnostic information obtained, is needed for optimum treatment or has important prognostic implications. Typical questions are: Is medical or surgical treatment indicated? Do these procedures have a realistic chance of being of benefit for the patient? Unfortunately often there are not enough data to answer these questions.

The basic scientist has a different attitude. He tries to understand the fundamental processes, the cause-effect relationships, without asking for

*J. Baan, A.C. Arntzenius, E.L. Yellin (eds.), Cardiac Dynamics, 333–338.*

their actual relevance. He can also apply techniques not justified for the investigation of patients. Nevertheless it is advantagous, even in experimental cardiology, to measure the phenomena in as noninvasive and undisturbed a manner as possible.

With respect to the applicability it can be stated in general, that noninvasive methods are always preferable to invasive ones, if the relevant information, the reliability and accuracy of the data obtained are the same. But it is quite clear that uncertain or questionable results obtained in a comfortable way may cause much more discomfort and risk at a later date. Efforts therefore should be made in two directions: (1), to improve reliability, accuracy and relevant information of noninvasive techniques, and (2) to reduce the risk and discomfort of the invasive techniques and to make them as safe and comfortable as possible.

Before discussing the validity of invasive and noninvasive techniques for the assessment of cardiac performance I would like to mention briefly some of the methods available for analysis of structure and function of the cardiovascular system (Figure 1). All classifications have their limitations, nevertheless we can separate methods which are recording biological signals produced by the heart itself. Among those which are strictly noninvasive the electrocardiogram, phonocardiogram, the various sphygmograms and the ballistocardiogram have different diagnostic values. The importance of the ECG is emphasized in the paper by Hugenholtz and Nelson (this volume). Recording of low, medium and high-frequency vibrations can give useful clinical information and thereby reduce the need for invasive procedures. The high diagnostic value of the audible vibration in particular in valvular

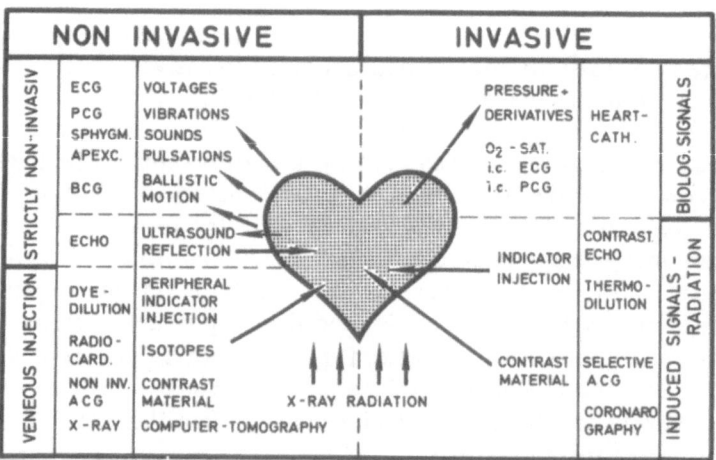

*Figure 1.* Survey on the invasive and noninvasive methods mainly used for measuring cardiac performance.

and congenital heart disease is well established. A more quantitative analysis of the vibrations would be possible, but I doubt if this would be a real step forward.

Not strictly noninvasive are those methods which introduce *indicators* into the circulation. But as long as the injection is made intravenously the classification of noninvasive may be used. Also on the noninvasive side of Figure 1 is contrast material; I will discuss briefly at the end of this presentation, how angiocardiography can be made noninvasive.

The classical invasive techniques are listed on the right side of Figure 1. There is no question about it that these methods are still a sine qua non in most of the patients who have to be considered for surgical treatment of their congenital defects or coronary heart disease. These methods will also serve as established references for other noninvasive approaches which aim at measuring fundamental parameters of cardiac performance quantitatively. But this situation may change during the next decade. In particular echocardiography and radionuclide techniques are very promising tools for the study of cardiac performance in a noninvasive way.

In *echocardiography* the combination of two-dimensional cross-sectional imaging with pulsed Doppler techniques is a very valuable diagnostic tool which allows the monitoring of the beating heart and circulation noninvasively (2). The accuracy of one or two-dimensional measurements for the determination of the ejection fraction, the end-systolic and end-diastolic volumes or dimensions and the wall thickness and heart motion is probably also useful in discriminating pathological cases and for follow-up.

Nuclear medicine, in spite of its lower spatial resolution when compared to angiocardiography, is also evolving rapidly and will be unrivalled if specific metabolic processes can be indicated by radio-pharmaceuticals. Positron emission tomography is in serious competition with similar, but presently much more expensive, radiological techniques for three-dimensional reconstruction of the heart (3, 4).

Tremendous efforts have been made, particularly by the Wood group (5, 6, 7) to arrive radiologically at a complete high-speed, high-resolution three-dimensional reconstruction of the beating heart. The planned unit, still under construction as a prototype, incorporates 28 rotating X-ray chains with the corresponding image-intensifier television units interfaced to a digital computer. On the other side, there are also possibilities to improve conventional two-dimensional "projection" angiocardiography by applying to it specific digital image processing techniques. Our approach is to digitize the whole video (or cine) angiocardiographic picture series, in real time with real-time subtraction of a corresponding background mass (7), or to store the angiocardiogram in the conventional way on magnetic tape and to digitize each video field in real time but to transfer it into the mass memory of a digital computer in a stroboscopic mode using a high-speed external

digital picture memory (8, 9). All relevant reference data are included in the
video pictures. The principle according to which the contrast is enhanced
and by which the information can be improved upon is demonstrated in
Figure 2. Several angiocardiographic pictures from the same phase of the
cardiac cycle are summed up *before* contrast is injected (but following
logarithmic conversion) and this noise-reduced "background" is substracted
from an equal number of contrast pictures obtained from the same cardiac
phase. By this procedure not only is the noise reduced but the contrast
material injected can be utilized much better than in conventional angiocardiography where we are used to looking for the single picture or cycle
with the highest contrast. The classical example of the procedure is demonstrated in Figure 3. On the left is the best opacified single video picture
from a conventional angiocardiogram after two injections of 4 ml

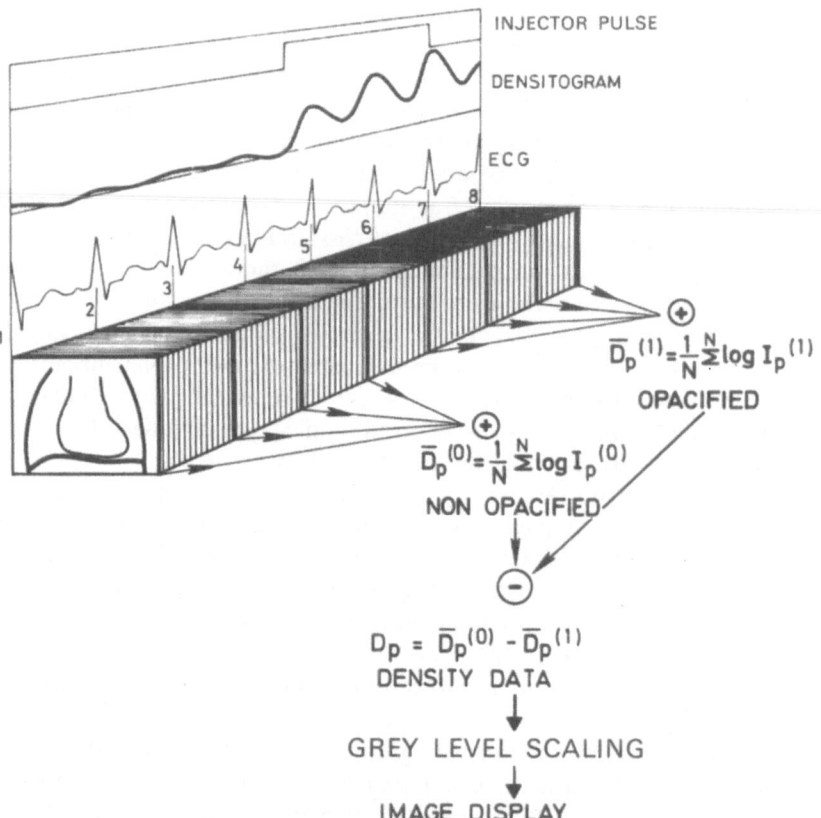

*Figure 2.* Principle of background subtraction and contrast image integration according to
which the contrast can be enhanced.

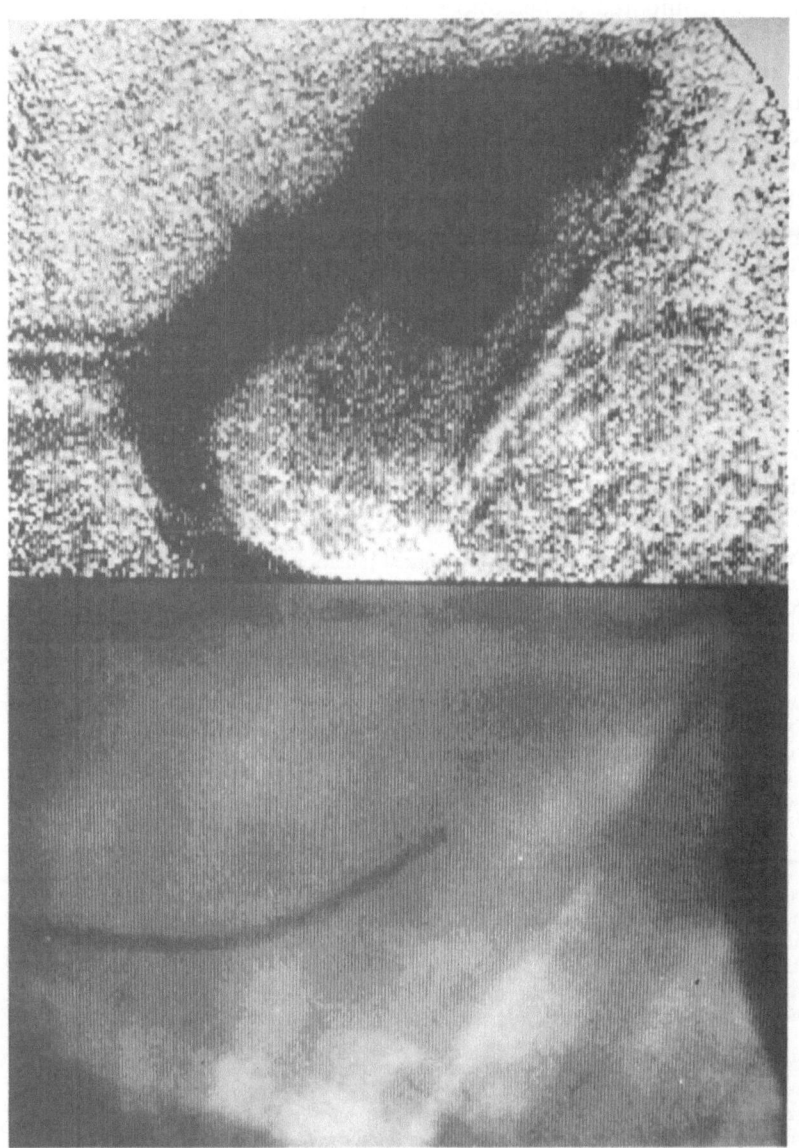

*Figure 3.* Example for contrast enhancement by computerized videoangiocardiographic image processing. *Left:* best opacified single videoangiocardiogram after injection of 2 × 4 ml of Urographin 76% into the left ventricle; *right:* result of digital image processing according to the principle demonstrated in Figure 2.

Urographin 76% into the left ventricle. On the right is the result of digital image processing with contrast subtraction and integration. The gain in contrast is such that the contrast material to be injected can be reduced by a factor of 10 compared to heretofore applied standard techniques.

With this enhancement and better use of contrast material even *non-invasive* angiocardiography with venous injections of small amounts of dye can provide the relevant diagnostic information in specific circumstances (10). For example in children with transposition of the great arteries the anteriorly located aorta can be clearly visualized using only 1–3 ml of contrast material which is injected peripherally. In addition, this technique can improve quantitative analysis of angiocardiograms for determination of size, shape and contraction of both ventricles (7, 10, 11, 12, 13, 14).

REFERENCES

1. Mirsky I, Ghista DN, Sandler H (eds): *Cardiac mechanics: physiological, clinical and mathematical considerations*, New York, John Wiley and Sons, 1974.
2. Griffith JM, Henry WL: An ultrasound system for combined cardiac imaging and doppler blood flow measurement in man. *Circulation* 57 (5):925–930, 1978.
3. Schelbert HR: Future trends in cardiac imaging: non-invasive measurement of myocardial perfusion and metabolism by emission tomography. Israel scientific research conference on cardiac imaging, Arad, Aug. 13–15, 1978.
4. Ter-Pogossian MM: Reconstruction using emitted radiation. Symposium on computerized 3-D reconstruction of structure and function of biologic objects, Anaheim, California, April 12–16, 1976.
5. Wood, EH: New vistas for the study of structural and functional dynamics of the heart, lungs, and circulation by noninvasive numerical tomographic vivisection. *Circulation* 56 (4):506–520, 1977.
6. Ritman EL, Sturm RE, Robb RA, Wood EH: Needs, requirements and design of a high temporal resolution synchronous cylindrical whole-body transaxial scanner for simultaneous study of the structure and function of the heart and circulation. In: *Roentgen-video-techniques*, Heintzen PH, Bürsch JH (eds), Stuttgart, G. Thieme, 1978.
7. Heintzen PH, Bürsch JH (eds): *Roentgen-video-techniques for dynamic studies of structure and function of the heart and circulation*. Stuttgart, G. Thieme, 1978.
8. Brennecke R, Brown TK, Bürsch J, Heintzen PH: Computerized video-image processing with applications to cardio-angiographic roentgen-image series. In: *Digital image processing*, Nagel HH (ed), Berlin, Springer, 1977.
9. Brennecke R, Brown TK, Bürsch J, Heintzen PH: Digital processing of videoangiocardiographic image-series using a minicomputer. In: *Computers in cardiology*, IEEE catalog no 76CH1160–1C, 1976, p 255–260.
10. Heintzen PH, Brennecke R, Bürsch JH: Computerized videoangiocardiography. In: *Coronary heart disease*, Kaltenbach M, Lichtlen P (eds), Stuttgart, G. Thieme, 1978, p 116–121.
11. Heintzen PH, Moldenhauer K, Lange PE: Three-dimensional computerized contraction pattern analysis. *Eur J Cardiol* 1 (3):229–239, 1974.
12. Heintzen PH, Brennecke, R, Bürsch JH, Lange P, Malerczyk V, Moldenhauer K, Onnasch D: Automated video-angiocardiographic image analysis. *Computer* 8:55–64, 1975.
13. Heintzen PH: Erfahrungen mit der quantitativen Analyse von Video-angiokardio-grammen. *Biomed Technik* 22:75–77, 1977.
14. Lange P, Onnasch D, Moldenhauer K, Malerczyk V. Farr EL, Hüttig G, Heintzen PH: The analysis of size, shape and contraction pattern of the right ventricle from angiocardiograms. *Eur J Cardiol* 4 (suppl): 153–164, 1976.

## 5.3. THE CLINICAL USEFULNESS OF NONINVASIVE AND INVASIVE TOOLS IN THE ASSESSMENT OF LEFT VENTRICULAR FUNCTION IN MYOCARDIAL INFARCTION

Paul G. Hugenholtz, Clifford V. Nelson

### 1. INTRODUCTION

First and foremost, as with all techniques in medicine, the assessment of the clinical value of any measurement, must be judged by four essential factors: the *sensitivity* of the method, its *specificity*, its *utility* and ultimately always its *cost*. I define here sensitivity as the chance of diagnosing correctly the disease when it is present, specificity as the chance of not diagnosing the disease when it is not there, utility as the ease with which a tool can be used under everyday "battlefield" conditions (and not therefore the utility in an isolated laboratory setting or in a research environment) and finally the cost, that is, the total expense needed for the purchase and maintenance of apparatus as well as the manpower and time needed for the performance of that test as well as its interpretation.

In coronary artery disease we have to put the central issue into perspective: as with the evolution of any branch of science, cardiac diagnostics too, has had to yield to the time-tested process which converts information to knowledge and hopefully knowledge to wisdom. Involved are familiar and accepted phases: posing the fundamental issue, conducting the initial experiments, preparing the reports, receiving review and criticism from peers, and finally, after some considerable delay, sometimes achieving acceptance of the new method or knowledge. As each new contribution passes into the literature it diffuses into general awareness and then may undergo further evaluation in a number of ways or even be lost, seemingly forever. Eventually, all of this will become the material for resynthesis along with all other, perhaps, newer knowledge. And then eventually, with even more time, some, or all of this may become doctrine and rest between the covers of some authoritative text to become standard practice.

You all have experienced this. The method is slow and tedious, but it is so for good reasons and cannot be replaced by any other. There are limits to its acceleration and one approaches cautiously any perturbation of the dynamics of a system that seems almost to derive from natural law. Yet, one hears continuously arguments today, as in the past, for modifying the traditional ways of handling information or thinking. The demand is rising for, if you wish, improved wisdom, or better-quality wisdom, served with

J. Baan, A.C. Arntzenius, E.L. Yellin (eds.), Cardiac Dynamics, 339–353.

shorter delays, particularly when the matter or question has important social dimensions. The latter is certainly the case when we talk about diagnosis in coronary artery disease. This demand is not only created by physicians and patients but also by others sometimes not even related to the field, yet who seem to have the most authoritative opinion of health technology. So, in a way, we are all more or less against our will getting involved in "technology management." And it is against this background that this presentation will advocate looking once more at an old and trusted signal, which was the first used in heart disease, the electrocardiogram. Why do I return to the electrical information? Because the heart provides it cheaply and continuously and we can obtain it by noninvasive means, and because I think it contains information also on the hemodynamic status of the heart, information which has thus far escaped the attention of most of us.

There are two different new avenues of using the electromotive information of the heart. The first is the prediction of left heart filling pressure and its sequential change in acute myocardial infarction from the terminal force of the P-wave. The second one is the influence of intracardiac blood on QRS, a topic we will deal with later.

Earlier clinical investigations have suggested that acute changes in the P-wave configuration give information of acutely developing left ventricular (LV) dysfunction in acute myocardial infarction (1). Therefore the reliability of this electrocardiographic indicator of left atrial overloading was examined for its ability to predict one major hemodynamic factor, the left heart filling pressure, by the correlation of serial changes of the P-wave with pressures simultaneously measured through a catheter in the pulmonary capillary wedge position. Severity of acute infarction was also assessed clinically, by auscultatory evidence for left ventricular failure, by the degree of pulmonary vascular congestion and heart size on the chest film, and by pulmonary arterial oxygen saturation measured intermittently. These parameters were likewise related to serially measured filling pressures.

## 2. TERMINAL FORCE OF THE P-WAVE

### 2.1. *Patients and methods*

The study comprised 40 acutely ill patients admitted to the coronary care unit of the University Hospital, Rotterdam. Thirty-six of them had acute ischaemic heart disease; 29 of these had acute myocardial infarction, and 7 prolonged angina pectoris. Four patients with, respectively, aortic stenosis, tight mitral stenosis complicated by acute pulmonary oedema, complete heart block, and noncardiac chest pains, were also included. There were 5 women and 35 men. The mean age was 57.2 years, with a range of 28 to 78 years.

In every patient a Swan-Ganz 5F flow-directed double-lumen balloon catheter was inserted on admission to the coronary care unit. The catheter was floated rapidly, without significant arrhythmias, into a peripheral branch of the pulmonary artery so that the pulmonary capillary wedge pressure could be measured whenever the balloon was reinflated (3). The pulmonary capillar wedge mean pressure from beats over several respiratory cycles was averaged. Serial pressure measurements were done every 1 to 2 hours in each patient. An average of 4 comparisons with simultaneous electrocardiograms were analysed per patient. The zero reference level was taken to be 5 cm below the sternal angle. A Statham 23dB pressure transducer, and a Philips or Hewlett-Packard preamplifier and ink-jet recorder were employed for these measurements and recordings. In this study pulmonary capillary wedge pressure was considered to be equivalent to the left heart filling pressure.

### 3. RELATION OF P TERMINAL FORCE TO LEFT HEART FILLING PRESSURE

Pulmonary capillary wedge and/or pulmonary arterial diastolic pressure were available in 77 instances from 27 patients in whom left ventricular dysfunction developed acutely (2). Comparison of mean pulmonary capillary wedge and P terminal force in this group had a correlation coefficient of $r = -0.82$, $P < 0.001$. The regression equation was: PCW $= 3.7 - 191$ PTF (mm sec) $\pm 4.0$ ($Sy$, $x$) mmHg. The electrocardiogram was always abnormal, i.e. P terminal force less than $-0.03$ mm sec, if pulmonary capillary wedge exceeded 12 mmHg. If it was below 10 mmHg, P terminal force remained either normal or occasionally was borderline abnormal, i.e. between $-0.03$ mm sec and $-0.04$ mm sec.

Five patients had long-standing hypertension and/or chronic heart failure and were admitted due to acute worsening of their clinical state. These 5 patients often had abnormal P terminal force despite normal filling pressure ($r = -0.63$; $P < 0.01$); the regression line was steeper than when left ventricular dysfunction developed acutely. Serial changes generally revealed a decrease in left ventricular filling pressure during treatment. In 46 comparisons the sequential pressure changes were associated with parallel changes in P terminal force. Discordant changes were only minor and were observed in 10 of 13 instances within the normal range for both these variables (Figure 1). In the 3 remaining observations the range of the pulmonary capillary wedge changes was only 3 mmHg or less. It was striking to observe that P terminal force paralleled acute variations in pulmonary capillary wedge over a wide range rapidly: this frequently occurred within a period of just a few hours. Compared to other bedside findings of left ventricular dysfunction, such as the onset or disappearance of pulmonary rales, the presence of atrial or ventricular gallop sounds, or the

RELATIONSHIP BETWEEN P TERMINAL FORCE AND PULMONARY ARTERY MEAN PRESSURE

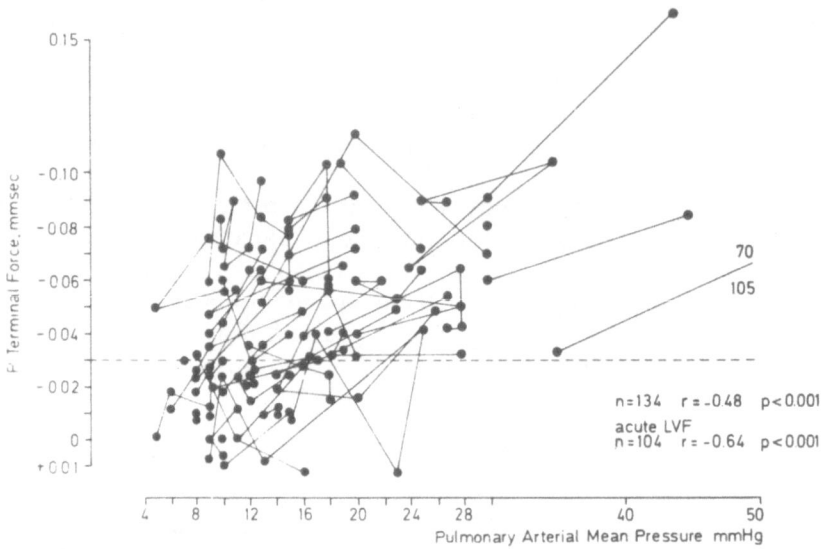

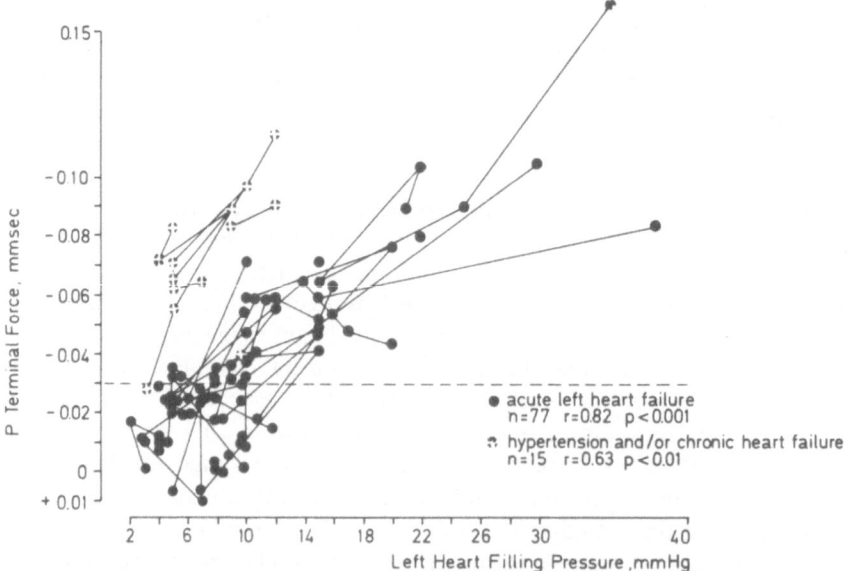

*Figure 1.* Variations in pulmonary capillary wedge pressure are predictable by electrocardiographic left atrial overload, particularly with high ranges of pulmonary capillary wedge pressure, within a few hours. (2)

radiological changes of pulmonary oedema, P terminal force demonstrated changes in LV filling pressure much more rapidly and accurately than did any other recorded variables.

The results appear to provide the clinician with an external noninvasive method as a useful tool for the sequential assessment of the hemodynamic state of the left ventricle. In acute myocardial infarction sequential changes in the LV filling pressure may occur over a wide range within a few minutes or hours. These changes in preload reflect rapid alterations in left ventricular contractile performance (4). Thus acute variations in the P-wave recorded from a standard precordial lead appear to relate quantitatively to the severity of acute changes in the state of cardiac function. Recent experimental evidence that acute changes in the electrical resistivity of left atrial blood are related to changes in peak spatial magnitude of the P-wave ($r = 0.89$; $P < 0.01$; Figure 2) and the fact that changes in the resistivity of ventricular blood have similar effects on the QRS spatial vector (5) have suggested that altered blood resistivity or its closely related causative factor, altered hematocrit, might be a pathophysiological mechanism for the observed alterations in P terminal force. Since the spread of atrial activation is largely tangential, increased hematocrit would tend to increase these tangential forces and thus P terminal force. The theoretical possibility that there are such sudden changes in hematocrit as a result of sequestration of the circulating body fluids in various compartments, e.g. pulmonary oe-

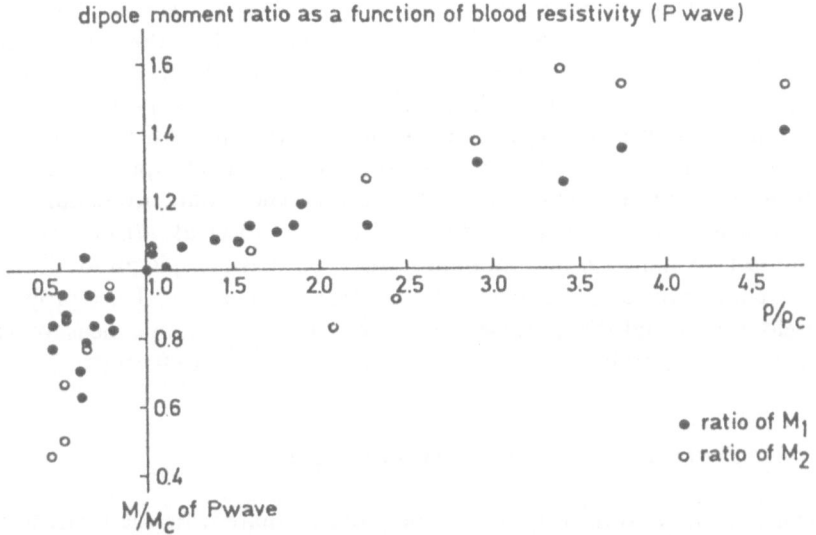

*Figure 2.* Relation between dipole moment $M/M_c$ of P-wave and blood resistivity ($\rho$), inside left atrium of dogs. As resistivity is augmented, P increases and vice versa. (2)

dema, warrants further investigation. Earlier observations on LV failure and on the influence of acute papillary muscle dysfunction in acute myocardial infarction, lend support to another explanation, that sudden increases and decreases in left atrial volume could be a relevant mechanism. Sudden increases in left atrial wall stretch by pressure rise could cause delayed activation and hence altered cancellation. This would tend to augment the influence of the left atrial vectors. However, a plot of the duration (0.04 to 0.08 sec) against the amplitude of the terminal deflection of the P-wave in $V_1$, i.e. the two components of P terminal force, failed to indicate that an increased duration (and hence decreased cancellation by right atrial depolarization) was the cause of the augmentation of P terminal force. Finally, the observation that the changes occur within hours clinically, and instantaneously in an experimental study, appears to exclude atrial muscle hypertrophy as a mechanism. Left ventricular dysfunction occurs in every patient with transmural acute myocardial infarction. The extent of this dysfunction is chiefly governed by the amount of muscle fibres destroyed, the degree of asynergy of ventricular contraction, the change in cardiac compliance, and the added burden of mitral regurgitation caused by papillary muscle dysfunction (6). All these acute changes contribute to the rise of LV filling pressure, and thus of left atrial pressure and may eventually lead to pulmonary congestion. As preload, reflected by pulmonary capillary wedge, is one of the most important determinants of the myocardial performance, frequent determination of LV filling pressure has great clinical importance in the evaluation of the adequacy of pump function in acute myocardial infarction. Since directly assessed LV filling pressure when the left ventricle is acutely damaged is the only correct determinant of left ventricular preload presently available at the bedside, the present electrocardiographic method is advocated as a possible adjunct or as an early-warning system in acutely ill patients where pulmonary pressure monitoring is not available. Its only drawback appears to be in patients with pre-existing atrial hypertrophy. These data from our laboratory have recently been confirmed by Kanemoto et al. (7) in Japan. In addition to confirming our data, they proposed that the magnitude PTF-$V_1$ was significantly correlated with Peel's prognostic index. They proposed therefore to extend the usefulness of this electrocardiographic measurement to prognosis in addition to the assessment of treatment efficacy.

4. INFLUENCE OF INTRACARDIAC BLOOD ON QRS

The next series of observations we would like to share with you relate to the influence of the intracardiac blood on the QRS complex of the electrocardiogram. The Brody effect (8) states that the presence of intracardiac blood strengthens the radial and weakens the tangential dipoles during depolarization. So, together with Nelson and Angelakos we have in the past looked into the relationships between the intracardiac blood mass and the surface electrocardiogram in animals (9). Both from the data obtained in dogs, which we will not discuss here, and from those obtained in monkeys, the suggestion is very strong that a relationship exists between the intra- cardiac blood mass and the appearance of the surface electrocardiogram. Particularly, now that recently attention has been refocused away from the continuous measurement of the ST segment or from precordial ST-segment mapping since it has been shown not to be a reliable measurement of infarct size, proposals have been made to measure the R-wave voltage, including the qR ratios, in the assessment of infarct size during various methods and medication schemes proposed in the treatment of evolving acute myocardial infarction. This could lead to considerable *mis*information.

In the earlier part of these studies it was shown that intracardiac blood had a significant effect on spatial dipole moment of the dog heart. When blood hematocrit was raised by exchange transfusion of packed cells for normal blood, the early parts of the spatial QRS-curves were reduced in magnitude while later portions of that same complex were increased. When hematocrit was reduced by transfusion of plasma opposite effects were observed. These findings are in keeping with the Brody effect. In the current observations we extended our studies to the rhesus monkey since the latter animal in many respects resembles the human species, particularly in terms of its torso configuration. The aim of the study therefore was to analyse to what extent changes in the intracardiac blood would influence the surface electrocardiogram.

Given the varying resistivities from the tissues between the centre of the heart and the surface of the chest, diverging results on the surface electro- cardiogram can be expected. In these studies all factors were considered to remain constant and the only two parameters that were changed were the end-diastolic volume and the hematocrit. If the Brody effect were to be physiologically active, the effects would be as illustrated in Table 1. In other words the apparent strength of the dipole moment on the surface of the chest is strongly altered by the intracardiac blood mass. Since the sequence

*Table 1.* Horizontal cross-section of a thorax model.

|                          | $\rho$(ohm/cm)            |
|--------------------------|---------------------------|
| Blood resistivity        | 160                       |
| Cardiac muscle           | 450                       |
| Pericardium              | 420                       |
| Lung                     | 2000                      |
| Rib, skin, outside world | $400 - 2.6 \times 10^{12}$ |

of depolarization shown for the animal as well as the human heart is, as shown by many workers, initially *radially* directed, that is from inside outwards, say up to the first one-third of the QRS-complex and tangentially directed, i.e. tangential to the heart wall, in the mid and later portions of the QRS-complex, the effects of the intracardiac blood should be opposite in these two periods of the total QRS-time.

## 5. METHODS

The measurements of the electromotive forces were made by the Nelson lead system of which the details are published elsewhere (5). It probably is the most ideal lead system to measure total electromotive force since it is adjustable for thorax shape and for thorax dimensions, and has been shown in other studies to provide great accuracy with a nearly linear relationship

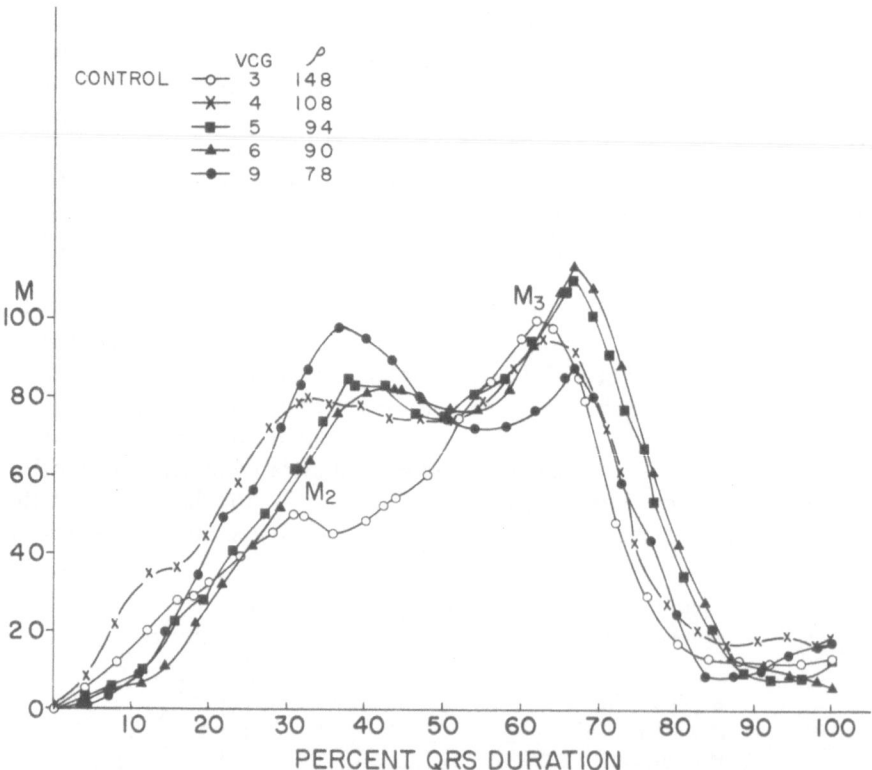

*Figure 3.* Curve of *M* for one monkey in whom blood resistivity was brought down from 148 to 78 ohm cm by exchange transfusions with rheomacrodex. (9)

between heart weight, expressed as a function of bodyweight and dipole moment, for various species ranging from the frog to the horse.

When one alters the hematocrit (Hct), and with it resistivity ($\rho$) and measures the spatial magnitude ($M$) and its peaks ($M_1$, $M_2$, $M_3$) at different successive time-points, with the spatial directions at those times – cephalad-caudad and posterior-anterior plotted against percent of total QRS time (PQD) – then variations in $\rho$ from 148 (in the normal) to 78 ohm cm (in anaemia) will result in the changes depicted in Figure 3, 4, and 5. A drastic change in the ECG indeed! In order to understand the rapidity with which such changes occur we will describe a typical experiment.

In this experiment, lasting six hours, there were first three exchanges of packed cells for whole blood, 130 cm³ in total; 40 cm³ of blood that had been withdrawn were then added. After this there were five exchanges of dextran 6% in saline, 290 cm³ in total. It was then tried to raise the hematocrit again by exchanges with concentrated blood. The results are shown in Figure 6. During the first packed cell exchanges up to 200 minutes, hematocrit increased from 42 to 55 (31%) and $\rho$ from 151 to 196 ohm cm (30%). During this period $M_2$ decreased by 10% and $M_3$ increased by 12%. The ratio $M_2/M_3$ fell by 21%. As SV and CO fell, heart rate

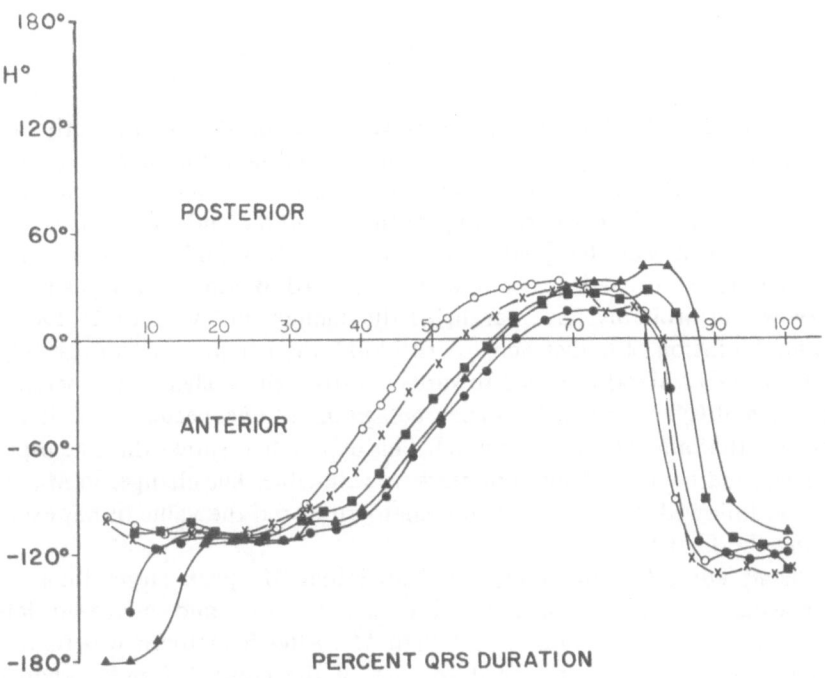

*Figure 4.* As Figure 3. Curve of $H^0$. (9)

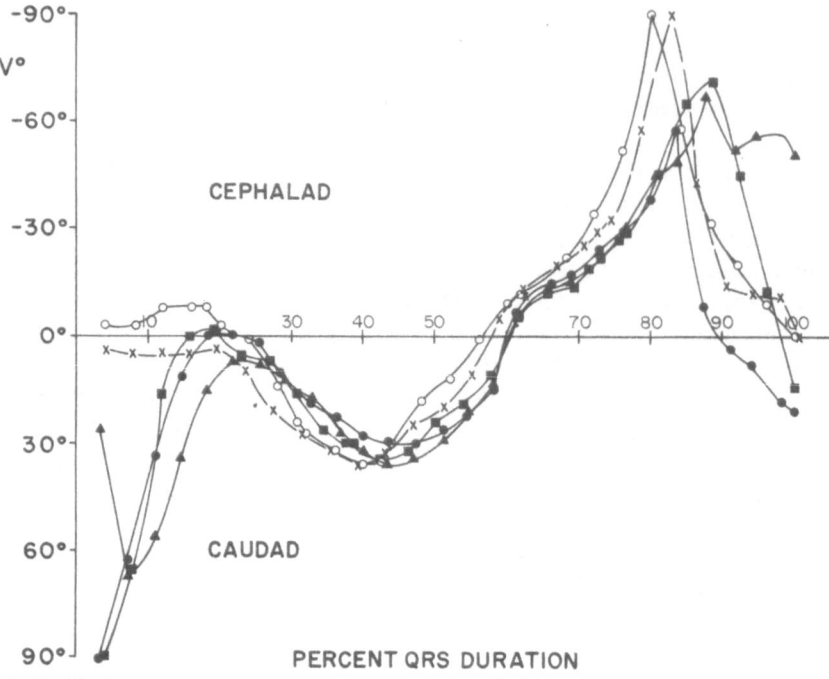

*Figure 5.* As Figure 3. Curve of $V^0$. (9)

increased. After the dextran exchanges were started, $M_2$ rose abruptly until 250 minutes in the experiment, whereas $M_3$ fell continuously by a fairly large amount (155 to 105 k mA/cm or 32%). $M_2/M_3$ increased markedly from 0.85 to 1.38. Hematocrit and $\rho$ both fell and SV and CO increased. As the experiment was designed to last over 4 hours and in order not to damage the left ventricle, EDV was not measured. Based on previous results EDV would probably have paralleled the changes in SV and CO. During the final infusion of higher hematocrit blood, the hematocrit and resistivity of the animal's blood returned towards control values. Heart rate increased and SV and CO both fell. $M_3$ increased again, but unexpectedly, so did $M_2$. Even so, the ratio $M_2/M_3$ decreased. This experiment shows that the dipole moment and hemodynamic changes were reversible. The changes in $M_3$ and $M_2/M_3$ followed the variations in hematocrit as did the value of $M_2$ except during the final portion.

The $M$ curve for this animal had an initial $M_2$ peak larger than $M_3$. Increasing the hematocrit reduced earlier voltages and increased later voltages so that $M_3$ became larger than $M_2$. After hematocrit was reduced again, the wave shape returned to that of the control. Similar changes occurred in the $M_z$ curve with $Q_z$ decreasing and $R_z$ increasing as hematoc-

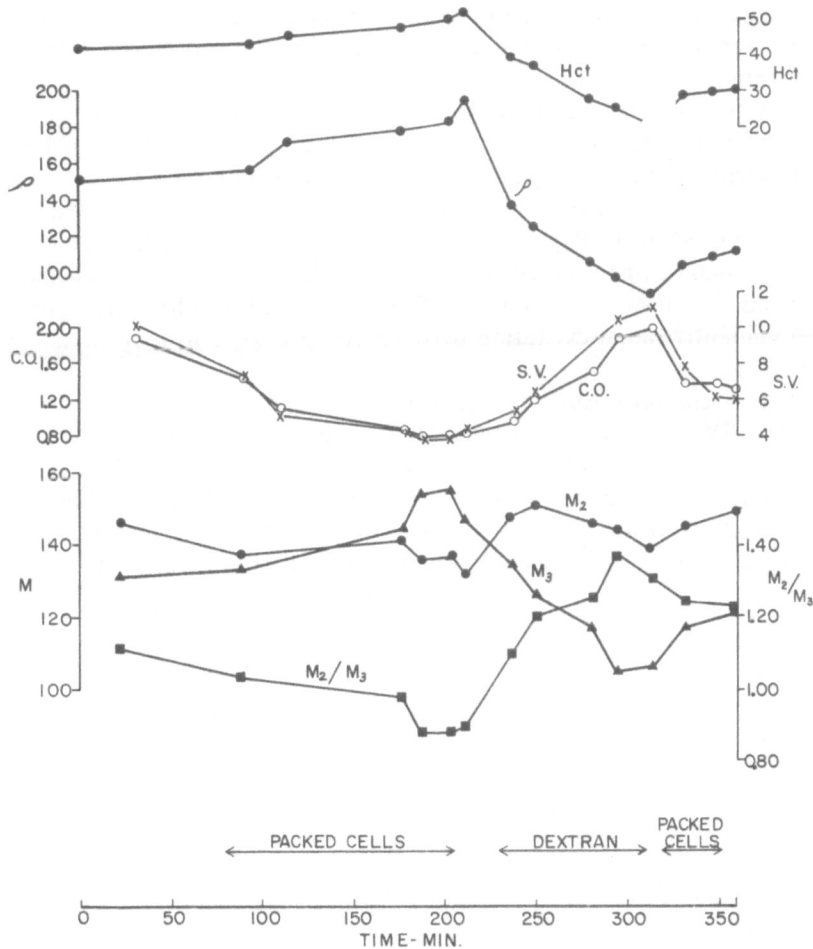

*Figure 6.* Time record of reversal experiment in one monkey. Blood resistivity was first increased by two exchanges with packed cells, then lowered again by exchanges with dextran. An attempt was then made to increase hematocrit again using packed cells.

rit was raised, reverting to near control values when hematocrit was reduced again. Increasing hematocrit, therefore, had the effect of making the absolute peak of $M$ occur later in time. The correlation coefficient between PQD of peak $M$ and $\rho$ was $r = 0.91$, $P < .001$. High correlation coefficients were found between the magnitude of $M_3$ and $\rho$ ($r = 0.96$, $P < .001$) and between $M_2/M_3$ and $\rho$ ($r = -0.98$, $P < .001$). For $M_2$ there was a good correlation ($r = -0.91$) for vectors 1–10 but after that, $M_2$ declined instead of increasing as $\rho$ decreased. At the time of vector 11, the experiment had been in progress for four hours and 40 minutes, so it is possible that the heart had begun to fail. The correlation between $M_2/M_3$ and $\rho$ remained high over the entire range and appears to be the most significant observation.

Since the influence of alterations in blood resistivity relates to successive vectors of the QRS complex, correlation coefficients and lines of best fit were calculated for each five percent of QRS duration. For 10 to 55 PQD, the slopes were negative, i.e. increasing $\rho$ gave smaller $M$ values. Maximum slope occurred at 35 PQD. From 60 to 90 PQD, the slopes were positive and maximum slope occurred at 70 to 75 PQD. Best correlation coefficients occurred at 30–40, 50, and 65–75 PQD. These results correspond to predominantly radial excitation between 10–55 PQD and tangential spread thereafter.

The correlation coefficient between CO and Hct was $r=0.75$, $P=.003$. CO and SV varied inversely with Hct because of blood viscosity changes. The correlation between blood $\rho$ and Hct was again very high ($r=-0.99$, $P<.001$). An inverse type of experiment, where $\rho$ was increased by hemoconcentration from 135 to 217, is shown in Figure 5. Again there was a dramatic change in $M_2$ inverse to that of $M_3$. In several experiments of this

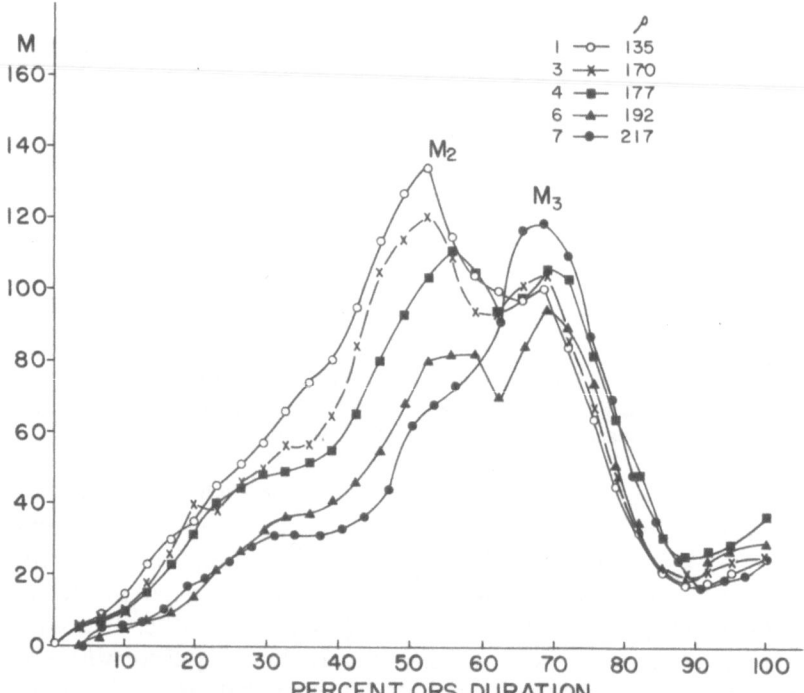

*Figure 7.* Typical experiment showing changes in $M_2$ and $M_3$ while hematocrit (not shown) and resistivity ($\rho$) is increased from 135 to 217 ohm/cm.

type, large drops in EDV were accompanied by a fall in $M_2$ and an increase in $M_3$. As $\rho$ remained fairly constant, this observation strongly supports the thesis that changes in $M_2$ were caused by the drop in EDV while the reverse also applied (Figure 8).

Correlation coefficients were also calculated for $\rho/\rho_{c'}$ $M_2/M_{2c}$, $M_3/M_{3c}$, and $M_2/M_3$ with EDV/EDV$_c$. For the individual monkeys, most correlation coefficients had $P$ values $\leq 0.10$. For one monkey the correlation between $M_2/M_{2c}$ with EDV/EDV$_c$ was 0.96, $P = 0.04$, but there were only four values. Combining data of the 19 measurements in monkeys 2, 5, 10 and 11, correlations of EDV/EDV$_c$ with $\rho/\rho_c$ were $r = -0.80$, $P < .001$ and

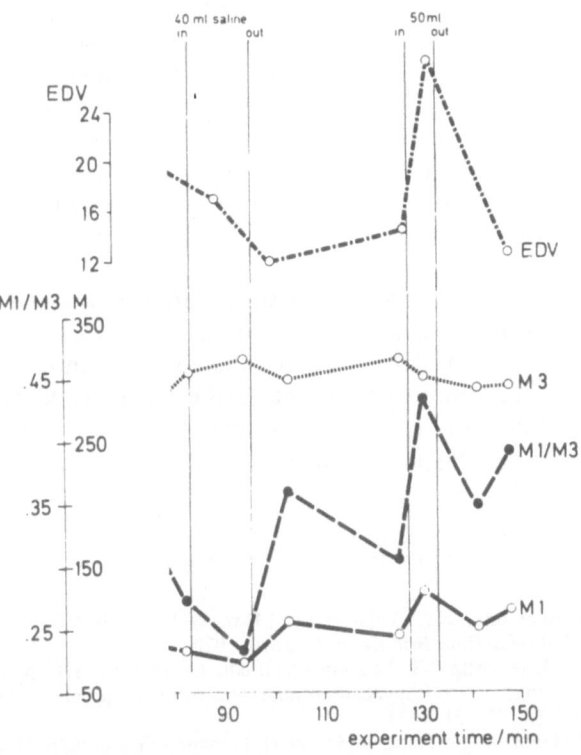

RELATIONSHIP OF DIPOLE MOMENT AND HEMODYNAMIC FACTORS
DURING ACUTE VOLUME CHANGES

*Figure 8.* Part of an acute experiment in which $M_1$ and $M_3$ were measured in close approximation to EDV. During rapid suction of 40 ml blood from the LA 95 minutes after onset of the experiment EDV dropped to 12 ml just before the ratio $M_1/M_3$ was 0.24. At 130 minutes with rapid infusion of 50 ml of saline, EDV rose to 28 ml and the ratio $M_1/M_3$ to 0.44, clearly showing the profound influence of diastolic blood volume on the ratio $M_1/M_3$. Since there were simultaneous changes in resistivity the ratio $M_1/M_3$ does not return to control values after each intervention.

with $M_3/M_{3c}$, $r = -0.77$, $P < .001$. There was no overall correlation between $M_2/M_{2c}$ and EDV/EDV$_c$ although it did exist in individual animals. Since for all monkeys taken as a group, the only electrical variable that correlated consistently with both $\rho/\rho_c$ and EDV/EDV$_c$ was $M_3/M_{3c}$, that regression equation was calculated: $M_3/M_{3c} = 1.31 - 0.33$ EDV/EDV$_c$.

Evidence to support this has appeared in humans. Rosenthal et al. (10) showed in some young humans that the left maximal spatial vector (LMSV) was smaller than RMSV. After erythrophoresis, LMSV increased and RMSV decreased so that LMSV became the larger vector. These peaks corresponded to our $M_2$ and $M_3$ peaks. In these patients with hypertrophy the results are consistent with the Brody theory. It appears that a given change in blood resistivity has a greater effect in the monkey than the dog and the potential influence of the intracardiac blood mass is such that it at least doubles the real value of $M_2$ and reduces $M_3$ by about one-third.

In conclusion, the data indicate that the magnitudes of cardiac dipole moments and surface potentials are profoundly influenced by the presence of intracardiac blood. As in the dog, voltages due to radial excitation during the early parts of the QRS complex of the monkey are enhanced while later forces, spreading predominantly in a tangential manner, are attenuated. Alterations in intracardiac blood volume and resistivity may explain the electrocardiographic changes observed by others during exercise (11), cardiac surgery (12), anaemia and polycythaemia (10) and may hinder measurement of infarct size. If a more accurate relationship between the measured dipole moment and the actual strength of cardiac excitation forces is desired, corrections must be made for the effects of intracardiac blood. It appears that further studies which could further elucidate their relationships in an effort to utilize the electrical information on the body surface as an indicator of the hemodynamic state of the heart are indicated.

REFERENCES

1. Heikkilä J, Luomanmäki K: Value of serial P-wave changes in indicating left heart failure in myocardial infarction. *Brit Heart J* 32:510, 1970.
2. Heikkilä J, Hugenholtz PG, Tabakin BS: Prediction of left heart filling pressure and its sequential change in acute myocardial infarction from the terminal force of the P-wave. *Brit Heart J* 35:142–151, 1973.
3. Swan HJC, Ganz W, Forrester J, Marcus H, Diamond G, Chonette D: Catheterization of the heart in man with use of a flow-directed balloon-tipped catheter. *New Engl J Med* 283:447, 1970.
4. Hood Jr WB: Pathophysiology of ischemic heart disease. *Prog Cardiovasc Diseases* 14:297, 1971.
5. Nelson CV, Rand PW, Angelakos ET, Hugenholtz PG: Effect of intracardiac blood on the spatial vectorcardiogram I: results in the dog. *Circ Res* 31:95–104, 1972.
6. Forrester JS, Diamond G, Freedman S, Allen HN, Parmley WW, Matloff J, Swan HJC: Silent mitral insufficiency in acute myocardial infarction. *Circulation* 44:877, 1971.

7. Kanemoto N, Akizuki T, Ogawa S, Oosuzo F, Nakamura Y: P-waves in acute myocardial infarction. *Jap Heart J* 17(2):172–179, 1976.
8. Brody DA: Theoretical analysis of intracavitary blood mass influence on the heart-lead relationship *Circ Res* 4:731–738, 1956.
9. Hugenholtz PG, Angelakos ET, Nelson CV; Effect of intracardiac blood on the spatial vectorcardiogram II: results in the monkey. *Circ Res* (Submitted).
10. Rosenthal A, Restieaux NJ, Feig SA: The influence of acute variations in hematocrit on the QRS complex of the Frank vectorcardiogram. *Circulation* 44:456–465, 1971.
11. Simoons ML, Hugenholtz PG: Gradual changes of ECG waveform during and after exercise in normal subjects. *Circulation* 52:570–577, 1975.
12. Nelson CV, Dowling JT, Sloman G: Changes in heart dipole moment after surgical correction of atrial septal defect. *Am Heart J* 91:766–782, 1976.

## 5.4. MODEL-BASED HEMODYNAMIC INDICATORS OF LEFT VENTRICULAR PERFORMANCE

J. Yasha Kresh, Walter Welkowitz, Byoung G. Min, Sylvan Fich, Casimir A. Kulikowski

### 1. INTRODUCTION

Quantitative evaluation of the intrinsic capability of the heart to pump blood as opposed to the actual pump output represents an important study. Thus, a need remains to determine the function of the underlying myocardium independent of the peripheral load changes and compensation which often obscure the presence of myocardial infarction in its early evolution (1, 2, 3, 4, 5, 6).

The present study was designed to explore the relationship between the extent of myocardial injury following coronary ligation and the resulting changes in left ventricular pump and myocardial muscle function. The left ventricle is mathematically modelled both as a pulsatile pump and as an integrated muscle unit. The principal objective was to determine the quantitative influence of left ventricular impairment on newly defined and analytically derived model-based pump and muscle performance indicators.

### 2. THEORETICAL ANALYSIS

In this analysis, the left ventricle is considered to be a pressure source with an internal impedance (7, 8). The computation of the equivalent source representation (Figure 1) is carried out in the frequency domain, where the equivalent source consists of the intrinsic pressure generator $P_g$ in series with an internal hydraulic impedance $Z_g$. The source parameters are computed from measurements of aortic flow and left ventricular pressure under two loading conditions: a physiological load impedance $(Z_L)$, and an externally modified load $(Z'_L)$. $Z_L$ is the lumped impedance for the aortic valve and arterial load impedance.

A quantitative assessment of left ventricular dysfunction, particularly the intrinsic pump condition following myocardial infarction, can be obtained if the effect of the afterload is eliminated. Referring to the equivalent hydraulic model (D in Figure 1) in the isovolumic condition, the load impedance $(Z_L)$ is infinite. The left ventricular pressure $(P_{lv})$ is equal to the source pressure $(P_g)$. Thus, $P_g$ represents the isovolumic equivalent pressure of the left ventricle throughout the cardiac cycle in the intact heart. In addition, the load condition $(Z_L=0)$ can be used to compute the short-circuited ventri-

J. Baan, A.C. Arntzenius, E.L. Yellin (eds.), Cardiac Dynamics, 355–368.

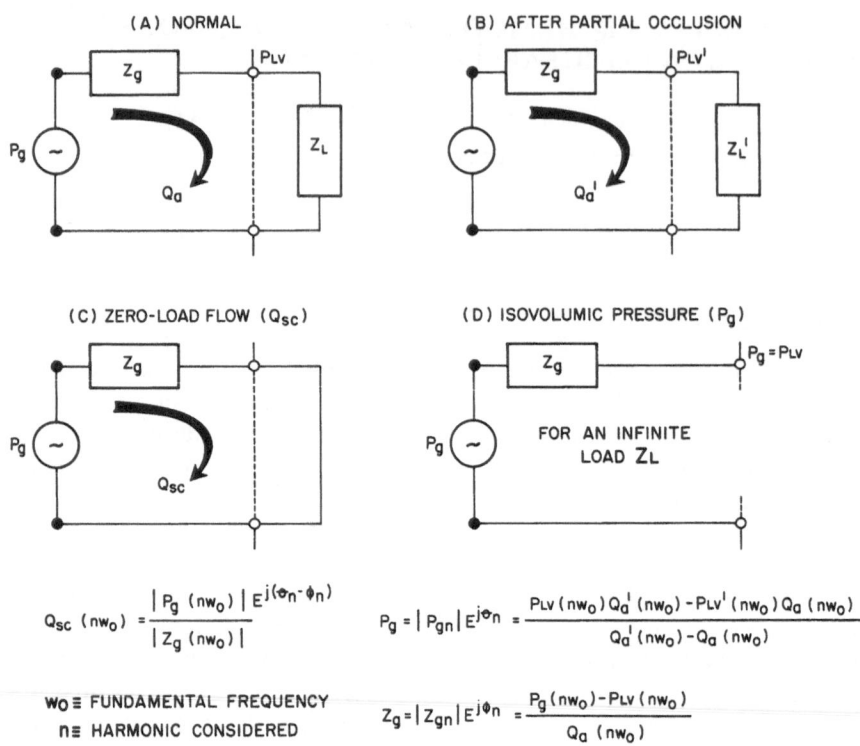

$$Q_{sc}(nw_0) = \frac{|P_g(nw_0)| E^{j(\Phi_n - \phi_n)}}{|Z_g(nw_0)|}$$

$$P_g = |P_{gn}| E^{j\Phi_n} = \frac{P_{Lv}(nw_0) Q_a'(nw_0) - P_{Lv}'(nw_0) Q_a(nw_0)}{Q_a'(nw_0) - Q_a(nw_0)}$$

$w_0 \equiv$ FUNDAMENTAL FREQUENCY

$n \equiv$ HARMONIC CONSIDERED

$$Z_g = |Z_{gn}| E^{j\Phi_n} = \frac{P_g(nw_0) - P_{Lv}(nw_0)}{Q_a(nw_0)}$$

*Figure 1.* Pressure source equivalent representation: (A) normal load impedance; (B) modified aortic impedance by partial occlusion; (C) analytically computed zero-load flow; (D) left ventricular pressure for an infinite aortic impedance.

cular flow (C in Figure 1) Zero-load flow simulates a hypothetical physiologic condition of zero aortic pressure, an idealized zero afterload.

The phasor components of the afterload independent flow are defined in Figure 1 (c) and are computed as the quotient of the source parameters, $P_g(nw_0)$ and $Z_g(nw_0)$. By definition, both the zero-load flow and the source pressure are independent of afterload changes and peripheral circulation. A steady-state instantaneous zero-load flow ($Q_{sc}(t)$) and the source pressure $P_g(t)$ can be computed by inverse Fourier series synthesis from the harmonic components.

Although the geometry of the intact heart is far more complex than that of a simple muscle fibre, myocardial muscle models have been developed, providing a working framework within which to derive indices of contractility and contractile state in terms of established cardiac muscle mechanics. For the intact left ventricle during the isovolumic portion of systole the contractile element velocity ($V_{ce}$) has been expressed as $V_{ce} = (dP_{lv}/dt)/28 \cdot P_{lv}$ where, $P_{lv}$ is the isovolumic intraventricular pressure (9).

The present investigation, having the analytical capability and means of mathematically reconstructing a complete isovolumic pressure contraction, has suggested the possibility of studying the contractile state or modified force-velocity relation of the intact heart. It was reasoned that the isovolumic index as defined could be analogously determined from the source pressure ($P_g$) and its corresponding rate of change ($dP_g/dt$). The maximum shortening velocity $(V_{ce})_{max}$ was defined and computed for the phase plane plot of $(dP/dt)/28 \cdot P$ versus $P$, linearly extrapolated to the $P = 0$ axis; where $P$ is the isovolumic intraventricular pressure (mathematically reconstructed or experimentally measured).

### 3 ANIMAL PREPARATION AND MEASUREMENT

Eight mongrel dogs weighing from 23–30 kg were anesthetized using sodium pentobarbital (25 mg/kg), intubated and artificially ventilated with room air, using a Harvard respirator (model 607). The heart rate was maintained between 150 and 180 beats/min using a Grass stimulator (SD-9). Pericardiotomy was performed and the exposed heart was cradled in the open pericardium. Ascending aortic flow was measured with a pulsed-logic Biotronex (BL-610) flowmeter. Left ventricular pressure was recorded using optimal techniques of catheter-tip transduction (frequency response is flat to 1.6 kHz, Millar). Aortic pressure was measured with an end-hole saline-filled 7-French catheter attached to a Stathan P23Db pressure transducer. Simultaneous hemodynamic recordings were made on a Gould Brush-400 recorder and a Hewlett-Packard (HP 3960) FM4 channel magnetic tape recorder.

For the determination of source parameters, two distinct peripheral loading states were required. The aortic load impedance was modified by partial occlusion of the descending aorta. A saline-filled vascular occluder (In-vivo Metric System, OC-20) was used to produce an instantaneous change in input impedance (changing aortic input resistance by 20% or more). The partial occlusion was maintained for two beats only, to avoid neural control effects.

Sequential ligation of the proximal and distal diagonal branches of the left anterior descending coronary artery (LAD) was performed to produce a progressively more severe myocardial infarction. The infarct area was localized at the anterolateral surface. Topographic left ventricular epicardial electrograms were obtained from 12 sites in the distribution of the LAD to delineate the ischaemic area. The average ST-segment elevation-quotient of the sum of elevation and the total number ($n$) of exploring sites ($\Sigma \, ST/n$) was used as an overall index of the extent of ischaemic injury (10).

The pressure and flow data were digitized (DEC-LPS-11 A/D converter) at a sampling rate of 250 samples/sec. Data reduction (Fourier transforms, frequency domain analysis) and model representation were carried out on a DEC PDP-10 computer (Figure 2).

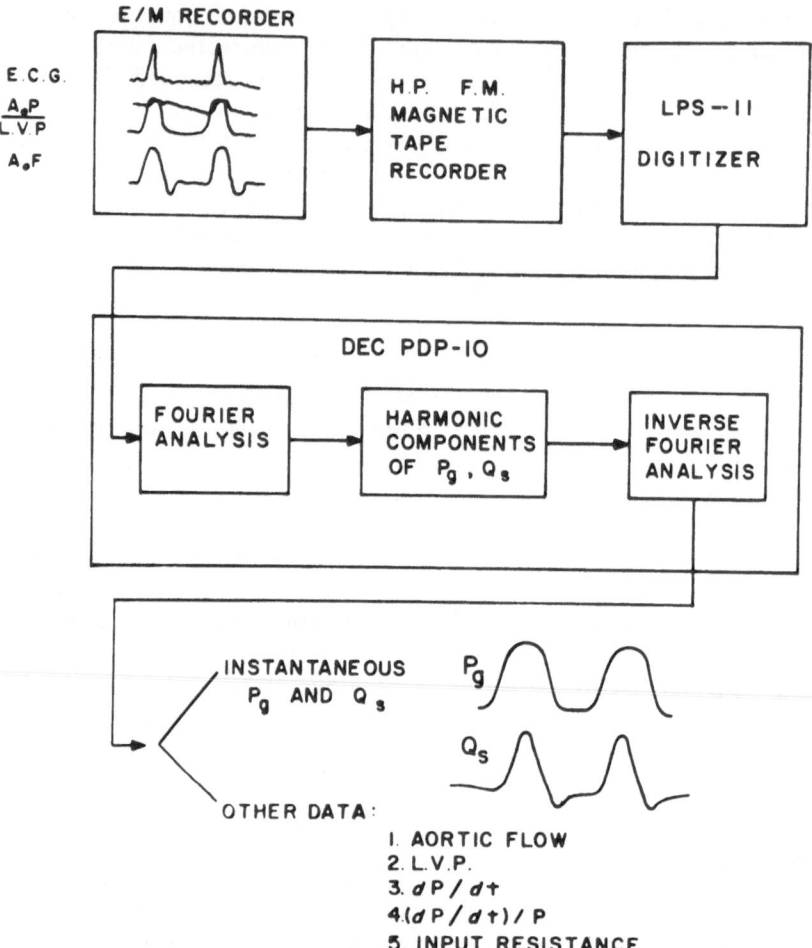

*Figure 2.* Hemodynamic data recording and computer analysis system. LVP is the left ventricular pressure: AoP is aortic pressure; AoF is the aortic blood flow.


4. RESULTS

Figure 3 summarizes 46 sets of results in 8 dogs. Included in the figure are measured and derived hemodynamic parameters, in addition to the analytically computed indices of ventricular function. Group 1 (G-1) combines all controls (pre-ligation); group 2 (G-2) combines all measurements after ligation of the proximal diagonal branch of LAD; and group 3 (G-3) includes measurements with one or two additional LAD branch ligations. Approximately one hour elapsed between G-2 and G-3 measurements.

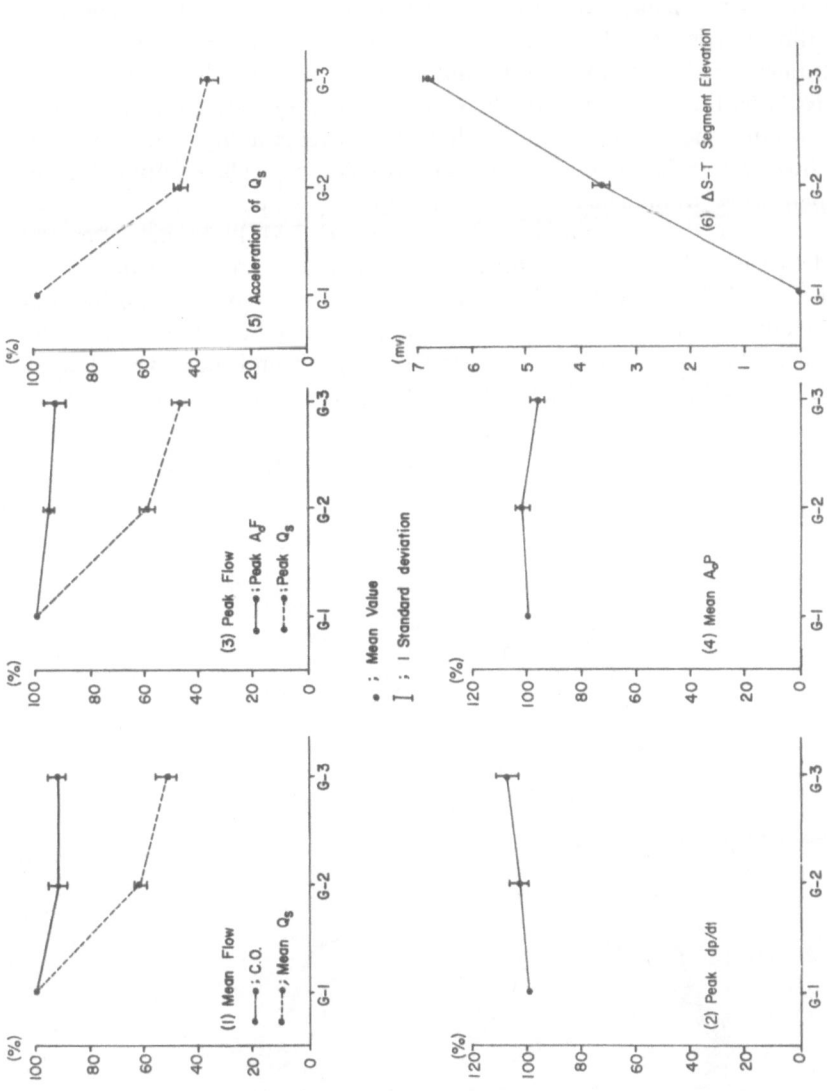

*Figure 3.* Summary of results in eight animals. Changes in hemodynamic parameters (solid lines), zero-load flow (broken line), and ST-segment elevation in three groups. Control is considered 100% level (G-1: control, G-2: measurement after single branch of LAD ligation, G-3: measurement after multiple ligations).

Statistical significance of the difference among the three groups was calculated by a paired *t*-test.

A typical instantaneous computed zero-load flow during the time course of a representative experimental procedure is shown in Figure 4. Figure 5 shows the peak, mean, and rate of change of zero-load flow. The corresponding aortic peak flow and cardiac output are included for the same time frames. Peak zero-load flow diminished from a pre-ligation value of 21.37 to 11.69 litres/min after the first ligation. It diminished further to 6.23 litre/min after the second ligation while the corresponding values of peak aortic flow were 5.9, 6.0 and 5.4 litres/min respectively. The computed mean zero-load flow diminished from a pre-ligation value of 11.56 to 4.98 litres/min after the first ligation, descending to 2.31 litres/min after the second ligation. The corresponding cardiac output measured values were 1.80, 1.83, and 1.74 litres/min for control, first ligation and second ligation respectively. The rate of change of ejection of zero-load flow reflects the directional changes observed in the respective peak and mean values (2.86 to 1.58 to 0.54 litres/sec$^2$). Figure 6 shows the time course of the extrapo-

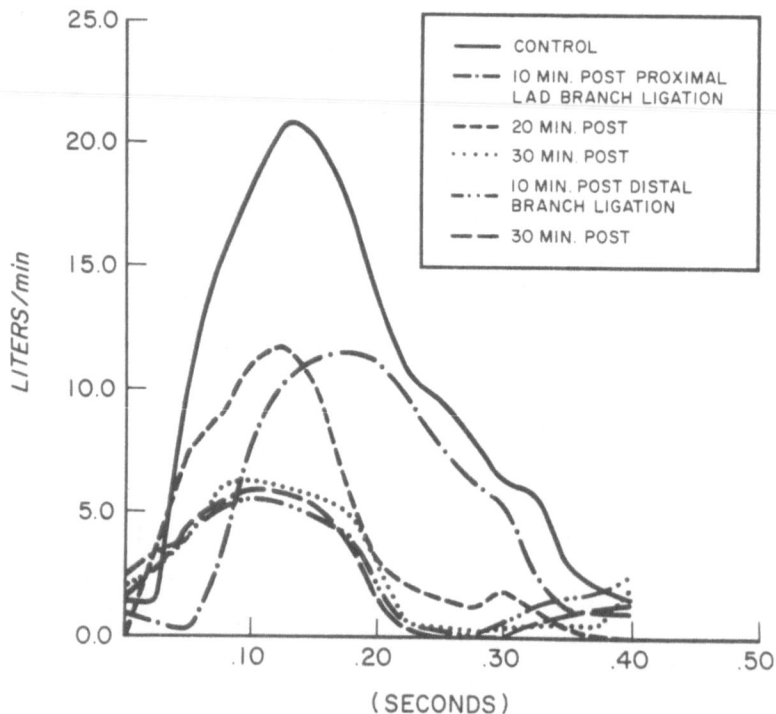

*Figure 4.* Instantaneous computed zero-load flow during sequential ligation of diagonal branches of left anterior descending coronary artery (LAD).

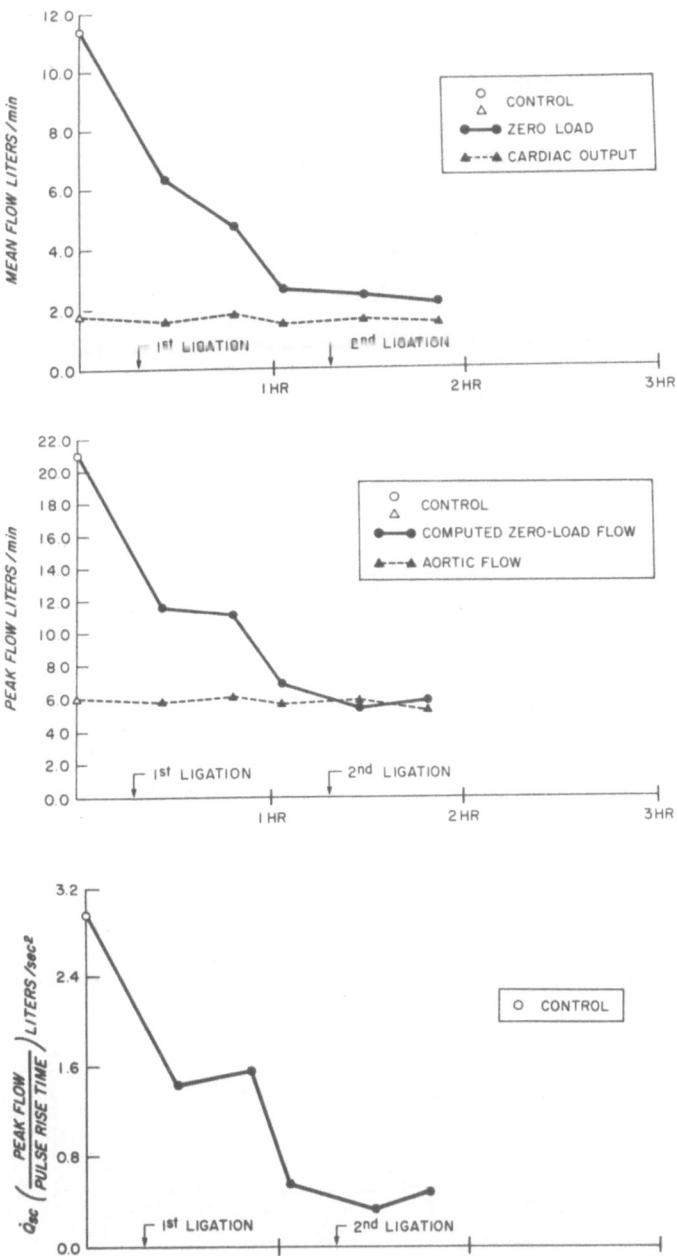

*Figure 5.* Mean, peak, and rate of change of computed zero-load flow during sequential coronary artery branch ligation (solid lines); accompanied by corresponding measured cardiac output and peak aortic flow (dashed lines).

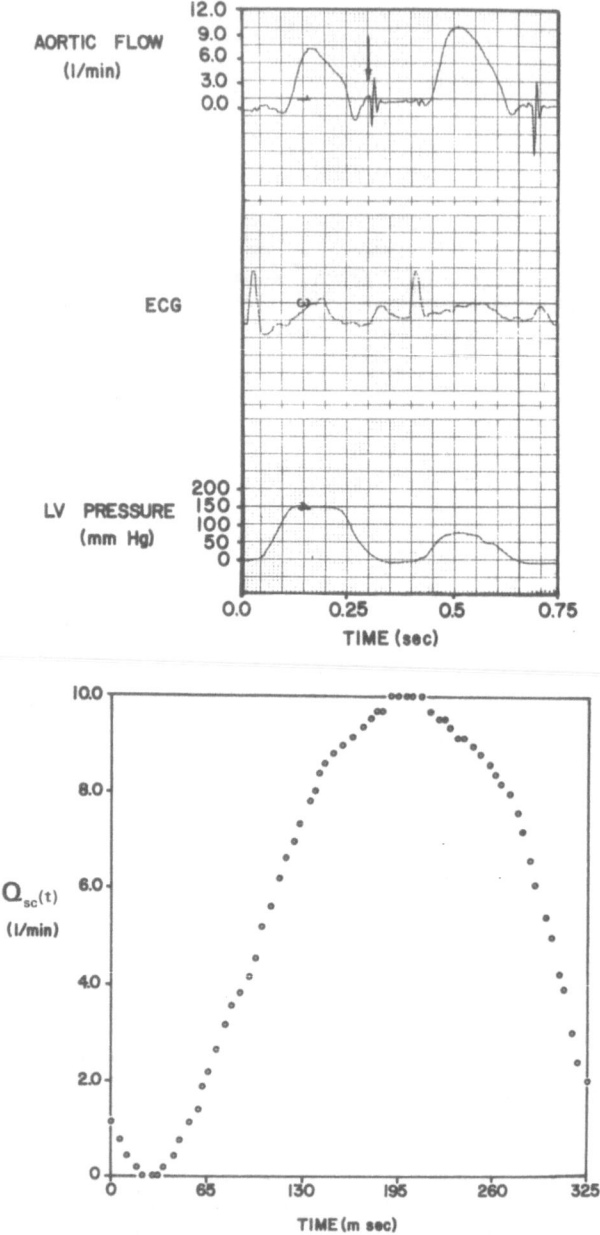

*Figure* 6. *Top:* isovolumic pressure-derived contractility index $V_{max}$ ($P_g$) and $V_{max}(P_{lv})$ for sequential coronary artery branch ligation; *bottom:* summary of results in eight animals; changes in $V_{max}$ ($P_g$) and $V_{max}$ ($P_{lv}$): G-1: control, G-2: measurement after single branch of LAD ligation, G-3: measurement after multiple ligation).

lated isovolumic index based upon normal intraventricular pressure, $V_{max}(P_{lv})$, and the analytically computed isovolumic beat, $V_{max}(P_g)$. Included in Figure 6 are also the results summarized for 8 dogs. A considerable deterioration of the performance parameters is shown, while $V_{max}(P_{lv})$ displays insensitivity to the impaired condition.

## 5. EXPERIMENTAL VERIFICATION OF SOURCE PARAMETERS

Experimentally, the actual zero-load flow can be measured at the first beat after transection of the aorta, during the diastolic phase (Figure 7). The waveform shape and peak amplitude of the computed zero-load flow agreed well with the experimentally measured zero-load aortic flow. In one experiment (a dog with moderate myocardial infarction), the measured value of peak flow was 9.85 litres/min and the peak value of the analytically predicted zero-load flow, $Q_{sc}(t)$ was 10.03 litres/min (Figure 7).

The instantaneous pulsatile source pressure can be measured by presenting an infinite load to the ejecting left ventricle, by cross-clamping the aorta (Figure 8), prior to ejection. The first post cross-clamping intraventricular pressure shown in Figure 8 is in reasonable agreement when compared (superimposed) with the analytically computed source pressure $P_g(t)$. The agreement between computed and measured source parameters is encouraging as it further supports the validity of the equivalent mathematical representation in modelling left ventricular pump function.

## 6. DISCUSSION

The most prominent feature that can be noted from both the sequential experimental measurements and the cumulative results of all the experiments (Figure 3, Table 1) is the difference in the changes in parameters and overall system performance that were observed between results for the normal and the impaired left ventricle. Furthermore, it can be seen from Table 1 that the set of standard hemodynamic indicators when compared to the model-based performance indicators show only small changes in cardiac output, peak aortic flow, mean left ventricular pressure, aortic pressure, peak $dP_{lv}/dt$ and extrapolated $(dP_{lv}/dt)\ 28 \cdot P_{lv}$ for the pre- and post-ligation conditions. The conventional hemodynamic performance parameters give little information concerning the effectiveness of the left ventricle as a pulsating pump or equivalent muscle unit independent of the peripheral vascular system.

A statistically significant diminution in peak zero-load flow, forward blood acceleration, mean zero-load flow and extrapolated isovolumic index

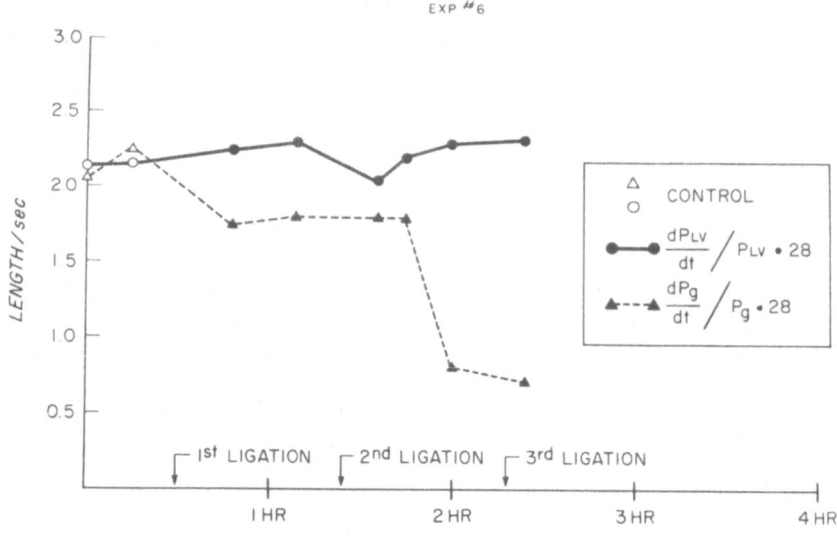

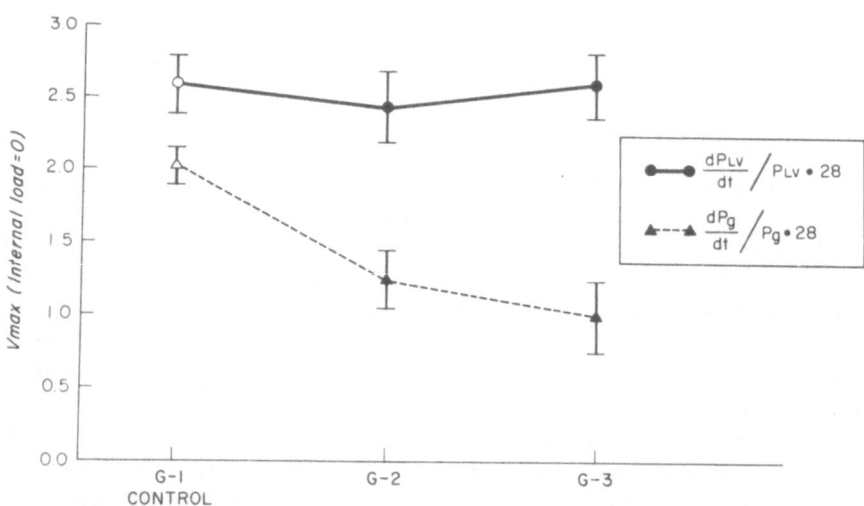

*Figure 7. Top:* measurement of zero-load flow during the first beat after transection of the aorta (indicated by an arrow); *bottom:* analytically predicted zero-load ($Q_{sc}$) for the same animal, calculated using the phasors of pressure and flow in two consecutive beats (see Figure 1) with different setting of the input impedance.

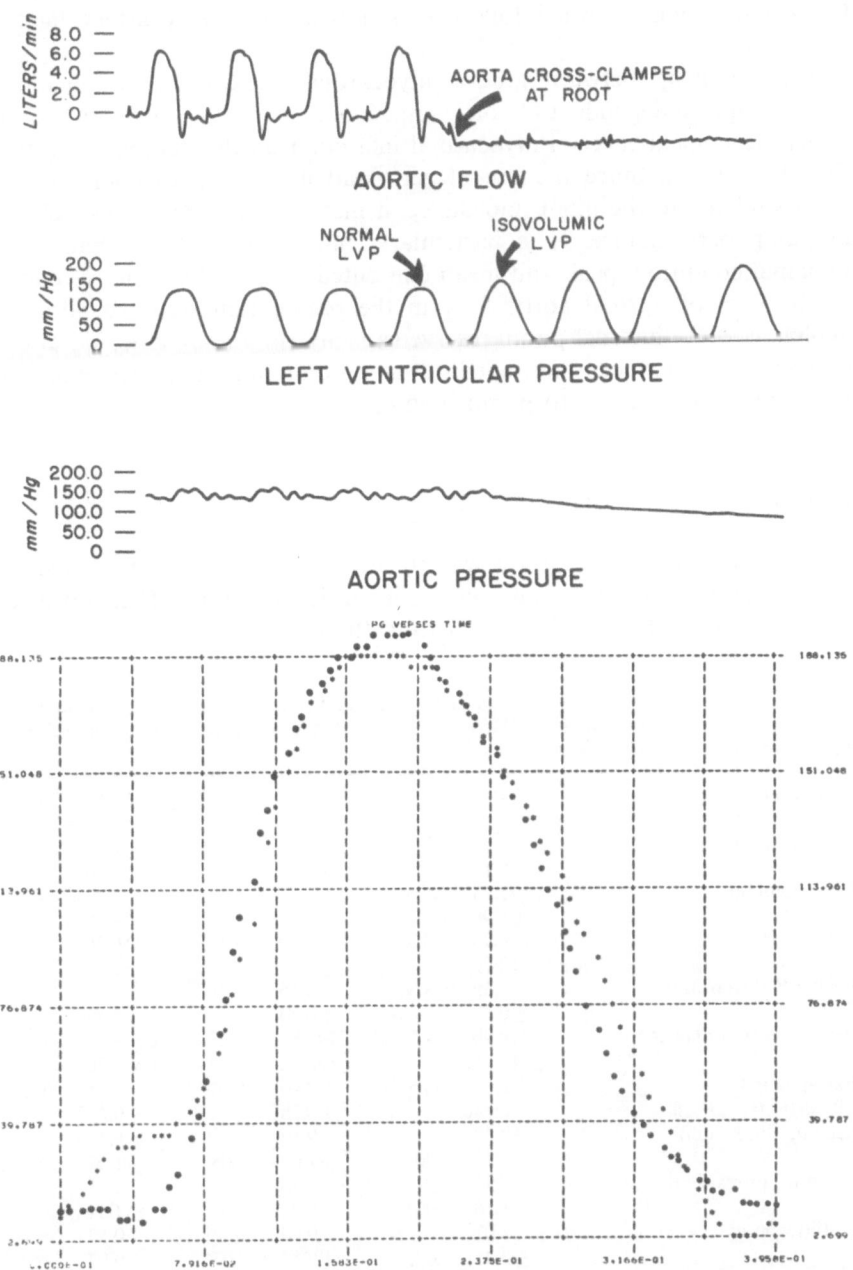

*Figure 8. Top:* measurement of the isovolumic pressure response (aorta is cross-clamped at the root); *bottom:* superimposed source pressure, $P_g$ (asterisks), and isovolumic left ventricular pressure, $P_{lv}$ (points), beat.

$V_{max}(P_g)$ was demonstrated following sequential coronary artery ligation (Table 1).

A relationship between graded myocardial impairment and hemodynamic output independent of aortic impedance enables the evaluation of the direct mechanical effect of myocardial infarction on the pumping ability of the intact heart. Since the use of zero-load flow excludes compensatory factors related to the input impedance, it may indicate the intrinsic change in pump performance. It is particularly interesting to note that in the impaired condition, peak and mean computed zero-load flow were reduced to the level of normal aortic flow in the pre-ligation state, suggesting a depletion of the internal pump reserve capacity (Figure 5). It would appear that zero-load flow can be singled out as a pump parameter expressing the true ability of the heart to pump blood.

SUMMARY

The aim of the present study was to assess quantitatively the effects of regional myocardial ischaemia on the intrinsic mechanical function of the intact left ventricle. In this investigation the left ventricle was mathemati-

Table 1. Summary of results in eight animals. The significance of change is calculated by a paired $t$-test. $P^1$; $P$ value comparing G-1 with G-2. $P^2$; $P$ value comparing G-2 with G-3. $P^3$; $P$ value comparing G-1 with G-3.

| Parameter | G-1 | $p^1_<$ | G-2 | $p^2_<$ | G-3 | $p^3_<$ |
|---|---|---|---|---|---|---|
| CO (litres/min) | 1.27 ±0.12 | N.S. | 1.15 ±0.14 | N.S. | 1.16 ±0.16 | N.S. |
| LVP (mmHg) | 73.14 ±6.06 | N.S. | 79.77 ±8.98 | 0.025 | 67.32 ±4.25 | N.S. |
| AP (mmHg) | 128.90 ±12.59 | N.S. | 131.70 ±6.44 | 0.025 | 116.36 ±1.87 | N.S. |
| Peak AF (litres/min) | 6.49 ±0.49 | N.S. | 6.16 ±0.30 | N.S. | 6.46 ±0.46 | N.S. |
| Peak $(dp/dt)$ mmHg sec$^{-1}$ | 2079.90 ±211.55 | N.S. | 2141.85 ±163.12 | 0.05 | 2353.92 ±390.56 | .05 |
| Extrapolated $dP_{lv}/dt/P_{lv}(V_{max}P_{1v}))$ | 2.55 ±0.186 | N.S. | 2.44 ±0.282 | N.S. | 2.55 ±0.237 | N.S. |
| Peak $q_{sc}$ (litres/min) | 17.34 ±2.10 | .001 | 9.19 ±1.0 | .005 | 6.565 ±1.04 | .001 |
| Mean $q_{sc}$ (litres/min) | 7.908 ±1.16 | .001 | 4.46 ±0.064 | .005 | 3.31 ±.064 | .001 |
| $q_{sc}$ (litres/min$^2$) | 2.02 ±0.25 | .005 | 0.90 ±0.12 | .005 | 0.57 ±0.07 | .001 |
| Extrapolated $dP_g/dt/P_g$ $(V_{max}(P_g))$ | 2.015 ±0.126 | .005 | 1.327 ±0.235 | .025 | 0.971 ±0.285 | .001 |
| ST-segment $(\Sigma ST/n)$ | | .001 | 3.66 ±0.27 | .001 | 6.84 +0.85 | .001 |
| Number of measurements | 14 | | 19 | | 13 | |

cally represented as an equivalent pressure source. The equivalent representation in the form of a pressure generator in series with an internal impedance provided a working framework for defining and computing a number of model-related performance indicators, such as non-ejecting intraventricular pressure and zero-load aortic flow. The computed zero-load flow was found to agree well with the experimentally measured flow following a total transection of the aorta. The equivalent pressure source time domain function is mathematically related to the isovolumic pressure variation of the left ventricle as experimentally measured by producing an infinite load (cross-clamping the aorta) for the ejecting left ventricle. The synthesized isovolumetric beat was used to construct a contractile state plane diagram based upon existing models of muscle mechanics.

The results presented examine the sensitivity of the traditional hemodynamic performance indicators such as cardiac output, peak aortic flow, left ventricle pressure and isovolumic contractility index ($V_{max}$). The study in 8 dogs showed that the model-based performance indicators consisting of pump and muscle parameters are sensitive indicators of the functional state of the myocardium. In addition, they proved to be more discriminating in detecting early impairment of left ventricular performance when compared to the traditional hemodynamic performance indicators. Thus, more precise and conceptually meaningful methods have been developed for quantitatively defining the changes in left ventricular function independent of the extrinsic compensatory effects that follow acute myocardial infarction.

ACKNOWLEDGEMENTS

This research was supported by the Department of Electrical Engineering, Rutgers University and in part by Grant 1R01MB00161, Bureau of Health Resources Development, Department of Health, Education, and Welfare.

REFERENCES

1. Swan HJC, Forrester JS, Diamond G, Chatterjee K, Parmley WW: Hemodynamic spectrum of myocardial infarction and cardiogenic shock, a conceptual model. *Circulation* 45:1097, 1972.
2. Lekven J, Mjos OD, Kjekhus JK: Compensatory mechanisms during graded myocardial ischemia. *Am J Cardiol* 31:467, 1973.
3. Rackley LE, Russell RO: Left ventricular function in acute myocardial infarction and its clinical significance. *Circulation* 45:231, 1972.
4. Smith ER, Redwood DR, McCarron WE, Epstein SE: Coronary artery occlusion in the conscious dog: effects of alterations in arterial pressure produced by nitroglycerine, hemorrhage and alpha-adrenergic agonists on the degree of myocardial ischemia. *Circulation* 47:51, 1974.
5. Peterson DR, Bishop VS: Reflex blood pressure control during acute myocardial ischemia in the conscious dog. *Circ Res* 34:226, 1974.
6. Leidtke AJ, Urschel CW, Kirk ES: Total systemic autoregulation in the dog and its inhibition by barroreceptor reflexes. *Circ Res* 32:673, 1973.

7. Fich S. Welkowitz W, Shastri S: An equivalent pressure source for the heart. *Int J Eng Sci* 11:601, 1973.
8. Kresh Y: Model-based hemodynamic indicators of left ventricular performance in acute myocardial infarction. PhD thesis, Department of Electrical Engineering, Rutgers University, New Brunswick, New Jersey, 1977.
9. Mason DT, Spann, Jr JF, Zelis R: Quantification of the contractile state of the intact human heart: maximal velocity of contractile element shortening determined by the instantaneous relation between the rate of pressure rise and pressure in the left ventricle during isovolumic systole. *Am J Cardiol* 26:248, 1970.
10. Moroko PR, Kjakshus JK, Sobol BE, Watanabe T, Covell JW, Ross Jr J, Braunwald E: Factors influencing infarct size following experimental coronary artery occlusion. *Circulation* 43:67, 1971.

## 5.5. COMPARATIVE EVALUATION OF MYOCARDIAL PERFORMANCE FACTORS

FRANCIS L. ABEL

### 1. INTRODUCTION

The manner in which the heart functions as a pump is of vital importance to maintaining an adequate flow of blood to the tissues of the body. Evaluation of its performance as a pump continues to be a serious problem in diseased states where that performance is compromised. Numerous variables have been proposed to evaluate pumping ability, hopefully related to inotropic changes such as can be described for the isolated papillary muscle fibre. These relate to the effect of a change in contractility on the relationship between velocity of contraction and force or pressure produced (afterload), velocity and initial length (preload) and the length-force relationship (work) (Figure 1). Many variables have been based on one plane of that diagram, with a shift to a different curve expected with a change in the inotropic state. Such variables, however, are often of limited value in the intact individual because of difficulty in making the measurements or because they are correlated with changes in preload, heart rate, or afterload. The desired variable would be independent of these factors but sensitive to changes in the inotropic state whether they are produced from extrinsic or intrinsic sources. The sensitivity of the various measurements utilizing pressure measurements alone have previously been described (1). This paper is an extension of those observations to include flow and impedance variables.

### 2. METHODS

The data were collected from 7 mongrel dogs weighing from 14 to 24 kg following anaesthetization with sodium pentobarbital, 30 mg/kg i.v. An endotracheal tube was inserted and attached to a positive pressure ventilator supplying an enriched oxygen mixture. The thorax was opened in the fifth intercostal space and a Konigsberg P-20 transducer inserted into the left ventricle via an incision in the apical dimple and retained by a purse-string suture. A small polyethylene tube attached to the transducer cable near the base of the transducer and connected to a Statham P23Db

J. Baan, A.C. Arntzenius, E.L. Yellin (eds.), Cardiac Dynamics, 369–379.

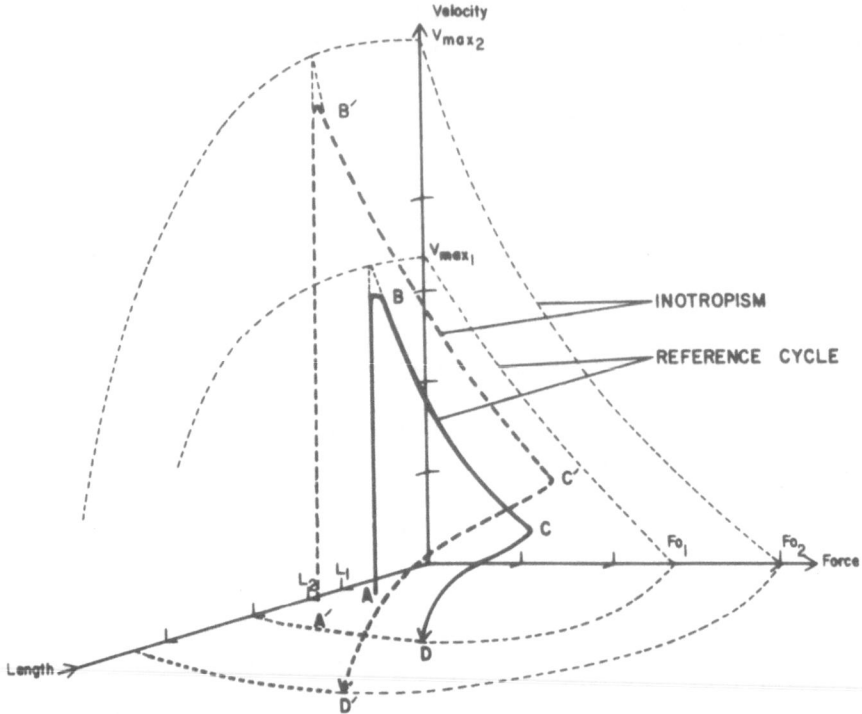

*Figure 1.* Schematic of length (volume), velocity, force (pressure) relation for the intact ventricle during a control cardiac cycle and after a positive inotropic change. Normal ventricle begins at length $L_1$ and follows path ABCD, then returns to length axis and fills to $L_1$.

transducer continuously monitored zero offset and calibration of the P-20 transducer while retaining the high-frequency characteristics (flat to 1.6 kHz) and immunity to catheter movement of the latter. Arterial pressure was measured via a catheter advanced through the left common carotid artery to the ascending aorta and attached to a Statham P23Db transducer. In 5 of the animals, a servo-controlled pump was connected to a cannula in the left subclavian artery to permit alteration and control of arterial blood pressure from a reservoir containing cross-matched heparinized dog blood. In some cases a bypass line was also connected to the left atrium to permit stepwise increases in left atrial pressure. Blood gases, pH, and body temperature was monitored; sodium bicarbonate was added to the perfusion system as required to maintain pH and $P_{CO2}$ within normal limits. The aorta was dissected free and an electromagnetic flow probe placed around the ascending aorta and connected to a square-wave electromagnetic flowmeter.

Following a control period of approximately 30 minutes, catecholamines were infused via a Harvard syringe pump and a polyethylene catheter inserted into the right femoral vein. Infusion rates were from 1.5 to 10 $\mu$g/kg/min depending on the particular drug. Each infusion was continued until several minutes of peak response level data were obtained. Five to ten minutes were allowed between infusions until return to control levels was judged to be complete.

The data were continuously recorded on a Hewlett-Packard 3960 tape recorder through RC filters that were down by 3 db at 120 Hz. These signals were then digitized at 200 samples per second per channel using a Nova 1200 minicomputer and 12-bit A-D converter. The computer was programmed to select one cardiac cycle, using end-diastolic pressure as a criteria of the beginning of the cycle, and the raw variables computed for each cycle. The data from 3 cycles were averaged together and stored for further analysis. End-diastolic pressure was defined by the computer program as the point where left ventricular pressure was less than 30 mmHg, and the difference in pressure between the sampled point and two samples previous was positive and less than 3 mmHg. This defined a flat pressure area which was usually short enough to accept an atrial kick but to reject aberrant noise.

Forty-one variables, along with Fourier power and $V_{max}$ terms, were computed from this data. This paper focuses on the flow data with sufficient pressure data to compare with previously presented information (1). The data were grouped by the computer into similar ranges of mean systolic arterial pressure (MSAP or afterload), heart rate (HR), and end-diastolic pressure (EDP or preload).


2. RESULTS

Figure 2 indicates the sensitivity to infusion of the catecholamines epinephrine, norepinephrine, and isoproterenol versus the variation of the control data as indicated by the standard errors. While the changes with the drugs in this group were small, it is apparent that most of the usable factors are those included within the circle shown on the figure. Other variables with considerably more sensitivity to drugs show such wide variability that it would not be possible to predict a change from the control state. It is also important to consider the undesirable correlation of a variable with preload, afterload, or heart rate (HR). The effects of two of these factors may be seen on cardiac work (Figure 3). Afterload had a marked influence principally on work at low preloads, and preload exerted its greatest effect at afterloads of less than 120 mmHg. Such effects are partly indicated by the variation in control data seen in Figure 2 and, where consistent, may also appear in the correlation function.

Since relatively small numbers are involved and the data is not nec-

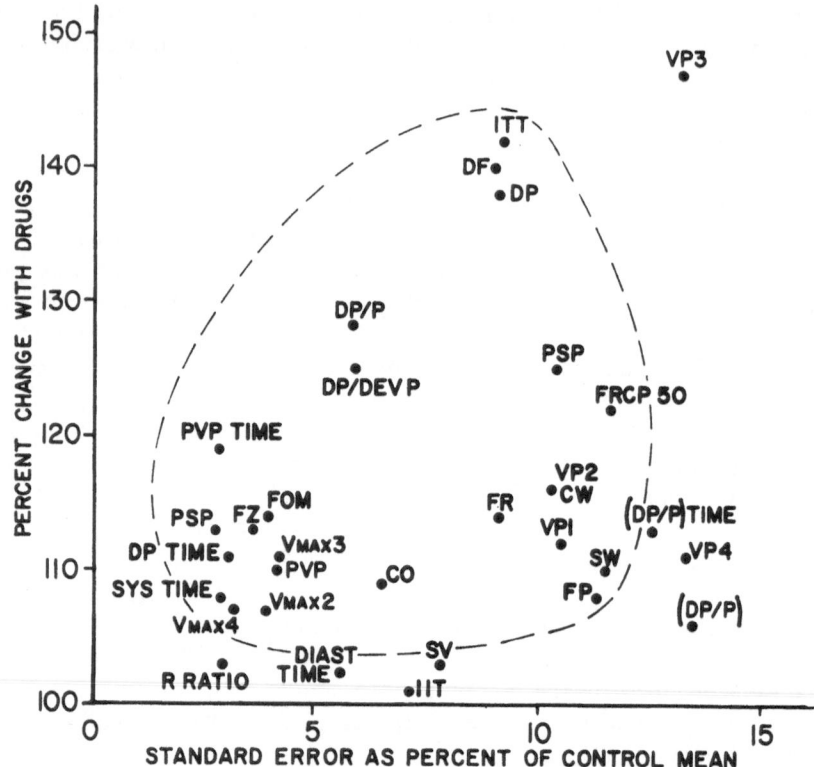

*Figure 2.* Sensitivity to catecholamines versus data variance for better variables. Circle outlines those most likely to be useful. VP3 = third harmonic of ventricular power; DF = max $df/dt$; DP = max $dp/dt$; IIT = integrated isometric tension; ITT = DP/IIT; PSP = peak stroke power; FRCP 50 = fractional rate of change of power at 50 mmHg, DEV P = P − EDP, FOM = PVP time × HR, $V_{max2}$ = second term in $V_{max}$ calculation from DP/28DEV P; SYS time = systolic time, DP time = time to max $dp/dt$, DIAST = diastolic, PVP = peak ventricular pressure, CO = cardiac output, SV = stroke volume, SW = stroke work, CW = cardiac work, FP = forcing (ventricular) power, FR = forcing resistance, FZ = forcing impedance, R ratio = FR/input (aortic resistance). Data obtained over HR range of 100–200, EDP of 0–20 mmHg, MSAP of 60–180 mmHg. PSP near DP time is PSP time.

essarily parametric, correlation coefficients were obtained using a Spearman correlation coefficient analysis. (This is a nonparametric method with a power near that of the Pierson product moment correlation procedure. The results were run both with the Pierson product moment and the Spearman method and were similar.) Table 1 presents the experimental data listing the major variables and the Spearman correlation coefficients with afterload, heart rate, and preload along with the control means, the means for a catecholamine group (consisting of norepinephrine, epinephrine, and isoproterenol), the standard errors for the control as a percentage of the control means, and the drug sensitivity as a percentage of the control mean.

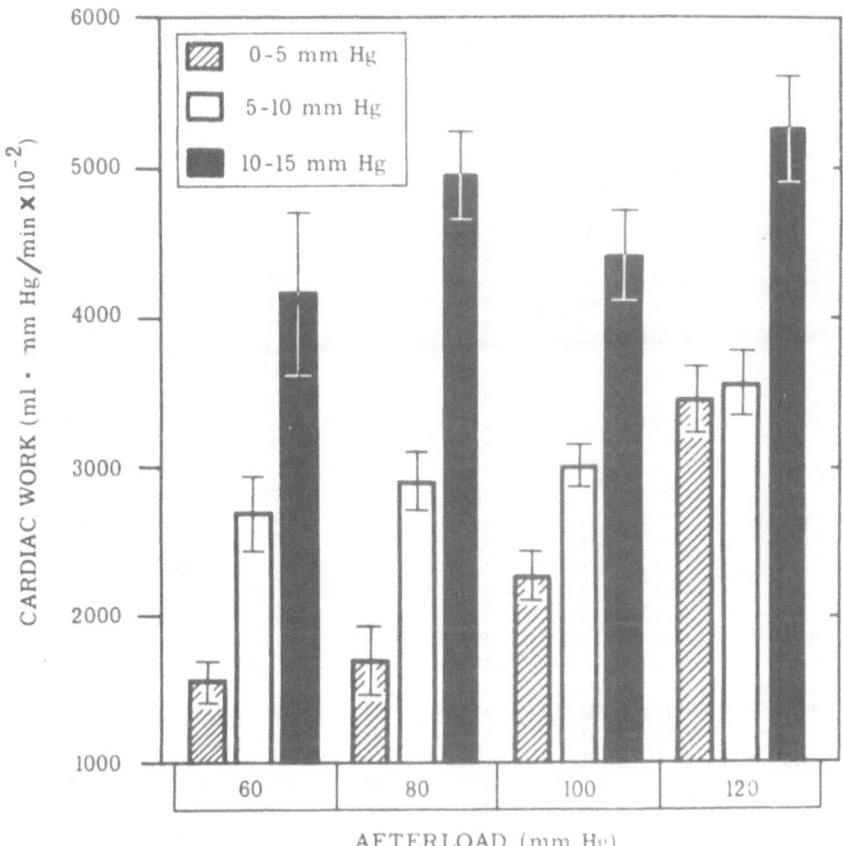

*Figure 3.* Alterations in cardiac work by preload and afterload. Means ± S.E.

A correlation index was derived by taking the square root of the correlation coefficients for preload, afterload, and HR following the squaring and summing of each coefficient. This would be equivalent to the length of the vector obtained if the correlation coefficients were mapped in three-dimensional space versus ordinates of preload, afterload, and heart rate. However, since a perfect correlation of unity for all 3 variables would result in a correlation index of 1.732 ($\sqrt{3}$), the resultant data were mapped into a 0 to 1 space by dividing by 1.732. Individual variables are plotted in Figures 4 and 5. A correlation index of 0.23 was arbitrarily chosen as a cutoff point, where no individual correlation could be greater than 0.4.

PVP time, while not an extremely sensitive variable, showed little control variability or undesired correlation aspects. In this regard it is more useful than either $dp/dt$ or $df/dt$. Of the flow-related variables the only ones that appear to be of possible useful value for evaluating ventricular performance are the forcing impedance, PSP time, and possibly two ventricular power

*Table 1.* Statistical analysis of the major variables.

| Variable | Spearman correlation coefficient with, | | | Control mean | Drug mean | Control variance (%) | Drug sensitivity (%)* |
|---|---|---|---|---|---|---|---|
| | MSAP | HR | EDP | | | | |
| VP 3 | 0.29 | −0.67 | 0.01 | 47.0 | 69.0 | 13.2 | 147 |
| VP 4 | 0.30 | −0.51 | −0.31 | 13.2 | 14.6 | 13.3 | 111 |
| PVP | 0.67 | −0.19 | 0.03 | 136.8 | 150.5 | 4.1 | 110 |
| PVP time | 0.13 | 0.15 | 0.32 | 87.7 | 73.8 | 2.8 | 119 |
| DP | 0.52 | −0.28 | −0.21 | 3.31 | 4.58 | 9.1 | 138 |
| DP time | −0.17 | 0.43 | −0.30 | 38.7 | 35.0 | 3.1 | 111 |
| SV | 0.06 | −0.68 | 0.20 | 0.88 | 0.90 | 7.8 | 103 |
| CO | 0.08 | −0.43 | 0.25 | 131.4 | 142.7 | 6.5 | 109 |
| SW | 0.19 | −0.58 | 0.29 | 1.17 | 1.28 | 11.5 | 110 |
| CW | 0.20 | −0.43 | 0.24 | 172.7 | 200.9 | 10.3 | 116 |
| DF | 0.35 | −0.57 | −0.26 | 3.21 | 4.50 | 9.0 | 140 |
| FOM | 0.06 | 0.69 | 0.11 | 13.6 | 12.0 | 4.0 | 114 |
| PSP | 0.30 | −0.53 | 0.07 | 1.39 | 1.74 | 10.4 | 125 |
| PSP time | −0.19 | 0.40 | 0.49 | 96.9 | 86.0 | 2.8 | 113 |
| SYS time | 0.02 | −0.25 | 0.46 | 154.6 | 142.8 | 2.9 | 108 |
| DIAST time | 0.06 | −0.92 | −0.05 | 194.6 | 190.5 | 5.6 | 102 |
| $FRCP_{50}$ | 0.47 | −0.11 | −0.23 | 7.59 | 9.23 | 11.6 | 122 |
| $FRCP_{75}$ | 0.22 | −0.01 | 0.18 | 3.50 | 5.88 | 20.9 | 168 |
| IIT | 0.25 | 0.18 | −0.41 | 2.50 | 2.51 | 7.1 | 101 |
| ITT | 0.11 | −0.41 | 0.30 | 1438. | 2038. | 9.2 | 142 |
| DP/P | 0.14 | −0.31 | −0.02 | 4.36 | 5.56 | 5.8 | 128 |
| (DP/P) | 0.25 | −0.18 | −0.79 | 8.84 | 8.33 | 13.5 | 106 |
| (DP/P) time | −0.14 | −0.06 | 0.52 | 15.7 | 17.7 | 12.5 | 113 |
| DP/DEV P | 0.12 | −0.30 | 0.29 | 5.11 | 6.38 | 5.9 | 125 |
| % Z Diff | 0.11 | −0.15 | −0.30 | 10.4 | 5.45 | 22.1 | 192 |
| R Ratio | −0.09 | 0.25 | 0.36 | 0.58 | 0.56 | 2.9 | 113 |
| FP | 0.22 | −0.57 | 0.28 | 113.8 | 123.4 | 11.3 | 108 |
| FZ | 0.53 | −0.10 | 0.11 | 11.8 | 10.4 | 3.6 | 113 |
| FR | 0.22 | 0.54 | −0.09 | 30.7 | 27.0 | 9.6 | 114 |
| $V_{max2}$ | −0.13 | 0.90 | −0.08 | 5.19 | 5.58 | 3.9 | 107 |
| $V_{max3}$ | 0.22 | 0.50 | −0.13 | 5.22 | 5.78 | 4.2 | 111 |
| $V_{max4}$ | 0.32 | 0.03 | −0.14 | 4.27 | 4.55 | 3.2 | 107 |

*Reciprocal used if less than 100%. See Figure 2 for abbreviations. Mean values for time in msec, pressures in mmHg, flow in ml/kg, derivatives in $^2/sec^{-1} \times 10^{-3}$. Means of 3 cardiac cycles, grouped for HR of 100–200, EDP 0–20, MSAP 60–80. $N$ is 32 for controls, 23 for drugs.

terms (VP1, VP2). However, it should be noted that $df/dt$ is approximately equivalent to $dp/dt$ although showing more correlation with HR than does $dp/dt$. This correlation was similar to that of stroke volume, indicating that the two variables measure the same factor, i.e., the rapidity at which blood flows from the heart is closely correlated to the total amount of flow that occurs and these are both inversely related to HR. Stroke work was similarly inversely correlated with HR; $dp/dt$, on the other hand, was more highly correlated with afterload. In this series these variables were more sensitive than PVP time although that was not consistently true in the previous series (1).

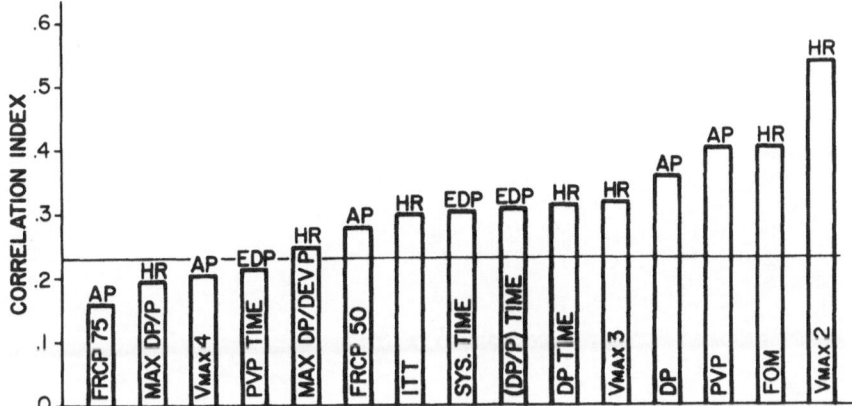

*Figure 4.* Pressure variables from Figure 2 as correlated with HR, MSAP (AP), and EDP.

The time variables, in general, show less change than do the derivative terms but they are also much more stable in terms of relative variation with changes in afterload, preload, and HR and show less undesired correlation with these variables than do the derivative variables. Attempts to compute other non-dimensional variables resulted in increased sensitivity to drugs but were associated with an increase in control variability. The percentage impedance difference (defined as the difference between the calculated forcing impedance and input impedance divided by the forcing impedance) was by far the most sensitive and was not significantly correlated with any variable (Table 1). The wide variability in this term however precludes its value as a performance indicator unless a specified state can be found where such variability does not occur.

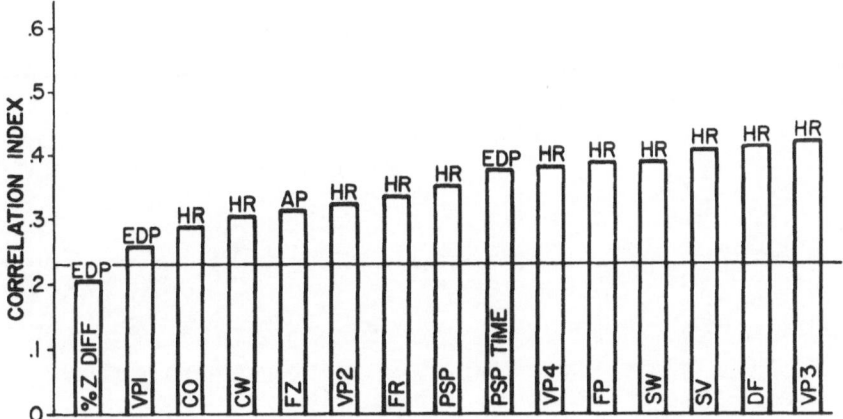

*Figure 5.* Flow and power variables from Figure 2. See text for definition of % Z difference.

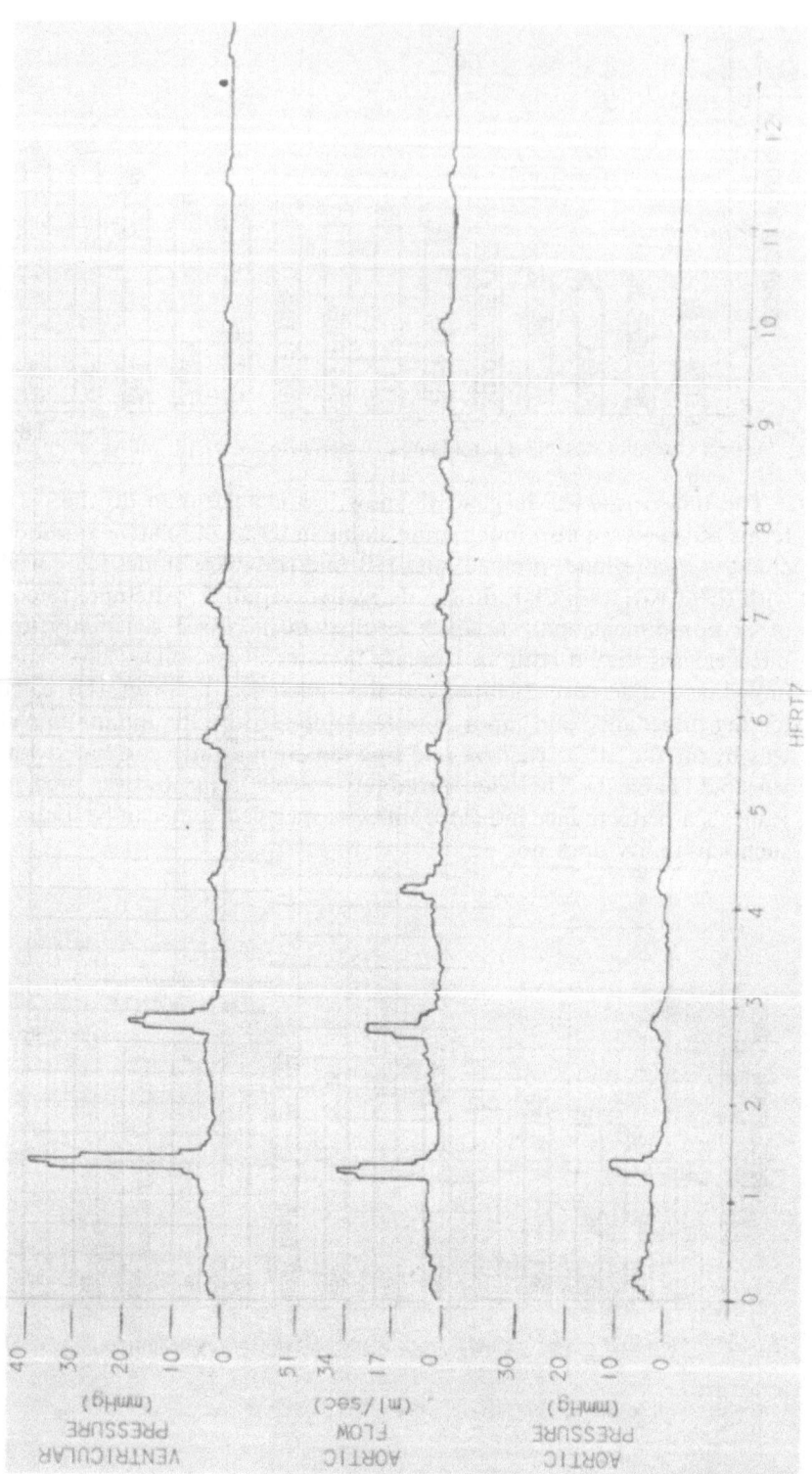

*Figure 6.* Power spectrum analysis of single cardiac cycle.

With each beat of the heart a power spectrum is generated with its fundamental at the heart rate. A spectral analyser (Honeywell 7900) was used to provide the sample spectrum shown in Figure 6. This is similar to previously presented Fourier analysis data (2) indicating particularly the shift in information to higher frequencies within the ventricle versus in the aorta. As a comparison between the Fourier series computed ventricular power and power error terms, the upper portion of Figure 7 shows the alteration in the normalized ventricular power terms with the infusion of different catecholamines. Again, the curves are similar to those previously presented (2). Norepinephrine, isoproterenol, and epinephrine shift the curves to slightly higher values whereas neosynephrine reduces the curve. The power error curves shown also indicate a similar relationship to that

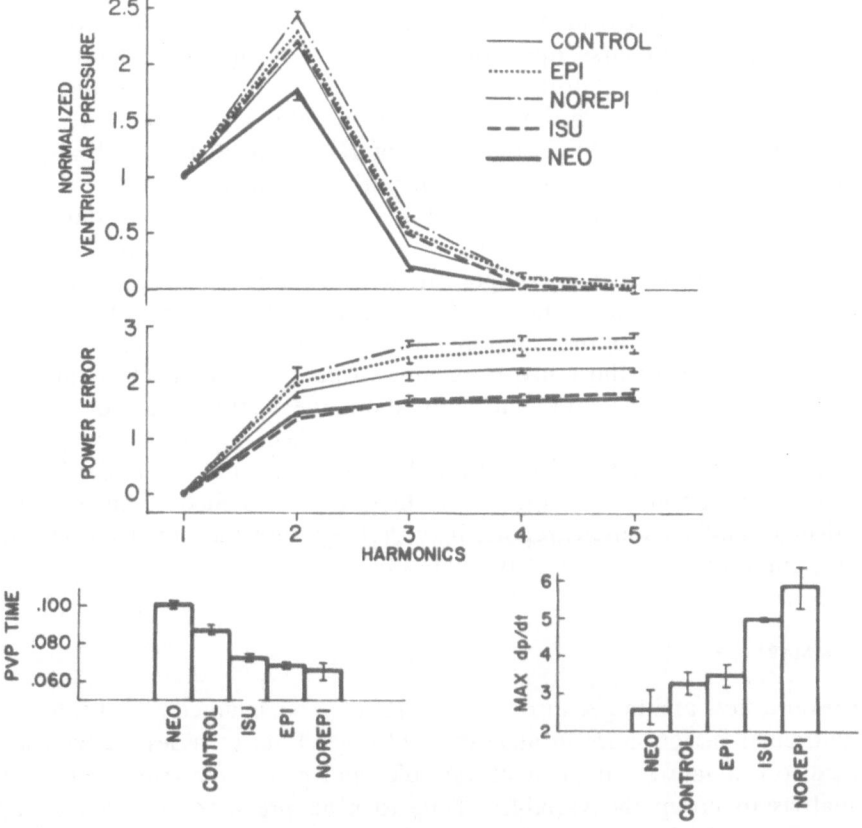

*Figure 7.* Normalized ventricular power harmonics from Fourier series analysis during control and catecholamine infusion. Normalized by dividing by first harmonic (DC term). Power error = normalized forcing power − normalized load power. At bottom PVP time in seconds, max $dp/dt$ in mmHg/sec $\times 10^{-3}$.

previously described. These are measures of the ability of the left ventricle as a pump to match load impedance. The corresponding changes in PVP time versus maximal $dp/dt$ are shown at the bottom of the figure. Again, PVP time appears to be an excellent measure of alterations in the contractile state produced by the catecholamines in a similar manner to $dp/dt$ but less sensitive to influences by preload, afterload, and heart rate. This variable remains as the best single variable yet determined for evaluating ventricular performance.

## 3. DISCUSSION

The use of Fourier analysis to analyse left ventricular impedance has been criticized because of the nonlinear nature of the aortic valves. However impedance is only calculable during the period of positive flow when the aortic valve is, of course, open. In an attempt to evaluate this factor, power terms were calculated from a Fourier series performed throughout the cardiac cycle and only during ventricular ejection. The results were essentially identical ($r = .989$) over a range of HR from 90 to 167 beats/min, during control and infusion of neosynephrine and isoproterenol.

Finally, principal component factor analysis was applied to the data in an attempt to distinguish groupings of variables which measure the same function. Four orthogonal components were identified comprising (a) components associated with the rate of pressure development; (b) those associated with flow; (c) those representing interactions of flow and pressure, i.e., power; and (d) those involving time to peak development. While it is difficult to make absolute statements about the relative value of a given group, the data appear to indicate that the last group, involving time variables, shows the most promise of freedom from undesired correlations and should be roughly comparable to time to peak isometric tension in the isolated papillary muscle, reportedly correlated with the time to attain the maximum intensity of the active state (3).

### SUMMARY

Pressure, flow and impedance variables have been evaluated as indicators of ventricular performance in anaesthetized dogs. Fourier series analysis was used to evaluate the impedance variables and power spectrum and factor analysis to group the variables. Time to peak pressure showed the best combinations of sensitivity, low control variability and lack of undesired correlations. None of the power variables were as good; there was an increase in the power error at higher frequencies with increased ventricular performance.

REFERENCES

1. Abel FL: Comparative evaluation of pressure and time factors in estimating left ventricular performance. *J Appl Physiol* 40:192–205, 1976.
2. Abel FL: Fourier analysis of left ventricular performance: evaluation of impedance matching. *Circ Res* 28:119–135, 1971.
3. Sonnenblick EH, Parmley WW: Active state in heart muscle: force-velocity-length relations and the variable onset and duration of the maximum active state. In: *Factors influencing myocardial contractility*, Tanz RD, Kavaler F, Roberts J (eds). New York. Academic Press, 1967, 65–83.

## 5.6. CIRCULATORY CHANGES DURING ISOMETRIC EXERCISE MEASURED BY TRANSCUTANEOUS AORTOVELOGRAPHY

D.S. BLOOM, L.H. LIGHT

### 1. INTRODUCTION

The use of Doppler ultrasound for the measurement of instantaneous blood flow velocity in the aorta has been described previously (1) and has also been used in clinical practice (2). It has been shown also that velocity is closely proportional to the volume of blood flow into the descending aorta over a wide range of conditions (3). Although the circulatory changes that accompany isometric exercise in man have been well studied, there is little data on the actual velocity of blood flow and also most of the studies have used invasive methods. We therefore have used transcutaneous aortovelography (TAV) to study the changes found during isometric stress in young individuals and have compared these to those found in older subjects as well as with some values found in dynamic exercise.

### 2. METHODS

Ten medical students aged between 18 and 23 were subjected to an isometric stress. This was done by asking them to raise the water level in a rubber bulb connected to a closed glass tube filled with water to a height of one-third of their maximum ability (4). Then they held this pressure for three minutes. Before the exercise they rested for ten minutes during which blood pressure and TAV recordings were done. The method for obtaining TAV readings is shown in Figure 1. These were repeated during the isometric stress. The identical protocol was followed in eight subjects aged between 50 and 63. In all subjects a Valsalva measure was carefully avoided during the stress. The TAV recordings were then measured by transferring the readings onto punched tape and the average of ten cycles at rest and during stress analysed by computer. Finally the results were compared with some data found using TAV in five subjects (aged 20–25) performing dynamic exercise on a bicycle ergometer sufficient to increase the heart rate to a similar level found during the isometric stress.

*J. Baan, A.C. Arntzenius, E.L. Yellin (eds.), Cardiac Dynamics, 381–386.*

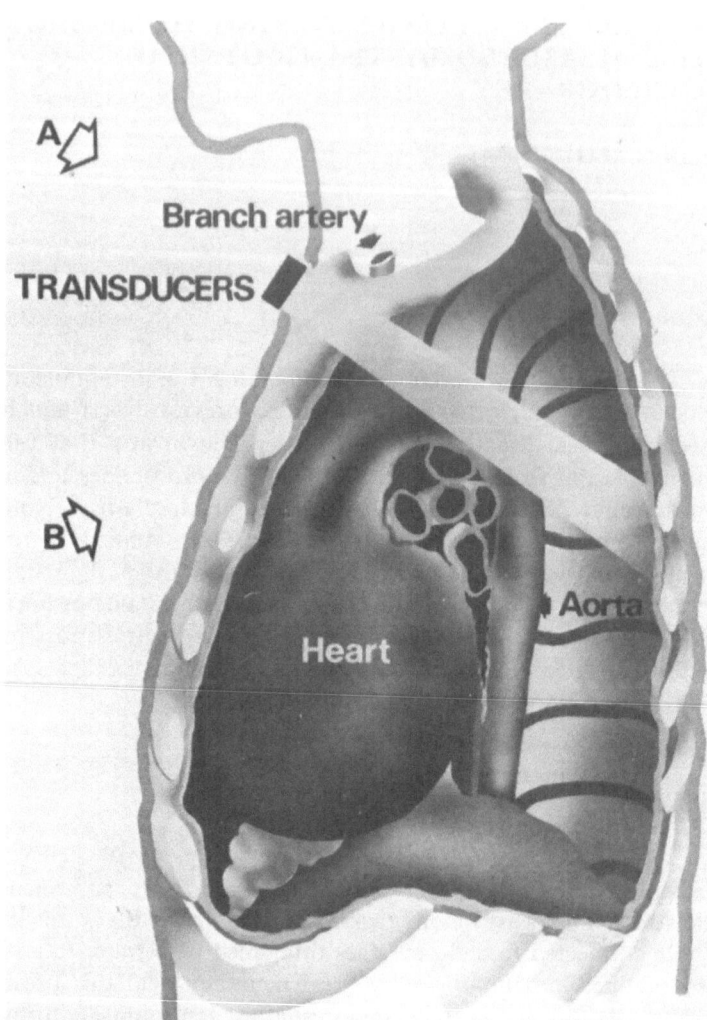

*Figure 1.* The method for TAV recording. An ultrasound beam is directed so that part of it intersects flow in a nearby in-line manner (residual angle $\theta$). This is apparent from the appearance of the grey-scale recording which presents the full spectra of Doppler shifts ($\Delta f$) backscattered by red blood cells moving away from the transducer. These Doppler shifts are related to blood velocity by $v = K\Delta f/\cos\theta$. Provided $\theta$ is less than 25 the highest instantaneous blood velocity can be deduced from the highest Doppler shift ($\Delta Fm$ by taking $\cos\theta$ equal to 0.95 so that $v = K\Delta Fm/0.95$.

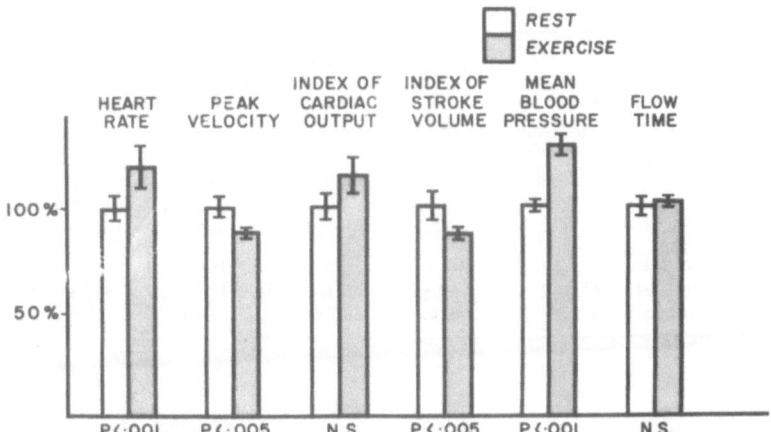

*Figure 2.* The changes found in 10 medical students subjected to an isometric stress of 3 minutes duration.

## 3. RESULTS

In the medical students the heart rate rose in all subjects ($21.5 \pm 9$ s.e.m., $p < 0.001$). This was accompanied by a significant increase in the mean blood pressure ($3.7 \pm 0.4$ Kpa, $p < 0.001$). The manner of systolic ejection also changed. There was a significant reduction in peak aortic blood velocity ($19.8 \pm 5.4$ cm/sec, $p < 0.005$). Flow time remained constant despite the increase in heart rate and there was a reduction in the index of stroke volume ($12.5 \pm 0.3$, $p < 0.005$). There was also a tendency to increase the cardiac output. In seven individuals the index of cardiac output increased (25%) but in three individuals it fell by 9%. This gave a mean increase in the whole group of $16 \pm 7\%$ ($p < .01$). These results are shown in Figure 2. After the stress the values returned rapidly to normal with a slight overshoot in peak flow velocity.

In the older individuals similar results are found but there was a lesser fall in peak velocity and stroke volume as well as a smaller increase in the index of cardiac output. The comparison with the younger individuals is shown in Table 1. Some of the results obtained in dynamic exercise are summarized in Table 2. Although the heart rate increased accompanied by an increase in peak velocity, there was a reduction in flow time.

## 4. DISCUSSION

Sustained isometric exercise has been shown by invasive methods to increase the mean arterial blood pressure, raise the heart rate and reduce the end-diastolic volume of the heart despite an increase in end-diastolic pressure

*Table 1.* Comparison between young and older age groups.

| | | Heart rate (beats/min) | Peak velocity (cm/sec) | Mean velocity (volume flow | Index of stroke volume | Flow time (m/sec) | Mean blood pressure (K/Pa) |
|---|---|---|---|---|---|---|---|
| Young age group (18–23) | Before test | 72.5 ± 4.3 | 156 ± 7.6 | 34 ± 2.3 | 28.3 ± 1.8 | 362 ± 11.6 | 13.19 ± 0.32 |
| | During test | 93.8 ± 6.7 | 136 ± 4.9 | 39.6 ± 4.2 | 25.1 ± 1.7 | 363 ± 12.5 | 17.16 ± 0.65 |
| | % Change | + 29.6 | − 12.5 | + 16.4 | − 12.5 | + 0.2 | + 29.2 |
| Older age group (60–63) | Before test | 65.2 ± 6.1 | 107.4 ± 9.8 | 20.4 ± 2.1 | 19.2 ± 1.9 | 358 ± 13.2 | 13.0 ± 0.4 |
| | During test | 73.0 | 97.0 ± 10.7 | 21.1 ± 3.0 | 17.4 ± 2.2 | 360 ± 16.7 | 16.23 ± 5 |
| | % Change | + 11.9 | − 9.4 | + 4.9 | − 9.3 | + 0.5 | + 25.1 |

within the heart (5, 6, 7). Left ventricular performance is improved with greater systolic emptying achieved from a smaller end-diastolic volume in the presence of a higher pressure load (6).

We have shown by a noninvasive method that in addition to the above there is a reduction in peak aortic blood flow and a fall in the index of stroke volume. Nevertheless, the index of cardiac output tended to rise due to the increase in heart rate. Although some of this reduction in peak blood flow velocity could be explained by aortic dilatation produced by the raised mean arterial blood pressure it is probable that this is an actual decrease in flow, since it occurred in older subjects as well, when the aorta would be expected to be much stiffer. We would expect the change in aortic diameter which is produced by the pressure changes to be in the order of 2.5% (8).

It would also seem that the manner of systolic ejection also changes. We found that on average flow time remained constant despite an increase in heart rate. This means that since the total cycle time is reduced, a greater proportion of that time is occupied by systole thereby reducing diastolic filling time. In dynamic exercise flow time is reduced in addition to a shortened diastolic filling time. Therefore at the increased heart rate there is less encroachment on diastolic filling compared with the isometric stress.

*Table 2.* Changes found in dynamic exercise.

| Subject | Δ heart rate (beats/min) | Δ peak velocity (cm/sec) | Δ flow time (m/sec) |
|---|---|---|---|
| 1 | + 25 | + 60 | − 40 |
| 2 | + 40 | + 22 | − 40 |
| 3 | + 50 | + 25 | − 70 |
| 4 | + 39 | + 40 | − 80 |
| 5 | + 18 | + 30 | − 20 |
| Mean | + 34.4 ± 5.7 | + 35.4 ± 6.8 | − 50 ± 10.9 |

This altered pattern of ejection could explain the fall in end-diastolic volume found in isometric exercise by workers using invasive methods (6).

In conclusion we have confirmed, using a noninvasive method, the alterations found in cardiovascular dynamics seen by workers using invasive techniques. We have also shown that the ejection pattern of the heart changes with lower peak flow rates and disproportionately reduced diastolic filling times. We have in addition demonstrated that although there is a similar alteration in blood pressure in isometric exercise in older individuals, the changes in cardiac dynamics are less than those seen in younger subjects.

SUMMARY

We have used Doppler ultrasound to measure instantaneous blood flow velocity into the descending aorta during isometric stress. We have compared the changes found in cardiovascular dynamics in young individuals with those found in older subjects. We found that there was an increase in blood pressure with an increased heart rate and index of cardiac output, but a fall in the index of stroke volume and a decreased peak aortic blood flow velocity. There was less change seen in older subjects and in both groups flow time remained constant compared to dynamic exercise when flow time is reduced. From this we conclude that there is a shorter diastolic time in isometric exercise than in dynamic exercise which could explain some of the findings found using invasive methods.

ACKNOWLEDGEMENT

We wish to thank Dr. R.J. Vecht and Dr. E. Besterman of St. Mary's Hospital, Paddington, for facilities provided for this work.

REFERENCES

1. Light H: Transcutaneous aortovelography: a new window on the circulation. *Brit Heart* 38:433–442, 1976.
2. Buchtal A, Hansen GC, Peisach AR: Transcutaneous aortovelography: potentially useful technique in the management of critically ill patients. *Brit Heart* 38:451–457, 1976.
3. Bilton AH, Brotherhood J, Cross G, Hanson GC, Light LH, Sequeira RF: Transcutaneous aortovelography as a measure of central blood flow. *J Physiol* (in press).
4. Vecht RJ: The grip test: a simple method for the assessment of left ventricular function. *Eur J Cardiol* 4:335–347, 1976.
5. Helfant RH, Devilla MA, Meister SG: Effect of sustained isometric handgrip exercise on left ventricular performance. *Circulation* 44:982–993.

6. Flessas AP, Connelly GD, Shunnosuke H, Tilney LR, Koster CK, Rimner RH, Keefe JF, Klein MD, Ryan TJ: Effects of isometric exercise on the end-diastolic pressure, volumes and function of the left ventricle in man. *Circulation* 53:839–993, 1976.
7. Lind AR, Taylor SH, Humphreys PW, Kennelly BM, Donald KW: The circulatory effects of sustained voluntary muscle contraction. Clin Sci 27:229–239, 1964.
8. Luchsinger PC, Sacks M, Patel DJ: Pressure radius relationship in large blood vessels of man. *Circ Res* 11:885–888, 1962.

## 5.7. VALIDITY OF PARAMETERS OF VENTRICULAR PERFORMANCE DETERMINED BY RADIOCARDIOGRAPHY IN PATIENTS WITH CORONARY ARTERY DISEASE

HARALD TILLMANNS, WOLFRAM H. KNAPP,
KLAUS VON OLSHAUSEN, HELMUTH C. MEHMEL,
JÜRGEN DOLL, WOLFGANG KÜBLER

### 1. INTRODUCTION

In 1962 Folse and Braunwald reported on determination of left ventricular (LV) ejection fraction, applying radionuclide indicator dilution (1). Since then, numerous investigators have evaluated central circulatory dynamics by means of radioisotope angiocardiography, either during the first passage of a radioactive bolus through the heart (2, 3, 4, 5, 6, 7, 8, 9), or after equilibrium of a tracer that remains within the circulation, using the gated cardiac blood pool technique (10, 11). Applying high time resolution, the first passage of a radioactive tracer allows estimation of ventricular performance by means of (a) time parameters, especially minimal cardiac transit times (MTT) reflecting the ratio of cardiac segmental volumes to cardiac output (2, 3, 6, 7, 8, 9) and (b) by means of the ratio of end-systolic and end-diastolic activities, according to the corresponding volume ratios (4, 5). This study was undertaken to test the validity of radiocardiographic parameters of ventricular performance, such as MTT as well as right and left ventricular ejection fraction (RVEF and LVEF), simultaneously measured by first-pass radionuclide angiography. Furthermore, the sensitivity and specifity of these noninvasive parameters with regard to identification of compromised RV and LV performance were determined in patients with coronary artery disease (CAD).

### 2. MATERIAL AND METHODS

Radionuclide angiocardiography was performed in 3 groups of 111 patients who all had undergone selective coronary angiography: (1) in 34 controls with normal coronary angiograms (group 1); (2) in 45 patients with angiographically proven coronary artery disease (1, 2 or 3-vessel disease, stenoses ≥ 75%, group 2); and (3) in 32 patients with CAD and LV aneurysm (group 3).

Within 24 hours following coronary angiography and cineventriculography, in 52 of 111 patients minimal cardiac transit times (MTT) as well as right and left ventricular ejection fraction (RVEF and LVEF) were simul-

*J. Baan, A.C. Arntzenius, E.L. Yellin (eds.), Cardiac Dynamics, 387–393.*

taneously determined by noninvasive radioisotope angiocardiography. In all patients, a bolus of 10–15 mCi technetium-99m-DTPA was rapidly injected into a large medial antecubital vein. As the tracer travelled through the cardiac chambers, precordial activity during the first passage was recorded for 60 seconds in 30° LAO projection with a gamma scintillation camera (Baird-Atomic) interfaced to a computer system. Image data were stored on magnetic disc and later transferred to a magnetic tape. High-frequency time-activity curves were generated from the regions of interest (RV and LV blood pool as well as the surrounding background area), and ventricular ejection fractions (first pass RVEF and LVEF) were determined from the cyclic fluctuations of the RV and LV time-activity curves which correspond to RV and LV volume changes during each cardiac cycle (12).

Image data from the same study were also used to measure MTT as the differences between arrival times of the radioisotope in consecutive cardiac compartments (8, 9). Total MTT (from the right atrium to the aortic root) and segmental MTT were determined over 8 regions of interest by means of their respective time-activity curves; all values were corrected for an arbitrary heart rate of 60 per minute. The results of both radiocardiographic methods were compared with each other and with those obtained from contrast angiography. Using the cineangiographic data, LV volumes and LVEF were determined according to standard procedures (13).

## 3. RESULTS AND DISCUSSION

### 3.1. Comparison between parameters of ventricular performance obtained by monoplane cineangiocardiography and by radionuclide angiography

LVEF obtained by monoplane cineangiography ($LVEF_{angio}$) in the control group ($n = 34$) averaged 75%. Patients with CAD (group 2, $n = 45$) exhibited a significant decrease in $LVEF_{angio}$ (mean = 58.2%), and a further decline in $LVEF_{angio}$ was noted in the 32 patients with CAD and LV aneurysm (mean $LVEF_{angio} = 42.9\%$).

Figure 1 shows the linear correlation between $LVEF_{angio}$ and the LVEF determined by first pass radionuclide angiocardiography (first pass LVEF). Both methods correlated well ($r = 0.88$); only in patients with poor LV performance documented by contrast angiography ($LVEF_{angio}$ below 35%) did the radionuclide method overestimate LVEF. This systematic error in the radiocardiographic determination of LVEF is probably due to the background subtraction which is influenced by the distribution of the tracer (9).

A decline in $LVEF_{angio}$ was associated with a prolongation of MTT from the right atrium to the aortic root ($MTT_{total}$); the relationship of these two

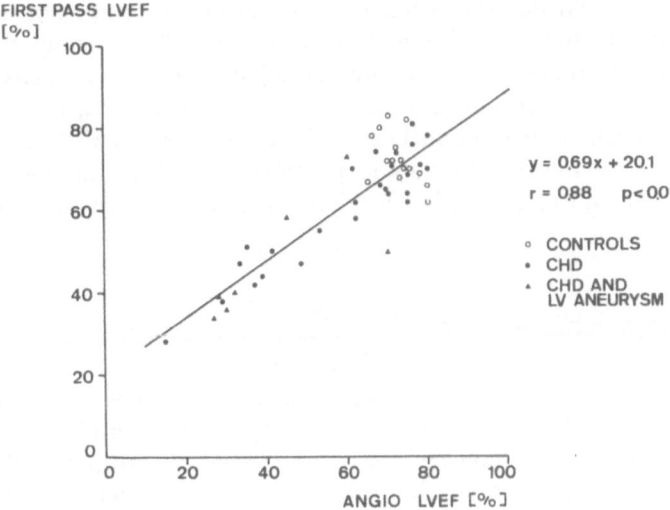

*Figure 1.* Correlation between LV ejection fractions obtained by contrast cineangiocardiography (ANGIO LVEF) and by first pass radionuclide angiography (FIRST PASS LVEF) in patients with coronary heart disease (CHD) and controls.

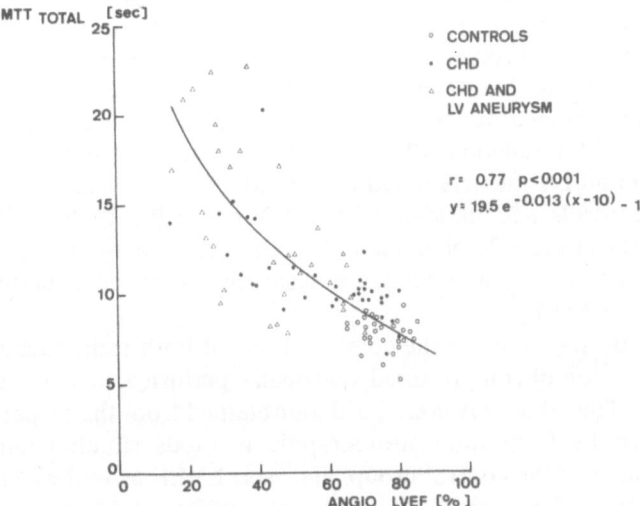

*Figure 2.* Correlation between LVEF obtained by contrast angiocardiography and $MTT_{total}$ (from the right atrium to the aortic root) in patients with coronary heart disease (CHD) and controls.

parameters could be approximated by an exponential function (Figure 2). The relatively low correlation coefficient ($r = 0.77$) as compared to our earlier results (6, 7), was probably caused by the heterogeneity of the 3 groups of patients examined in this study. A slightly better correlation was noted between both radionuclide methods, first pass LVEF and $MTT_{total}$ ($r = 0.86$). The radiocardiographic parameters of RV function, first pass RVEF and $MTT_{RV}$, correlated relatively poorly (correlation coefficient $r = 0.66$).

## 3.2. Sensitivity and specifity of the radiocardiographic parameters

Because of the assumptions which are required with respect to LV geometry, in patients with segmental ventricular dysfunction (hypokinesia, akinesia, or dyskinesia), the contrast-angiographic determination of LVEF may be influenced by considerable methodological errors. For this reason, the clinical validity of the radiocardiographic parameters of ventricular performance was also tested by evaluation of their sensitivity and specificity in monitoring compromised ventricular function. In Figure 3 the $MTT_{total}$ of all 111 patients are listed. Both groups of patients with CAD showed a significant prolongation of $MTT_{total}$ by 39% ($p < 0.01$) or 73% ($p < 0.01$). respectively. The existence of an LV aneurysm resulted in an additional increase in $MTT_{total}$ ($p < 0.05$). Only in 8 of 45 patients of group 2 and in 5 of 32 patients of group 3 was no prolongation of $MTT_{total}$ seen. Similar results were obtained by using the LV minimal transit time: the prolongation of $MTT_{LV}$ in both groups of CAD averaged 71% ($p < 0.01$) and 118% ($p < 0.01$), respectively. Despite the slightly more pronounced increase in $MTT_{LV}$ as compared to $MTT_{total}$ in patients with CAD, the segmental LV transit time seemed to be less suitable for individual identification of compromised LV function: 18 of 45 patients with CAD and 8 of 32 patients with CAD and LV aneurysm had normal $MTT_{LV}$. The worst discrimination between controls and patients with CAD was achieved by using the RV minimal transit time: 29 of 45 patients with CAD and 14 of 32 patients with CAD and LV aneurysm exhibited normal right ventricular performance as measured by $MTT_{RV}$.

The diagnostic value of the combined use of both radionuclide methods for the detection of compromised ventricular performance in CAD is shown in Table 1. The table only contains data obtained from the 52 patients being investigated by both radiocardiographic methods simultaneously. In all but 1 member of the control group, first pass LVEF as well as $MTT_{total}$ and $MTT_{LV}$ were within normal limits. Only 1 patient exhibited a prolongation of $MTT_{RV}$. In 13 of 30 patients with CAD, but without LV aneurysm, a decline in LVEF was noted; in 24 patients of this group, $MTT_{total}$ were prolonged. Applying both criteria, 25 patients with compromised LV

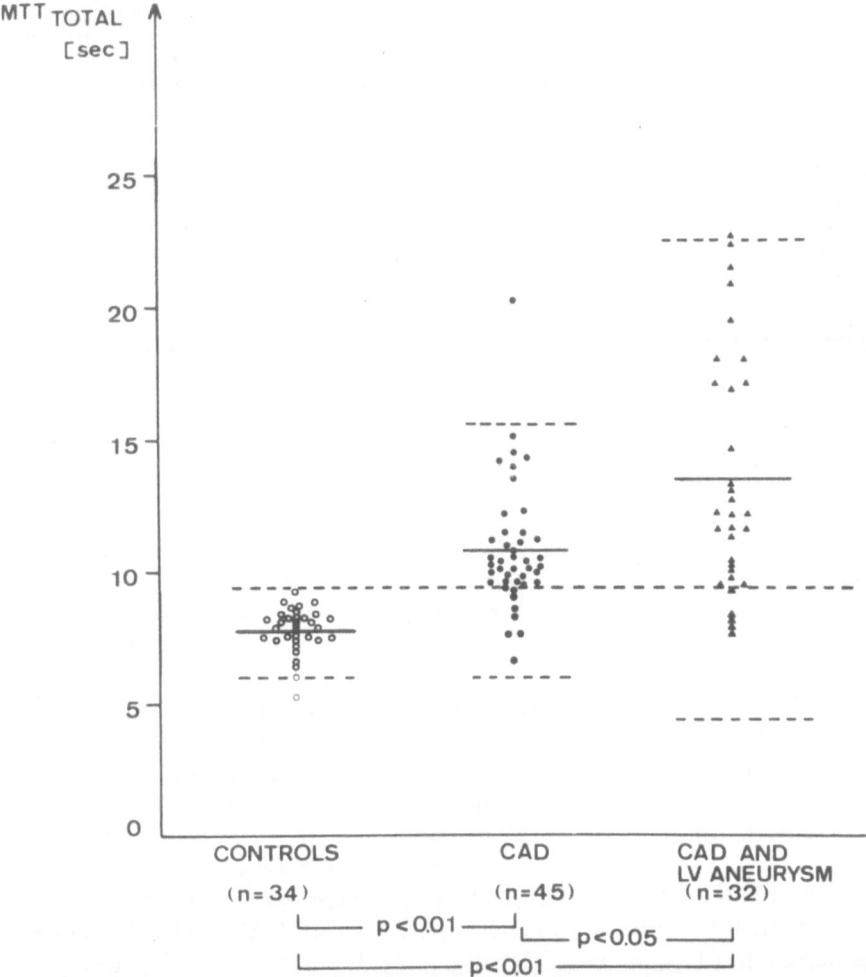

*Figure 3.* Total minimal cardiac transit times (MTT$_{total}$) in 34 controls, 45 patients with coronary artery disease (CAD), and 32 patients with CAD and LV aneurysm. In all groups, mean values (solid lines) and confidence limits ($\pm 2$ SD, dotted lines) are shown. The shaded area represents the confidence limit of the control group.

function were identified; this number increased to 27 (of 30) by additional consideration of the RV minimal transit time. Six of 7 patients with CAD and LV aneurysm exhibited a decrease in first pass LVEF; in only 5 patients a prolongation of MTT$_{total}$ was noted. Both parameters together helped to identify all 7 patients with disturbance of ventricular performance.

*Table 1.* Behaviour of radiocardiographic parameters of LV and RV performance.

| Parameter | Controls $(n = 15)$ | CAD $(n = 30)$ | CAD + LV aneurysm $(n = 7)$ |
|---|---|---|---|
| First pass | | | |
| LVEF ↓ | 0 | 13 | 6 |
| MTT$_{total}$ ↑ | 0 | 24 | 5 |
| First pass LVEF ↓ | | | |
| and/or | | | |
| MTT$_{total}$ ↑ | 0 | 25 | 7 |
| MTT$_{LV}$ ↑ | 0 | 17 | 3 |
| MTT$_{RV}$ ↑ | 1 | 10 | 4 |
| First pass LVEF↓ | | | |
| and/or MTT$_{total}$↑ | | | |
| and/or MTT$_{LV}$ ↑ | | | |
| and/or MTT$_{RV}$ ↑ | 1 | 27 | 7 |

SUMMARY

The validity of noninvasive radiocardiographic parameters of ventricular performance was tested in 45 patients with angiographically proven CAD, in 32 patients with CAD and LV aneurysm, and in 34 controls. Within 24 hours following the contrast-angiographic examination, precordial activity during the first passage of an intravenously administered bolus of 10–15 mCi $^{99m}$Tc-DTPA was recorded with a gamma scintillation camera, and minimal cardiac transit times (MTT) as well as right and left ventricular ejection fraction (first pass RVEF and LVEF) were determined. There was a close linear correlation between first pass LVEF and LVEF$_{angio}$ $(r = 0.88)$. The correlation between MTT$_{total}$ and first pass LVEF $(r = 0.86)$, or LVEF$_{angio}$ $(r = 0.77)$ respectively, exceeded that between MTT$_{RV}$ and first pass RVEF $(r = 0.66)$. MTT$_{total}$ and MTT$_{LV}$ were significantly prolonged in patients with CAD (group 2) and in patients with CAD and LV aneurysm (group 3): MTT$_{total}$ increased by 39% and 73%, MTT$_{LV}$ by 71% and 118%, respectively. Discrimination between controls and patients of groups 2 and 3 was best achieved by MTT$_{total}$, less so when using MTT$_{LV}$ and MTT$_{RV}$, as well as first pass LVEF. Combining both radionuclide methods, the best noninvasive procedure for evaluation of ventricular performance of patients with CAD was obtained.

REFERENCES

1. Folse R, Braunwald E: Determination of fraction of left ventricular volume ejected per beat and of ventricular end-diastolic and residual volumes. *Circulation* 25:674-685, 1962.
2. Schicha H, Vyska K, Becker V, Seipel L, Feinendegen LE: Minimale kardiale Transitzeiten (MTT's) in der Herzdiagnostik, Messungen mit der Gamma-Retina und Indium-113m II:

MTT's bei verschiedenen Herzklappenfehlern. *Z Kreislaufforsch* 60:947–957, 1971.

3. Vyska K, Schicha H, Becker V, Seipel L, Feinendegen LE: Minimale kardiale Transitzeiten (MTT's) in der Herzdiagnostik, Messungen mit der Gamma-Retina V und Indium-113m: MTT's bei Myokardschädigung und nach Digitalisierung. *Z Kreislaufforsch* 61:820–827, 1972.

4. Van Dyke D, Anger HO, Sullivan RW, Vetter WR, Yano Y, Parker HG: Cardiac evaluation from radioisotope dynamics. *J Nucl Med* 13:585–592, 1972.

5. Schelbert HR, Verba JW, Johnson AD, Brock GW, Alazraki NP, Rose FJ, Ashburn WL: Nontraumatic determination of left ventricular ejection fraction by radionuclide angiocardiography. *Circulation* 51:902–909, 1975.

6. Tillmanns H, Knapp WH, Mehmel HC, Kübler W, Doll J, Schömig A: Regionale Myokardperfusion und Myokardfunktion: Ergebnisse eines neuen nuklearmedizinischen Verfahrens. *Verh Dtsch Ges Inn Med* 82:1141–1145, 1976.

7. Tillmanns H, Knapp WH, Mehmel HC, Kübler W, Doll J, Olshausen K von, Schömig A: Regionale Myokardperfusion und Myokardfunktion bei Myokardinfarkt mit normalem Koronar-Angiogramm. *Verh Dtsch Ges Inn Med* 83:249–252, 1977.

8. Knapp WH, Doll J: Eine automatisierte Methode zur Bestimmung von Kreislaufzeiten in der nuklearmedizinischen Herzdiagnostik. *Nucl Med* (in press).

9. Knapp WH, Tillmanns H, Doll J, Mäurer K, Georgi P: Radiokardiographie während der ersten kardialen Indikatorpassage: Vergleich zweier Prinzipien im Hinblick auf ihre Bedeutung für die quantitative Erfassung der Myokardfunktion. (In press).

10. Mason DT, Ashburn WL, Harbert JC, Cohen LS, Braunwald E: Rapid sequential visualization of the heart and great vessels in man using the wide-field Anger scintillation camera. *Circulation* 39:19–28, 1969.

11. Strauss HW, Zaret BL, Hurley PJ, Natarajan TK, Pitt B: A scintiphotographic method for measuring left ventricular ejection fraction in man without cardiac catheterization. *Am J Cardiol* 28:575–580, 1971.

12. Baird-Atomic: *System seventy-seven, user handbook 1*, vol 2.

13. Greene DG, Carlisle R, Grant C, Bunnell IL: Estimation of left ventricular volume by one-plane cineangiography. *Circulation* 35:61–69, 1967.

# 5.8. ASSESSMENT OF THE DYNAMICS OF CARDIAC RESPONSES TO POSITIVE INOTROPIC AGENTS

Louis C. Sheppard, Bruce McA. Sayers,
Wilfred F. Holdefer, H. Cecil Coghlan

## 1. INTRODUCTION

The decision by the physician to employ pharmacologic intervention is based upon patient management programs which are composed of structured rules designed to aid in systematic decision making (1). The infusion of positive inotropic agents in the treatment of patients following open intracardiac operations is administered manually by the bedside nurse. The principal objective of this research was to determine to what extent the techniques of computer-based control of interventions could be applied in the management of epinephrine and dopamine in the clinical environment.

The multiple actions and subsequent effects of these drugs on hemodynamic variables and the performance of various organ subsystems dictated that the dynamics of the physiological responses to these agents be investigated.

## 2. METHODS

Five healthy mongrel dogs were anaesthetized with intravenous Diabutal (25 mg/kg) by continuous infusion and endotracheal ventilation was maintained by a Harvard respirator. Heart rate (HR), mean arterial pressure (MAP), mean left atrial pressure (LAP) and mean coronary (COR FLO), aortic (AOR FLO) and femoral (FEM FLO) blood flow rates were measured using appropriate techniques (2).

The characteristics of the dynamics of the response of a linear system (e.g., network, animal, patient) are contained in the impulse response. In biological terms, the impulse response is similar to the response of a physiological variable to a bolus injection of energy, pharmacological agent, or indicator. However, the bolus response method may drive the organism beyond the range of linear behaviour because of the large quantity of agent which must be injected to obtain an observable response (2). It is theoretically feasible to obtain the impulse response by using a cross-correlation method, which relies on the fact that for random signal excitation, the cross-correlation function (CCF) of the input and output signals is directly

J. Baan, A.C. Arntzenius, E.L. Yellin (eds.), Cardiac Dynamics, 395–404.

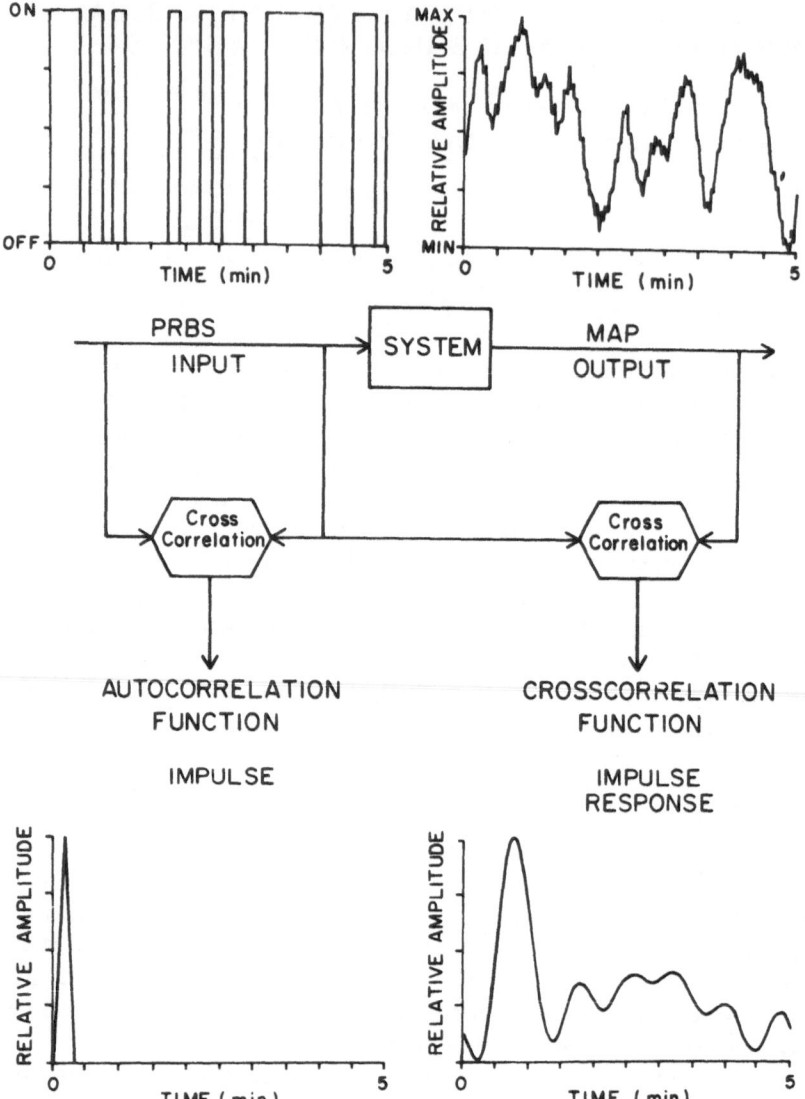

*Figure 1.* The PRBS programmed infusion of *dopamine* (ON = 4 μg/kg/min, OFF = zero μg/kg/min) is shown in the upper left corner and the MAP response is at the upper right. Illustrated in the centre is the autocorrelation function of the PRBS input to the dog (system) which is the impulse shown at the lower left. Correlation of the MAP output with the PRBS input yields the impulse response (cross-correlation function) at lower right.

proportional to the impulse response (3). Thus the system can in principle be evaluated within the linear range near its operating state without introducing an unacceptably large disturbance.

We have applied pseudo-random binary signals (PRBS) in conjunction with the cross-correlation method to the assessment of the dynamic effects of positive inotropic agents on cardiovascular control (Figure 1). This class of signals is repetitive, behaves predictably, meets the criteria of randomness over the sequence length, and possesses properties that are well known and fully described mathematically.

During PRBS programmed infusion of the inotropic agents, the preprocessed physiological signals and the PRBS level were digitzed in real time on line or from the FM tape at one sample per second per signal using a DEC PDP 8/I minicomputer. The data were transmitted by common carrier to an XDS Sigma 7 for storage and analysis. The PRBS level was normalized to zero for pump off and to plus one ($+1$) for pump infusing. Analytically, each subject was treated as a single input (programmed agent) and multiple output system. The input signal was cross-correlated individually with each output on the Sigma 7 computer to determine the subject's transfer characteristics (impulse responses equivalent to a response to a bolus injection) for each recorded output.

## 3. RESULTS

### 3.1. Mean arterial pressure (MAP)

For the 0.10 $\mu$g/kg/min dose ($1\times$) of epinephrine (Table 1) the peak of the MAP response occurred at 38.82 sec and the peak occurred 1.85 sec earlier at 36.97 sec for the 0.15 $\mu$g/kg/min ($1\frac{1}{2}\times$) dose. In the same animal, dopamine exhibited a more significant change than epinephrine even

Table 1. The time of the occurrence of the maximum or minimum of the MAP impulse response is tabulated for epinephrine and dopamine at the standard dose ($1\times$) and at 150% of standard ($1\frac{1}{2}\times$) along with the change in the time of occurrence ($\Delta t$) as the dose was increased.

| Experiment number | Time of occurrence (sec) Dose level | | Difference (sec) | |
|---|---|---|---|---|
| | $1\times$ | $1\frac{1}{2}\times$ | $\Delta t$ | Agent |
| 77-1DE | 38.82 | 36.97 | 1.85 | Epinephrine |
| 77-1DE | 47.95 | 42.20 | 5.75 | Dopamine |
| 77-2D | 46.59 | 36.46 | 10.13 | Dopamine |
| 78-3D | 44.70 | 34.60 | 10.10 | Dopamine |

though the epinephrine produced high-dose-related alpha-adrenergic ($\alpha$) responses and the dopamine responses were consistent with low dosages, i.e., beta-adrenergic ($\beta$) or dopaminergic ($\delta$) action (4). The minimum of the MAP excursion was at 47.95 sec for 4 $\mu$g/kg/min (1 $\times$) and 5.75 sec earlier at 42.20 sec for 6 $\mu$g/kg/min (1$\frac{1}{2}$ $\times$).

### 3.2. Heart rate

The elapsed time between the main vasoactive effect and the maximum of the vagal response is tabulated (Table 2) at each dose along with the difference in seconds. For epinephrine the time interval increased 3.54 sec from 11.15 sec at 0.10 $\mu$g/kg/min (1 $\times$) to 14.64 sec at 0.15 $\mu$g/kg/min (1$\frac{1}{2}$ $\times$). In the same animal increasing the dopamine from 4 $\mu$g/kg/min (1 $\times$) to 6 $\mu$g/kg/min (1$\frac{1}{2}$ $\times$) decreased the time interval 7.08 sec from 25.32 sec to 18.24 sec. No change in the elapsed time was observed in another animal; the interval was 8.11 sec at both dosages.

### 4. DISCUSSION

### 4.1. Epinephrine impulse responses

Both low-dose ($\beta$) and high-dose ($\alpha$) pressor impulse responses were observed (Figure 2). The vasodilatation, as evidenced by a rapid decrease in MAP (A in Figure 2) was associated with a corresponding increase in AOR FLO which correlated with the reduced afterload. The MAP returned toward baseline in the first minute as the $\beta$ effect quickly receded causing a decrease in AOR FLO. Concurrently the positive inotropic (INO) action of the epinephrine produced a more slowly acting increase in AOR FLO which was dissipated by the end of the fourth minute. The cardiac response

Table 2. The elapsed time is tabulated for the delay between the time of occurrence of the main feature of the vasoactive response (as shown in Table 1) and the time of the occurrence of the baroreceptor evoked vagal response at the standard dose (1 $\times$) and at 150% of standard (1$\frac{1}{2}$ $\times$) along with the change ($\Delta t$) in the time delay.

| Experiment number | Time delay (sec) Dose level | | Difference (sec) | Agent |
|---|---|---|---|---|
| | 1 $\times$ | 1$\frac{1}{2}$ $\times$ | | |
| 77-1DE | 11.15 | 14.64 | −3.54 | Epinephrine |
| 77-1DE | 25.32 | 18.24 | 7.08 | Dopamine |
| 77-2D | 8.11 | 8.11 | 0.0 | Dopamine |

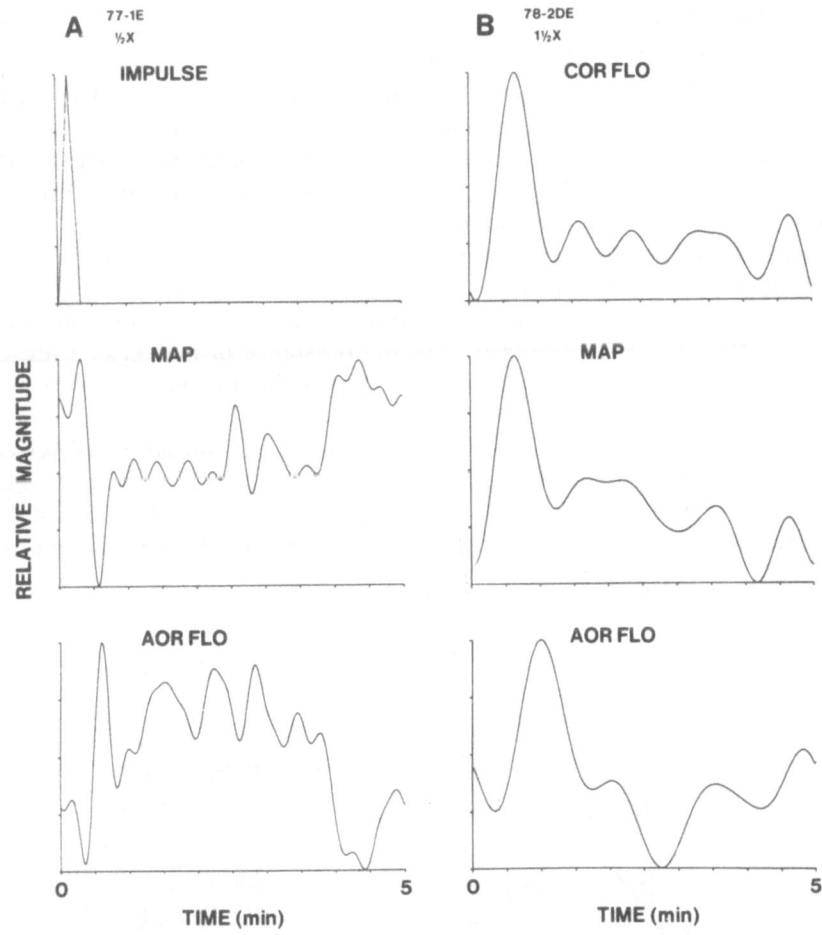

*Figure 2.* A: From top to bottom are the impulse for *epinephrine* (0.05 μg/kg/min) followed by the MAP impulse response (centre) and the AOR FLO impulse response; B: impulse responses for *epinephrine* (0.15 μg/kg/min) illustrated with COR FLO at top, MAP center, and AOR FLO bottom.

to the low dose was composed of two features: the faster component, associated with the fall and recovery of MAP and its effect on afterload, and the slower component, produced by the positive inotropic action of the drug.

The COR FLO analysed in a dog exhibiting an α epinephrine response (B) was observed to increase in phase with the MAP; after a delay of 30 sec the increase in AOR FLO occurred indicating that the COR FLO was closely correlated in time with the MAP increase and recovery rather than with AOR FLO.

### 4.2. *Dopamine impulse responses*

Dopamine elicited δ, α, and β adrenergic pressor responses in the dogs studied. Figure 3 illustrates a combined δ and α response. The MAP increase was caused by the receptor pressor effect. The initial decrease in aortic flow was caused by the elevated MAP; the high afterload negated the inotropic (INO) action. Blood flow redistribution was reflected by a momentary increase in femoral blood flow rate. The dopaminergic effect increased renal and mesenteric capacitance (CAP) causing the decrease in LAP after one circulation time. The effect was more dominant than the α effect as demonstrated by the peak of the increase in femoral flow followed by a gradual decrease. Restoration of the resistance of the skeletal muscle bed restored LAP and the α effect dissipated. Spontaneous activity was restored within 2.5 min.

The reflex fall in heart rate was caused by vagal inhibition (VAGAL) from increased baroreceptor activity mediated by the MAP increase. This chronotropic effect although low in magnitude, perhaps because of the barbiturate anaesthesia, was consistently organized in phase in the animals

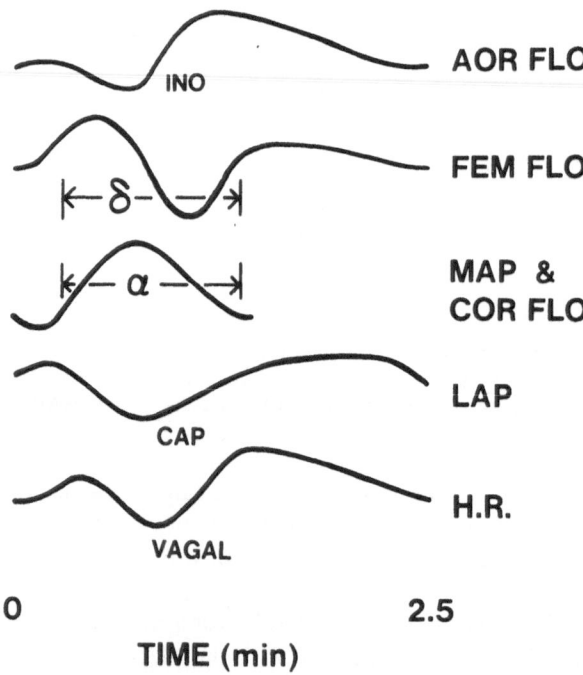

*Figure 3.* Retraced impulse responses for the five variables AOR FLO, FEM FLO, MAP, LAP, and HR from dog 77-2D at 4 μg/kg/min *dopamine*; COR FLO from dog 77-2DE at 4 μg/kg/min *dopamine* overlays the MAP response.

studied. Coronary artery flow impulse reponses were positively correlated with the MAP impulse responses, and the transient increase in COR FLO may have been caused totally by the MAP increase. Whether coronary vascular impedance was a factor cannot be stated with certainty because measurement of this variable was not feasible. However, since the onset of the response occurred before the onset of the positive inotropic effect (INO), increased myocardial oxygen demand is unlikely to have elicited the increase in flow.

### 4.3. *Time dependence of response to dopamine dose level*

Increasing the magnitude of the dose of dopamine produced an earlier onset of the MAP impulse response (Figure 4). This phenomenon was much more

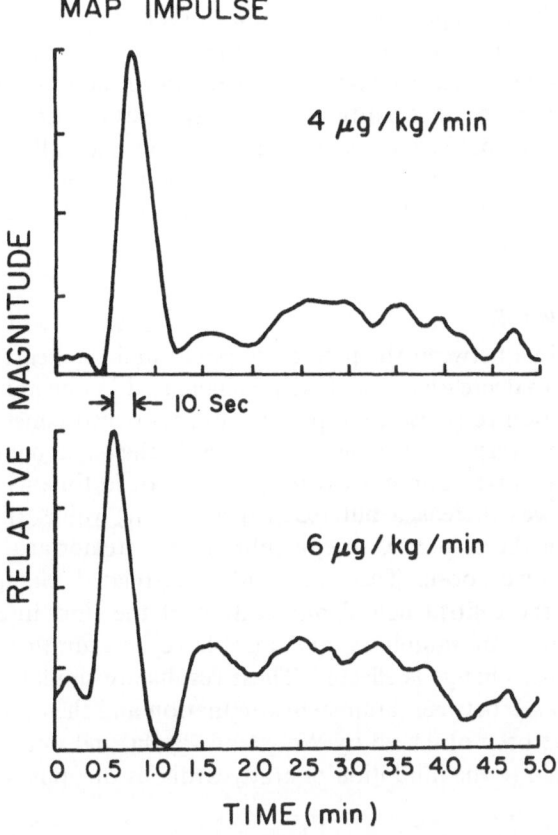

*Figure 4.* These two dopamine impulse reponses exhibit at 10.13 sec difference in the times of occurrence of the peaks of the responses. The maximum appears at 46.59 sec for 4 $\mu$g/kg/min in the upper impulse response and at 36.46 sec for 6 $\mu$g/kg/min in the lower impulse response.

pronounced in the dogs exhibiting α MAP response (MAP increase) than in the dog wherein the MAP response was β or δ (MAP decrease).

Comparison of epinephrine and dopamine response times at different dose levels in the same dog showed that the time of the occurrence of the response was significantly advanced by increasing the dopamine dose, but was barely modified with epinephrine. The hypothesis that the effect is mediated peripherally or by decreased circulation time due to increased cardiac output is unlikely to be supported by these observations; we propose that the dose dependence of the time of the response onset originates centrally.

Ample evidence for central nervous system modulation of cardiovascular responses has been reported. Both inhibition and augmentation of the sympathetic and para-sympathetic nervous systems have been documented. For example, Klevans and Gebber observed significant interaction between carotid sinus baroreceptor activation and forebrain stimulation (5).

In their experiments, only the modulation of the amplitudes of the responses was discussed. However, expansion of the concept that the central nervous system modulates cardiovascular responses to include variable time delay seems reasonable and bears consideration. Actually, central neural modulation of delay may be the hypothesis required to interpret our observations properly, but these results do not preclude the presence of a direct peripheral effect.

### 4.4. *Vagal response*

The elapsed time between the pressor response and the heart rate response was observed to decrease as the dose was increased in one animal exhibiting the vasodilatation response to dopamine, but remained constant in the dog which had the α response (Table 2). Apparently the vagal component of the baroreceptor reflex response was brought forward in time as the dose level of dopamine was increased but reached a limiting value. In contrast, the lapsed time for the responses to epinephrine was greater at the higher dose than at the lower dose. The dose and drug-related changes in timing indicate that the central neural modulation of the time intervals may be either facilitatory or inhibitory and may have a saturation limit beyond which no further change is effected. These results are similar to the variable delays of 2–14 sec between brainstem stimulation and the onset of tachycardia which have been observed by Weiss and Priola, and were reported to be inversely related to the inhibition of bradycardia by atropine (6).

### 4.5. *Central neural modulation*

The ultimate cardiovascular responses depend upon the hypothalamic integration of afferent stimuli from many facilitatory and inhibitory sites. It can be argued that dopamine acted centrally (7) to alter the interneuronal transmission along these multiple pathways to produce dose-dependent variable delays in the onsets of the pressor and vagal responses. Subsequently, the magnitudes of the time delays were determined by the interplay of competing central neural levels of augmentation and inhibition.

Although the onsets of both sympathetic and parasympathetic effects appear to be facilitated by increasing the dose level of dopamine, the modulation of the reflex vagal response to baroreceptor activity seems to be largely independent of the modulation of sympathetic activity. Hence the facilitatory relationships between central neural control and the time delays (sec) are likely to differ quantitatively for pressor, vagal, and central cardiac effects. By such a mechanism a variety of integrated responses may be produced.

## 5. CLINICAL IMPLICATIONS

The management of these interventions by a stepwise procedure seems advisable. The starting dose and incremental changes should be small. Bearing in mind that increased sympathetic drive may be elicited at higher rates of dopamine infusion, a modest increase in cardiac output at a low dose may be more beneficial hemodynamically than the integrated response produced by a higher dose of dopamine.

The multiple and variable pharmacological actions of dopamine (or epinephrine) dictate comprehensive assessment of several clinical parameters during the administration of the agent in the clinical setting. Whether the pressor response is dominated by $\alpha$, $\beta$, or $\delta$ activity determines the direction of the vagal response. However, in the dog studies the magnitude of the chronotropic effect has been no greater than the spontaneous fluctuation of cardiac rate.

Obviously, when viewed in the context of computer-based care, enormous potential for a comprehensive structured cardiovascular system management program is afforded by the automated measurements, automatic control of nitroprusside or trimethaphan, automated blood infusion to maintain LAP, and cardiac output (CO, CI) measurement by thermodilution (8). The following procedure is proposed for the management of epinephrine or dopamine by semi-automatic control of the drug infusion pump. After measurement of CO and CI the particular drug and initial dose are specified according to the desired effect – vasoconstriction or dilatation. At one-minute intervals the rate of infusion is increased using an increment of 10% of the desired dose. If the MAP or HR violates an upper or lower limit the rate of infusion is decremented and the decision is made to modify the limits, change agents, increase or decrease the dose, start nitroprusside, or an appropriate combination of these actions. Otherwise when the specified dose is reached the CI is measured again after an additional 5–10 min of constant infusion; the dose is then increased, decreased, or held constant depending on whether the desired level of performance has been achieved.

SUMMARY

The systemic and cardiac effects of dopamine and epinephrine were studied in open-chest dogs. The response dynamics of mean aortic blood flow, mean femoral blood flow rate, mean aortic pressure, mean left atrial pressure, mean coronary artery blood flow and mean cardiac rate were characterized using pseudo-random programmed infusion and correlation methods. The nature of the responses was related to the magnitude of the dose and the net effect of the hypothalamic integration of the diverse actions of each drug. However, dopamine, administered in increasing doses, consistently produced a response which suggests neural modulation of the cardiovascular control centres as demonstrated by a marked reduction in the time of occurrence of the maximum or minimum mean aortic pressure. Similarly, dopamine modulated the observed time interval between the pressor (or dilator) response and the vagal component of the baroreceptor reflex response. Based on these studies, structured rules were developed for the clinical use of these agents in management of patients in the Cardiac Surgical Intensive Care Unit following open intracardiac operations.

REFERENCES

1. Kirklin JW: Systems analysis in surgical patients with particular attention to the cardiac and pulmonary systems. 15th Macewen Memorial Lecture, University of Glasgow, 1970.
2. Sheppard LC, Sayers BMcA: Dynamic analysis of the blood pressure response to hypotensive agents, studied in postoperative cardiac surgical patients. *Comp Biomed Res* 10:237–246, 1977.
3. Schultz WC, Rideout VC: Control system performance measures: past, present, and future. *IRE Trans Automatic Control* AC-6:22–35, 1961.
4. Goldberg LI, Hsieh Y, Resnekov L: Newer catecholamines for treatment of heart failure and shock: an update on dopamine and a first look at dobutamine. *Prog Cardiovasc Diseases* 19:327–340, 1977.
5. Klevans LR, Gebber GL: Facilitatory forebrain influence on cardiac component of baroreceptor reflexes. *Am J Physiol* 219:1235–1241, 1970.
6. Weiss GK, Priola DV: Brainstem sites for activation of vagal cardioaccelerator fibers in the dog. *Am J Physiol* 223:300–304, 1972.
7. Abboud FM, Heistad DD, Mark AL, Schmid PG: Reflex control of the peripheral circulation. *Prog Cardiovasc Diseases* 18:371–403, 1976.
8. Sheppard LC, Kouchoukos NT: Automation of measurements and interventions in the systematic care of postoperative cardiac surgical patients. *Med Instrumentation* 11:296–301, 1977.

# 5.9. ASSESSMENT OF CARDIAC FUNCTION IN THE DOG BY CROSS-SECTIONAL ECHOCARDIOGRAPHY

Samuel Meerbaum, H.L. Wyatt, Ming Heng, Julio Cobo, Eliot Corday

## 1. INTRODUCTION

Experimental studies of cardiac function in normal states and during myocardial derangements have played an important role in providing an undertanding of physiologic mechanisms and formulating a rational basis for treatments. Fundamental to such studies are measurements of ventricular dimensions, volumes and segmental wall dynamics, all of which serve to define global and regional cardiac function. These measurements are essential to the assessment of progressive alterations such as the loss of contraction and increased myocardial stiffness which may supervene with ischaemic injury and infarction.

Animal models have ranged from open-chest procedures, frequently employed for exploratory investigations, to sophisticated comprehensively instrumented closed-chest or conscious animal preparations. Whenever logistics permit, the most valid simulation of physiologic states should clearly be aimed at, and it is often important to avoid thoracotomy and pericardiotomy which are known to result in substantial experimental artifacts. One of the limitations in deciding on preparations has been the unavailability of quantitative noninvasive measurements for the study of function and to reponse to reduced interventions. While recent application of M-mode echocardiography, cardiokymography and nuclear imaging have contributed useful data, these methods do not provide the desired simultaneous visualization or dynamic mapping of myocardial mechanics within all the segments of the left ventricle.

Tomographic real-time measurements by means of cross-sectional echocardiography (CSE) promises to overcome the above deficiencies. This technique should open up new vistas for experimental as well as clinical studies, and may bring about an improved understanding of factors related to evolvement and treatment of ischaemic heart disease (1, 2, 3). Serial and sequential CSE short and long-axis sections allow reconstruction of left ventricular volumes as well as detailed study of segmental wall motions throughout the ventricle (4, 5, 6, 7, 8, 9, 10, 11). The technique is totally noninvasive, atraumatic, readily repeatable and economical, but it remains to be validated as a quantitative methodology. A number of problems,

J. Baan, A.C. Arntzenius, E.L. Yellin (eds.), Cardiac Dynamics, 405–415.

errors or inadequacies of present imaging have already been pointed out (12) and major bioengineering advances in the ultrasound systems may be anticipated in the future. Our objective was to develop the use of CSE in the experimental animal, and to validate currently representative CSE against direct measurements of volumes and regional cardiac function.

## 2. THE CSE SYSTEM

Our studies were performed with the commercial Varian V-3000 ultrasonic real-time phase-array sector scanner. The engineering characteristics of this cross-sectional echocardiography system have been described (13). The ultrasonograph features an 84° sector angle, 30 frames/sec, a range up to 21 cm and a 64 lines/frame presentation. The unit consists of a videorecorder and monitor. There is an ECG display Polaroid and 90 mm photography with stills triggered by the ECG, as well as M-mode recording at selected sites and periods. The transducer has 32 active elements, array length and width are 13 and 12 mm respectively, lens focal length is 80 mm, and the frequency range is 2–3 mHz. The ultrasonic beam from this transducer is directed through intercostal spaces at different levels and in various directions for short-axis and long-axis cross-sectional visualization of the heart.

## 3. THE CSE DOG MODEL

In the past, echocardiographic studies in the dog were considered difficult, largely because of the dog's chest configuration. For studies of myocardial ischaemia, echocardiography was unable adequately to visualize the anterior left ventricular wall which is frequently studied for its reponse to partial and total occlusions of the left anterior coronary artery. In contrast with other attempts (14) the closed-chest model developed in our laboratory does not necessitate prior surgical intervention or instrument implantation. The dog is simply normally laid on its right side onto a table equipped with appropriate cutouts through which the CSE transducer is directed upward against the dog's chest at the fourth or fith intercostal level (Figure 1). Presumably, lung tissue which impedes echocardiographic imaging is sufficiently displaced to provide good definition of the dog's endocardial and epicardial left ventricular interfaces, including the anterior region which is most distant from the transducer. With this closed-chest model, satisfactory visualization in several short and long-axis cross-sectional views has been obtained by us in about 90% of the approximately 200 dogs studied so far. Most recently, similar quality CSE images were demonstrated in our laboratory in conscious animals trained to lie on their side on the above table.

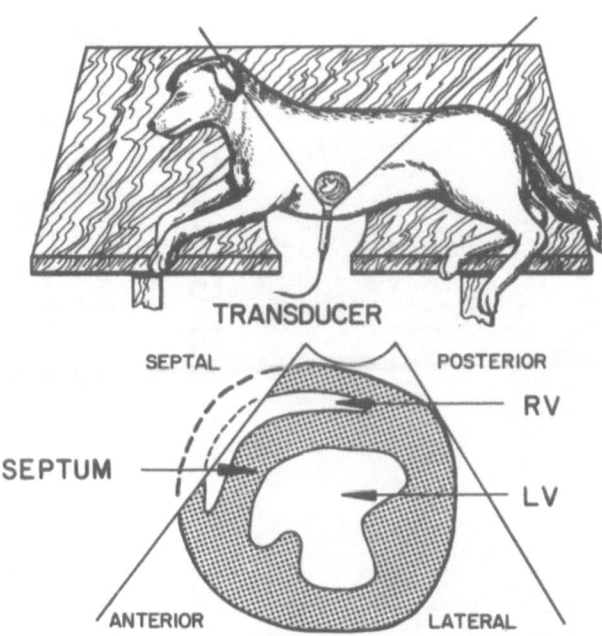

*Figure 1.* Examination table equipped with window and transducer location for noninvasive cross-section echocardiography (CSE) in dogs. The dog is laid on its right side onto the table and the transducer is pointed upward through the table window onto the chest wall, in the fourth or fifth intercostal space about 2–6 cm from the sternum. A CSE schematic short axis view at the papillary muscle level is indicated below, showing the visualized anatomic configuration, including septum, anterior, lateral and posterior walls of the left ventricle.

## 4. SHORT AND LONG-AXIS CSE CROSS-SECTIONS

Polaroids in Figure 2 illustrate a typical CSE definition of endocardium and epicardium achieved with our dog model. Delineation of endocardial and epicardial surfaces is actually greatly enhanced by video observations of real-time dynamics of the ventricular walls (demonstrated in a film presentation of the real-time contractile motions of ventricular sections before and after coronary occlusion as well as reperfusion). Nevertheless, questions remain with regard to image uncertainties of the exact position of the cardiac interfaces and some echo "dropouts" along the endocardial or epicardial contour requiring interpolation. In vitro calibrations of the CSE system with an array of discrete wires of known dimensions and distances have provided clues as to the position of the CSE signature which actually represents the interfaces, while in vivo confirmation is accomplished by intraventricular infusions and microbubble delineation of the acoustic echo from the endocardial interface. For dogs larger than 30 kg, we often found it necessary to extrapolate the long-axis section in order to estimate the

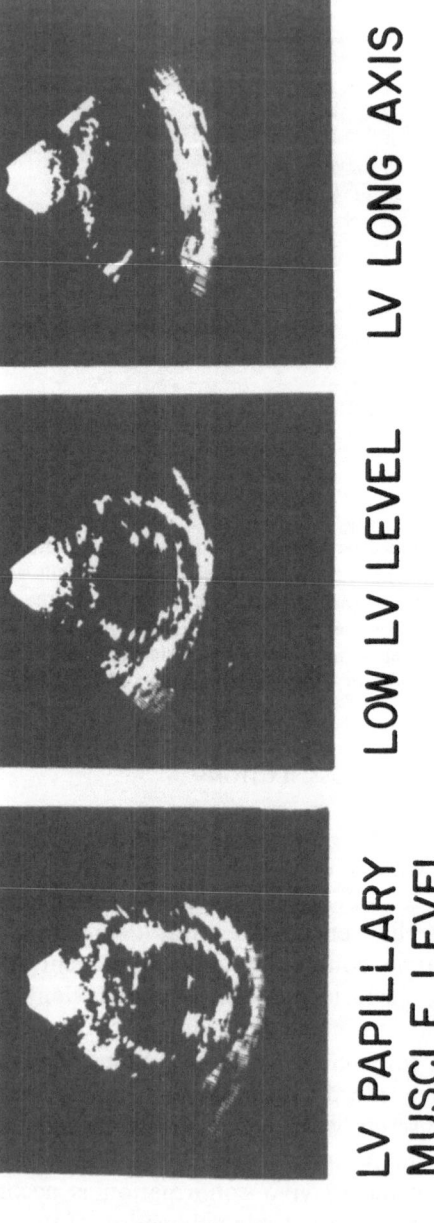

LV PAPILLARY MUSCLE LEVEL    LOW LV LEVEL    LV LONG AXIS

*Figure 2.* Typical polaroids of images obtained with cross-sectional echocardiography (CSE) in closed-chest dogs. Two left ventricular short axis sections (one at the papillary muscle level and another at a lower level of the ventricle) as well as a long axis section are shown. The quality and reproducibility of endocardial and epicardial interface definition was found to be very good in 90% of the dogs, based on analysis of videotapes of geometry and motions of left ventricular walls. The long axis view demonstrates the difficulty of imaging the ventricular apex in large dogs.

portions of the apex or else combine two long-axis CSE views so as to reconstruct the left ventricular length.

Both ventricular length and several short-axis cross-sections were normally obtained for volume reconstruction by means of Simpson's rule, the basis of which is indicated in Figure 3. It should be noted that tomographic CSE sections allow Simpson volume reconstruction of left ventricles even in the presence of significant and highly regional asymmetries; such may be

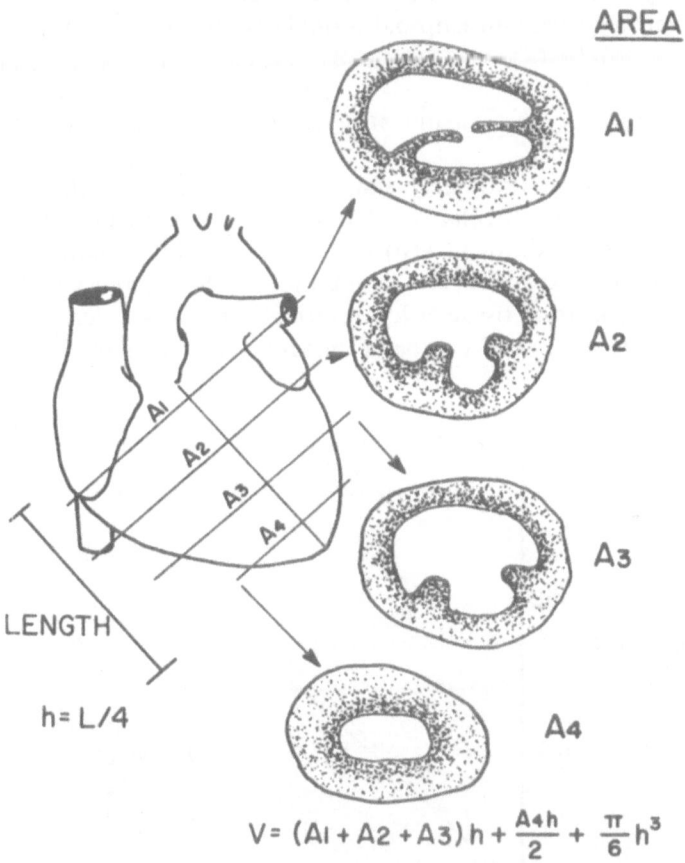

$$V = (A1 + A2 + A3) h + \frac{A4h}{2} + \frac{\pi}{6} h^3$$

*Figure 3.* Volume reconstruction from cross-sectional echocardiography (CSE) measurements of short and long-axis sections. Shown here are short-axis sections at the level of the mitral valve, high and low papillary regions, and the apical segment of the left ventricle. A long section view (not shown) is used to derive the apex to mitral-aortic junction length, which is divided by the number of short-axis sections to give "slabs" of equal height. Short-axis lumen area (regardless of asymmetry) is multiplied by the cylindrical slab height except for the apical segment where an ellipsoidal formula is employed (last two terms of the summation formula for left ventricular volume).

encountered with profound segmental ischaemia, and myocardial infarction. Section areas can be obtained by planimetry or more economically with a digitized pen allowing direct computerized analysis. The intraobserver, independent interobserver and beat-to-beat reproducibility of such measurements was found by us to range from 2.5% to 7.5%, indicating that these determinations are an acceptable basis for quantitative reconstruction. The left ventricle length is subdivided into short-axis "slabs" on the basis of the number of CSE sections. The mathematical model indicated in Figure 3 employs cylindrical slabs of CSE-derived sections except at the lower level of the ventricle where an ellipsoid formula is used for the apical region.

## 5. VALIDATION OF CSE MEASUREMENT OF VENTRICULAR VOLUMES

Utilizing the above extremely simple computational methods, we have performed a left ventricular validation study in closed-chest dogs. CSE assessment was made of in vivo end-diastolic volumes contained by endocardium and epicardium, and by multiplying the difference by the specific gravity of myocardial tissue, a left ventricular mass was derived. The CSE measurements were then compared against the weight of the excised left

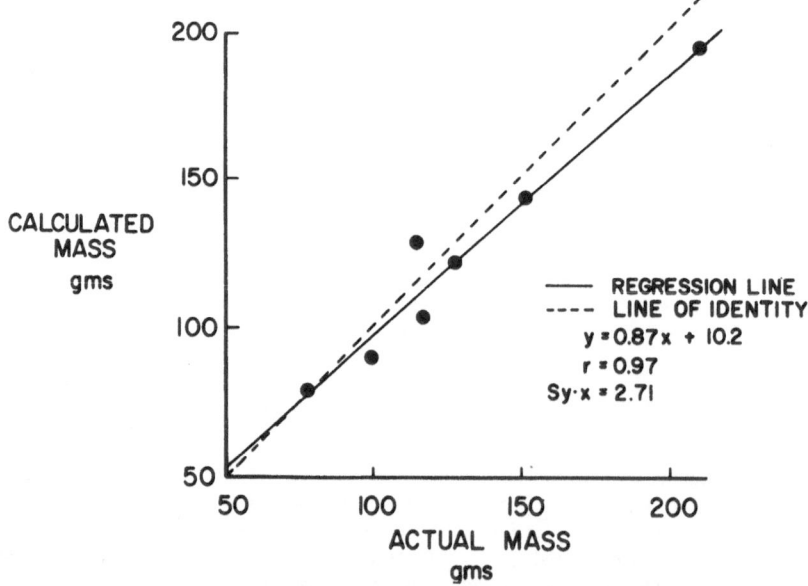

*Figure 4.* Correlation in seven closed-chest dogs between cross-sectional echocardiography derived mass of the left ventricle vs. measured weight of the excised ventricles. Linear regression and identity lines are indicated. $S_{yx}$ is the standard error of estimate.

ventricles. Figure 4 indicates a good correlation observed in this preliminary study.

Basic validation of left ventricular volumes was approached by us through in vitro studies of excised hearts. Formalin-fixed hearts of a variety of sizes and of geometric configurations were immersed in oil. CSE studies were then performed to obtain a series of short and long-axis cross-sections for volume reconstruction. The actual ventricular volume was determined accurately by fluid filling up to the valve ring. Figure 5 shows our early results and, again, indicates excellent correlation with the Simpson CSE reconstruction. Since it will be desirable, in many studies, to estimate ventricular volumes with procedures involving the least possible number of cross-sectional views, other mathematical model were also examined. Thus, the in vitro CSE validation allowed direct volume comparisons and also provided useful information on possible models which might be employed for left ventricular volume measurements. A study of in vivo CSE versus contrast left ventriculography is also being performed by us in a series of closed-chest dogs since cineangography is a standard procedure employed for determining left ventricular volumes.

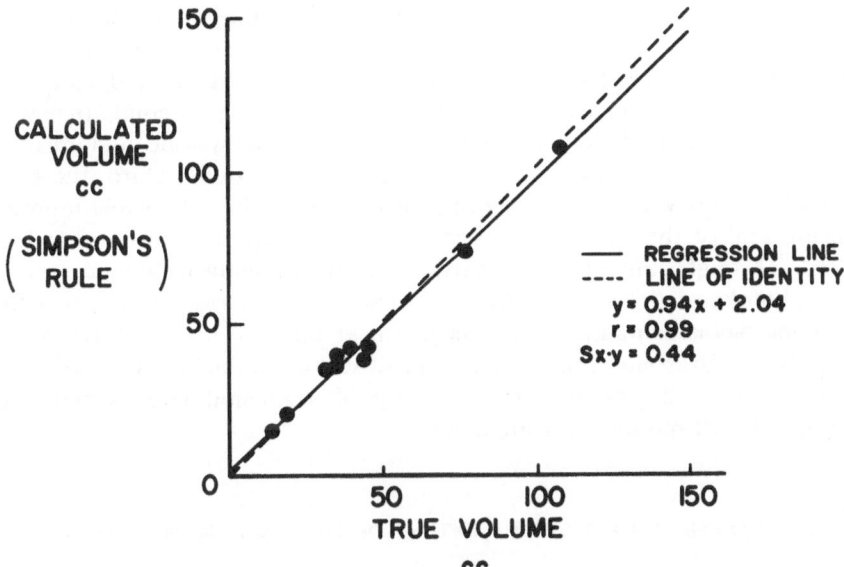

*Figure 5.* Correlation of left ventricular volumes in formalin-fixed canine hearts measured with cross-sectional echocardiography (CSE) and direct fluid filling of the ventricle. Simpson's rule reconstruction from CSE views was employed analogous to the procedure employed in closed-chest dogs. Linear regression and identity lines are shown. $S_{xy}$ represents the standard error of estimate.

## 6. CSE MEASUREMENT OF VENTRICULAR SEGMENTAL WALL MOTIONS

Noninvasive quantitation of segmental wall motions is a fundamental requirement for CSE. Global and segmental cardiac function should be accurately assessed in normal states and during derangements caused by myocardial ischaemia and infarction, leading to regional dyssynergy, scar tissue or aneurysm. As already indicated, real-time tomographic presentation with CSE has the potential of providing satisfactory noninvasive measurements in every segment of the left ventricle, i.e. the free walls, papillary muscles, interventricular septum and intracardiac structures. The effects of acute coronary occlusions or interventions on segmental function can, for example, be studied in short-axis cross-sections in terms of the individual or interrelated response of directly ischaemic, adjacent and remote zones. Frame-by-frame analysis of diastolic and systolic CSE views provides a basis for documenting the contractile dynamics in ischaemia, i.e. whether a particular segment exhibits normal or hyperfunction, hypokinesis, akinesis, or paradoxical dyskinesis. The question is, of course, to what extent these CSE derived measurements of segmental wall motions are a quantitative representation of actual cardiac mechanics.

The CSE procedure employed by us in delineating wall motions and segmental derangements of function was as follows: first, the videotape was played back at normal and slow speed to make a qualitative judgement as to the site and extent of the contractile dysfunction. Second, this was assessed more objectively by superimposing traced systolic and distolic epicardial and endocardial outlines of individual sections. Third, the borders of the dyssynergic area were confirmed by holding the superimposed tracing against the video image and running the tape several times at low speed. Through computerized analysis, signal averaging techniques and a new photokymographic monitoring of cardiac interfaces, the above CSE methodology is being made more economical and less subjective. However, more basic ultrasound image enhancement will undoubtedly be required to ensure a high degree of reproducibility of segmental endocardial and epicardial wall motion measurements.

## 7. CSE DETERMINATIONS OF THE EXTENT OF DYSSYNERGIC MYOCARDIUM

One of our CSE animal studies of myocardial ischaemia compared echo-derived contractile derangements with direct measurements using myocardial gauges applied in corresponding segments. Based on observed correspondence of sites and function in several dogs, we performed a comparison between force gauge mapping (20–25 sites) of an acutely ischemic

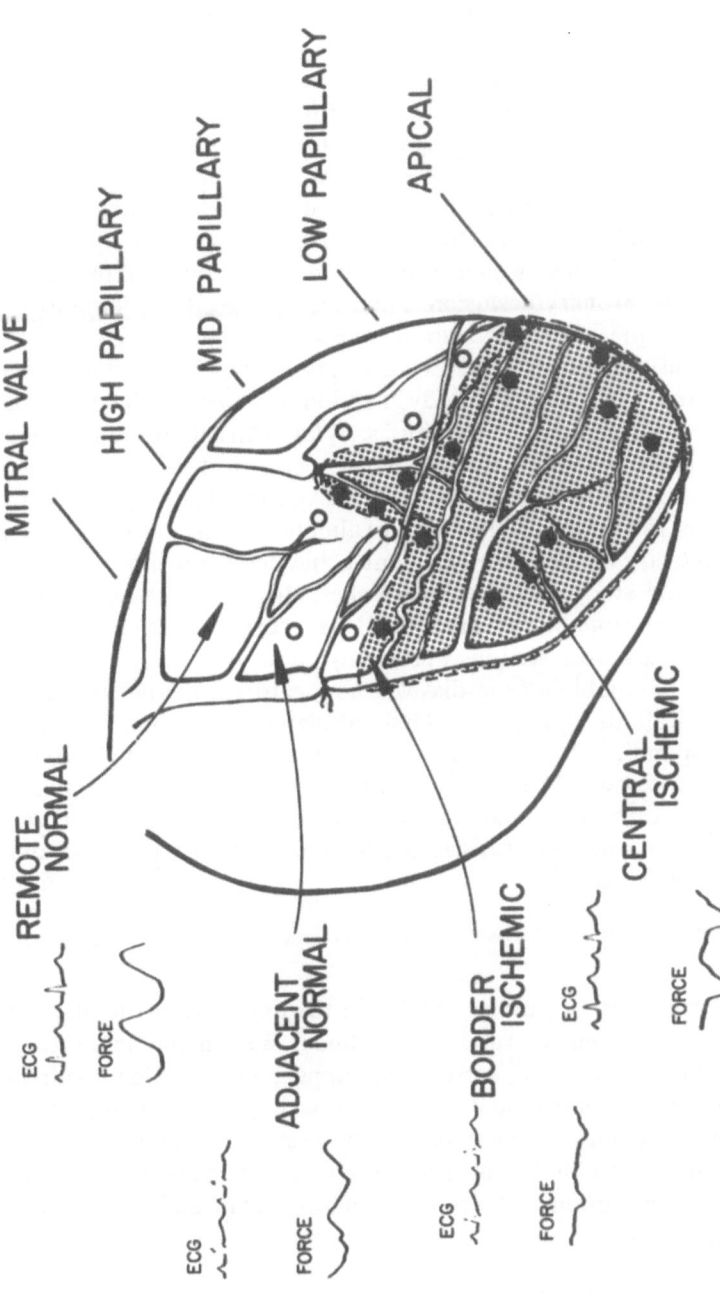

*Figure 6.* This schematic illustrates force gauge mapping of the anterior left ventricular wall in dogs and approximate location of short-axis cross-sections at which two-dimensional echocardiographic views were obtained. Coronary ligations are indicated, and the speckled area represents the ischaemic dysfunctioning area determined by extensive and repeated gauge mapping at many sites, particularly at the margins of the injured zone. ECG and myocardial force recordings are shown on the left of the figure for specific regions of the left ventricle. Normal function was defined as positive systolic force development, and ischaemic dysfunction was defined as either zero or negative force development. The latter has been shown to correspond to segmental dyskinesis in the region of the gauge and loss of contractile force to the point where mural tension prevails.

zone versus CSE cross-sectional analysis of the extent of dysfunction. In this initial study, dogs were placed on their right side and CSE was performed in a manner analogous to our other canine studies, however, the left side of the chest was opened to permit mapping of the ischaemic zone. A piezoresistive gauge developed in conjunction with the Jet Propulsion Laboratory of the California Institute of Technology, was found to be suitable for essentially atraumatic and rapid mapping at as many as 25 sites. The myocardial gauge tracing exhibits a characteristic positive upward stroke during normal contraction, and clearly portrays regional akinesis and dyskinesis (negative downward stroke) which ensue in most instances immediately following an acute coronary occlusion. Figure 6 indicates the procedure of gauge mapping of the ischaemic zone in one dog. Based on prior verification studies and anatomic landmarks, corresponding CSE sections were used to reconstruct the size of the dysfunctioning zone of the ventricle exhibiting segmental akinesis or dyskinesis. While satisfactory correlation ($r = 0.95$) was noted of these independently performed ischaemic zone delineations, performed in 8 cases, more extensive investigation and reproducibility studies will clearly be needed to validate fully the ability of CSE to quantitate the size of the zone with contractile derangements.

A second animal study involved closed-chest dogs with 48-hour intracoronary plug occlusion of the proximal LAD coronary artery. In this study, CSE short-axis cross-sections were analysed for dyssynergy using the above procedure of combining end-diastolic endocardial superposition with observation of wall dynamics. Nitro-blue-tetrazolium staining was employed in corresponding slabs of excised left ventricles to delineate infarcted and noninfarcted zones. The CSE-derived mechanical dyssynergy consistently exceeded the size of infarction, and correlation between these two measurements was found to be satisfactory ($r = 0.89$). Further studies of this type are being implemented.

## 8. COMMENT

The described experimental studies of CSE in the dog were preliminary in character and more extensive validation is under way in our laboratory. However, the initial data and correlations appear encouraging, both in terms of ventricular volume and segmental wall motion quantitation. Reliable noninvasive measurement of regional as well as global cardiac function or dysfunction in ischaemic syndromes and following interventions will constitute an important advance in the management and treatment of ischaemic heart disease.

REFERENCES

1. Birnholz J, Wynne J, Finberg H, Alpert JS: Two-dimension echocardiography in acute myocardial infarction. *Circulation* 55/56 (suppl: 3–827:158, 1977.
2. Wynne J, Birnholz J, Finberg H, Alpert JS: Regional left ventricular wall motion in acute myocardial infarction as assessed by two-dimensional echocardiography. *Circulation* 55/56 (suppl 3–152):583, 1977.
3. Heger J, Weyman AE, Noble RJ, Dillon JC, Feigenbaum H: An analysis of the site, extent, an hemodynamic consequences of acute myocardial infarction by cross-sectional echocardiography. *Circulation* 55/56:584, 1977.
4. Wyatt HL, Heng MK, Meerbaum S, Davidson R, Lee SS, Corday E: Quantitative left ventricular analysis in dogs with the phased array sector scan. *Circulation* 56:(4, suppl 3)3:152, 1977.
5. Wyatt HL, Heng MK, Meerbaum S, Davidson R, Corday E: Noninvasive two-dimensional echocardiography: quantitative analysis of the left ventricle. *Physiologist* 20:103, 1977.
6. Wyatt HL, Heng MK, Meerbaum S, Davidson R, Corday E: Evaluation of models for quantifying ventricular size by 2-dimensional echocardiography. *Am J Cardiol* 41:369, 1978.
7. Kohm MS, Schapira JN, Beaver WL, Popp RL: In vitro estimation of canine left ventricular volumes by phased array sector scan. *Clin Res* 26(3):244A, 1977.
8. Charuzi Y, Davidson RM, Barrett MJ, Swan HJC: Segmental wall motion in acute myocardial infarction determined by wide angle 2-dimensional echocardiography. *Amer Fed Clin Res* 26:223A, 1978.
9. Schiller N, Botvinick E, Cogan J, Greenberg B, Acquatella H, Glantz S: Noninvasive methods are reliable predictors of contrast angiographic left ventricular volumes. *Circulation* 55/56 (suppl 3–221):857, 1977.
10. Chaudry R, Ogawa S, Pauletto FJ, Hubbard FE, Dreifus LS: Biplane measurements of left and right ventricular volumes using wide angle cross-sectional echocardiography. *Am J Cardiol* 41:391, 1978.
11. Kisslo JA, Robertson D, Gilbert BW, et al: A comparison of real-time, two-dimensional echocardiography and cineangiography in detecting left ventricular asynergy. *Circulation* 55:134–141, 1977.
12. Roelandt J, Van Dorp WG, Bom N, Laird JD, Hugenholz PG: Resolution problems in echocardiography: a source of interpretation errors. *Am J Cardiol* 37:256, 1976.
13. Anderson WA, Arnold JT, Clark D, et al: A new real-time phased array sector scanner for imaging the entire adult human heart. In: *Ultrasound in medicine*, vol 3A, New York, Plenum, 1976.
14. Franklin Jr TD, Weyman AE, Egenes KM: A closed-chest canine model for cross-sectional echocardiographic study. *Am J Physiol* 233(3):H417–H419, 1977.

## 5.10. DYNAMICS OF THE LEFT VENTRICULAR CENTRE OF MASS IN INTACT UNANAESTHETIZED MAN IN THE PRESENCE AND ABSENCE OF WALL MOTION ABNORMALITIES

Neil B. Ingels, Jr., Carol Mead,
George T. Daughters II,
Edward B. Stinson, Edwin L. Alderman

### 1. INTRODUCTION

Over the past two decades there has been increasing interest in quantifying the motion of the left ventricular centre of mass throughout the cardiac cycle.

Noordergraaf (1) first attempted to estimate longitudinal left ventricular centre of mass dynamics in his studies on the theoretical basis of the ballistocardiogram. Later, he and van de Weerd (2) extended these studies to predict the lateral displacement of the centre of mass as well. Morse and Longoria (3) measured longitudinal and anterior-posterior displacement of the centre of gravity of the whole heart in dogs and stressed the importance of measuring such dynamics along both axes.

Pearlman et al. (4) suggested recently that the human left ventricular walls might contract symmetrically towards the centre of mass of the chamber. Heintzen et al. (5), in describing a computerized system for contraction pattern analysis, suggested that the left ventricular centre of gravity might be a stable and useful point for such analysis. Rickards et al. (6) extended this work and showed that the average rotation of a line through the midpoint of the aortic valve and the centre of gravity from systole to diastole was minimal in the human ventricle as determined by contrast angiography.

In spite of this interest, however, no detailed studies of the motion of the left ventricular centre of mass throughout the cardiac cycle have been reported. The present study was therefore designed to measure these dynamics in intact unanaesthetized man, both with and without wall motion abnormalities, using computer-processed fluoroscopy of radiopaque markers implanted into the left ventricular myocardium at the time of cardiac surgery.

*J. Baan, A.C. Arntzenius, E.L. Yellin (eds.), Cardiac Dynamics, 417–431.*

## 2. METHODS

### 2.1. Patient groups

A total of nineteen patients was studied, divided into two groups: a "normal" group consisting of ten patients with normal volumetric parameters and wall dynamics, and an "abnormal" group consisting of nine patients with abnormal volumetric parameters and at least one akinetic wall segment as measured in the 30° right anterior oblique plane. Studies were conducted 0.4 to 4.6 months after surgery (cardiac transplantation in 8 patients and coronary artery bypass surgery in 11 patients). Summary data for the two patient groups, calculated as previously described (7, 8), are given in Table 1.

Table 1. Summary data for two patient groups studied: TX = cardiac transplant recipient; CABG = coronary artery bypass graft patient.

|  | Normal | Abnormal |
|---|---|---|
| Patients (surgery) | 10(6TX, 4 CABG) | 9(2TX, 7 CABG) |
| End-diastolic volume | $133 \pm 22$ ml | $139 \pm 37$ ml |
| End-systolic volume | $51 \pm 9$ ml | $72 \pm 24$ ml $(p < .02)$ |
| Stroke volume | $82 \pm 16$ ml | $67 \pm 15$ ml |
| Heart rate | $74 \pm 16$ beats/min | $84 \pm 13$ beats/min |
| Cardiac output | $6.0 \pm 0.9$ l/min | $5.6 \pm 1.2$ l/min |
| Ejection fraction | $62 \pm 5\%$ | $49 \pm 5\%$ $(p < 10^{-4})$ |
| Contraction velocity | $1.07 \pm 0.08$ circ/sec | $0.77 \pm 0.16$ circ/sec $(p < 10^{-4})$ |

### 2.2. Marker implantation

At surgery, as previously described (7, 8) and with informed consent, each patient had seven tantalum markers implanted into the left ventricular midwall; three in the anterior wall, three in the inferior wall, and one in the apex, so as to silhouette the left ventricular chamber in the 30° right anterior oblique projection (Figure 1). An additional pair of silver tantalum clips was affixed to the adventitia of the ascending aorta, at a location 2 cm above the aortic valve ring (Figure 1, bottom) in order to delineate the position of the aortic valve.

Figure 1. Top: right anterior oblique aspect of the heart showing marker sites ( × ) lying in the projection plane; bottom: cross-section of the left ventricle showing midwall markers, aortic valve defined by translated aortic markers, and seven triangles used to calculate areas in the RAO projection.

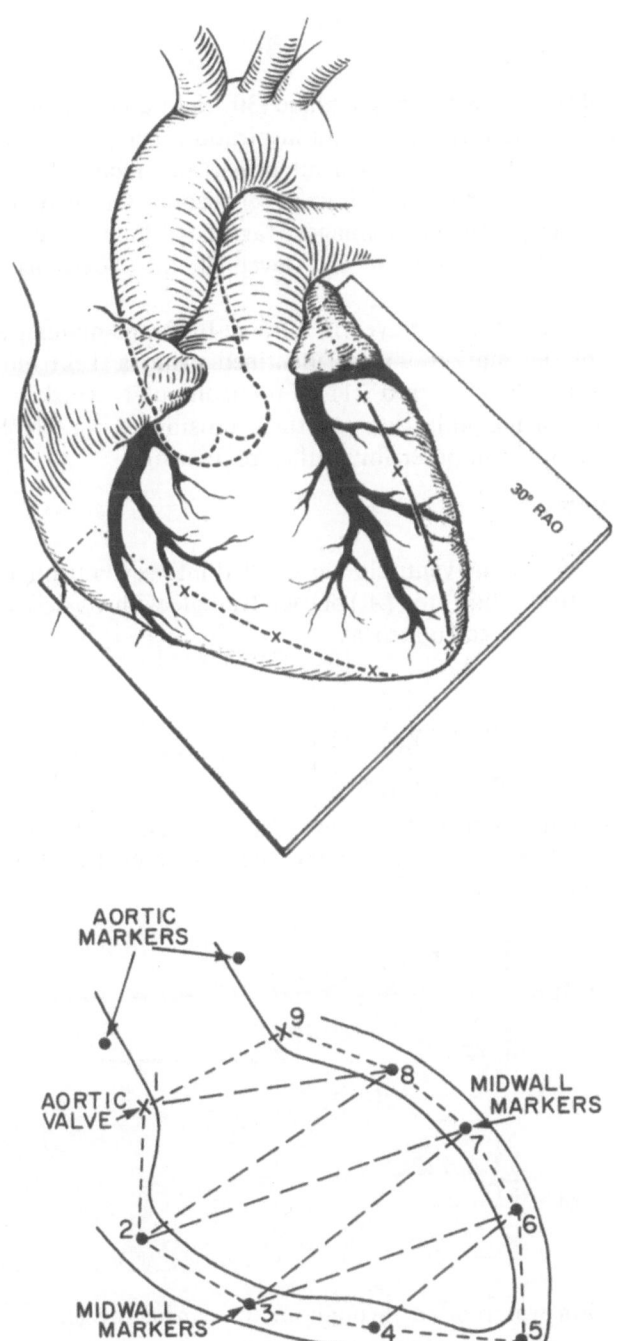

## 2.2. Data acquisition

At the time of study, resting single-plane (30° right anterior oblique) cardiac fluoroscopy was performed at end-inspiration using a Philips 300MA generator with a Philips nine-inch intensifier and recorded on an Ampex DR10A video disc recorder at 30 frames per second. The lead-II ECG signal was superimposed on the video image. Magnification factor was determined by imaging a 1 cm grid at the level of the heart as determined echographically.

Video recordings were replayed in a frame-by-frame manner and the $X$-$Y$ coordinates of the marker images identified using a Tektronix light pen coupled to a Hewlett-Packard 2115A minicomputer. Marker coordinates were corrected for magnification and then transmitted via telephone line to a CDC6400 digital computer for further processing.

### 2.3. DATA ANALYSIS

At each sample time, the ventricle was divided into seven triangles as shown in Figure 1 (bottom). The area ($A_i$) of each triangle with vertices ($X_l$, $Y_l$), ($X_m$, $Y_m$), and ($X_n$, $Y_n$), was calculated as

$$A_i = \pm \tfrac{1}{2} \begin{vmatrix} X_l & Y_l & 1 \\ X_m & Y_m & 1 \\ X_n & Y_n & 1 \end{vmatrix} \qquad [1]$$

and the coordinates of its centre of area ($XCA_i$, $YCA_i$) from the intersection of its medians. The coordinates of the ventricular centre of mass ($XCM$, $YCM$) were calculated as

$$XCM = \frac{\sum\limits_{i=1}^{7} A_i\, XCA_i}{\sum\limits_{i=1}^{7} A_i}, \qquad [2]$$

and

$$YCM = \frac{\sum\limits_{i=1}^{7} A_i\, YCA_i}{\sum\limits_{i=1}^{7} A_i} \qquad [3]$$

and the position was plotted throughout the cardiac cycle.

In addition, the centre of mass coordinates were plotted at end-diastole and end-systole along with the positions of the midwall and (translated) aortic markers plotted at 33 millisecond intervals from end-diastole to end-systole. The total path length traversed by the centre of mass at end-diastole and end-systole was calculated, as was the distance between the centre of mass at end-diastole and end-systole. The distance from the midpoint of the aortic valve to the centre of mass was also calculated and plotted as a function of time from end-diastole to end-systole.

The maximum energy expenditure ($E$) to translate the centre of mass in systole was calculated for each beat from its position at end-diastole ($ED$) to its position at end-systole ($ES$) as

$$E = p \sum_{j=ED}^{ES} V_{t_j} \, a_{t_j} \, \Delta S_{t_j} \qquad [4]$$

joules, where $p$ is the volume density of blood and muscle (assumed equal), $V_{t_j}$ is the total volume of the ventricular myocardium and its contents at time $t_j$, $a_{t_j}$ is the acceleration of the centre of mass of the ventricle at time $t_j$, and $\Delta S_j$ is the distance travelled by the centre of mass from $t_{j-1}$ to $t_j$.

3. RESULTS

Representative segmental, aortic, and centre of mass dynamics for three patients in the group with normal dynamics and three patients in the group with abnormal dynamics are shown in Figures. 2 and 3, respectively.

In the patients with normal wall motion, translations of the centre of mass were small relative to the motions of the ventricular midwall segments. In the normal group as a whole, the total centre of mass path length was $6.0 \pm 1.3$ mm from end-diastole to end-systole, which resulted in a net translation of the centre of mass of $2.6 \pm 1.2$ mm for the group over this interval. In general, although still small, centre of mass translations were greater in the patients with wall motion abnormalities. For this group, average centre of mass path length was $7.6 \pm 1.8$ mm and net translation was $4.6 \pm 1.3$ mm from end-diastole to end-systole.

The centre of mass vector from end-diastole to end-systole tended to be directed toward akinetic segments although this tendency did not achieve statistical significance in the present study, with the angle between this vector and the ventricular long axis being $83° \pm 28°$ in the group with anterior wall motion abnormalities and $51° \pm 47°$ in the group with normal segmental dynamics. Thus, in both groups, this vector was rotated clockwise (toward the anterior wall) from a reference vector at $0°$ pointed at the aortic valve midpoint.

The nearly invariant centre of mass position throughout systole was brought about by midwall segmental dynamics which were not directed at the centre of mass. Illustrated in Figure 2 are the typical inward and

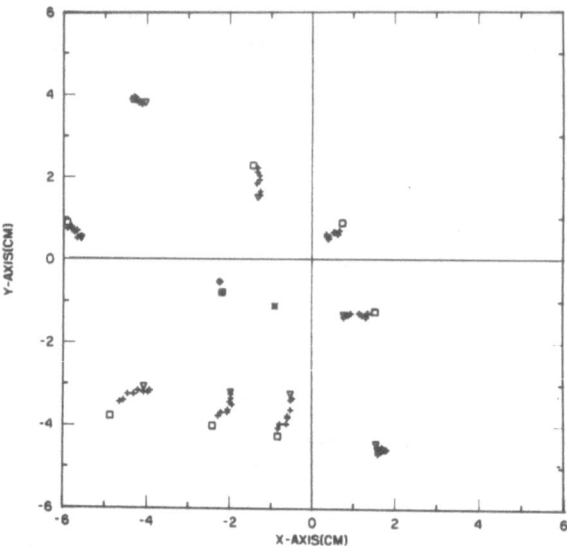

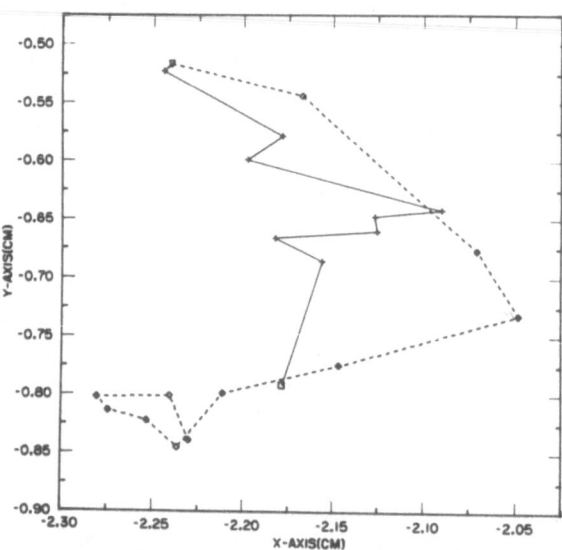

*Figure 2. Upper panels*: Segmental and aortic dynamics at 33 msec intervals from end-diastole to end-systole for three patients in the group with normal dynamics; □: end-diastolic position; ▽: end-systolic position; ⊞: centre of mass at end-diastole; ◆: centre of mass at end systole; ▩: centre of strain representing that point toward which, to best approximation, segmental

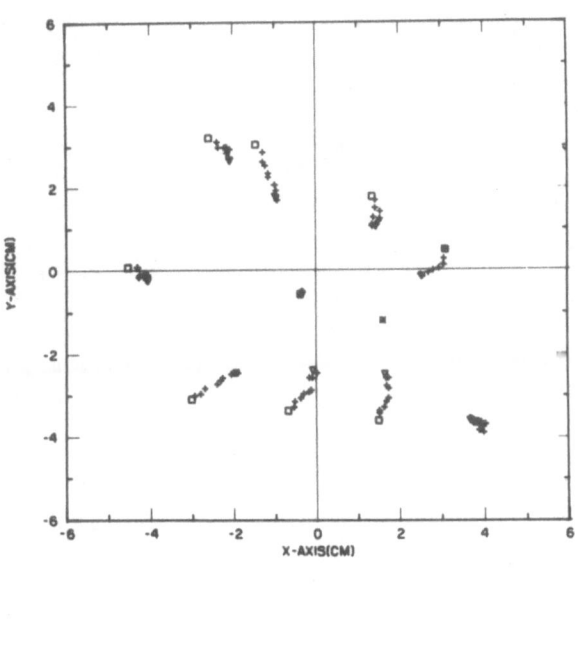

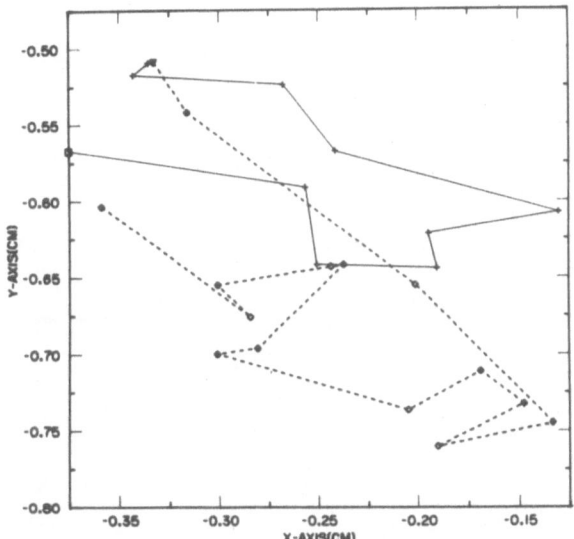

*Figure 2.* Continued
motion is directed; *lower panels*: motion of the centre of mass at 33 msec intervals throughout
the cardiac cycle for the beat shown in the panel directly above; □: end-diastole; ▽: end-
systole; Solid line: motion during systole; dashed line: motion during diastole.

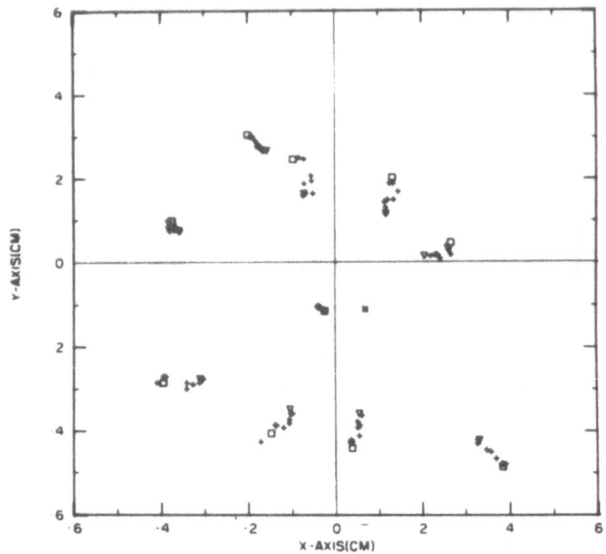

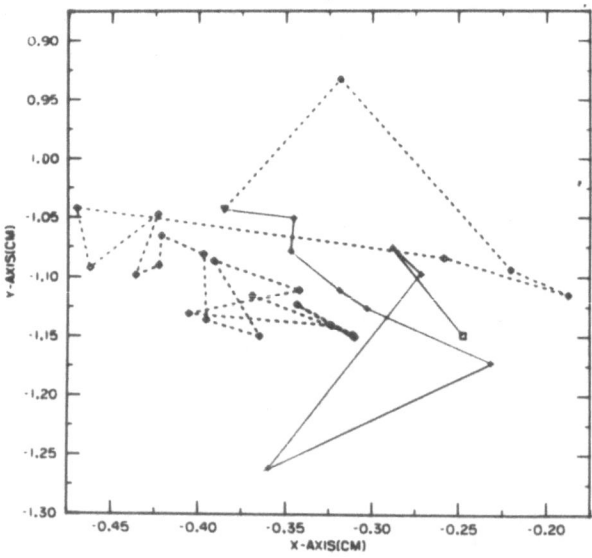

*Figure 2.* Continued

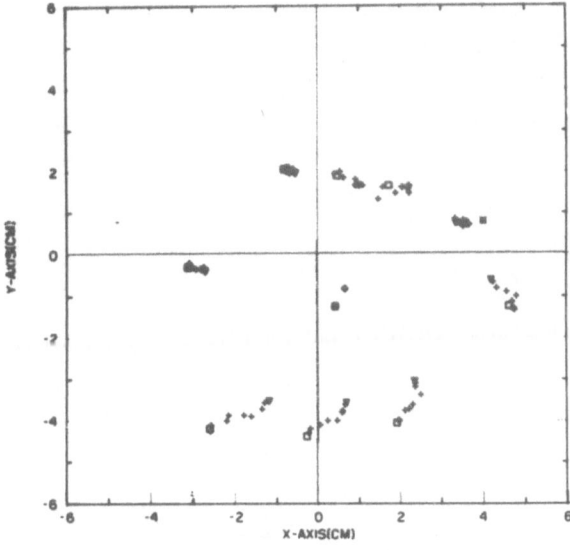

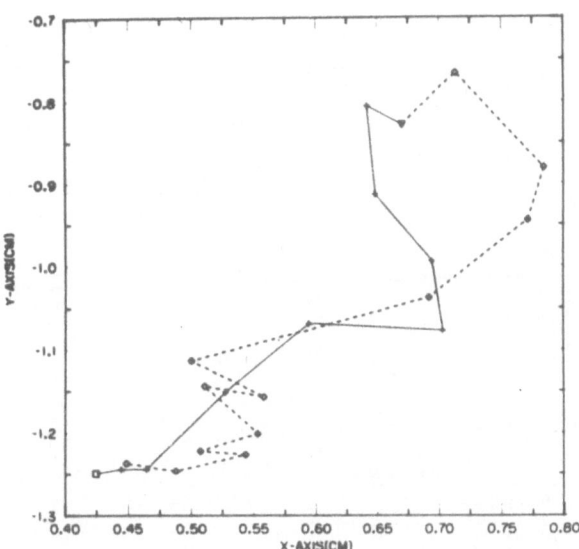

*Figure 3.* Segmental, aortic, and centre of mass dynamics for three patients in the group with wall motion abnormalities. Key as in Figure 2.

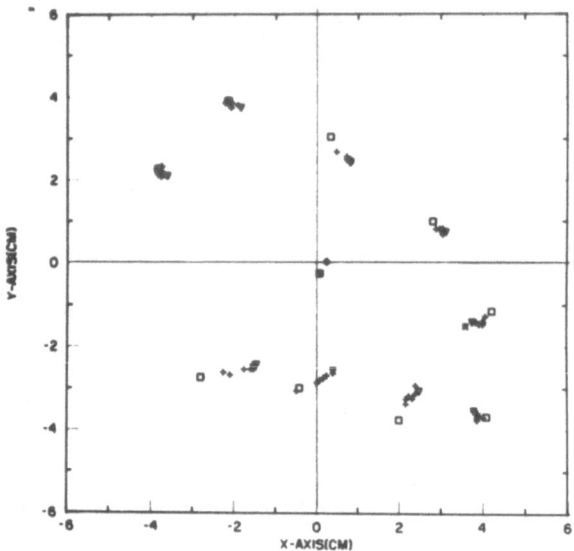

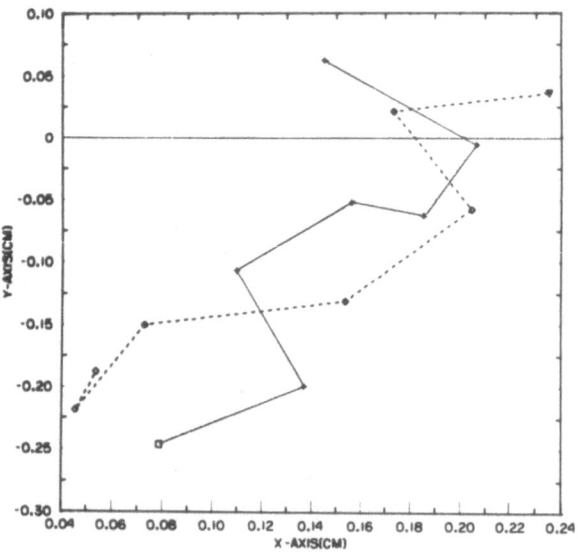

*Figure 3.* Continued

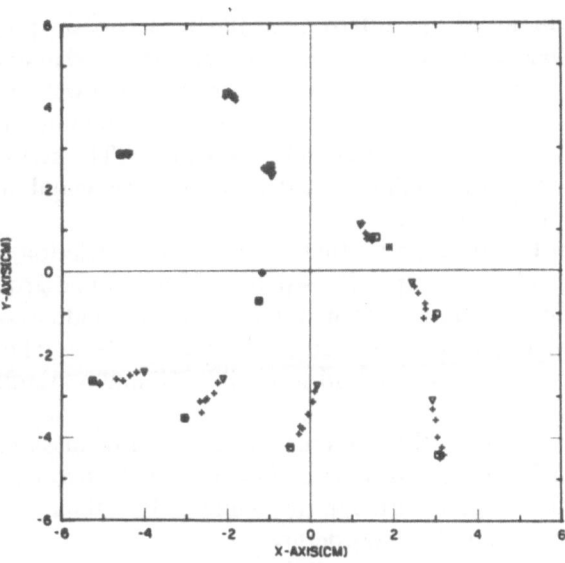

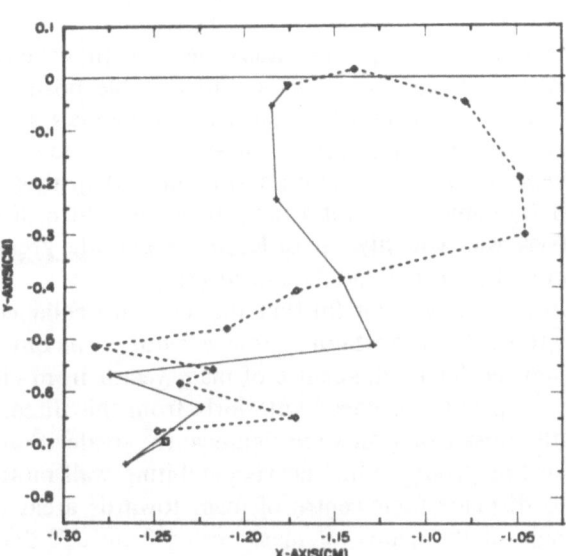

*Figure 3.* Continued

downward motions of the anterobasal and posterobasal points (points 2 and 8), the inward and upward motions of the anteroapical and posteroapical segments (points 4 and 6), and the almost purely inward motions of the midbase-apex segments (points 3 and 7), a common finding in our previous studies of midwall segmental dynamics in man (9). The resulting centre of strain, representing that point toward which the segmental vectors appear to be moving, is also shown.

Note also in Figures 2 and 3 that mean apical translation is nonzero. In fact, by end-systole, mean apical translation in the normal group as a whole was not significantly different from anteroapical and midbase-apex segmental translation in the 30° right anterior oblique plane. The aortic valve midpoint, not the apex, was found to exhibit minimum systolic translation in these patients.

The distance between the left ventricular centre of mass and the aortic valve midpoint for the first 400 msec of systole for the two patient groups is plotted in Figure 4. Also plotted in this figure is the estimate of this distance as calculated originally by Noordergraaf (1).

The energy expenditure in translating the left ventricular mass in systole was found to be $0.4 \pm 0.2$ millijoules in the group with normal dynamics and $0.5 \pm 0.3$ millijoules in the group with abnormal dynamics.

4. DISCUSSION

The principal findings in the present study were: (1) that the centre of mass of the left ventricle is maintained at a rather stable position throughout systole in patients with normal left ventricular dynamics and, (2) that the path length traversed by the centre of mass during systole, while small, is greater in patients with wall motion abnormalities than those with normal left ventricular dynamics. The total motion of the centre of mass in both groups, however, was roughly an order of magnitude greater than that measured in dogs by Morse and Longorio (3).

Rickards' group's suggestion (6) that the left ventricular centre of mass moves directly towards the aorta in systole was not borne out in the present study. In the normal heart, the centre of mass vector from end-diastole to end-systole was typically displaced anteriorly from this direction, since the excursions of the posterior wall were significantly greater than those of the anterior wall in this group. While hearts exhibiting wall motion abnormalities tended to displace their centre of mass towards areas of akinesis in systole, the angle of the centre of mass vector from end-diastole to end-systole relative to the ventricular long axis did not, in itself, prove reliable in differentiating the two groups. The two groups could be perfectly discriminated, however, by several indices taking both magnitude and direction of centre of mass translation into account, simultaneously.

The suggestion of Pearlman et al. (4) that left ventricular segmental shortening is directed toward the centre of mass is not supported by the results of the present study. The apparent focus of segmental shortening vectors was always found closer to the apex than the centre of mass (Figure 2), a finding we have recently corroborated in a study of 173 cardiac cycles in 40 patients with markers (9).

Noordergraaf's estimate (1) of the distance between the aortic valve and the centre of mass throughout the cardiac cycle (Figure 4) proved surprisingly good, especially since data available at that time indicated that the descent of the base of the heart towards the apex was twice the ascent of the apex towards the base at systole, which was not found in the present study.

To good approximation, the hydraulic work associated with ejection is 1 joule per beat. Our calculations showed that the work which goes into moving the centre of gravity of the left ventricle was only 0.04% of this work in the normal heart and 0.05% of this work in the hearts with wall motion abnormalities, an apparently trivial amount in either case. This finding, coupled with the results of our earlier studies showing very small rotations in systole about either the major or minor axes (7, 10), suggests that the left ventricle ejects blood with a minimum of wasted motion and energy.

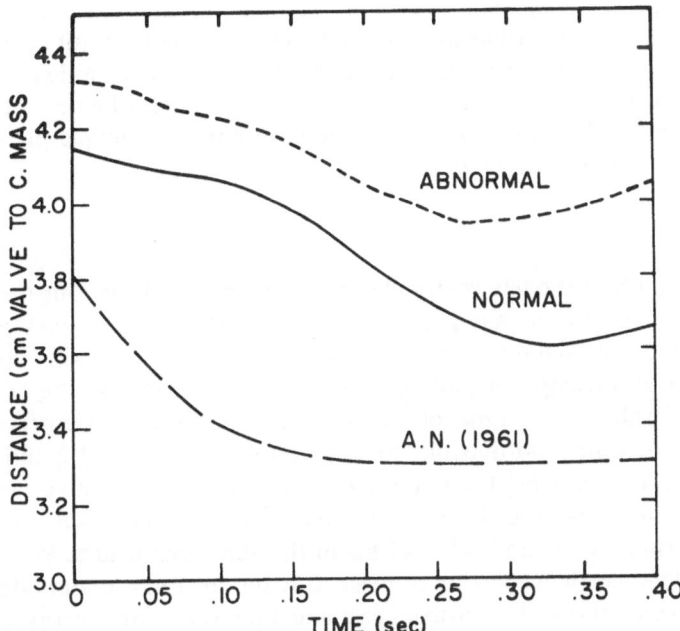

*Figure 4.* Distance between the left ventricular centre of mass and the aortic valve midpoint for the first 400 msec of systole. Solid line: normal group; short dashes: abnormal group; long dashes: as originally calculated by Noordergraaf(1).

The marker method used in this study has the advantage that left ventricular myocardial sites can be identified accurately and reproducibly (7, 8) without the need for premedication, catheterization, or injection of contrast agents. It further avoids the effects of dye exclusion by papillary muscles and myocardial trabeculations which confound studies of wall motion using contrast angiography, particularly those of the anterior wall.

There are, however, two disadvantages associated with this method, the first being that studies are performed only in the 30° right anterior oblique plane, which, while measuring two components of centre of mass dynamics, ignores that component along an axis perpendicular to this plane. In previous biplane studies, we have shown that left ventricular minor axis rotations are small (7), but the 30° right anterior oblique plane translates slightly toward the sternum in systole, so further studies will be needed to describe the motion of the centre of mass perpendicular to this plane.

The other disadvantage of the method is that only patients having prior cardiac surgery are available for study. This makes the definition of "normal" left ventricular dynamics somewhat tenuous. Those patients having left ventricular function deemed "normal" exhibited normal values of volumetric and ejection phase velocity indices (Table 1), and all myocardial segments under study were contracting vigorously inward. Those identified as having abnormal segmental dynamics showed almost no shortening (akinesis) in at least one segment in the ventricular wall as visualized in the 30° right anterior oblique plane. Thus, until such time as truly normal hearts can be studied by noninvasive techniques, we feel justified in suggesting cautious use of these data to describe the dynamics of the left ventricular centre of mass in the right anterior oblique projection in intact unanaesthetized man.

SUMMARY

The dynamics of the left ventricular centre of mass throughout the cardiac cycle were studied in ten patients with normal hemodynamics and wall motion and nine patients with wall motion abnormalities using computer-processed fluoroscopy of tantalum markers implanted into the left ventricular midwall at the time of previous cardiac surgery Centre of mass translations from end-diastole to end-systole were $2.6 \pm 1.2$ mm in the normal hearts and $4.6 \pm 1.3$ mm in the abnormal hearts ($p < .01$). The energy expended in translating the left ventricular mass in systole was $0.4 \pm 0.2$ mJ in the normal hearts and $0.5 \pm 0.3$ mJ in the abnormal hearts. We conclude that the left ventricular centre of mass is maintained in a remarkably stable position throughout the cardiac cycle and thus very little energy is wasted during contraction in hearts with either normal or abnormal contractile dynamics.

REFERENCES

1. Noordergraaf A: Further studies on a theory of the ballistocardiogram. *Circulation* 23 (3):413, 1961.
2. Weerd JM van de, Noordergraaf A: Prediction of the human lateral ballistocardiogram. *Proc. 1st world congr. ballistocard. cardiovasc. dynamics, Amsterdam* 1965, Basel, Karger, 1966, p 281–284.
3. Morse RL, Longoria RN: Mass movement in the region of the heart of the dog. Proc. 13th ann meeting ballistocardiograph res soc, Atlantic City, N.J. 1968, *Bibl Cardiol* 22:18–21 1969.
4. Pearlman AS, Clark CE, Henry WI, Morganroth J, Itscoitz SB, Epstein SE: Determinants of ventricular septal motion: influence of relative right and left ventricular size. *Circulation* 54 (1):83, 1976.
5. Heintzen PH, Moldenhauer K, Lange PE: Three-dimensional computerized contraction pattern analysis: description of methodology and its validation. *Eur J Cardiol* 1 (3):229–239, 1974.
6. Rickards A, Seabra-Gomes R, Thurston P: The assessment of regional abnormalities of the left ventricle by angiography. *Eur J. Cardiol* 5(2):167–182, 1977.
7. Ingels Jr NB, Daughters II GT, Stinson EB, Alderman EL: Measurement of midwall myocardial dynamics in intact man by radiography of surgically implanted markers. *Circulation* 52:859, 1975.
8. Daughters II GT, Ingels Jr NB, Stinson EB, Alderman EL, Mead CW: Computation of left ventricular dynamics from surgically implanted markers. *Proc San Diego Biomedical Symp*16:97, 1977.
9. Ingels Jr NB, Mead CW, Daughters II GT, Stinson EB, Alderman EL: A new method for assessment of left ventricular wall motion. *Comput Cardial*:p 57–61, 1978.
10. Daughters II GT, Ingels Jr NB, Jang GC, Alderman EL, Stinson EB: Left ventricular long axis rotation assessed by cinefluoroscopy of implanted myocardial markers. *Fed Proc* 36:447, 1977.

## 5.11 CARDIAC PUMP FUNCTION BY BALLISTOCARDIOGRAM: NORMAL STANDARDS AND COMPARISON WITH CORONARY ARTERIOGRAMS

A. G. DINABURG, W.H. BANCROFT, JR.,
E.E. EDDLEMAN, JR.

### 1. INTRODUCTION

Aortic flow acceleration has been used to evaluate myocardial performance by invasive (1, 2, 3), or by non-invasive means (4) using the acceleration ballistocardiogram (BCG). Comparisons of the two methods in animals and man (5, 6, 7, 8, 9) have shown fairly good fits. Also, ejection fraction by ventriculogram could be estimated closely from BCG measures (10, 11). However, suggestive as these experimental and limited studies are, the widespread clinical use of the BCG has been hampered by lack of large-scale comparison with accepted clinical measures of pump function, by only a recent appreciation of aortic flow acceleration as a sensitive measure, and by lack of broadly acceptable clinical standards based on data with ultra-low frequency beds. Previous work with various beds, showing decline of BCG measures with increasing age, was reported by Starr and Noordergraaf (5), Moss (12), Proper (13) and Zuiderveld (14). A committee on clinical standards was appointed by the 4th World Congress on Ballistocardiography in 1975. The present paper, a contribution to that effort, derives standards for normal males, then applies them to post-infarct patients, and those having diagnostic coronary angiography.

### 2. MATERIALS AND METHODS

Subjects came from Herrick Hospital, Berkeley, California, or the Veterans' Administration Hospital in Birmingham, Alabama. The Berkeley series included two groups: normals, and those with coronary artery disease. Normals included 102 males, 19–66 years old, with no known history of heart disease, sitting blood pressures less than 140/90 mmHg, smokers and nonsmokers, and those with varying levels of obesity and physical activity. The cardiac group totalled 16 men, 38–71 years old, with documented myocardial infarctions, 14 of whom were studied 10 to 23 days after the onset of the infarction. Basic data recorded for each subject included age, weight, height, blood pressure, pulse rate, cardiac history, if any, smoking habits, time from the previous meal, and medications taken, if any.

*J. Baan, A.C. Arntzenius, E.L. Yellin (eds.), Cardiac Dynamics, 433–440.*

The Birmingham series included a control group of 108 males, aged 30–74 years, who had been in a physical fitness program for several years. The cardiac group totalled 811 males, aged 23–70 years, clinically thought to have ischaemic heart disease, who had coronary arteriography because of chest pain or electrocardiographic suggestion of myocardial infarction. These had both coronary arteriograms and ballistocardiograms. Basic data analysed in both groups included age, weight, height, blood pressure, pulse rate, and when arteriograms were done, the artery or arteries obstructed, their location (proximal or distal) and degree (below 50% 50–70%, 71–85%, 86–99%, and 100%) of obstruction.

The Berkeley data was obtained on a ULF air bearing bed weighing 4.88 kg and meeting international standards. Technical details are given in Dinaburg et al. (15). IJ amplitudes were measured for two full normal respiratory cycles, and averaged. The Birmingham catheterization series was recorded with a ULF air bearing bed weighing 4.8 kg, while the normals were recorded on a swing bed weighing 5.2 kg. Details of this sytem, recording and computer data analysis, are given by Bancroft et al. (16) and Jackson et al. (11). An average of held inspiration and held expiration for each of two beats was used. Card-punched data on the two sets of subjects, including age, weight, height, blood pressure, pulse rate, IJ and HI amplitudes, and coronary arteriogram data were sent to Berkeley for analysis by the senior author. BCG amplitues were corrected for bed weights by the factor:

$$BCG_{adjusted} = \frac{(Pt.\ Wt. + Bed\ Wt.) \times BCG,}{Pt.\ Wt.}$$

then multiplied by 10.

Statistical analyses were done an a Control Data 6400 computer, using either the SPSS (17) or Fortran programs. Statistical methods used are described in Zar (18).

3. RESULTS

The Berkeley normal group of 102 males had the following means and standard deviations: age: $37.4 \pm 11.7$ yrs; weight, $77.1 \pm 9.7$ kg; height, $177.9 \pm 6.5$ cm; systolic pressure, $119.4 \pm 11.2$ mmHg; diastolic pressure $77.0 \pm 7.4$ mmHg; pulse rate $68.8 \pm 10.5$ beats/min; $IJ_{adj}$, $43.1 \pm 11.3$ mG $\times$ 10. A multivariate stepwise linear regression program (17) produced age and weight as the most efficient predictors: $IJ_{adj}$ (mG $\times$ 10) $= 81.94 - 0.514$ Age (yrs) $- 0.254$ Wt. (kg). The multiple correlation coefficient was 0.595, and multiple $R^2$ was 0.354, indicating 35% of total IJ variance was attributable to age and weight. The $F$ ratio, (regression/residual mean square) 27.2, was highly significant. The interaction of age and weight and predicted $IJ_{adj}$ is shown in Figure 1.

The 95% prediction interval was computed from: predicted $IJ_{adj} \pm t \times$ (standard error of predicted $IJ_{adj}$) where $t = 0.05$ (2-tailed) $= 1.984$ for 100 subjects (18). A nomogram for the lower limit of the prediction interval is shown in Figure 2. Any observed $IJ_{adj}$, for a test individual, given his age and weight, below these prediction limits, is considered abnormal, with a 2.5% chance of a misclassification.

Fourteen Berkeley cardiac males had BCGs taken 10 to 23 days after the onset of a myocardial infarction, of which 3 were subnormal. The maximum creatine phosphokinase level, a measure of myocardial damage in the early period, plotted against the difference between predicted and observed IJ, is shown in Figure 3. The three patients with a subnormal BCG also had high CPK values over 1965 units, compatible with a major infarction.

The Birmingham exercise series of 108 males had mean and standard deviation values for age, $52.0 \pm 11.6$ yrs; weight, $78.9 \pm 8.5$ kg; height,

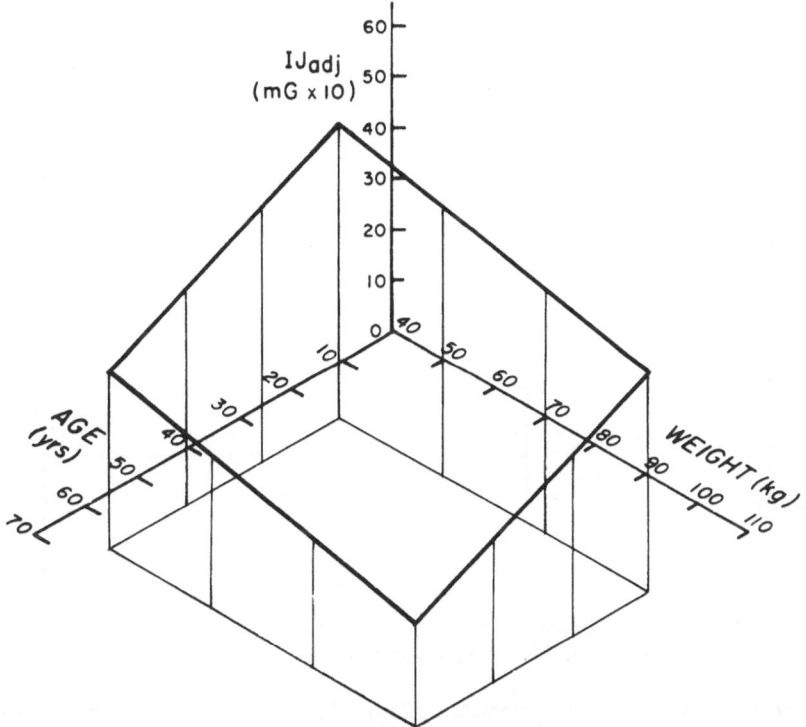

$$IJ_{adj}\ (mG \times 10) = 81.94 - 0.514\,Age(yrs) - 0.254\,Weight(kg)$$

*Figure 1.* Influence of age and weight on ballistocardiogram. Predicted $IJ_{adj}$ (mG × 10) given age and weight, based on multiple regression equation. Note greater change due to age.

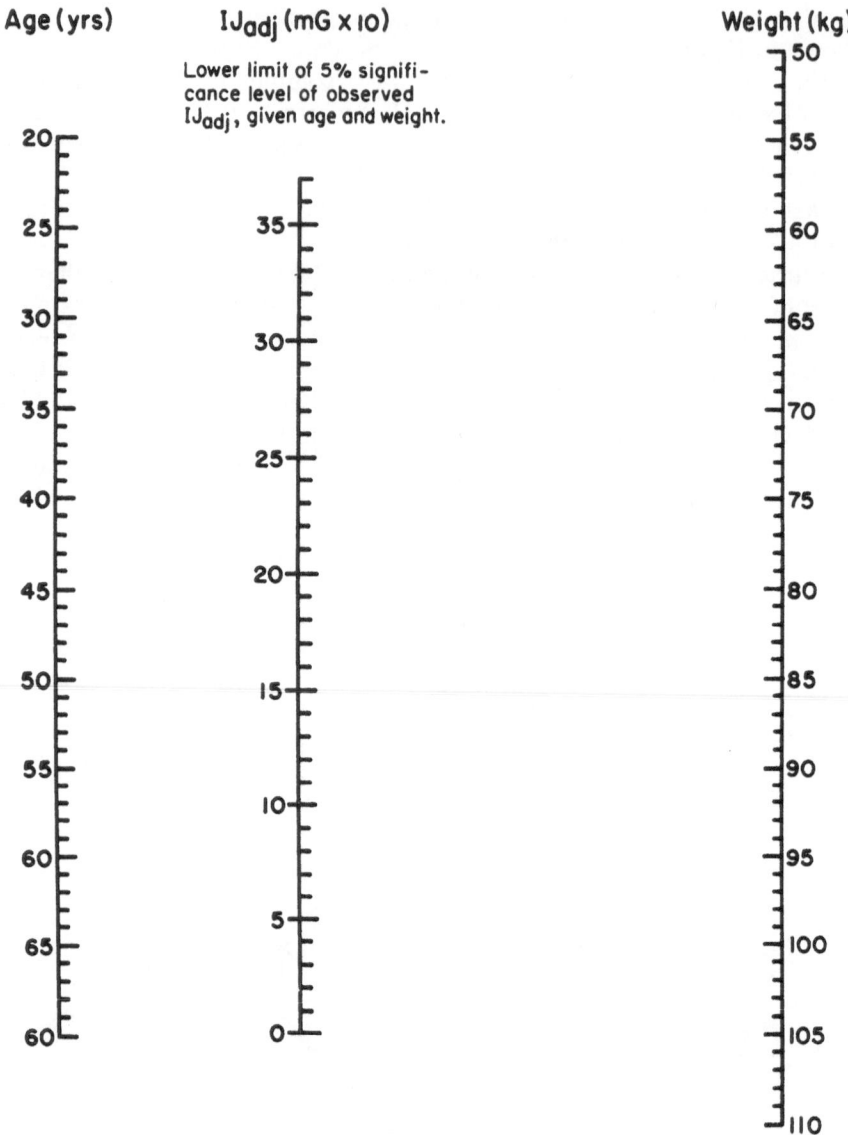

*Figure 2.* Nomogram to calculate predicted IJ$_{adj}$ from age and weight. Lower prediction limits for IJ$_{adj}$ (mG × 10), based on 95% prediction intervals are given.

177.9 ± 5.5 cm; systolic pressure, 123.8 ± 11.5 mmHg; diastolic pressure, 80.0 ± 7.5 mmHg; pulse rate 64.9 ± 9.8 beats min; IJ$_{adj}$ 35.9 ± 11.6 mG × 10. This group was not combined with the Berkeley normals because it was a selected one.

The 811 males with coronary angiograms included 79 with no arterial

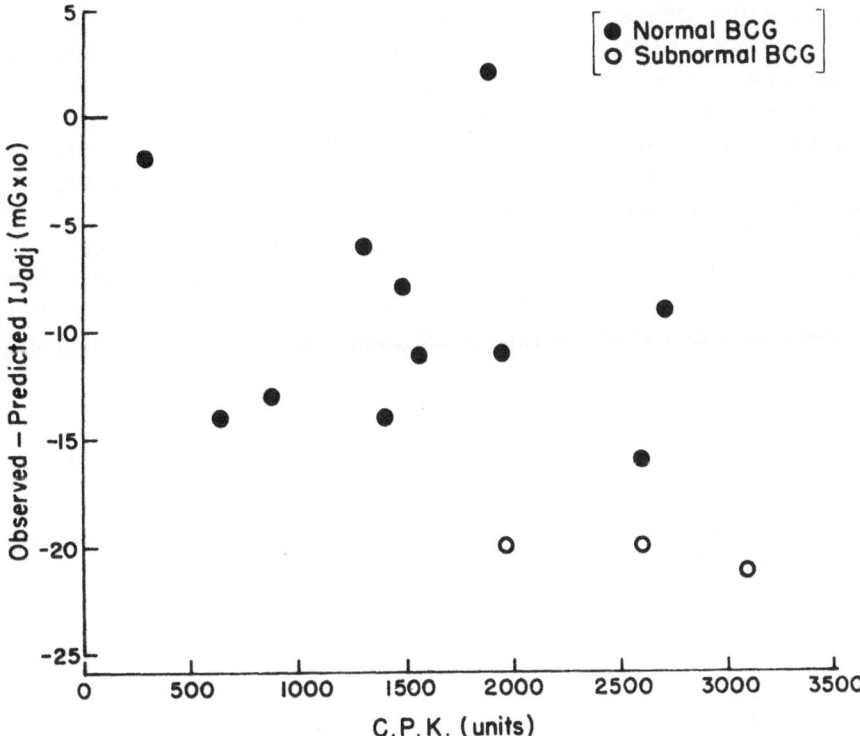

*Figure 3.* Comparison of BCG and enzyme elevations in myocardial infarction. Observed minus predicted $IJ_{adj}$ values in patients 10 to 23 days after onset of a myocardial infarction plotted against maximum creatine phosphokinase level observed during the infarction.

obstruction, and 649 with some proximal and 83 with distal obstruction (under 50 to 100%) of the four major arteries, singly or in combination. The mean IJ adjusted for arteries obstructed over 86% was 21.8 mG × 10 (526 men), no obstruction, 25.9 (79 men), and the control exercise group, 35.9 (108 men). 297 men had 1 artery restricted over 86%; 171, 2 arteries and 55, 3 arteries. The left anterior descending was the most frequent, followed by the right coronary.

To analyse the many combinations of arteries involved, level of restriction, age, and weight and their effects on the $IJ_{adj}$, a three-way analysis of variance (18) was done. To simplify the analysis, only proximal arterial restrictions in 649 men were included. This analysis indicates that age and weight have highly significant effects on $IJ_{adj}$ while coronary artery restrictions, when classified by artery involved, did not.

Since the overall effect on $IJ_{adj}$ of the artery involved (left anterior descending, circumflex, or right coronary), was not significant, the effect of similar degrees of restriction in one or more arteries was studied. Seven groups with proximal coronary arterial restrictions ranging from 0 to 100%, in 1 or more arteries, were sorted, and their mean $IJ_{adj}$ computed. No significant differences were found among the 7 groups' means, despite the large range of arterial restrictions. Each group was then tested individually by the Berkeley standards, producing a subgroup of normals and sub-normals. The details are presented in Figure 4, where the subgroup $IJ_{adj}$ means for each combination of arterial restriction is presented. Again, it is noteworthy that there is no trend in the mean $IJ_{adj}$ values in either the normal or subnormal subgroups with increasing proximal arterial re-striction. Subnormals ranged from 20 to 37% of the total in the 7 artery groups, with an overall average of 25%, and were also younger than their corresponding normals.

## 4. DISCUSSION

The present data indicate that not only is age an important factor influenc-ing the BCG, (as have previous studies), but weight as well. Age is 2.4 times

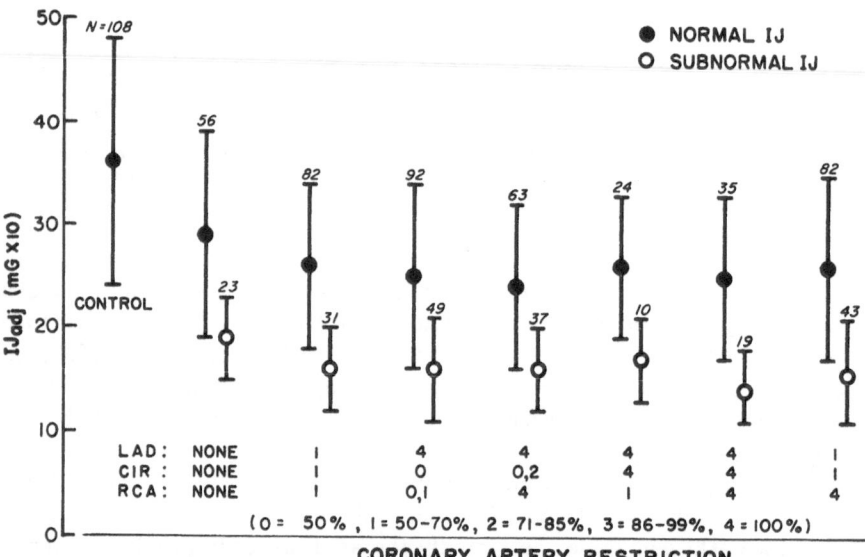

Figure 4. Comparison of ballistocardiogram and coronary arteriography. Mean $IJ_{adj} \pm$ S.D. in different groups, classified by arteries involved and degree of restriction on coronary arterio-grams. The first number of the three-number artery code refers to the left anterior descending; the second, the circumflex; and the third, the right coronary artery. Degree of restriction is indicated by the value of the number: 0 under 50% 1, 51–70%; 2, 71–85%; 3, 86–99%; 4, 100%. For comparison, values for 108 normal males in the exercise group, and 79 males with no arterial restrictions (blank).

more important than weight in this series. While the physiological explanation is not clear, it is important to adjust for weight in computing standards.

In the present study, the low $IJ_{adj}$ values associated with the high CPK enzyme values during acute infarction suggest the use of the BCG for monitoring recovery of pump function, after the acute phase is over.

As for the physiological significance of coronary artery restrictions, Kent et al. (19) indicate that adequate basal myocardial perfusion is possible with marked narrowing, with ischaemia developing under stress. This should be considered in comparing coronary arteriograms and the resting BCG.

Schöttelndreier and Rodrigo (20) found a semi-quantitative correlation between coronary arteriography and BCG. Goedhard and Norro (21) found a correlation of $-0.34$ ($P = 0.05$) between IJ and narrowing of two coronary arteries in 35 men and women, of which 26% had subnormal BCGs. However, the present larger series found no regular trend in group mean IJ values in various combinations of coronary artery restriction. In each group, patients with normal and subnormal $IJ_{adj}$ values were found, indicating varying levels of pump performance. This indicates the additional physiological noninvasive information provided by the BCG.

SUMMARY

Normal standards for the ULF BCG were derived from 102 normal males, given age and weight: $IJ_{adj}$ (mG × 10) = 81.94−0.514 Age (yrs) − 0.254 Weight (kg), and the 95% prediction intervals calculated. In 14 males with recent myocardial infarctions, lower IJ values were found with higher creatine phosphokinase levels. In 649 males with proximal coronary arterial restrictions by catheterizations, and with BCGs taken, the group mean IJ value did not change significantly with number, type or degree of restriction of the coronary arteries. However, within each group there was a fraction with subnormal IJ values, with an overall average of 25% of the total tested, and with no trend between degree of arterial restriction and subgroup mean IJ. The BCG may be useful for serial monitoring, or for separating patients with subnormal pump function, where the coronary arteriogram alone does not.

ACKNOWLEDGEMENTS

The authors wish to thank Richard M. Cummings for his invaluable help with the engineering and electronics problems; Lorna Wunderman and Paul C.C. Wang for statistical help, and Frank Todd for the graphics.

REFERENCES

1. Rushmer, RF: Initial ventricular impulse: a potential key to cardiac evaluation. *Circulation* 29:268–283, 1964.
2. Noble MIM, Trenchard D Guz A: Left ventricular ejection in conscious dogs. *Circ Res* 19:139–147, 1966.
3. Jewitt D, Gabe I, Mills C, Maurer B, Thomas M, Shillingford J: Aortic velocity and acceleration measurements in the assessment of coronary heart disease. *Eur J Cardiol* 1 (3):299–305, 1974.
4. Starr I: Studies made by simulating systole at necropsy XII: estimation of the initial cardiac forces from the ballistocardiogram. *Circulation* 20:74–87, 1959.
5. Starr I, Noordergraaf A: *Ballistocardiography in cardiovascular research*, Philadelphia, Lippincott, 1967.
6. Winter PJ, Deuchar DC, Noble MIM et al: Relationship between the ballistocardiogram and the movement of blood from the left ventricle in the dog. *Cardiovasc Res* 1:194–200, 1967.
7. Harrison WK, Friessinger GC, Johnson SL: Relation of the ballistocardiogram to left ventricular pressure measurements in man. *Am J Cardiol* 23:673–678, 1969.
8. Smith NT, Citters RL van, Verdouw PD: The relation between the ULF-BCG, the acceleration pneumocardiogram and ascending flow acceleration in the baboon. *Bibl Cardiol* 26: 189–205, 1970.
9. Baan J, Manchester JH, Shelburne JC: A quantitative relationship between the H-I slope of the head-foot BCG and the initial acceleration of flow in man. *Bibl Cardiol* 29:55–69, 1972.
10. Jackson DH, Eddleman Jr EE, Bancroft Jr WWT, Swatzell Jr RH: Ventricular function in idiopathic hypertrophic subaortic stenosis. *Am J Cardiol* 28, 641–647, 1971.
11. Jackson DH, Bancroft Jr WH, Tucker M3, Eddleman Jr EE, Bookin RN: Relationship of angiographic ejection fraction to ballistocardiographic parameters in coronary disease. *Ala J Med Sci* 13, 396–398, 1976.
12. Moss AJ: Ballistocardiographic evaluation of the cardiovascular aging process. *Circulation* 23:434–451, 1961.
13. Proper R: Age-related changes in professional pilots as defined by the Klensch-Schwarzer ultra-low frequency ballistocardiogram. *Bibl Cardiol* 20:50–56, 1968.
14. Zuiderveld V: *Honderd gezonde mannen*, Amsterdam, Excerpta Medica, 1974.
15. Dinaburg AG, Cummings RC, Heinzer W: Improved diagnosis of myocardial dysfunction by a stress test during ballistocariogram. *Bibl Cardiol* 34:94–104, 1974.
16. Bancroft Jr WH, Tucker M, Jackson DH, Eddleman Jr EE: Automatic computer processing of ultra-low frequency ballistocardiograms. *Bibl Cardiol* 32:1–10, 1973.
17. Nie NH, Hull CH et al: *Statistical package for the social sciences*, New York, McGraw-Hill 2nd ed 1975.
18. Zar J: *Biostatistical analysis*, Englewood Cliffs, NJ, Prentice Hall, 1974.
19. Kent KM, Borer JS, Green MV, Bacharach SL, McIntosh CL, Conkle DM, Epstein SE: Effects of coronary revascularization on left ventricular function during exercise. *New Engl J Med* 298 (26):1434–1439, 1978.
20. Schöttelndreier MAHW, Rodrigo FA: Correlation between ergometry, ballistocardiography and coronary angiography in 267 patients. *Bibl Cardiol* 29:35–43, 1972.
21. Goedhard, WJA, Norro G: Ballistocardiographic findings in relation to the coronary arteriogram, *Bibl Cardiol* 35, 123–128, 1976.

SECTION 6

# ENERGY LOSSES:
# HEMODYNAMICS OF VALVES

## 6.1. KONRAD WITZIG MEMORIAL LECTURE: SOME FLUID MECHANIC THEORIES AND THEIR APPLICATION TO THE DESIGN OF HEART VALVES AND MEMBRANE LUNGS

BRIAN J. BELLHOUSE

### 1. INTRODUCTION

As a research student in Switzerland, Konrad Witzig solved the complex mathematical problem of calculating the pressure and velocity distributions of pulsatile flow in elastic tubes (1). Womersley (2) subsequently extended Witzig's work, which, until recently rediscovered by Professor Noordergraaf, has been buried in the library of Berne University.

This paper also concerns the study of pulsatile blood flow, but is confined to flows which separate and re-attach to form convective vortices. These vortices occur in the sinuses of the aortic valve and exert a powerful influence on cusp movements; they occur in the left ventricle and help close the mitral valve during diastole; and they provide the secondary flows which are responsible for the high efficiency of the Oxford membrane lung.

This paper is concerned with our attempts at Oxford, over the last ten years, to understand the fluid mechanics of the natural heart valves and to exploit this knowledge to design better prosthetic valves and membrane lungs. It covers experiments with hydraulic models, testing of devices in animals and numerical solutions of vortex flows.

### 2. THE AORTIC VALVE

A photograph of a human aortic valve is shown in Figure 1. The diameter of the aorta is about 25 mm; the ventricle is marked $V$, the aorta $A$, the non-coronary sinus $S$ and its corresponding cusp $C$. The left coronary ostium is marked $O$ and the distal end of the sinus is marked $R$. The right coronary ostium lies within the unmarked sinus close to the distal end of the sinus, where it joins the aorta. The cusps are very thin (0.1 mm) and flexible; they drape across the sinuses when relaxed. Reinforcing bands of collagen in the cusps loop from commissure to commissure to support the valve when closed and under load. When the aortic valve is open, the cusps probably remain furled, because the force required to extend them in an axial direction is large relative to the integrated shear stresses at peak systole.

Leonardo da Vinci made anatomical studies of the aortic valve (3) and (in 1513) suggested that vortices would form in the aortic sinuses, and that

J, Baan, A.C. Arntzenius, E.L. Yellin (eds.); Cardiac Dynamics, 443–46 l.

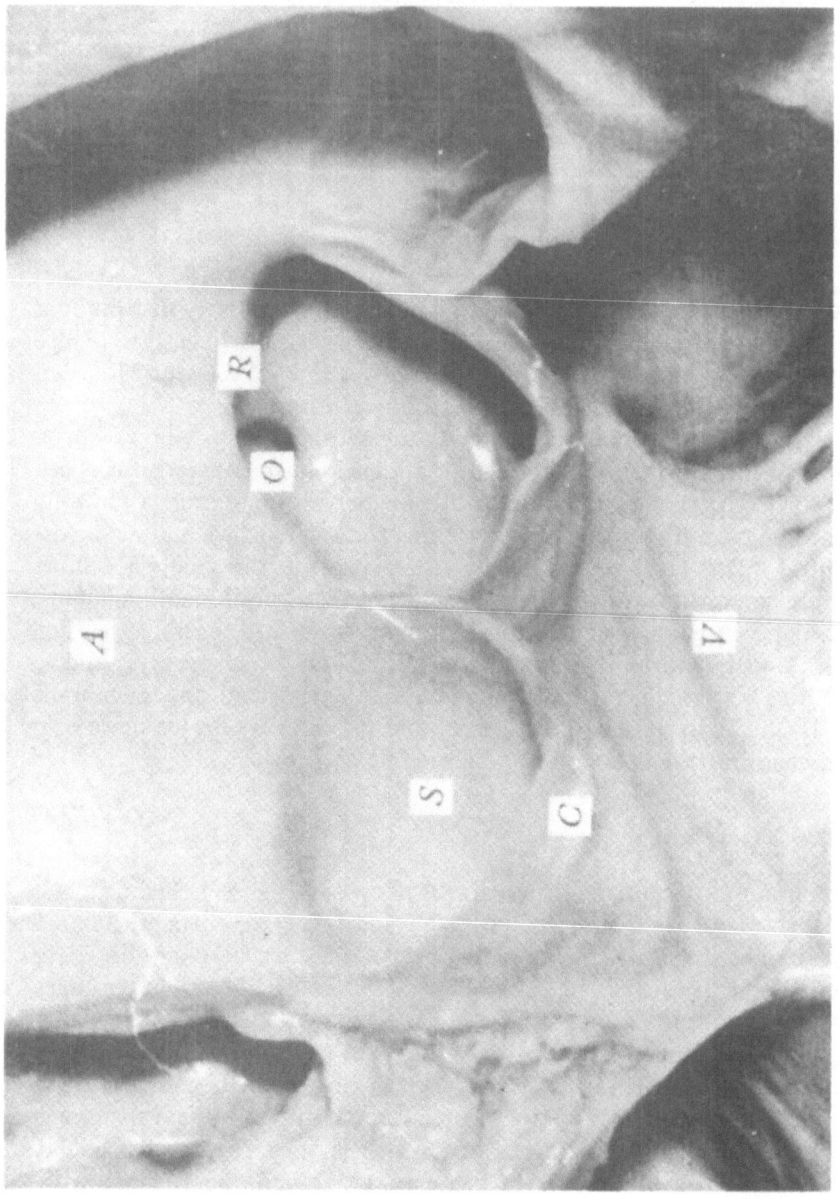

*Figure 1.* Photograph of a human aortic valve. The outflow tract of the left ventricle is marked *V*, the non-coronary sinus *S*, its corresponding cusp *C*, the left coronary ostium *O* and the distal end of the sinus *R*. Note the "furled-up," relaxed position of the cusps.

these vortices would move the cusps towards closure. It is hard to believe that he was unaware of the circulation of blood. However, he was mistaken in his view that vortices shed from the aortic sinuses would serve to warm the blood by viscous action. An alternative explanation of both aortic and mitral valve closure was suggested by Henderson and Johnson (4) in 1912; they called it the "breaking of the jet." The effect they described appears to be related to the adverse pressure gradient associated with decelerating flow through the valve.

In 1968, measurements of blood velocity in the ascending aortas of dogs was undertaken in Oxford (5). We observed that blood flow was laminar, despite a peak Reynolds number of 10,000, and that reversed flow was barely measureable. It was clear that the aortic valve had to open wide for much of systole (or turbulence would have resulted) and yet be almost-closed by the end of systole (or reversed flow would have been much larger).

The cusps were too thin for elastic recoil to be important, and no muscular control was evident. This left us only a fluid mechanic explanation of aortic valve behaviour. To investigate this a model aortic valve was constructed (6). It consisted of a rigid aortic root made of perspex with three sinuses and three cusps made of silicone rubber reinforced with nylon net. The cusps were 0.1 mm thick and assumed the fully-open position when no forces were applied to them. The model valve was placed in a pulse duplicator in which sinusoidal flow pulses could be superimposed on a chosen mean flow. It was seen that the valve opened wide early in systole and that strong vortices formed rapidly in the aortic sinuses (Figure 2, top). At mid-systole the cusps were balanced between the flows in the sinuses and in the aorta. As the aortic flow began to decelerate, the aortic pressure level with the distal end of the sinus exceeded the pressure in the aorta at the

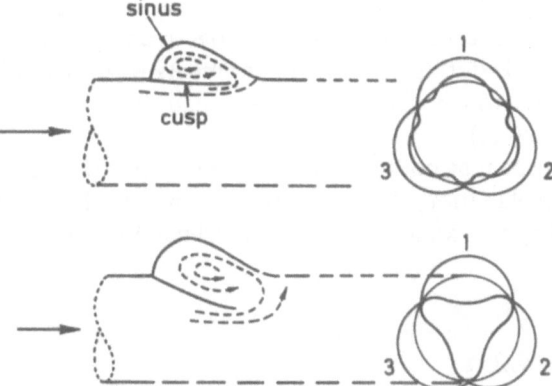

*Figure 2.* Diagrams of the flow patterns in the aortic sinuses at mid-systole (*above*) and late-systole (*below*). End views of the valve are shown on the right.

proximal end of the sinus. But since the sinuses were fed from the distal end, mean sinus pressure exceeded the mean pressure on the aortic side of the cusps and the aortic valve began to close. The vortex pattern and position of the cusps is shown in the lower part of Figure 2. By the end of systole the valve was three-quarters closed, and a small amount of reversed flow was required to seal the valve.

The sinus vortices reach their maximum strength at peak-systole and their chief role is to act as a control mechanism to synchronize the closure of the fragile cusps, and to harness the adverse axial pressure gradient (associated with decelerating aortic flow) in the latter part of systole. It is important to appreciate the effect of late closure of one or more cusps-large shock loads would be experienced when the late-closing cusps were caught by reversed flow, and valve lifetimes would be severely compromised. Since the cusps differ in size and stiffness, and aortic velocity is non-uniform (5), it is essential to have a synchronizing mechanism to ensure valve lifetimes of 70 years, or 2800 million cycles.

When the control mechanism is disrupted, by the blocking of a sinus, the corresponding cusp fails to close (Bellhouse, this volume). When sinus geometry is altered to improve vortex strength, the corresponding cusp closes earlier. Thus sinus geometry has an important effect on vortex strength and consequently on valve closure.

The vortices have two other roles, apart from controlling cusp closure. Firstly, the vortices scour the sinuses to prevent the formation of stagnant regions of blood behind the cusps, with consequent thrombus formation. Secondly, the vortices recover dynamic head within the sinuses, particularly at the distal end of the sinuses where the coronary ostia are located. Almost all the dynamic head is recovered at the ostia, and this contributes to systolic coronary flow, particularly in exercise, when peak velocity in the aorta is increased (7). It is likely that systolic coronary flow is stored in the epicardium and superficial coronary arteries ready for discharge into the endocardial vessels during diastole. Experiments with hydraulic models and with animals in which the aortic valve had been rendered insufficient support this view (8).

It would appear that both Leonardo da Vinci and Henderson were partly right in their explanation of aortic valve closure, but that the two hydraulic mechanisms they invoke are so closely interlinked it is not easy to separate them.

## 3. THE MITRAL VALVE

The anatomy of the mitral valve differs greatly from that of the aortic valve. It has two major cusps: the anterior (on the left of Figure 3(a) and the posterior. The mitral annulus is kidney-shaped and deforms during ventri-

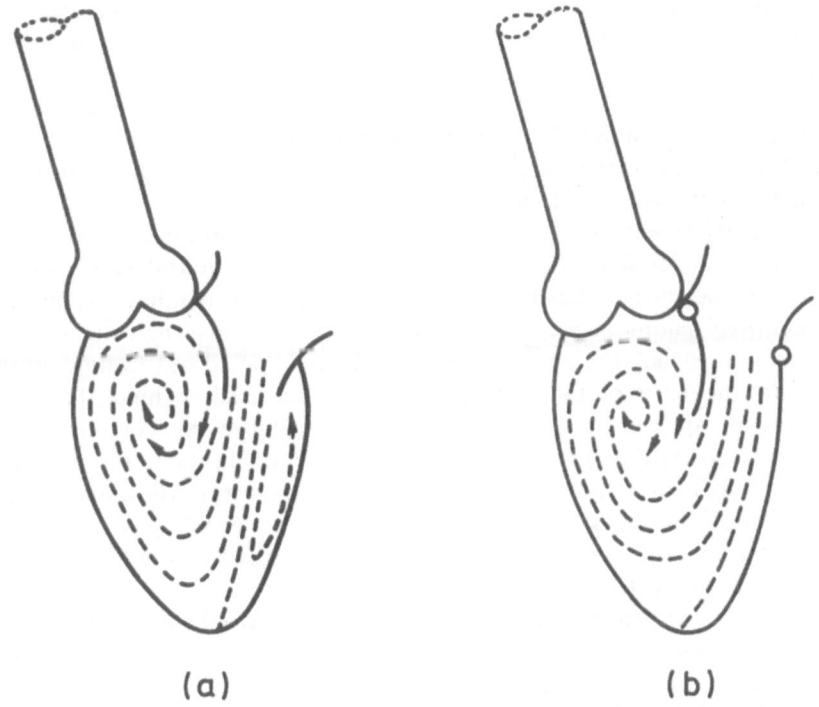

(a)                                                              (b)

*Figure 3.* Diagrams of flow patterns in the left ventricle with (a) a natural mitral valve and (b) the Oxford prosthetic mitral valve. In both cases, a strong vortex is formed with its main strength in the outflow tract of the left ventricle.

cular systole. The free margins of the cusps are connected by inextensible chordae tendineae to papillary muscles at the apex of the left ventricle. The cusps are thin and flexible.

One requirement for the left ventricle to work effectively is that it must fill rapidly from the left atrium. This requires that the mitral valve should offer minimal resistance to blood flow during diastole. It is important, too, that the mitral valve should close at the end of diastole with minimal reversed flow and that it should remain competent throughout systole, or ventricular stroke volume would be reduced.

To see if the mitral valve could be controlled by fluid mechanic forces similar to those which control the aortic valve, a model mitral valve and left ventricle was built (9). The base of the ventricle was rigid, and incorporated a mitral and an aortic valve; a transparent rubber bag simulated the remainder of the ventricle. The model ventricle was fixed inside a perspex tank, which was filled with water and connected to a piston pump to actuate the ventricle. The aortic valve was connected to a header tank from which water overflowed to a lower tank which discharged through a viewer and the mitral valve into the left ventricle.

The model mitral valve consisted of a sleeve of nylon net coated with silicone rubber, shaped to make two equal cusps 0.1 mm thick and 28 mm long. The sleeve was shaped on a divergent-cone mould (semi-angle 14°) with the narrower end attached to the mitral annulus. The free margins of the cusps were connected by threads to a fixed support 45 mm from the mitral ring, to prevent prolapse of the valve during systole. The diameter of the mitral annulus was 25 mm.

The ventricle was driven by a piston pump, which produced a sinusoidal flow, one half for diastole, the other for systole. The mitral valve opened rapidly at the start of diastole, but it did not open to its fullest extent, and the chordae tendineae were slack. After the mitral valve had opened, the incoming jet struck the apex of the ventricle and spread out to flow up the walls to the base of the ventricle, then turned back behind the cusps towards the apex again, to form a ring vortex (Figure 3a). The vortex was asymmetrical, with its greatest strength concentrated in the outflow tract of the ventricle, behind the anterior cusp. After peak diastole, the anterior cusp moved steadily towards closure, and before ventricular filling was complete the posterior cusp started to close also. Only a small amount of reversed flow was required to seal the valve.

Cine film of the mitral valve was taken from the atrial side. The film was projected frame by frame and the outline of the cusp-free margins, the supporting bar for the chordae tendineae (conveniently bisecting the mitral annulus), and the mitral annulus were traced onto white paper. The areas between the anterior cusp and the bar ($A_1$) and between the posterior cusp and the bar ($A_2$) were measured with a planimeter. In addition, the area of the mitral annulus ($A_0$) was measured. Velocity at the mitral annulus was measured with a thin-film gauge and was correlated with the cine film by means of a triggered light bulb.

In an attempt to obtain dynamic similarity the end-systolic volume was set at 107 ml, the stroke volume at 173 ml and the pulse rate at 24 beats/min. The performance of the mitral valve under these "normal" operating conditions is shown in Figure 4. Velocity at the mitral annulus is shown in (a), the area of the mitral cusp orifice divided by the area of the annulus is drawn in (b). The opening-areas of the anterior cusp ($A$) and the posterior cusp ($P$) are plotted non-dimensionally ($2A_1/A_0$ and $2A_2/A_0$, respectively) in (c). Time is plotted along the abscissa, with zero time corresponding to zero velocity at the centre of the mitral annulus.

These results show that both cusps open wide early in diastole, that the anterior cusp moves steadily towards closure throughout the latter three-quarters of diastole and that the posterior cusp stays wide open until the last quarter of diastole when it, too, moves towards closure. At the end of diastole the anterior cusp is closed and the posterior cusp is almost closed. The last 10–15% of valve closure is achieved by reversed flow.

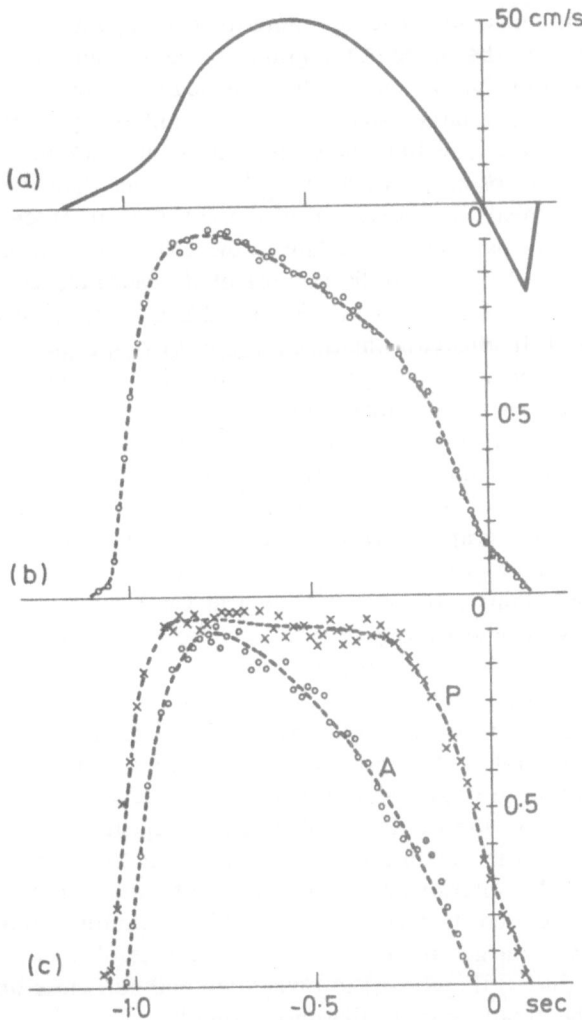

*Figure 4.* Graphs of opening area of a model mitral valve with a "normal" ventricle. (a) velocity through the mitral annulus; (b) valve opening area divided by annulus area; (c) individual opening areas (divided by half the valve annulus area), where A refers to the anterior cusp and P to the posterior cusp. All parameters are plotted as a function of time. The mitral valve is almost closed at the end of diastole (time zero), and the anterior cusp closes preferentially (end-systolic volume 107 ml, stroke volume 173 ml, frequency 24 beats/min).

The difference between the closure rates of anterior and posterior cusps was due to the difference in vortex strength behind the cusps. This was confirmed by pressure measurements (9). An alternative explanation of differential cusp movements would be differences in cusp stiffness. However, this was easily excluded by rotating the mitral valve so that the equal-sized cusps were interchanged. The new anterior cusp again closed earlier than the posterior, and the shape of the graph in Figure 4(c) was unchanged. As a further proof of the influence of the ventricular vortex, the ventricle was deformed so that a larger space existed behind the posterior cusp than behind the anterior. This time the vortex had its main strength concentrated behind the posterior cusp, which then closed earlier than the anterior.

These experiments indicated that, if the vortex were absent, the anterior and posterior cusps would close late in diastole and at an equal rate. To investigate this, the end-systolic volume of the ventricle was increased to 1216 ml, but the stroke volume (173 ml) and heart rate (24 beats/min) were left unchanged. In this case the incoming jet of blood failed to generate a strong vortex, since its energy was dissipated in mixing with the large volume of stagnant water already in the ventricle.

With the control mechanism destroyed, the cusps were slow to harness the decelerating stream through the mitral annulus, and the cusps were caught-out almost fully-open at the end of diastole. This is shown in Figure 5, where the three graphs correspond to those in Figure 4.

It would be unrealistic to claim that the huge end-systolic volume (1216 ml) was representative of any physiological ventricle, but it was a simple and effective way of disrupting the vortex without changing either the mitral valve or the diastolic flow through it. It was confirmed that intermediate. and more realistic, end-systolic volumes produced intermediate closure rates between those shown in Figures 4 and 5. Thus the ventricular vortex plays an important part in normal mitral valve closure, and ensures that flow deceleration through the mitral annulus is harnessed effectively so that the mitral valve is almost closed at the end of diastole.

One defect of the model mitral valve was that the cusps were of equal size, and that the anterior cusp could cover little more than half the mitral annulus when closed. It is no surprise that, in the natural mitral valve, the anterior cusp is larger than the posterior, 'and is able (with its superior closure rate due to the vortex) to open wide and still close during diastole and cover the greater part of the mitral annulus.

## 4. PROSTHETIC MITRAL VALVE

It is so difficult to copy the natural mitral valve that it seems inconceivable that either a tissue mitral valve (as opposed to a stented aortic valve in the mitral position) or a prosthetic valve of the same design as the natural mitral valve will be used clinically in the foreseeable future. Mitral valve replacement with either tissue valves or prosthetic valves has not been as successful as in the aortic position. Prosthetic valves are usually durable but cause greater energy losses than the natural mitral valve (which causes

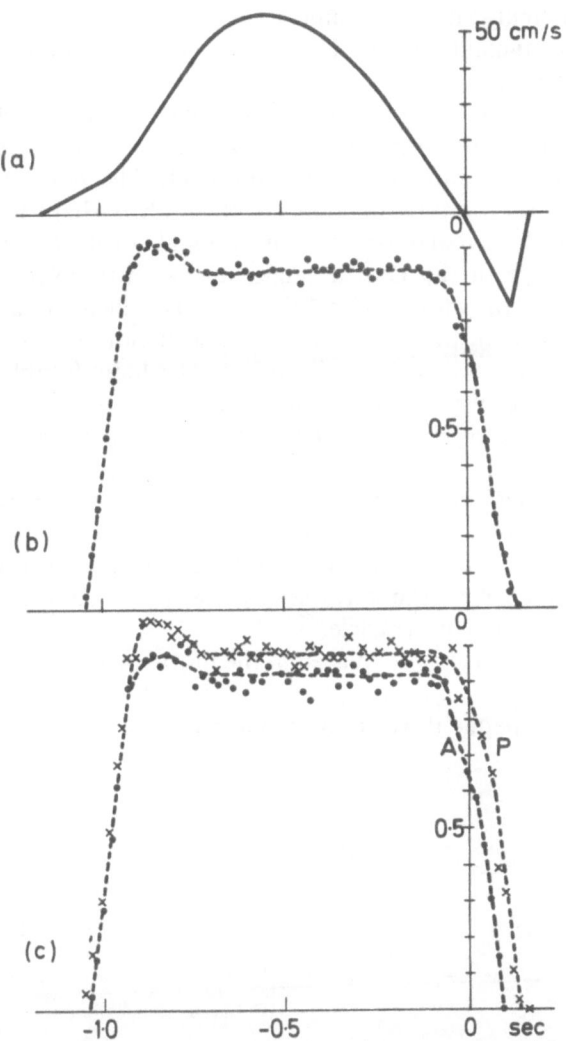

*Figure 5.* Graphs of opening area of a model mitral valve with a greatly dilated ventricle. The three parts of the figure correspond to Figure 4. The mitral valve is nearly open at the end of diastole (time zero) and most of its closure is achieved with reversed flow through the mitral annulus (end-systolic volume 1216 ml, stroke volume 173 ml, frequency 24 beats/min).

almost none) and are invariably thrombogenic unless anticoagulant therapy is used. They work better in the aortic position than in the mitral, partly because the left ventricle is a high-pressure pump and can cope with the extra pressure drop across the valve, while the left atrium, which produces much lower pressures, cannot cope with the extra pressure drop and ventricular filling is impaired. Gluteraldehyde-fixed, porcine, aortic valves, mounted on stents, are used clinically in both aortic and mitral positions without anticoagulant therapy. However, their long-term durability remains to be proven (10).

In an attempt to exploit the control and closure mechanism of the natural mitral valve in a prosthetic design, we have designed a single-cusp valve which has a number of novel features (11). The valve seat is D-shaped, which is a better approximation to the kidney-shaped natural mitral annulus than the circular ring of conventional prosthetic valves. Attached to the long edge of the D is a single, hinged cusp corresponding to the anterior cusp of the mitral valve (Figure 6). The cusp contains a rigid disc, which is concave on the ventricular side and perforated to allow keying to the polyurethane with which it is coated. The long, flexible, polyurethane hinge permits the cusp to open until it is at 180° to the valve seat. When the valve is closed the rigid disc locates on the rigid valve seat and the hinge is unstressed.

In model experiments with the prosthetic monocusp valve, it was seen that a strong vortex formed in the outflow tract behind the cusp and that much of valve closure occurred during diastole (Figure 3b). The cusp never opened beyond 90° to the valve seat, since it was controlled by the flow patterns within the left ventricle.

Six monocusp valves were placed in the mitral position in goats. Since the metal disc in the valve cusp and the metal reinforcement in the valve seat were both radiopaque it was easy to observe valve movements in the intact

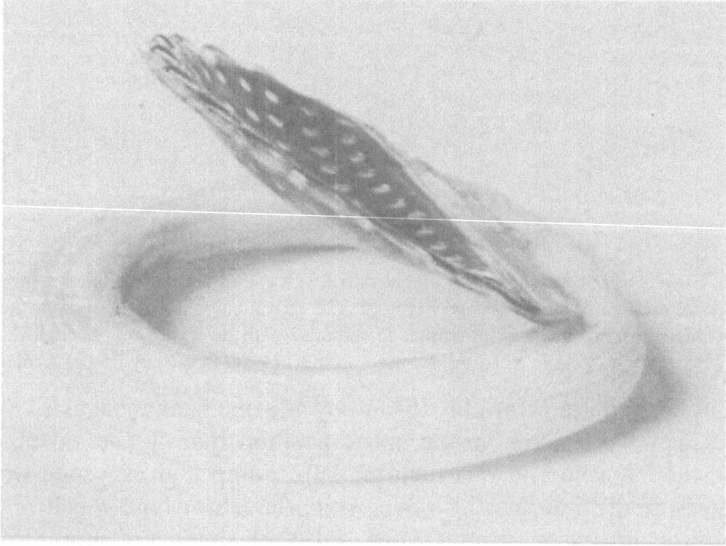

*Figure 6.* Photograph of the Oxford monocusp mitral valve. The valve seat is D-shaped, and the cusp is hinged along the straight edge of the D.

animal. The cusp opened wide (90° to the seat) early in diastole, moved gently towards closure until it was nearly shut at the end of diastole. When radiopaque dye was injected into the left ventricle a strong vortex behind the cusp was observed. Backflow on valve closure was negligible. Accelerated fatigue tests with this mitral valve in saline indicate fatigue lifetimes in excess of 650 million cycles.

The six valves implanted in goats have functioned satisfactorily for extended periods without anticoagulant therapy (11). Three goats are alive and well at 12 months, 6 months and 2 months after implantation. One goat was sacrificed at 6 months, one died at 3 months and one died at 1.5 months during catheterization. Tissue growth on the hinge has been a problem in some goats, particularly in those with the smallest-sized mitral valve where the ratio of valve orifice area to tissue annulus area was smallest.

## 5. MEMBRANE LUNG

Simple and efficient bubble oxygenators are widely used in open-heart surgery, but they cause significant blood trauma if perfusions last for more than a few hours. Although membrane oxygenators are sufficiently atraumatic to blood to permit prolonged perfusions, viscous boundary layers within the blood channels and oxygen concentration gradients at the membrane surfaces limited oxygen transfer rates in earlier designs. Oxygen has low solubility in plasma and consequently diffuses very slowly in blood. One way of overcoming this problem is to use narrow blood channels in the membrane oxygenator, but this produces high hydraulic resistance unless the channels are very short, and then flow distribution is a major problem.

A much better way of enhancing oxygen transfer is to stir the blood, transporting oxygen-poor red blood cells from the centre of each blood channel to the membranes and displacing oxygen-rich red cells from the membrane surface into the mainstream. In Oxford we used pulsatile blood flow over a furrowed membrane surface to generate secondary flows which mixed the blood and greatly enhanced gas transfer (12, 13). Membrane lungs were built with silicone rubber membranes, and oxygen and carbon dioxide transfer rates of 160 ml/min·m$^2$ of membrane were attained in prolonged animal experiments in new-born lambs. These transfer rates should be compared with 50 ml/min·m$^2$ in an efficient membrane oxygenator of conventional design which does not use secondary flows.

More recently, Spratt et al. (14) have reported on a version of the Oxford membrane lung which employed a microporous Teflon membrane and with which gas transfer rates of 420 ml/min·m$^2$ of membrane were achieved during extra-corporeal circulation of calves.

The membrane lung consisted of four blood channels and had a membrane surface area of 0.3 m². A section through two of the blood channels is shown in Figure 7. Furrowed microporous polytetrafluoroethylene membranes separated the blood and gas phases and were mounted on rigid plastic support plates. The gas flowed in the space provided between the membranes and the support plates, at right angles to the direction of blood flow. The blood channel spacing was 0.5 mm, furrow depth was 0.6 mm and furrow pitch was 2.2 mm.

Flexible bladders were mounted at each end of the membrane lung, and were actuated mechanically, in anti-phase, to provide a pulsatile component of blood flow. Mean blood flow was provided by a conventional roller pump on the inlet (venous) side of the membrane lung.

As blood accelerated from left to right across the furrows, strong vortices formed within the hollows as in Figure 7. When the flow reversed, these vortices were ejected and were replaced by a set of contra-rotating vortices. This mechanism provided sufficiently high shear stress at the membrane, combined with good exchange of blood between the hollows and the mainstream to ensure high efficiency in gas transfer.

The performance of the membrane lung in transferring both oxygen and carbon dioxide is shown in Figure 8. Blood flow rate through the membrane lung is plotted along the abscissa, and gas transfer rate divided by blood flow rate is plotted along the ordinate. The reference blood flow (14, 15) for oxygen was 2.9 l/min and for carbon dioxide it was 2.8 l/min. Since the membrane area was 0.3 m², the oxygen transfer rate under reference flow conditions was $(45 \times 2.9)/0.3 = 435$ ml/min·m². The corresponding transfer rate for carbon dioxide was $(45 \times 2.8)/0.3 = 420$ ml/min·m².

To see if the secondary blood flows enhanced gas transfer only at the expense of blood trauma, comparative studies were undertaken between

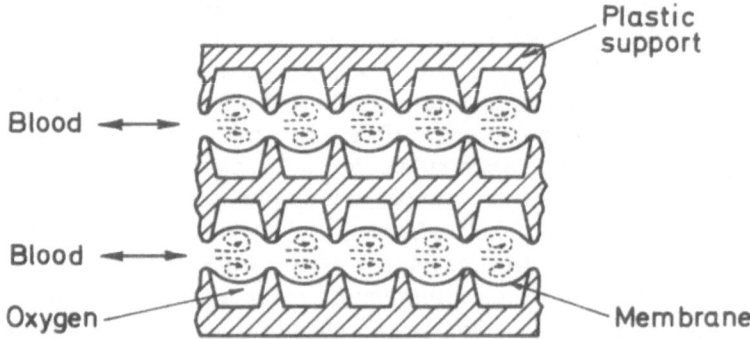

*Figure 7.* Cross-section of the furrowed membrane lung. The microporous membrane is supported on a plastic plate. Oxygen passages lie between membrane and the support plate in a direction perpendicular to the plane of the figure. Vortices are formed in the hollows as blood is pulsated back and forth across the furrows.

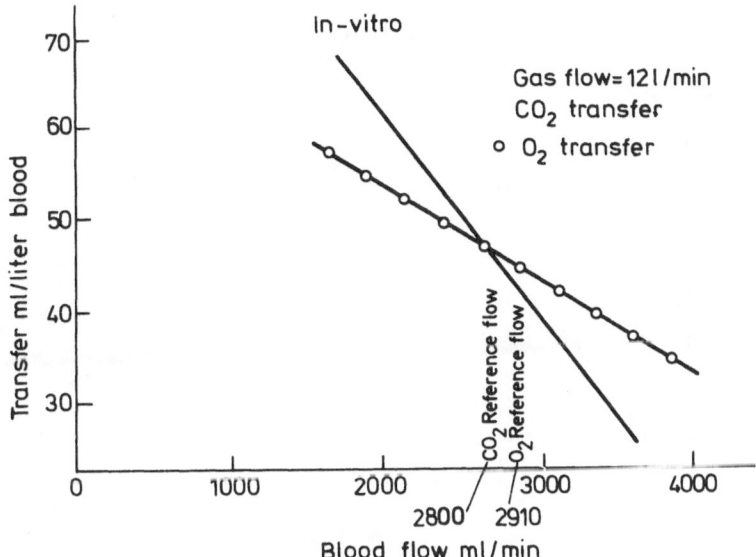

*Figure 8.* Performance of a furrowed membrane lung with 0.3 m² surface area. Blood flow rate is plotted along the abscissa and gas transfer rate divided by blood flow rate is plotted along the ordinate. The rated blood flow corresponds to a value of 45 on the ordinate (14, 15). The rated blood flows for $O_2$ and $CO_2$ were 2.9 and 2.8 l/min respectively.

extracorporeal circuits which contained the membrane lung and those in which it was absent (14). Plasma hemoglobin levels remained low throughout 6-hour perfusions (Figure 9), and although levels in the control circuit were always lower than when the oxygenator was included, there was no difference between them at the end of 6 hours. Platelet numbers fell rapidly immediately after bypass was begun, but these levelled off at about 70% of their initial values and remained stable throughout the 6-hour bypass (Figure 10). There was no significant difference in the platelet loss between the circuits with and without the membrane lung.

## 6. FLUID MECHANICS OF VORTICES IN TWO DIMENSIONS

We have made hydraulic models of the furrowed channels used in the membrane lung, and have tracked particle paths by means of high-speed cine film (17). Although these studies permitted us to visualize the process of vortex formation and ejection in pulsatile flow, and were useful in obtaining empirical design criteria, they were of little help in predicting the effects of changes in scale or geometry on flow patterns and mass transfer.

An alternative approach, undertaken in Oxford by Sobey (18), was to solve the equations for fluid flow (Navier-Stokes equations) numerically.

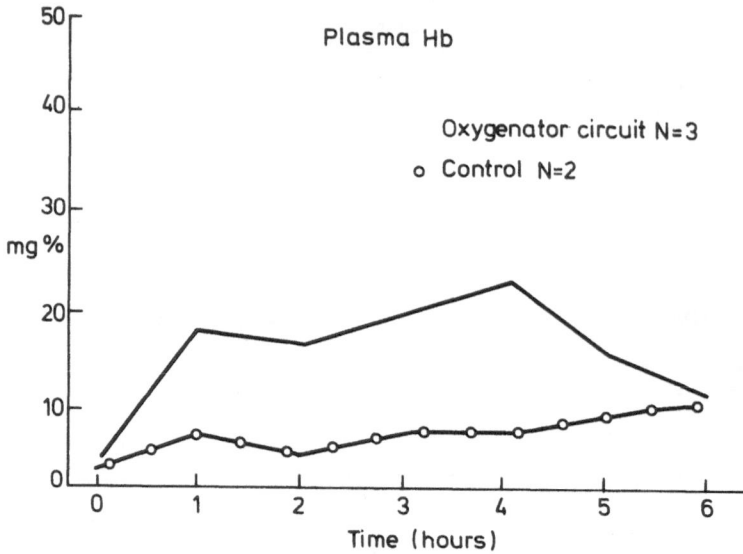

*Figure 9.* Plasma hemoglobin measurements during animal trials with the furrowed membrane oxygenator. The graph compares plasma hemoglobin levels in extra-corporeal bypass with and without (control) oxygenator in the circuit over 6-hour perfusions.

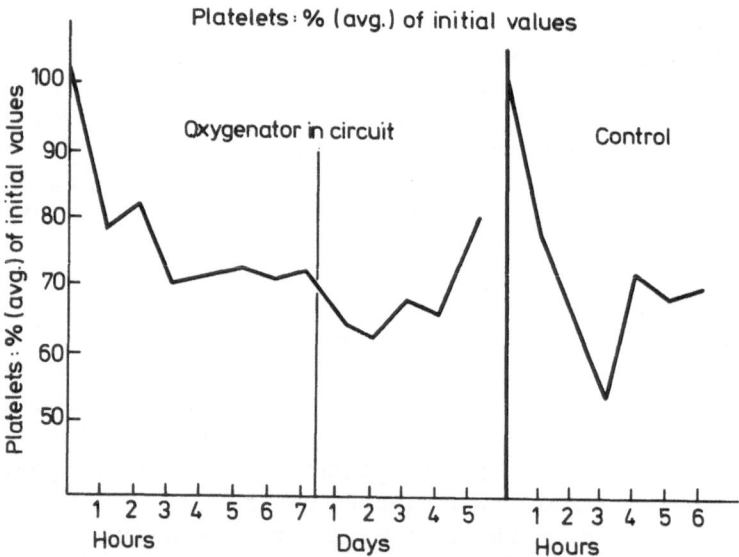

*Figure 10.* Platelet counts during animal trials with the furrowed membrane oxygenator. The graph compares platelet numbers in extra-corporeal bypass with and without (control) oxygenator in the circuit over 6-hour perfusions.

Sobey considered sinusoidal flow in a furrowed channel which was long enough for the velocity distributions at the inlet and outlet ends of a furrow to be identical. His calculated solutions agreed well with experimental observations. Typical results are shown (Figure 11) for sinusoidal flow in furrows of the same proportions as those used in the membrane lung. The time is given non-dimensionally, so $t = 0$ corresponds to flow in the mainstream accelerating from rest to the right, $t = 0.5$ corresponds to mainstream flow accelerating from rest to the left, and peak forward flow occurs when $t = 0.25$. The cycle period is unity.

In Figure 11, at $t = 0.225$, the flow has separated at the upstream lip of the hollow and reattached at the furrow bottom to form a small, strong vortex. Outside the vortex the streamlines expand to sweep the furrow bottom. At $t = 0.250$, the vortex has increased in size and mainstream flow is at its maximum value. As the mainstream decelerates, the vortex grows rapidly, $t = 0.323$, 0.400, until it bulges out into the mainstream at $t = 0.469$, just before the mainstream comes to rest. During the initial reverse flow phase

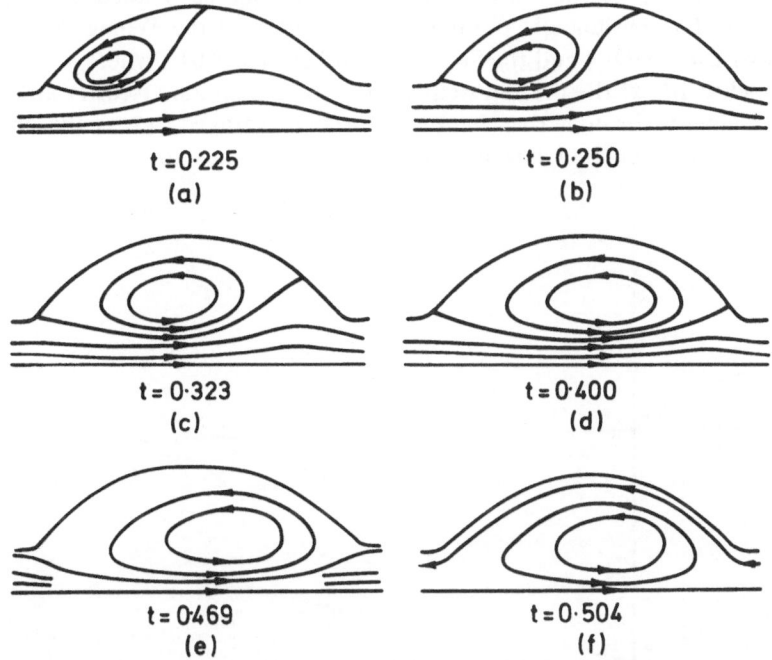

*Figure 11.* Computed streamlines for pulsatile flow in a part-circular hollow. The mainstream flow is sinusoidal. The time scale is non-dimensional, with the mainstream at rest at $t = 0$, and the period of oscillation unity. Peak forward flow occurs at $t = 0.25$. The vortex grows during forward flow until it bulges into the mainstream at $t = 0.469$. Just after the mainstream reverses the vortex is ejected from the hollow by fluid passing between the vortex and the hollow wall ($t = 0.504$).

the fluid then flows between the vortex and the furrow wall, $t = 0.504$, and displaces the vortex into the channel. The vortex is then washed away by the backward-flowing mainstream. Separation then occurs again at the right-hand lip of the furrow and a counter-rotating vortex is established in the furrow during the reversed-flow phase of the cycle. Sobey calculated vortex strength for hollows with different chord-to-depth ratios and concluded that 4:1 (the value chosen empirically for the oxygenator) was optimal. He was able to show, also, that flow patterns in channels with sinusoidally-varying walls were qualitatively the same as those in channels with sharp-lipped hollows. He concluded that vortex formation was caused by inertial effects, not by the generation of vortex sheets at the hollow lips.

When designing mass-transfer devices which exploit these secondary flows it is important to know what operating parameters apply. Sobey calculated a demarcation line between the regions in which "strong" vortices are present (above the line in Figure 12) and where they are absent (below the line). The circles are obtained from flow visualization experiments, using pulsatile flow of water containing suspended polystyrene particles. The parameters plotted are the square of the Witzig-Womersley number $\alpha = h\sqrt{(\Omega/\gamma)}$ and the Strouhal number $St = h\Omega/U$, where $h$ is half the channel width, $\Omega$ the driving frequency, $\gamma$ the kinematic viscosity and $\upsilon$ the peak velocity through the channel (spatially averaged across the channel width). The calculated line in Figure 12 corresponds to a peak Reynolds number $Uh/\gamma$ of 5.

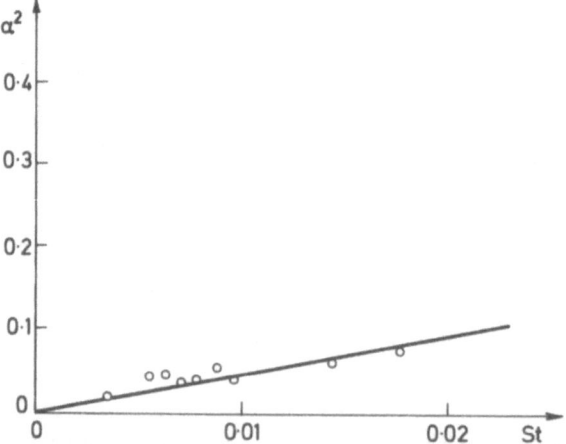

*Figure 12.* Graph of $\alpha^2$ against $St$ showing the demarcation line between the regions where vortices are predicted (above the line) and where they are not (below the line). The open circles correspond to experimental observations of transition to vortex patterns. The Witzig-Womersley parameter $\alpha$ is defined as $h\sqrt{(\Omega/\gamma)}$ and the Strouhal number $St$ is $h\Omega/U$ where $h$ is half the channel width, $\Omega$ the driving frequency, $\gamma$ the kinematic viscosity and $U$ the peak velocity through the channel (spatially averaged across the channel width).

We plan to use these computational methods to gain a better understanding of the complex vortex flows, and also to help us optimize designs of membrane lungs, dialysers and ultrafilters.


7. CONCLUSIONS

Vortices generated by unsteady flows control the function of the natural aortic and mitral valves, the Oxford prosthetic mitral valve and our high-performance membrane lung.

In both mitral and aortic valves, vortices ensure that when the flow through the valve decelerates, the cusps move towards closure. Another function of the vortices is to mix the blood within the aortic sinuses to prevent stasis and thrombosis. It is no accident that the coronary ostia lie within the sinuses of the aortic valve, since this permits the coronary circulation to benefit, in systole, from pressure recovery within the vortices. A single-leaflet prosthetic mitral valve, operated by a mechanism similar to that used by the natural valve has shown considerable promise in prolonged animal trials without the use of anticoagulant therapy.

Convectively-formed vortices are used to provide excellent mixing in the blood channels of the Oxford membrane lung, and they greatly enhance gas transfer without damaging the blood.

Sobey's theoretical and computational work on unsteady vortices gives us a new insight into vortex growth and structure, and also provides us with valuable design information for artificial lungs and kidneys.


SUMMARY

The role of vortices in the natural aortic and mitral valves, in prosthetic replacement valves and in a compact membrane lung, is the theme of this paper.

The natural aortic valve opens wide early in systole and strong vortices form rapidly in the aortic sinuses. The vortices help position the valve cusps and, together with the pressure gradient produced by aortic flow deceleration during the latter part of systole, move the cusps towards closure. Thus the valve is almost closed by the end of systole.

The natural mitral valve exploits a similar closure mechanism, despite the very different anatomy of the two valves. During diastole, the incoming jet of blood entering the left ventricle strikes the apex of the ventricle and forms a ring vortex with its main strength in the outflow tract. This vortex acts principally on the anterior cusp, moving it towards closure. Flow deceleration is again an important aid to diastolic closure movements of the mitral valve. Recent results of animal trials with a prosthetic mitral valve, consisting of a rigid D-shaped sewing ring and a single, hinged disc, are encouraging. Cusp movements and vortex patterns which were recorded radiographically, accorded well with model experiments.

Membrane lungs cause much less blood trauma than bubble oxygenators, when used for extracorporeal circulation of blood, but suffer from poor performance because boundary layers inhibit oxygen transfer. The use of pulsatile blood flow over furrowed membrane surfaces causes vortices to be formed in the hollows. The vortices disrupt the boundary layers and greatly enhance gas transfer. Animal experiments with the furrowed membrane lung have demonstrated that high rates of gas transfer can be maintained, provided blood flow is pulsatile, without significant blood trauma.

Numerical solutions of the Navier-Stokes equations, for pulsatile blood flow in the furrowed membrane lung, were undertaken by Dr. I.J. Sobey in Oxford. His solutions show good agreement with model experiments, and provide a new insight into vortex growth and structure in unsteady flow.

REFERENCES

1. Witzig K: *Über erzwungene Wellenbewegungen zäher, inkompressibler Flüssigkeiten in elastischen Röhren,* Bern, Ph.D. Thesis, 1914.
2. Womersley JR: Method for the calculation of velocity, rate of flow and viscous drag in arteries when the pressure gradient is known. *J Physiol* 127:553–563, 1955.
3. Vinci L da: *Quaderni d'Anatomica* 2:9, 1513.
4. Henderson Y, Johnson FE: Two modes of closure of the heart valves. *Heart* 4:69–82, 1912.
5. Schultz DL, Tunstall Pedoe DS, Lee G de J, Gunning AJ, Bellhouse BJ: Velocity distribution and transition in the arterial system. In: *CIBA foundation symposium on circulatory and respiratory mass transport,* London, 1968, p 172.
6. Bellhouse BJ, Bellhouse FH: Fluid mechanics of model normal and stenosed aortic valves. *Circ Res* 25:693–704, 1969.
7. Gregg DE: Physiology of the coronary circulation. *Circulation* 27:1128–1137, 1963.
8. Cornhill JF: Haemodynamic studies of coronary arteries. D Phil thesis, Oxford University, 1976.
9. Bellhouse BJ: Fluid mechanics of a model mitral valve and left ventricle. *Cardiovasc Res* 6:199–210, 1972.
10. Spray TL, Roberts WC: Structural changes in porcine xenografts used as substitute cardiac valves. *Am J Cardiol* 40:319–330, 1977.
11. Williams WG, Bellhouse BJ, Bellhouse FH, Haworth WS, Kent G, Lewis RWH: A single-leaflet mitral valve: its design, development and evaluation in long-term animal trials. *Trans Am Soc Artif Int Organs* 24, 1978.
12. Bellhouse BJ, Bellhouse FH, Curl CM, MacMillan TI, Gunning AJ, Spratt EH, MacMurray SB, Nelems JM: A high efficiency membrane oxygenator and pulsatile pumping system, and its application to animal trials. *Trans Am Soc Artif Int Organs* 19:72–79, 1973.
13. Nelems JM, Bellhouse BJ, Curl CM, MacMillan TI, MacMurray SB: Prolonged pulmonary support of new-born lambs with the Oxford membrane oxygenator. *Trans. Am Soc Artif Int Organs* 20:293–298, 1974.
14. Spratt EH, Edmunds J, Badolato A, Servas FM, Bellhouse BJ: Design and performance of high efficiency pulsatile membrane lung. *Proc Eur Soc Artif Organs* 3:123–126, 1976.
15. Standard for blood gas exchangers: draft proposal. *Trans Am Soc Artif Int Organs* 22:734, 1976.

16. Bellhouse BJ, Bellhouse FH, Snuggs TA, Aggarwal JK: Fluid mechanics of the Oxford membrane oxygenator and its evaluation in animal experiments. In: *Physiological and clinical aspects of oxygenator design.* Dawids SG, Engell HC (eds), Amsterdam, North-Holland, 1976, p 91–104.
17. Bellhouse BJ, Snuggs TA: Augmented mass transfer in a membrane lung and a haemodialyser using vortex mixing. In: *INSERM-Euromech* 92, Cardiovascular and pulmonary dynamics 71, 1977, p 371–384.
18. Sobey IJ: Fluid mechanics of the Oxford oxygenator. In *Conference digest of 1st international conference on mechanics in medicine and biology*, Aachen, Witzstrock, 1978, p V-183.

## 6.2. FLUID DYNAMICS IN THE AORTA

G. DE J. LEE

> "*Let no man read me who is not
> mathematician to my principles.*"
> Leonardo da Vinci.
> "*Be sure to approach your delibe-
> rations together in a truly integrated
> way.*"
> D.J. Kuenen.

This 1978 meeting of the international Cardiovascular System Dynamics
Society has provided a large number of papers on current endeavour
relating to the study of muscle and chamber function of the heart, especially
its left ventricle. I suspect, however, that the clinical members of the society
in particular will consider that we are still quite far from understanding how
best to study myocardial performance in man. Indeed the presence of so
many reports to the society at this meeting on attempts to arrive at the
truth through modelling experiments suggests that the basic scientists as
well as the more applied of us still just do not know the answers in the
intact healthy heart, let alone one affected by disease.

Even less sure are we of means to assess myocardial function in the face
of complicated loading conditions imposed on the heart ventricles as a
consequence of valve disease. That is why, in Oxford, Dr. Schultz and I
have developed such a deep interest in the possibility of defining the inate
pumping function of the heart independent of changes imposed upon it by
alterations in its load (Schultz et al., this volume). Our scientific relationship
first developed because I found as a cardiologist and clinical investigator
that, although I had unique opportunities to study man, because of the need
for pathophysiological diagnosis, I was not intellectually or professionally
competent to do so in terms of modern fluid dynamics. In short I failed full
intellectual entry to a society such as this whose language of fraternity has
such close affinity with that of my first quotation, "Let no man read me who
is not mathematician to my principles." This remarkable statement by
Leonardo da Vinci is made in the introduction to his collection of anatomical drawings. Dr. Schultz, on the other hand, clearly saw the scientific
opportunities offered by applying fluid dynamic principles to the study of

J. Baan, A.C. Arntzenius, E.L. Yellin (eds.), Cardiac Dynamics, 463–475.

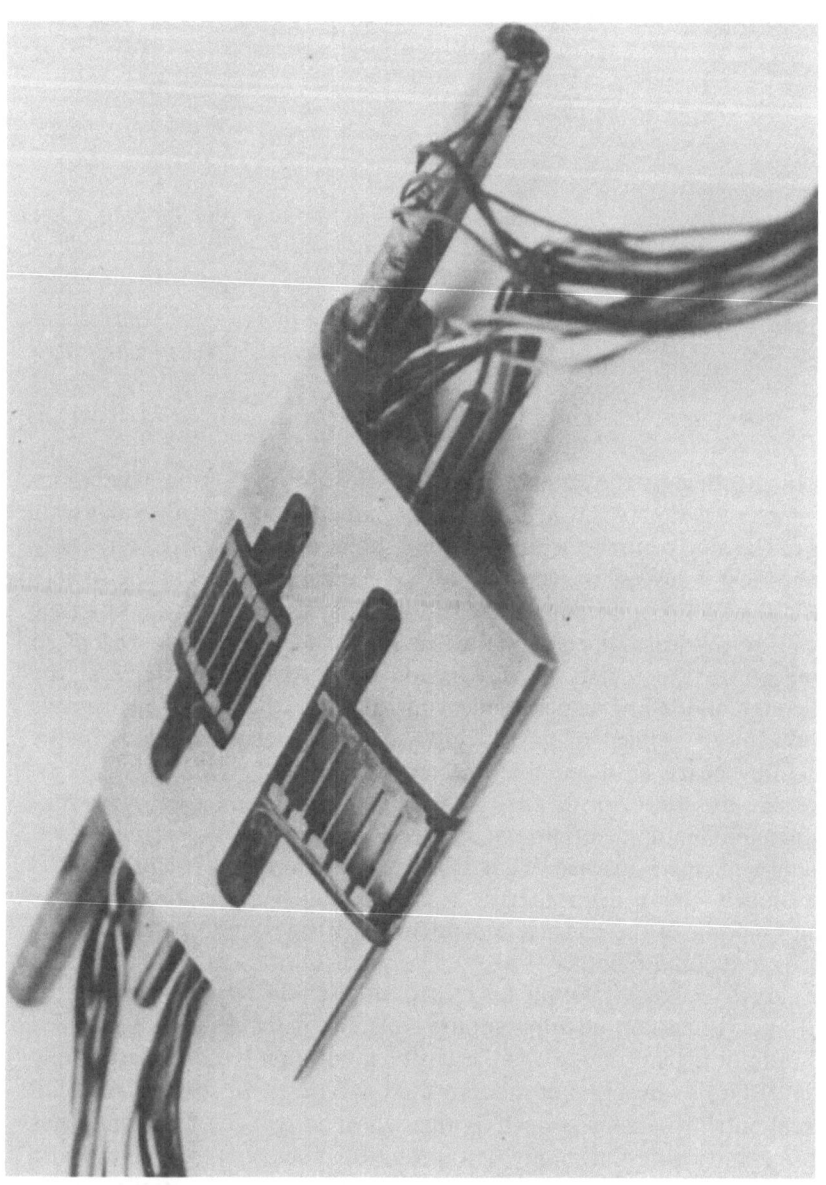

*Figure 1.* Photograph of platinum thin films mounted upon a jet engine turbine blade to measure heat transfer (by courtesy of Dr. D.L. Schultz, Univeristy of Oxford).

the human circulation. Hence our common purpose and a personal feeling of security at this conference that we are following the wisdom provided in my second quotation, "Be sure to approach your deliberations together in a truly integrated way," which was some of the wise counsel of Professor Kuenen in his rectorial address to us when he opened this conference.

The heat/velocity sensors that Dr. Schultz had been using for aerodynamic research (Figure 1) were ideal for our initial studies together; for even the velocity profile in the ascending aorta and main pulmonary artery were unknown when we started. The devices consist of thin gold or platinum films painted on small glass beads which are mounted in appropriate needles or catheters (Figure 2) to map velocities in vessels. This was first done in animals and then in man. The thin film is heated to maintain a constant temperature some 5°C above blood temperature, using a feedback bridge circuit. The frequency response of the device is limited only by that of the high-frequency amplifier driving it (1). Additional elements can also be incorporated on either side of the heated film to sense direction of flow as well as magnitude of velocity (Figure 3).

Figure 4 shows data obtained from the dog showing that the velocity profile in the ascending aorta is virtually uniform across its full cross-sectional diameter in the antero-posterior dimension throughout the cardiac cycle. This was also the case in the lateral dimension. Figure 5 shows velocity profiles from the human ascending aorta and main pulmonary artery obtained from needle traverses during open-heart surgery. Uniform velocity profiles were again found (1, 2). This information provided the necessary basis to allow calculations of bulk flow in both vessels from catheter-tip velocity measurements and a knowledge of the diameter of the vessels (3, 4).

Early clinical studies using a catheter-tip thin-film velocity meter enabled us to sense the importance of the pump function of the heart in the assessment of prognosis, even survival, particularly when selecting patients with valve disease for surgery. Figure 6 is an example of this in a patient with chronic heart failure from mitral incompetence in spite of obsessional medical management. At cardiac catheterization peak velocity in the ascending aorta was 40 cm/sec. The patient was next confined to bed for one month, all other treatment remaining the same. At open-heart surgery needle measurement from the ascending aorta showed that the patient's left ventricle could now eject blood with a peak velocity of 130 cm/sec.

We were next joined by Dr. Tunstall Pedoe who began to study the effects of valve disease upon aortic blood flow (5). I began to become somewhat dispirited about hopes that studies of fluid dynamics in the aorta would ever allow the clinical investigator to obtain useful information of myocardial function in the face of aortic valve disease. Not only is there the intuitively simple concept of increased ventricular load imposed either by

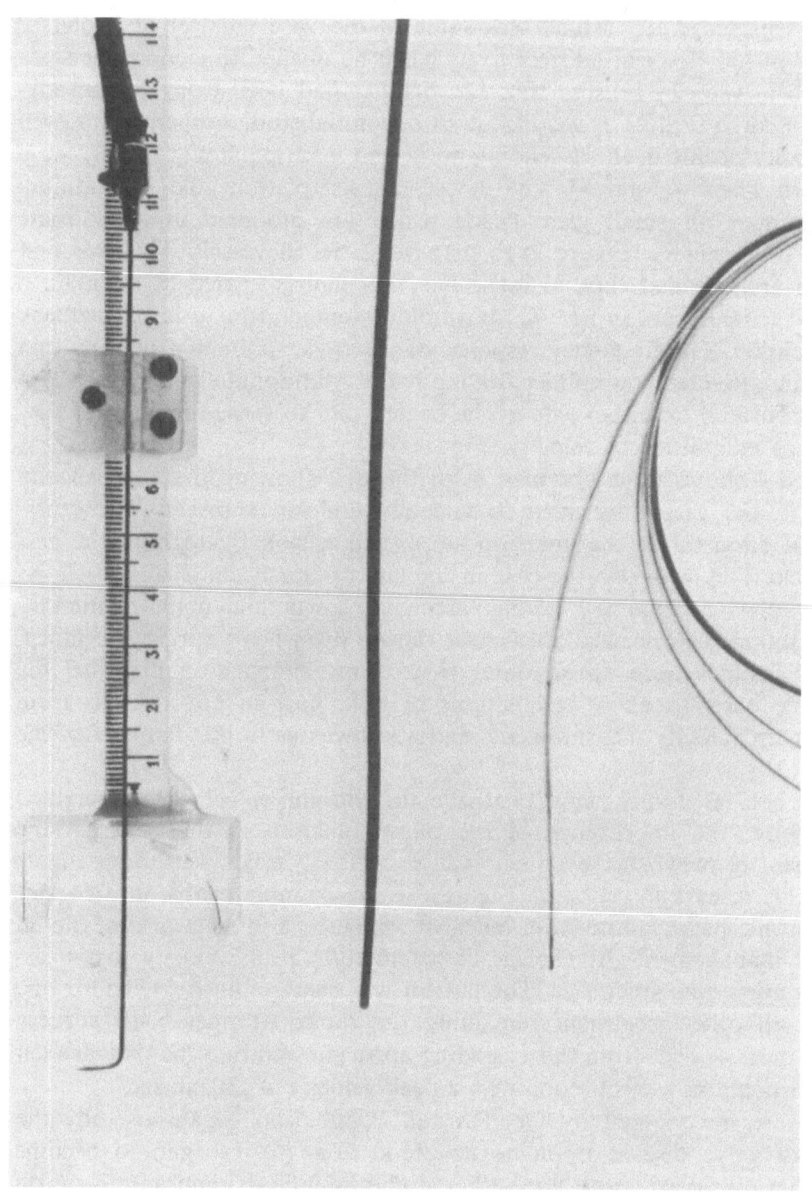

*Figure 2.* Photograph of a velocity sensing needle and its mount, used to map velocity profiles in the aorta and pulmonary artery. Velocity sensors mounted in the tip of a cardiac catheter and a fine nylon "float" catheter are also shown.

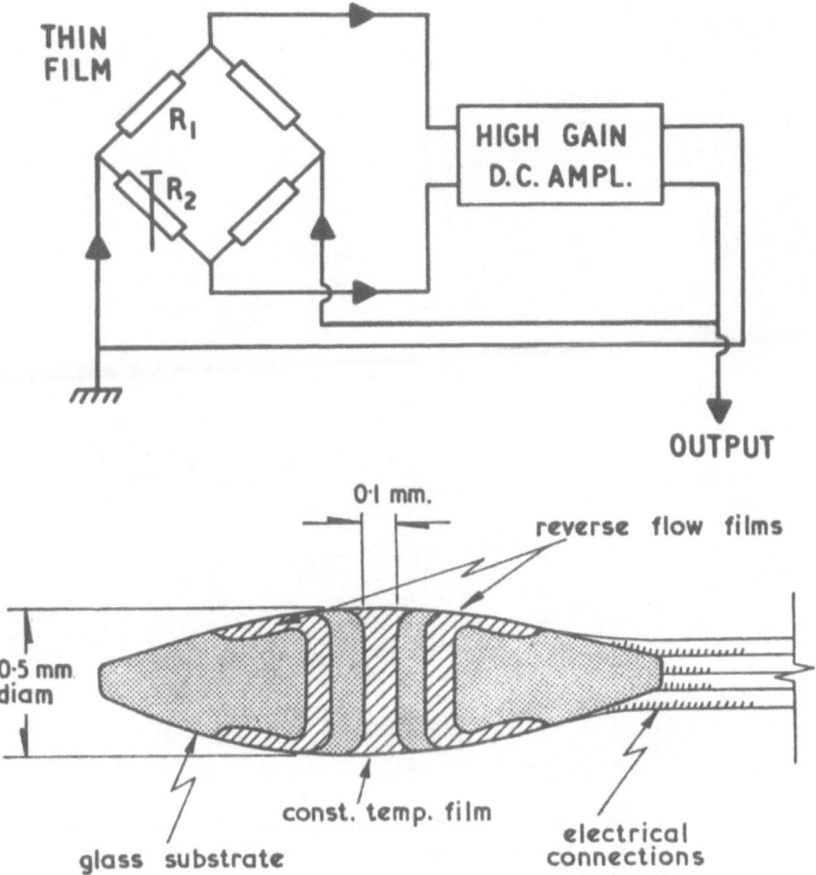

*Figure 3. Top*: design of a triple element thin-film probe for insertion in a catheter or hypodermic needle; *bottom*: diagram of feedback bridge to achieve operation at constant resistance of thin-film velocity probe. The bridge circuits for the direction sensitive films on either side of the velocity sensor are not shown.

obstruction or leakage of the valve; but, in addition, there are much more complex energy losses imposed by the transformation of laminar outflow from the heart to highly disturbed blood flow, often so great that red cell hemolysis occurs. It is about these energy losses that we are to learn today from some of our speakers. They arise from the disturbed flow which Dr. Tunstall Pedoe first described qualitatively in his work on aortic stenosis and incompetence (5). Figure 7 shows examples from this work of velocity profiles in the human ascending aorta in aortic stenosis and aortic incompetence.

I would now like to remind you again of my second quotation, taken

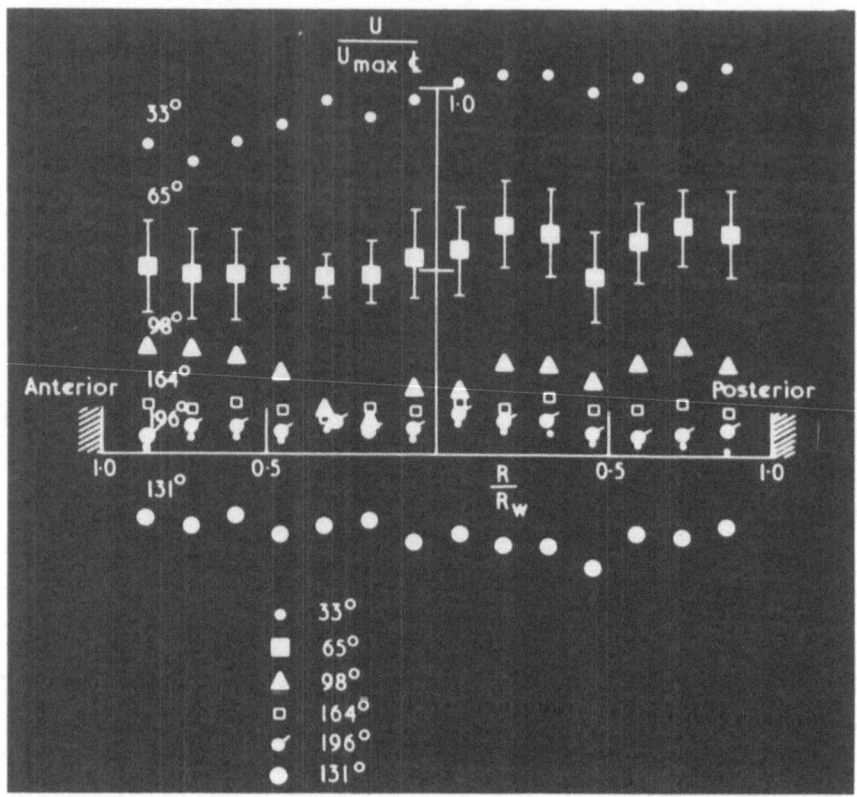

*Figure 4.* Velocity profile ($U/U_{max}$ at centre line) in dog ascending aorta. 1 cardiac cycle = 360°. Values averaged from 10 cardiac cycles are shown. Maximum divergence from average occurs during deceleration at 65°.

more or less directly from the lips of Professor Kuenen in his rectorial address to this conference: "Be sure to approach your deliberations together in a truly integrated way." May we try hard to follow his instructions, for rarely do applied mathematicians, physicists, engineers, physiologists, clinical investigators and conventional practicing physicians have the opportunity to meet together for long enough truly to assist one another in acquiring the necessary understanding of each other's disciplines. For this reason I hope we can make a beginning in learning how and how not to tackle the problems posed by human valve disease. This is important not merely as an academic exercise in applied fluid dynamics. For instance we need to develop reliable ways of assessing the strain imposed on the heart as a pump by the valve disease. We need to know for how long the heart pump can safely sustain this added load, for ideally, the clinician needs to select patients for valve surgery only when the pump is beginning to decide

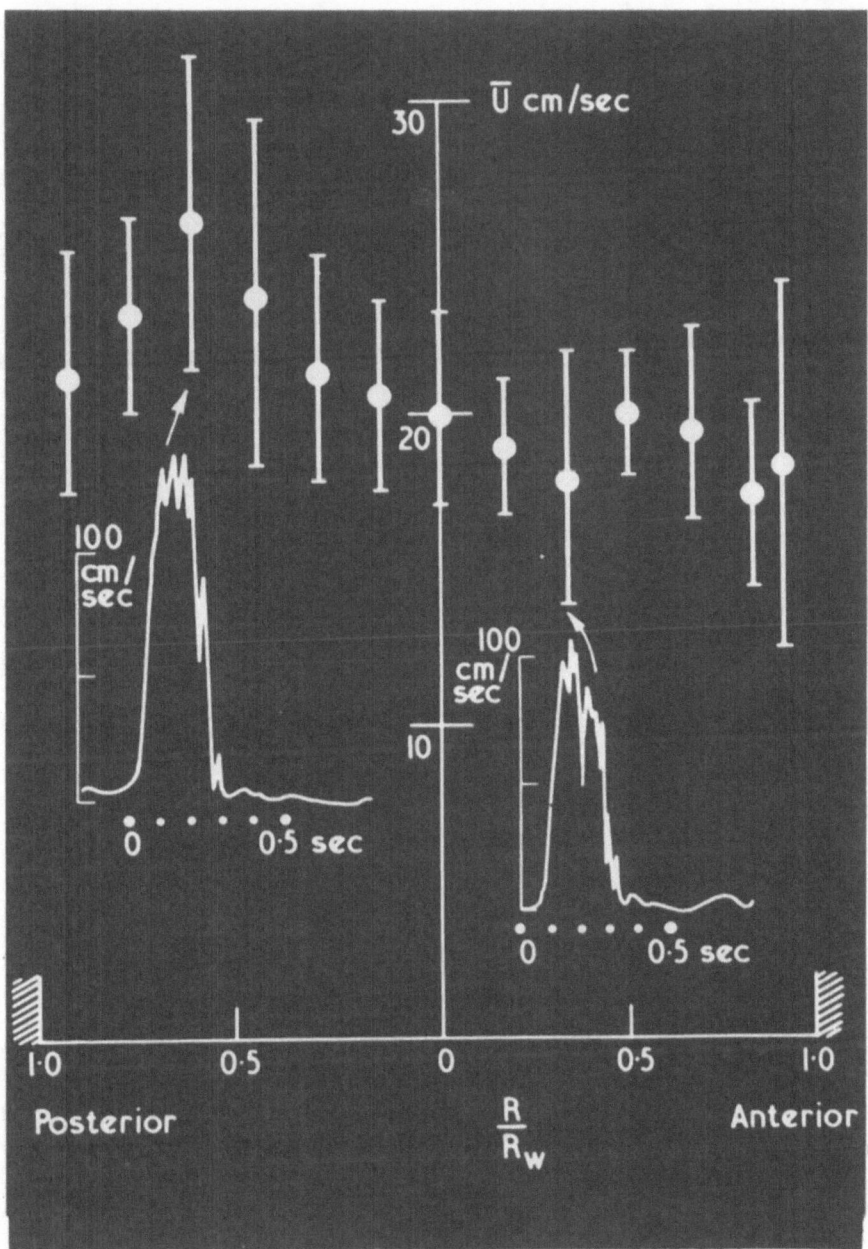

*Figure 5a.* Velocity profile in the normal ascending aorta of man obtained at the time of surgery for mitral incompetence. Time-averaged velocity V at each radial station ±1 standard deviation. Inserts show instantaneous velocity records from 2 stations with some turbulence. Maximum velocity 130 cm/sec.

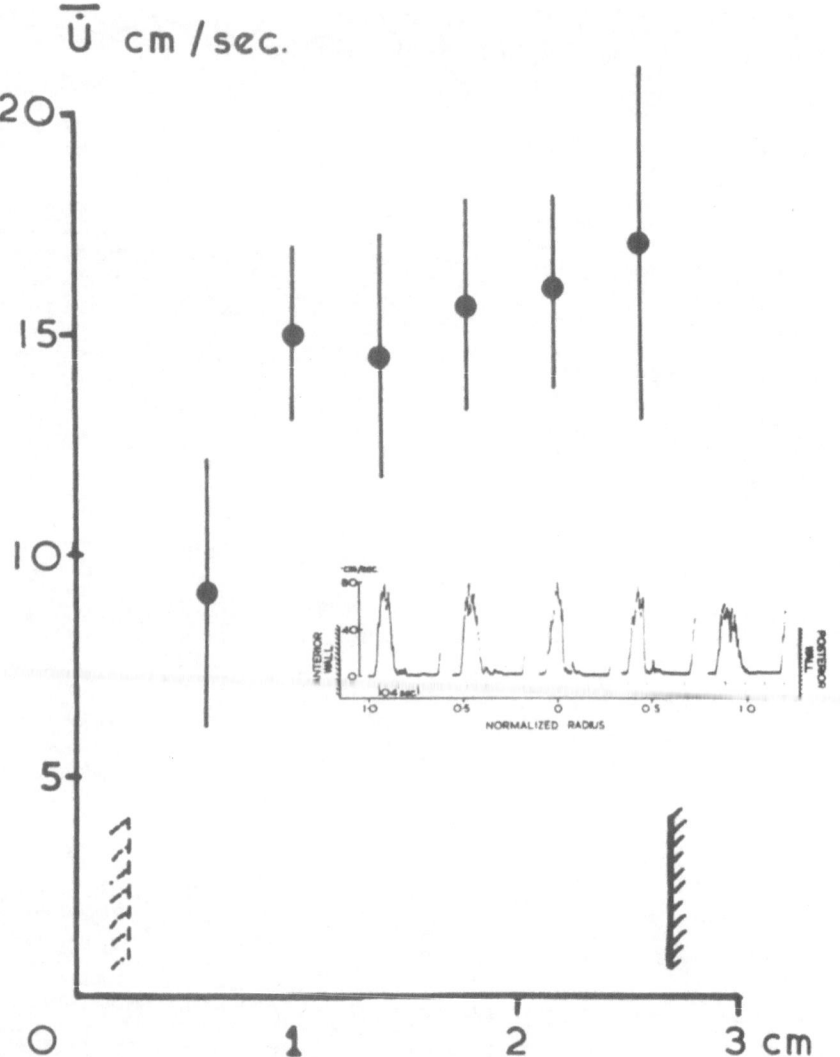

*Figure 5b.* Velocity profile in the normal main pulmonary artery of man obtained at the time of surgery for mitral incompetence. The instantaneous velocity trace at several stations is shown as well as the time-averaged velocity and its variation over 10 cardiac cycles.

to fail to respond to the added load. My reason for this cautious attitude to valve surgery is that I believe that we shall learn in this session about the necessary fluid dynamic requirements for optimal valve opening and closure in the aorta in particular. This is virtually impossible to achieve with

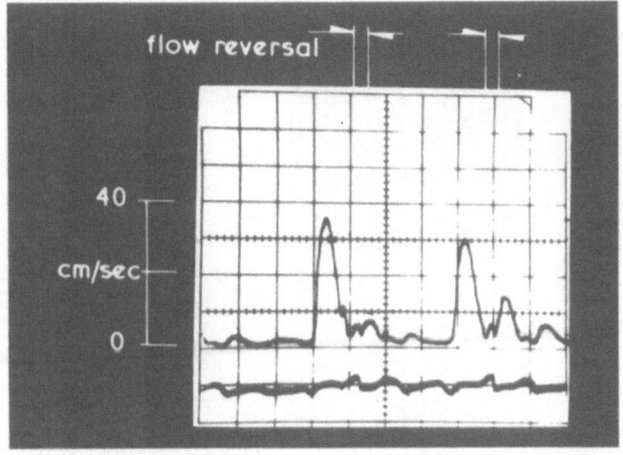

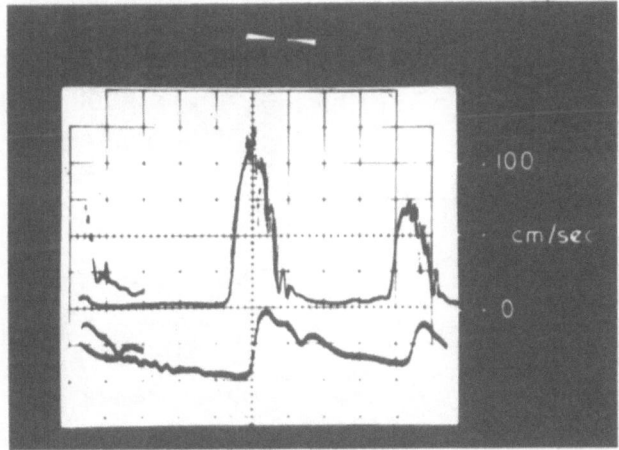

*Figure 6. Top:* aortic velocity recorded with catheter-tip probe, male 42 years, mitral incompetence, heart failure. Maximum velocity cm/sec. (Lower trace: signal from flow reversal detection system). *Bottom:* aortic velocity, same patient one month later after bed rest. Maximum velocity 130 cm/sec showing some turbulence (lower trace: femoral artery pressure).

current artificial devices, or even with graft valves, partly because of anatomical distortion produced by the disease process itself. Hence the likelihood that mortality and morbidity risks associated with valve implants will occur not only from immediate surgery but from long-term factors such as valve disintegration, embolism and infection. These events may well have a large component of their cause provided purely from fluid dynamic perturbations.

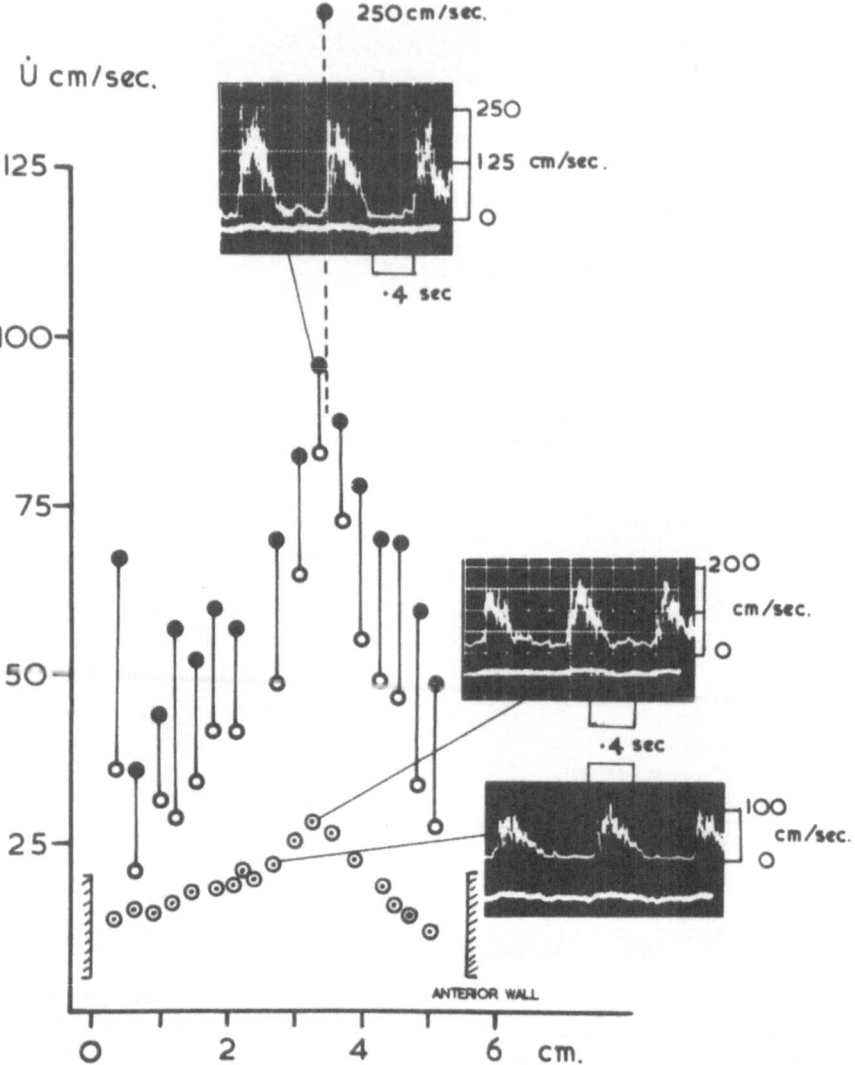

*Figure 7a.* Pre-operative aortic traverse in patient with aortic stenosis. Maximum and minimum systolic instantaneous velocities and time-averaged velocities are shown.

Dr. Bellhouse in his work on the fluid dynamics of the aortic valve (this volume) and in his Witzig lecture (this volume) shows us how important vortex formation can be for the normal behaviour of heart valves. He has also exploited vortices to increase gas and solute exchange efficiency of artificial membrane oxygenators and artificial kidneys. His detailed studies of the importance of vortices in the circulation link him across the centuries

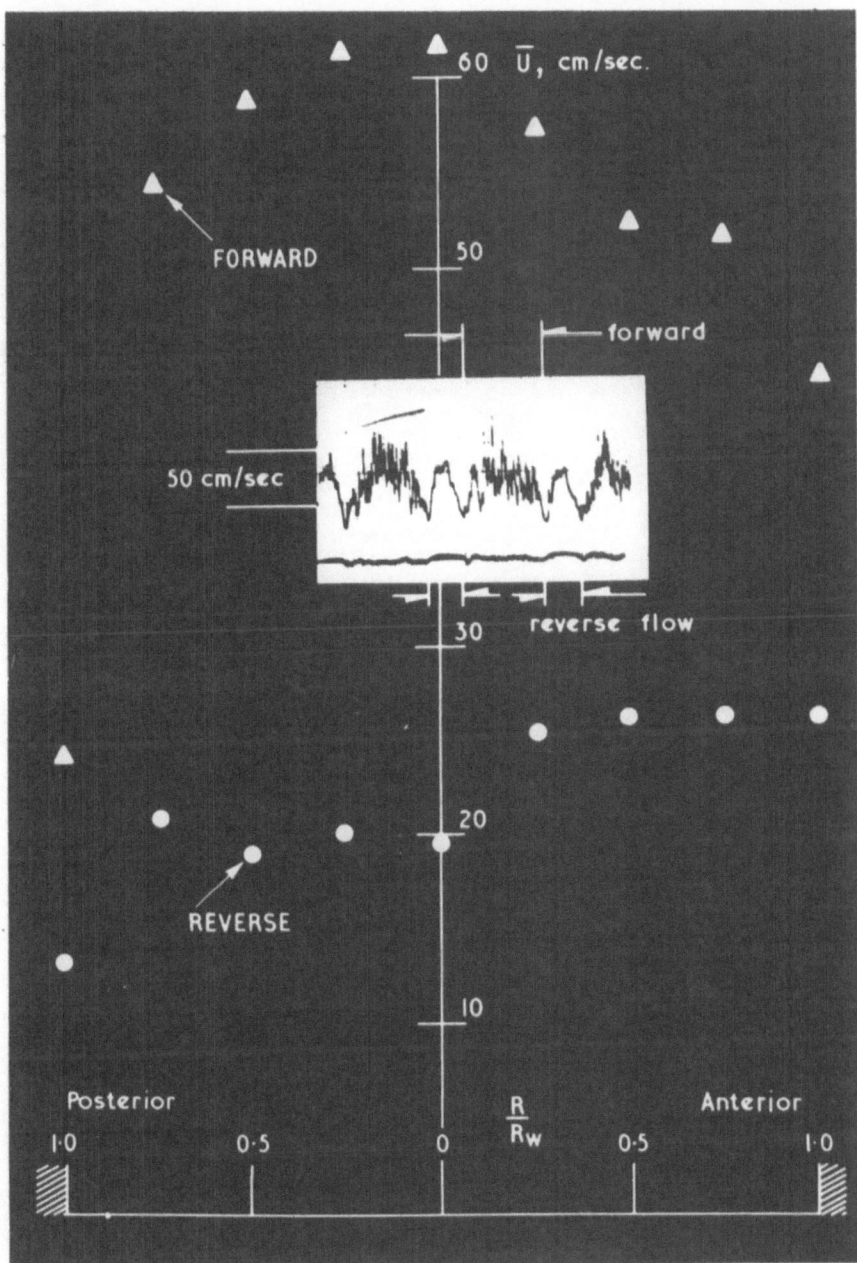

*Figure 7b.* Pre-operative aortic traverse in patient with aortic incompetence. Profiles of forward and reverse flow shown separately. *Insert*: catheter probe signal showing turbulent flow through perforated valve cusps followed by laminar regurgitation.

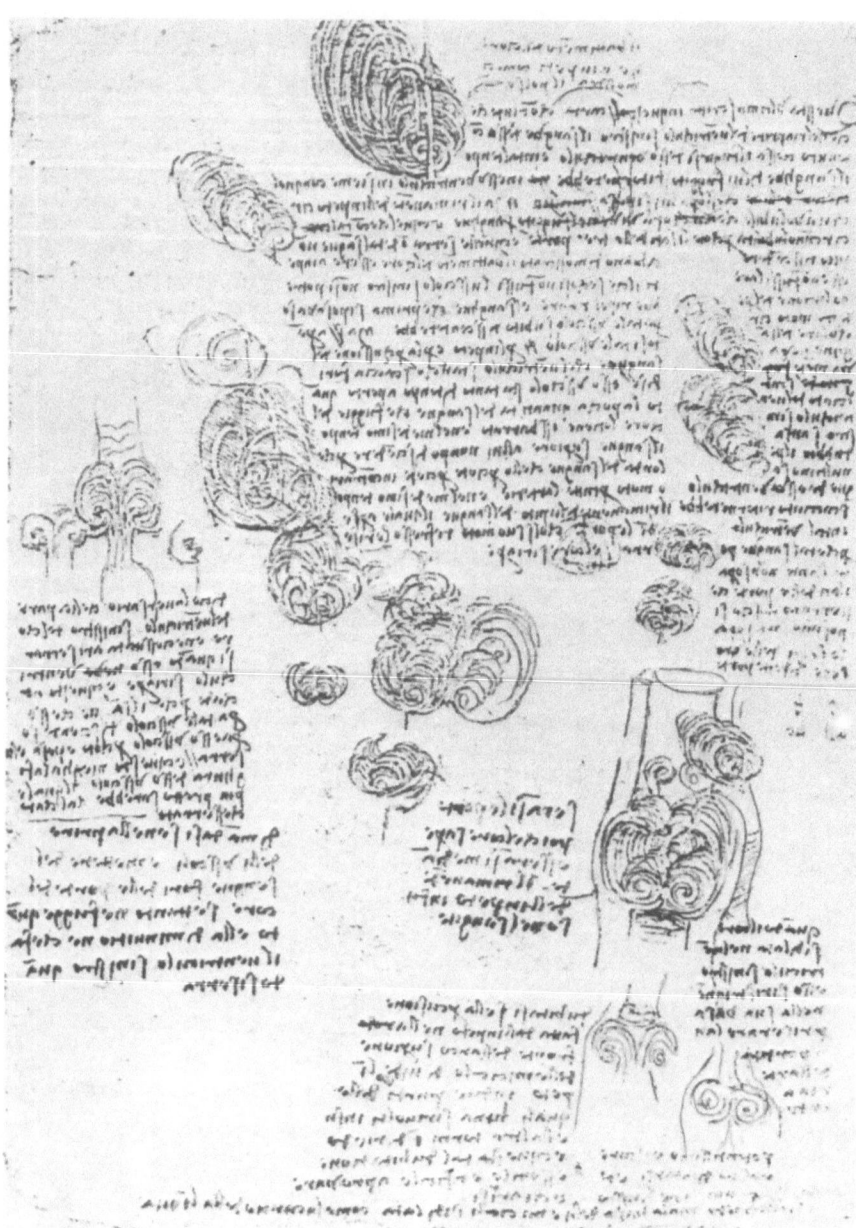

*Figure 8.* Reproduction of anatomical drawings by Leonardo da Vinci showing his concepts of vortices assisting closure of the aortic valve. Note also his drawing of a uniform velocity distribution in the ascending aorta (middle drawing in the left-hand margin).

with the originator of my first quotation, Leonardo da Vinci. Figure 8 is a rather poor reproduction of one of Leonardo da Vinci's many anatomical drawings devoted to this phenomenon. Most of the drawings in this illustration show how vortices within the aortic sinuses could assist in closing the aortic valve. I have chosen this particular folio for reproduction because the group of figures occupying the middle of its left margin also show something deeply interesting to me personally. Besides illustrating the circular motion of the vortices in the sinuses of Valsalva, Leonardo drew the flow distribution that he considered to be likely in the ascending aorta. Notice how he has shown this to be virtually uniform across the full diameter of the vessel. Some four hundred years later we, in Oxford, have been able to verify this concept by direct measurement.

ACKNOWLEDGEMENTS

I am grateful to Dr. D.L. Schultz for his illustration of thin film sensors mounted in a turbine blade of a jet aero engine. I am indebted to Dr. Tunstall Pedoe for illustrations of disturbed flow in the ascending aorta of patients with aortic stenosis and aortic incompetence. The illustration from Leonardo da Vinci's anatomical drawings is copied from O'Malley and Saunders's book entitled *Leonardo da Vinci on the human body*, New York, Schuman, 1952, p 266–267. Work undertaken with Dr. D.L. Schultz and Dr. Tunstall Pedoe was part of M.R.C. Project, Later Programme, grants.

REFERENCES

1. Schultz DL. Tunstall Pedoe DS. Lee G de J. Gunning AJ, Bellhouse BJ: Velocity distribution and transition in the arterial system. In: *Ciba foundation symposium on circulatory and mass transport*. Wolstenholm GEW, Knight J (eds), London, J & A Churchill. 1969, p 172–199.
2. Reuben SR, Swadling JP, Lee G de J: Velocity profiles in the main pulmonary artery of dogs and man, measured with a thin film resistance anemometer. *Circ Res* 27:995–1001. 1970.
3. Mills CJ: Measurement of pulsatile flow and flow velocity. In: *Cardiovascular fluid dynamics*. Bergel DH (ed) New York, Academic Press, 1972.
4. Firth BG: Studies of left ventricular mechanical function. D Phil Thesis, University of Oxford, 1975.
5. Tunstall Pedoe DS: Velocity distribution of blood flow in major arteries of animals and man. D Phil thesis, University of Oxford, 1970.

## 6.3. THE CLOSING BEHAVIOUR OF THE NATURAL AORTIC VALVE

Anton A. van Steenhoven, Cees W.J. Verlaan, Pieter C. Veenstra, Robert S. Reneman

### 1. INTRODUCTION

As discussed in earlier work (1), proper understanding of natural aortic valve closure is essential for the design of artificial triple leaflet valve prostheses. Some insight in valvular closing during deceleration of the main stream has been obtained from model studies (2, 3, 4). The present study was conducted in order to investigate this closing behaviour in animal experiments and to compare the results with those obtained from the theoretical model designed on the basis of the fluid behaviour in the analogue (5). Aortic valve movements were studied in open-chest dogs using direct high-speed cinematography. The aortic valve is schematically shown in Figure 1; it has three leaflets and behind each leaflet there is a half-spherical cavity, the sinus of Valsalva.

### 2. ANIMAL EXPERIMENTS

For an optically clear image of the aortic valve, perfusion of the heart with a transparent liquid is required (6). Under these circumstances the heart has to rely on the small oxygen content in a hemoglobin-free solution. Therefore, the duration of observation of the aortic valve is limited. In this technique reliable physiological recordings of the valve can only be made

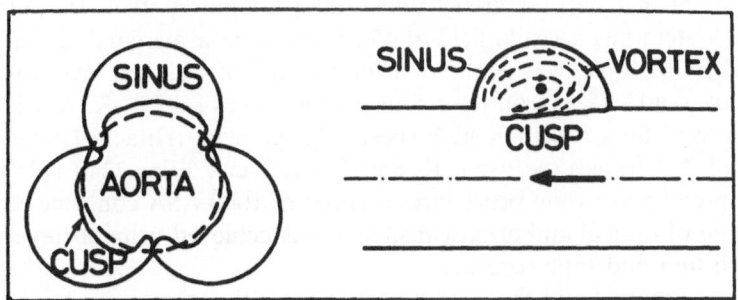

*Figure 1.* Diagram of the aortic valve and the sinuses of Valsalva (9).

J. Baan, A.C. Arntzenius, E.L. Yellin (eds.), Cardiac Dynamics, 477–488.
Copyright © 1980 by Martinus Nijhoff Publishers bv, The Hague, Boston, London. All rights reserved.

during the first six minutes following the start of perfusion. Separate coronary perfusion with blood (7) provides a much longer period of time for observation (three hours). In this technique, however, small quantities of blood enter the left ventricular chamber, causing a decrease in light transmission within the liquid and therefore a reduction in film speed. Methods applied to the intact animal (8) only give information about the valve in the closed position. For high-speed in-vivo recording of aortic valve movement only the first method can be used.

## 2.1. Methods and materials

Experiments were performed on mongrel dogs of either sex, unknown age, and ranging from 25 to 45 kg. The animals were premedicated with Hypnorm (1 ml/kg body mass i.m.). Anesthesia was induced with sodium pentobarbital (10 ml/kg body mass i.v.) and, after endotracheal intubation, was maintained with oxygen-nitrous oxide. Ventilation was kept constant during the experiment with a positive pressure respirator (Bird).

The ECG was derived from the limb leads. The chest was opened through the left fifth intercostal space and the heart was suspended in a pericardial cradle. Left atrial pressure was measured through a pulmonary vein with a polyethylene catheter connected to a pressure transducer (Ailtech). Millar catheter-tip micromanometers (PC 470) were used to measure aortic and left ventricular pressures. An electromagnetic flow probe was placed on the ascending aorta and connected to a sine-wave electro-magnetic flowmeter with a carrier frequency of 600 Hz and an upper frequency response of 100 Hz, – 3 dB (Transflow 600). The determined variables were recorded on a multi-channel physiological recorder (Schwarzer) and on an electromagnetic tape recorder (Ampex PR 2230). The upper frequency response of the whole recording system was 280 Hz, – 3 dB.

For direct cinematographic recording of aortic valve movement, a thin (4 mm) flexible fiberscope (Olympus BF 4C2) was placed in front of the valve through the left carotid artery under fluoroscopic control. In water the optical system has a visual field of 45°. Light from a mercury vapour lamp (ACMI-FCB 1000) was emitted from the tip of the lens system at an intensity of 400,000 lux and a colour temperature of 5000° K. Aortic valve motion was filmed with a high-speed film camera (Hitachi-Himac) at a speed of 200 frames/sec using Kodak Video News Film 7240 (125 ASA). With special processing procedures a speed of 1000 ASA could be reached. Coupling of optical and electrical signals was achieved using a timer signal on both film and tape recorder.

After the animal was thus instrumented, the pulmonary veins were ligated and the blood was replaced by a transparent Tyrode solution either with

(3.3 gram per cent) or without gelatine (UCB). The liquid perfusion was done with two roller pumps, one connected to the left atrium and the other to the femoral artery. The second connection appeared to be necessary for maintaining peripheral arterial blood pressure at physiological levels. Free outflow occurred through a cannula in the pulmonary artery. After the experiment the heart was removed and the valve geometry measured. The schematical representation of the experimental setup is given in Figure 2.

Analysis of the film was performed with an analysing projector (analector, Old Delft). The cusp positions were drawn frame by frame and the valve opening area was measured with a planimeter (OTT-31). A digital computer system (B 7700) was used for comparison between the optical and electrical signals. This system also determines from five heart beats the average curves for the aortic volume flow and the valve opening area. The fluid velocity in the ascending aorta was calculated by dividing the flowmeter reading by the aortic cross-sectional area. For coupling of the aortic valve motion to the calculated flow velocity between the leaflets as an instantaneous function of time, the measured flow signal was shifted by about 8 msec according to the position of the flow probe on the ascending aorta and the electronic delay in the flowmeter system.

## 2.2. Experimental results

In general less than one minute elapsed between the start of perfusion and the beginning of filming aortic valve movements. In 13 dogs a regular heart rhythm as well as relatively normal cardiac outputs and aortic and intraventricular pressures were maintained during the filming period.

The aortic valve movements were studied under various hemodynamic circumstances. The following variables were changed: fluid viscosity, mean left atrial pressure and aortic pressure. Two extreme situations will be discussed here. Figure 3 shows an experiment performed under rather physiological conditions. In this experiment the viscosity of the perfusion liquid was similar to that of blood ($\eta = 3.10^{-3}$ Ns.m$^{-2}$), mean left atrial pressure ($\bar{P}_{la}$) was 13 mmHg and systolic aortic pressure ($P_{ao}^s$) was 90 mmHg. In Figure 4 an experiment is shown in which both the fluid viscosity ($\eta = 10^{-3}$ Ns m$^{-2}$) and systolic aortic pressure were low ($P_{ao}^s = 55$ mmHg), and mean left atrial pressure was high ($\bar{P}_{la} = 30$ mmHg).

From these two experiments the valve-closing behaviour was compared with the corresponding aortic flow velocity signal. Figures 5 and 6 show the average curves of these signals as derived from five heart beats. The aortic flow signal, expressed in terms of fluid velocity as a function of time is shown in the top panel and the closing behaviour of the valve in the bottom panel. The closing parameter $\lambda^2$ shown in Figures 5 and 6 is defined as the ratio of the instantaneous and the maximum area of valve opening. If the

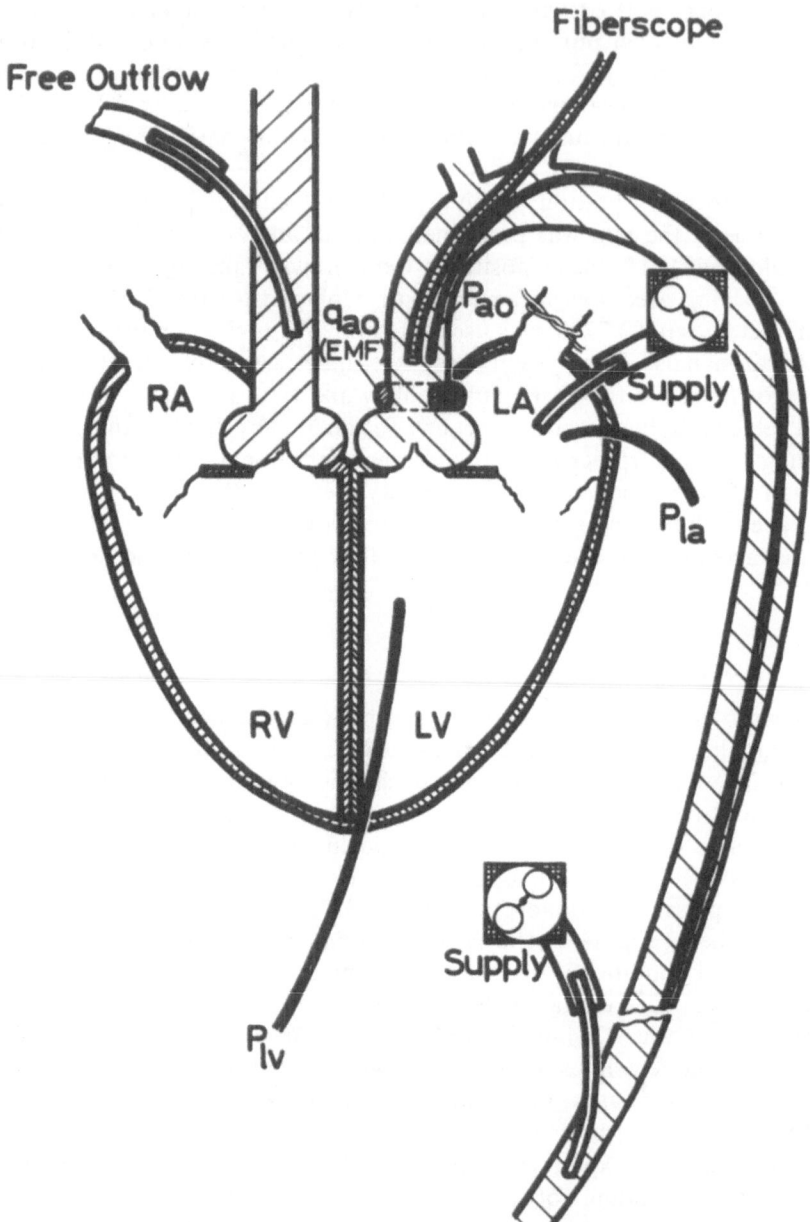

*Figure 2.* Diagram of the position of the measuring devices.

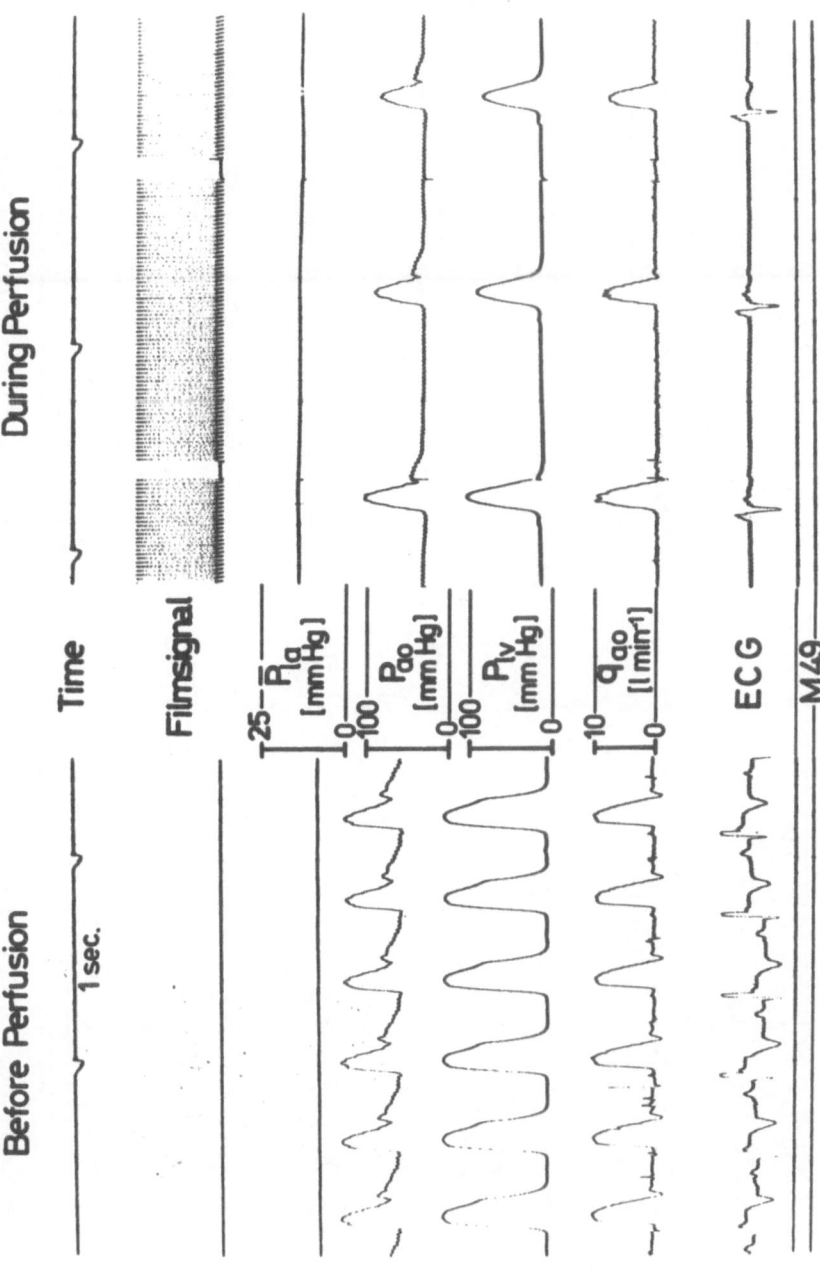

*Figure 3.* Recorded tracings of ECG, ascending aortic flow ($q_{ao}$), left ventricular pressure ($P_{lv}$), aortic pressure ($P_{ao}$), mean left atrial pressure ($P_{la}$) and the film signal under rather normal physiological hemodynamic conditions, before and during perfusion.

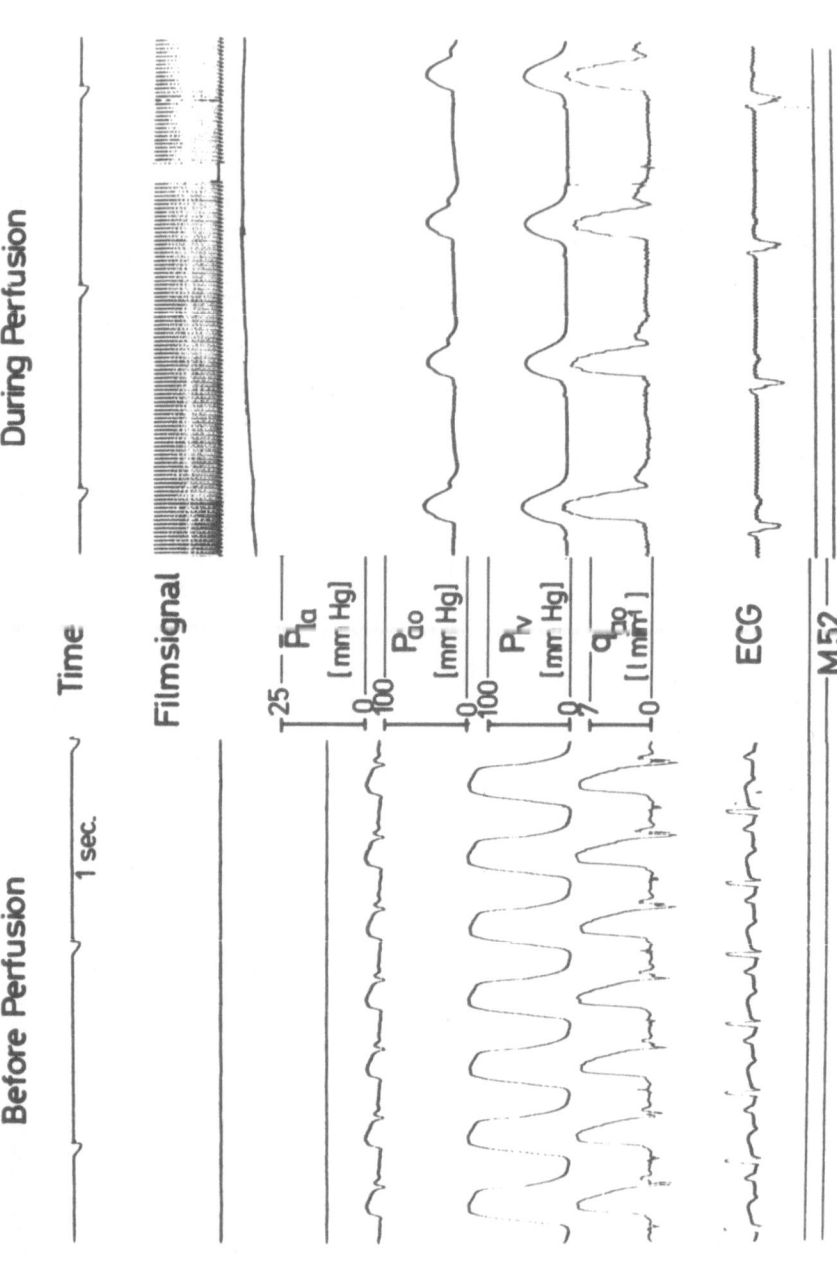

*Figure 4.* Recorded tracings of ECG, aortic ascending flow ($a_{ao}$), left ventricular pressure ($P_{lv}$), aortic pressure ($P_{ao}$), mean left atrial pressure ($\overline{P}_{la}$) and the film signal, with high left atrial pressure and low arterial pressure and viscosity, before and during perfusion.

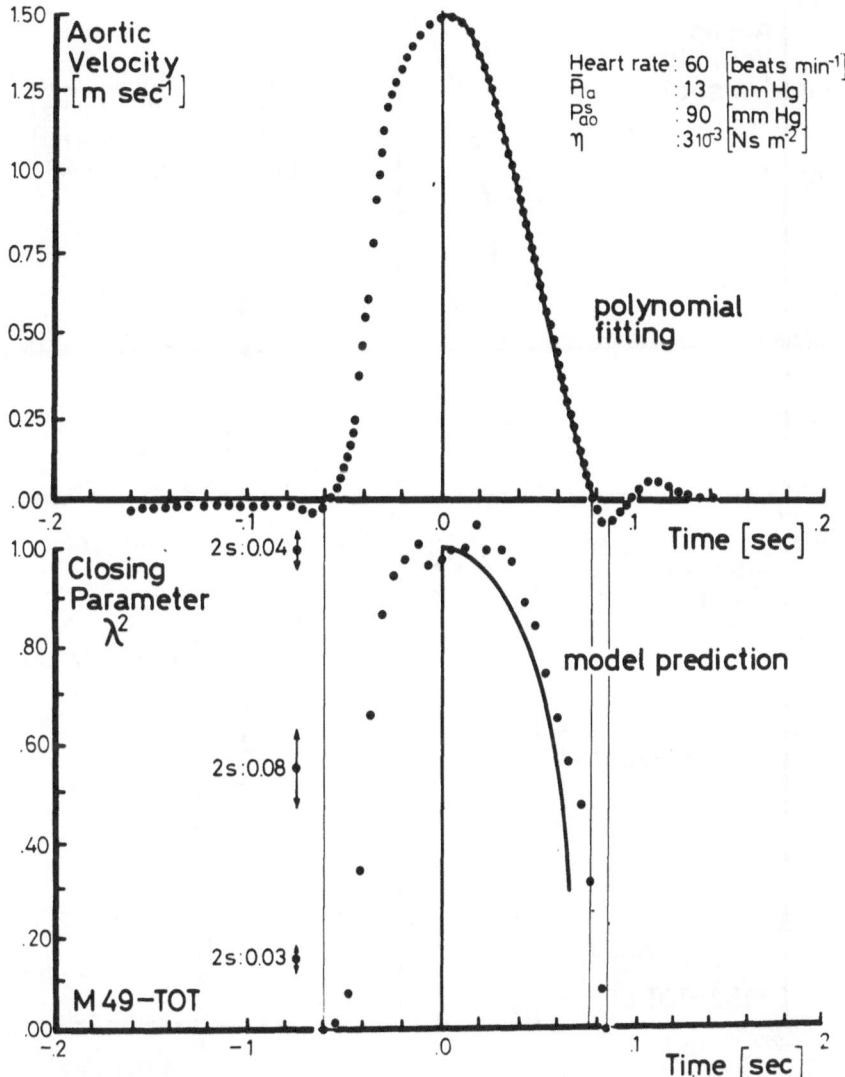

*Figure 5.* The relation between aortic fluid velocity (*top*) and closing behaviour of the aortic valve (*bottom*) under relatively normal physiological hemodynamic circumstances.

closing parameter equals 1, the valve is completely open and if this parameter equals zero, the valve is closed. In both graphs the dotted points represent the experimental results. The method used for describing valve movements is subject to some inaccuracy, especially when the valve is completely open. In this situation the image of the leaflet is often vague and

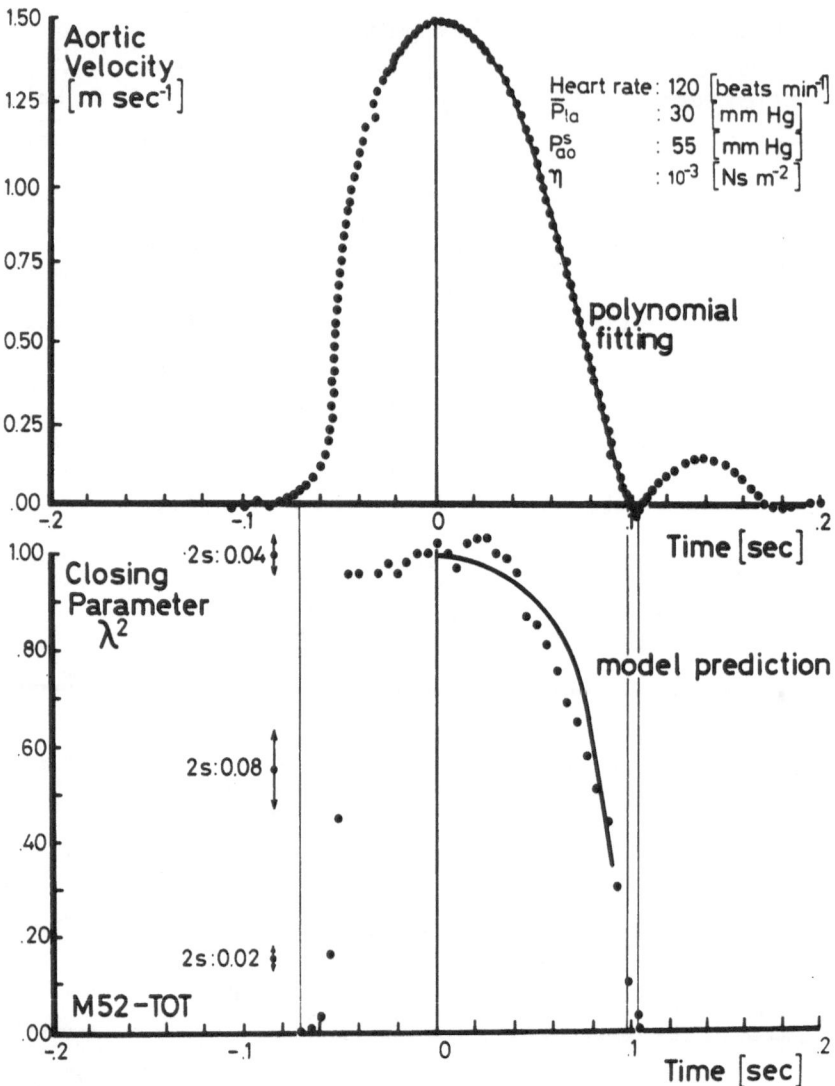

*Figure 6.* The relation between aortic fluid velocity (*top*) and closing behaviour of the aortic valve (*bottom*) at relatively high left atrial pressure ($P_{la}$) and low systolic arterial pressure ($P_{ao}^s$) and viscosity ($\eta$).

sometimes only parts of the leaflets can be seen. The missing parts then have to be geometrically reconstructed. Because of this procedure the closing behaviour was averaged over five heart beats, which is probably allowed since mainly random errors are involved. The 95% reliability intervals for some of the mean values of the closing parameter during the deceleration phase of systolic aortic flow are also shown in the graphs of

Figures 5 and 6. From these graphs it can be concluded that, under the different hemodynamic circumstances mentioned, the aortic valve starts to close during the deceleration phase of systolic aortic flow and that at least 80% of the closure is completed before aortic flow becomes zero. These and other experiments indicate that the moment of maximum backflow in the valve coincides with the moment of complete closure of the aortic valve.

### 3. MODEL STUDIES

The mechanism of the onset of valve closure during deceleration of the main flow is not yet fully understood. Bellhouse and Talbot (9) suggested that the trapped vortex within the sinus interacts with the decelerating flow field and thus pushes the leaflets into the aorta. However, their description of this interaction is not entirely satisfactory. Their theoretical model predicts pressure differences across the cusps which seem to be quite large considering the small mass of the leaflets.

Recent experimental studies (2, 3, 4) in a two-dimensional analogue of the aortic valve (Figure 7) have shown that during deceleration of the main stream:

1. The shape of the cusp does not change very much; it rotates around its attachment line.
2. The main stream velocity profile beneath the cusp remains nearly flat.
3. A region of recirculation is clearly visible behind the cusp. The flow pattern shows some resemblance with the phenomenon of boundary layer separation.
4. A vortex is present in the sinus during the stationary phase. The maximum velocity in the sinus seems to be much lower than that in the aorta.

These observations are illustrated in Figure 8.

On the basis of these experimental results a simplified theoretical model was designed (4) in which the pressure on the sinus side of the leaflet is assumed to be constant and equal to the pressure underneath the free edge

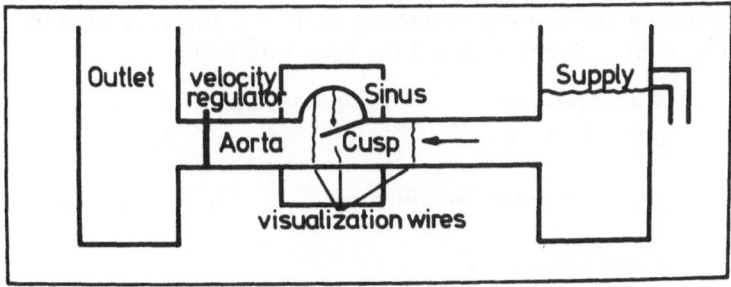

*Figure 7.* Diagram of two-dimensional analogue of the aortic valve.

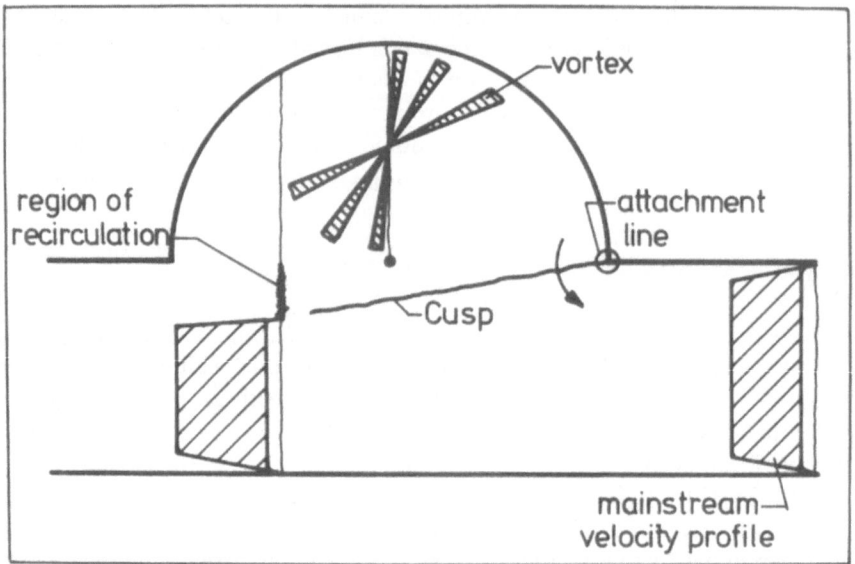

*Figure 8.* Diagram of the visualized fluid behaviour during deceleration of the main stream, as observed in model studies.

of the cusp. Two additional assumptions were made. the leaflet is straight and the mean pressure difference across the leaflet, because of its negligible mass, is equal to zero. From this model an equation is obtained which directly relates the aortic fluid velocity within the valve to the displacement of the leaflet.

### 3.1. *Application of model findings to animal experiments*

For comparison of the theoretical model with the animal experiments, the model has to be extended to the three-dimensional situation. For this purpose the cusps are assumed to be shaped as a truncated cone and the aorta to be a rigid tube. Using the same assumptions as in the two-dimensional model, after onset of deceleration ($t = 0$) the following relation is found between the closing parameter ($\lambda^2$) as a function of time ($t$), the measured aortic velocity ($u_0$) and the cusp length ($L$):

$$\frac{d^2\lambda}{dt^2} + \frac{16}{3}\frac{u_0}{L}\frac{d\lambda}{dt} - (1-\lambda)\left(4\frac{u_0^2}{L^2} + \frac{8}{3}\frac{1}{L}\frac{du_0}{dt}\right) = \frac{2}{L}\frac{du_0}{dt}$$

for $|(1-\lambda)| \ll 1$, with initial conditions:

$$t = 0 : \frac{d\lambda}{dt} = 0,\ \lambda = 1.$$

To be able to compare the results of this theoretical model with the experimentally observed closing behaviour, shown as the points in the bottom panels of Figures 5 and 6, a polynomial curve was fitted to the experimental flow velocity signal. This curve is shown as a solid line in the top panel. Then the equation was solved numerically for this time-dependent velocity. The closing behaviour thus obtained agrees fairly well with the results of the animal experiments as evidenced by the similarity of the theoretical lines and experimental data points in Figures 5 and 6 (bottom).

## 4. DISCUSSION

In spite of the improvement of the experimental setup by using two roller pumps to maintain peripheral arterial blood pressure at approximately physiological levels, the hemodynamic variables during perfusion changed as compared to the control situation. Variation in these variables depends among other factors on the inflow rate in both the left atrium and the femoral artery. Therefore, aortic valve closing behaviour could be studied under various hemodynamic circumstances. Occasionally during perfusion mean left atrial pressure was found to be high compared with diastolic left ventricular pressure. It is likely that these high pressure readings result from either a too high inflow rate or an unfavourable position of the pressure catheter in relation to the inflow cannula.

The results of the animal experiments indicate that aortic valve closure already starts during the deceleration phase of systolic aortic flow and that approximately 80% of the closure is completed before aortic flow becomes zero. The moment of onset of closure of the valvular leaflets, however, is difficult to determine because the changes in valvular opening during the first part of the closing curve may be due to constriction of the aortic wall, closing of the leaflets or both. Further investigations are required to distinguish between these two phenomena. Complete aortic valve closure probably coincides with the moment of maximum backflow in the valve. This is supported by the findings in model studies which show a close relationship between the time derivatives of the closing parameter and the mainstream velocity. Moreover, the present findings are in agreement with the qualitative behaviour of valve closure as observed in model experiments reported by Bellhouse and Talbot (9).

The similarity between the closing behaviour under different hemodynamic conditions as observed in the experiment and as predicted by the theoretical model suggests that the latter describes the natural valve closure fairly well. These findings, however, should be interpreted with some caution because of the simplified model assumptions.

SUMMARY

In open-chest dogs cinematographic high-speed recordings of aortic valve movement were made using a thin flexible fiberscope. Simultaneously ECG, ascending aortic flow and the pressures in aorta, left ventricle and left atrium (LA) were recorded. Replacement of blood by a transparent liquid (Tyrode solution) was done with two roller pumps, one connected to the LA and the other to the femoral artery. Free outflow occurred through a cannula in the pulmonary artery.

Comparison of the film frames with the aortic flow signals revealed that aortic valve closure starts during the deceleration phase of systolic aortic flow and at least 80% of the closure is completed before aortic flow becomes zero. Moreover, the results of a theoretical model of closure, based upon the presence of a region of recirculation behind the moving cusps as observed in model studies, agree fairly well with the experimental results.

ACKNOWLEDGEMENTS

We are greatly indebted to Th.J.A.G. van Duppen, J. Jacobs and the Audio-Visual Centre of the Eindhoven University for their technical assistance and to Drs. N.A.L. Touwen for his aid in the computer work. We wish to thank Dr. M.E.H. van Dongen for his hydrodynamic advice and A.M.P. Barts, A.J. Manders and H.G. Sonnemans for their help in preparing the manuscript.

REFERENCES

1. Spaan JAE, Steenhoven AA van, Schaar PJ van der, Dongen MEH van, Smulders PT, Leliveld WH: Hydrodynamical factors causing large mechanical tension peaks in leaflets of artificial triple leaflet valves. Trans Am Soc Artif Int Organs 21:396–403, 1975.
2. Steenhoven AA van, Dongen MEH van, Spaan JAE: Two-dimensional model experiments on the closing of the aortic valve. Trans Eur Soc Artif Organs 3:127-131, 1978.
3. Steenhoven AA van, Dongen MEH van, Vaessen ECJ, Wasser AAM: Model experiments on the closing behaviour of the natural aortic valve. Biomed Technik 22:135–136, 1977.
4. Steenhoven AA van, Dongen MEH van: Model studies on the closing behaviour of the aortic valve. J Fluid Mech 90(1):21-32, 1979.
5. Steenhoven AA van, Schaar PJ van der, Veenstra PC, Reneman RS: The closing behaviour of the natural aortic valve: abstract. Fed Proc 37:217, 1978.
6. Hider CF, Taylor DEM, Wade JD: Action of the mitral and aortic valves in vivo studied by endoscopic cine photography. Quart J Exper Physiol 51:372–379, 1966.
7. Padula RT, Cowan GSM, Camishion RC: Photographic analysis of the active and passive components of cardiac valvular action. J Thorac Cardiovasc Surg 56:790–798, 1968.
8. Dee P, Crosby I: Fibre optic studies of the aortic valve in dogs. Brit Heart J 39:459–461, 1977.
9. Bellhouse BJ, Talbot L: The fluid mechanics of the aortic valve. J Fluid Mech 35:721–735, 1969.

## 6.4. FLUID MECHANICS OF THE AORTIC VALVE

Brian J. Bellhouse

## 1. INTRODUCTION

The aortic valve consists of three thin (0.1 mm) cusps and three matching sinuses. The cusps are reinforced with collagen strands running from commissure to commissure. Under no load the cusps furl up in the axial direction. When closed, the cusps are stretched out and are supported by the underslung loops of collagen. A photograph of a human aortic root is shown in Figure 1 of chapter 6.1. The left ventricle is marked $V$, the aorta $A$, a cusp $C$ and its corresponding sinus $S$. The diameter of the aorta is approximately 25 mm. In measurements of instantaneous velocity in the ascending aortas of dogs, using heated thin-film gauges (1), it was shown that aortic blood-flow was laminar, that there was no central jet and that reversed flow at the end of systole was very small. These measurements showed, however, that velocity was not uniform across the aorta. These results were surprising, because they implied that the valve was open wide at mid-systole, otherwise the flow would have been turbulent (since the peak Reynolds number was 10,000), but that the valve closed, or nearly closed, during systole with flow still going forwards through the valve. Since the thin-film gauge responds to velocity fluctuations of frequencies well in excess of 10kHz, turbulence would certainly have been detected had it existed.

Anatomists have long been aware of the existence of the aortic sinuses, and Leonardo da Vinci (2) postulated (in 1513) that vortices were generated within them and that these vortices urged the cusps towards closure. The existence of the vortices, and the rapid clearance of radiopaque dye within them is readily apparent from cineangiograms of the aortic root.

In 1912, an alternative explanation of valve closure was given by Henderson and Johnson (3). They gave it the quaint title "the breaking of the jet," an effect depending on deceleration of the aortic flow.

Based on model experiments a fluid mechanic explanation of aortic valve closure was postulated (4). In the model valve, which had three natural rubber cusps (0.1 mm thick) and a rigid aortic root and sinuses, the cusps opened wide early in systole, vortices formed in the sinuses, and the cusps moved towards closure, under the action of the vortices together with the

*J. Baan, A.C. Arntzenius, E.L. Yellin (eds.), Cardiac Dynamics, 489–496.*

adverse pressure gradient associated with decelerating aortic flow, in the latter part of systole. A small amount of reversed flow (2%–5% of stroke volume) was required to seal the valve.

The relative importance of the sinus vortices and the adverse axial pressure-gradient in effecting valve closure has been difficult to determine, because they are so closely interrelated. The purpose of the work reported here was to attempt to separate the two hydraulic effects by varying the geometry of the aortic sinuses.

## 2. METHODS

A model of the aortic root was made (Figure 1), which consisted of a rigid perspex case into which the cusps were glued. The sinuses were made of perspex also, and were detachable, The cusps were made of uniform sheets of natural rubber 0.1 mm thick, and were glued with silicone rubber adhesive into the aortic root. The model valve was placed in a pulsatile flow rig (4) which could produce sinusoidal pulses, of frequences up to 10 Hz, superimposed on a steady flow. A viewer was placed downstream of the valve so that the cusps could be photographed with a cine camera at 50 frames per second.

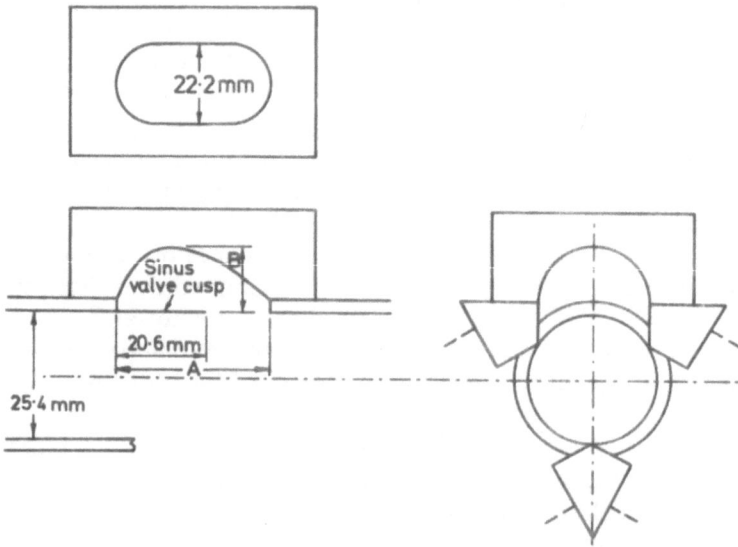

*Figure 1.* Scale drawing of a model of the aortic root with interchangeable sinuses of various geometries (side view on the left and end view on the right). Both sinus length (*A*) and sinus depth (*B*) were varied.

Velocity in the aorta was measured with a heated thin-film gauge (5). A microswitch, triggered by the piston of the pulsatile flow rig, controlled a light bulb which was visible on the cine film of the valve. The voltage pulse to the bulb was recorded simultaneously with aortic velocity. Thus movements of the valve cusps could be coordinated with instantaneous velocity in the aorta.

Dimensions of the model valve are shown in Figure 1. The internal diameter of the aorta was 25.4 mm, the length of the cusps was 20.6 mm, and the "normal" sinus (based on casts of human aortic roots) was 31.8 mm long, 22.2 mm wide and 12.7 mm deep. An end view of the valve is shown on the right of Figure 1.

Apart from the "normal" sinus, a blocked sinus (level with the aortic wall) and an elongated sinus (41.2 mm long, 22.2 mm wide and 12.7 mm deep) were tested. The cine film was analysed frame by frame by projecting it onto a screen and tracing out (onto white paper) the free margins of the cusps and the circumference of the aorta. Radial lines were then drawn from the centre of the aorta to the valve commissures and the individual cusp opening areas were measured with a planimeter.

3. RESULTS

When all sinuses were "normal" the valve opened wide early in systole and water entered the sinuses at the distal end to establish strong vortices in all the sinuses (Figure 2, top). At peak systole the central portions of the cusps

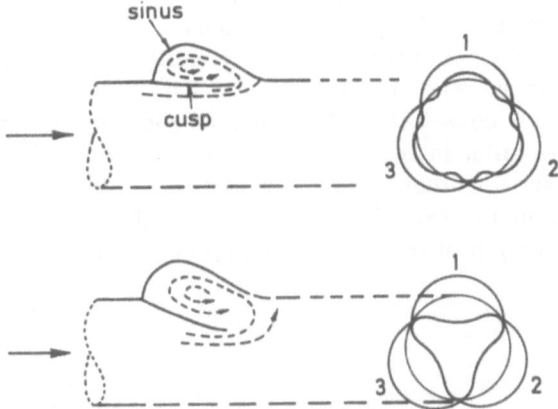

*Figure 2.* Drawing of vortex patterns in the sinuses of the model aortic valve. Mid-systole is shown above, late systole below (side view is shown on the left, the end view on the right). The sinuses are numbered 1–3. (Also illustrated in chapter 6.1 of this book.)

projected slightly into the sinuses; the commissure portions projected slightly into the aorta. In the latter part of systole the cusps moved towards closure, with the vortices persisting and enlarging (Figure 2, bottom). The cusps were well synchronized and were nearly closed before the end of systole, requiring very little backflow to seal the valve.

Dye injected at the aortic wall just upstream of the valve, at a point corresponding to the midpoint of a cusp, was swept into the corresponding sinus as soon as the cusp opened, early in systole. When dye was injected downstream of the valve, reversed flow at the wall was seen in the last quarter of systole. This reversed flow contributed to vortex growth as the valve closed.

When sinuses 1 and 2 were blocked (labelled as in Figure 2), but sinus 3 remained "normal", the performance of the valve was altered dramatically. This is shown in Figure 3, where measured valve-opening areas for cusps 2 and 3 are shown. The measured cusp-opening area, $A$, is divided by $A_0$, one third of the cross-sectional area of the aorta. In Figure 3 (bottom) cusp 3 (with its "normal" sinus) opened rapidly until it projected slightly into its sinus ($A/A_0 > 1$), then moved gradually into the aorta before moving rapidly towards closure in the latter part of systole. The aortic flow reversed just before cusp 3 closed.

The measured opening area of cusp 2, subjected to the same aortic flow, but with its sinus blocked, is shown in the top diagram of Figure 3. It can be seen that this cusp made only belated and ineffective movements towards closure, and then only after aortic flow had reversed. The broken line in Figure 3 (top) refers to cusp 3 and is transposed from Figure 3 (bottom) for comparison.

In the next test, sinus 1 was elongated and sinuses 2 and 3 were "normal". Figure 4 shows the comparative performance of cusps 1 and 3. Cusp 3 (Figure 4, bottom) performed as before (Figure 3, bottom), although the duration of systole was slightly longer. Cusp 1, however, closed much sooner, although considerable fluttering of the cusp free-margins (with corresponding scatter in the measurements) was observed (Figure 4, top). Dye studies showed that strong vortices were generated in both the "normal" and in the extended sinuses, although it was not possible to measure the strength of the three-dimensional vortex.

## 3. DISCUSSION

These experiments show that, if the sinuses are blocked, the model valve will not close until the flow reverses. They also show that cusp closure is affected by sinus geometry. By elongating the sinus, the gap between the cusp free-margin and the distal (downstream) end of the sinus is increased,

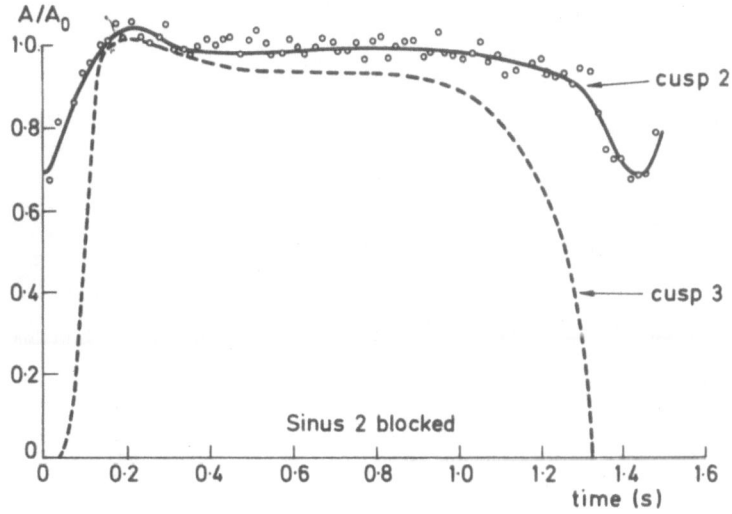

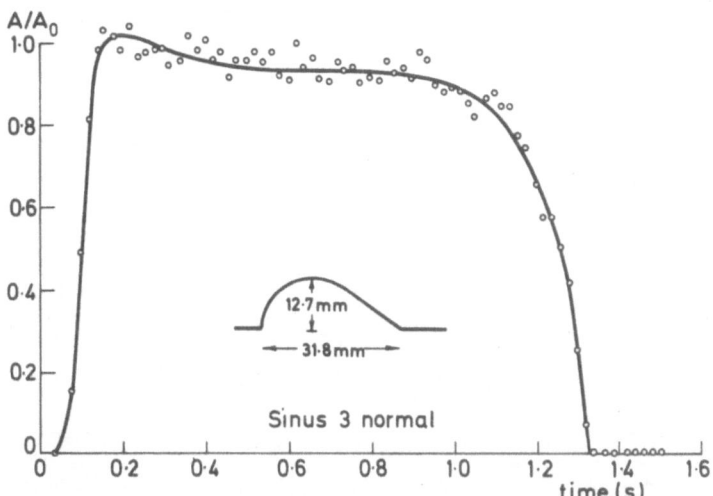

*Figure 3.* Graphs of valve opening area for cusp 2 (*above*), which had a blocked sinus, and for cusp 3 (*below*), which had a "normal" sinus. (See text for definitions of $A$ and $A_0$.)

permitting easier ingress and egress of water to generate the vortex. Thus the vortex would be stronger, thus causing the more rapid closure rate of cusp 1.

The improved performance of cusp 1 when the "normal" sinus is replaced with an elongated sinus does not suggest that man has evolved inefficient

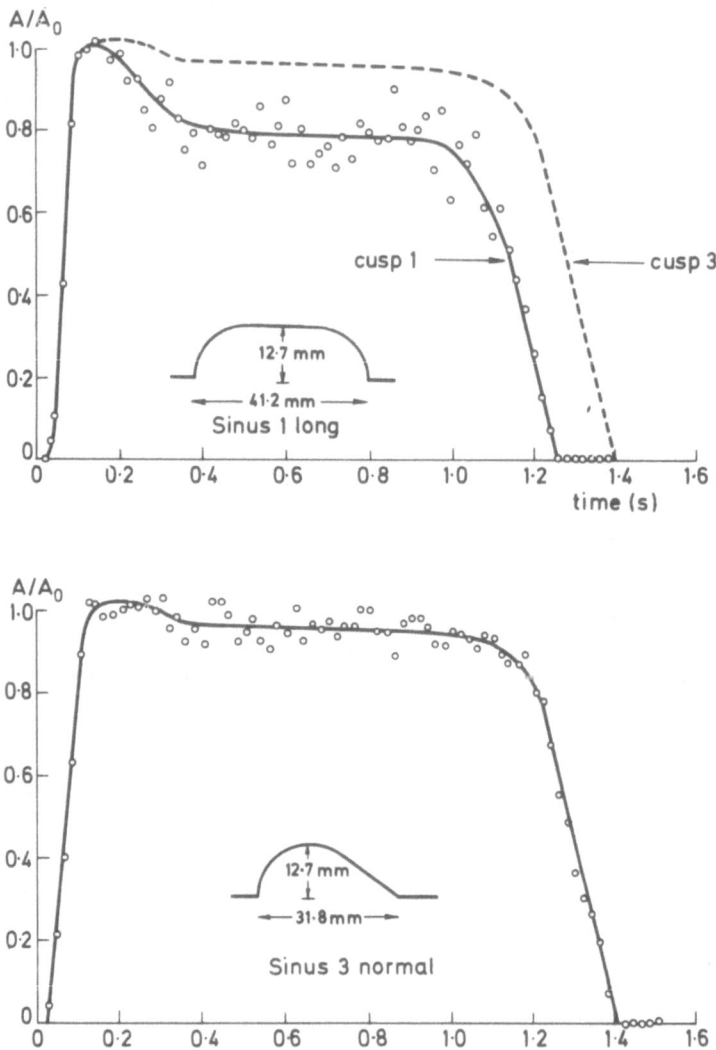

*Figure 4.* Graphs of valve opening area for cusp 1 (*above*), which had an elongated sinus, and for cusp 3 (*below*), which had a "normal" sinus. (See text for definitions of *A* and $A_0$.)

sinuses, rather that he has evolved cusps which furl up in systole to provide sufficient clearance between the cusp free-margins and the distal end of the sinuses to generate vortices of optimal strength. The simple rubber cusps used in the model experiments reported here have no such furling mechanism, and are just long enough to seal in diastole without prolapse, but too long for optimal vortex formation with "normal" sinuses. The vortices within the sinuses are formed rapidly, by convection, and are much stronger at peak systole in pulsatile flow than they would be in steady flow with the same aortic velocity. This is because, in pulsatile flow, viscous drag on the vortex has insufficient time to slow it down. However, since the vortex is formed convectively, its greatest strength is at peak systole, and the vortex strength decays in the latter part of systole. Thus an explanation of valve closure which relies solely on vortex thrust is incomplete. On the other hand, an explanation which relies solely on flow deceleration (which is maximal when the valve is moving at its fastest rate towards closure, at the end of systole) ignores the existence of sinuses and the vortices within them The evidence of this paper is that the sinuses are essential, that the geometry of the sinuses is important, and that the valve works best when the vortex is strongest.

This new evidence suggests that the vortices have a complex role to play in controlling the aortic valve during systole. The vortices provide both a control mechanism for the valve and additional thrust to aid closure in the latter part of systole. At peak systole, blood flowing into the sinuses is matched by blood flowing out, and the aortic pressure-gradient vanishes. Thus the cusps are balanced between the sinus vortices and aortic flow. When the aortic flow decelerates, pressure in the aorta at the level of the distal end of the sinuses exceeds that at the proximal end. Since blood enters the sinuses from the distal end, the average pressure in the sinuses exceeds that in the aorta, and the cusps respond to this pressure-difference by moving slowly towards closure, with blood flowing into the sinuses, but no longer out.

In addition to helping close the aortic valve, the vortices scourout the sinuses to prevent stagnation of blood and thrombus deposition behind the cusps, and they also help to recover dynamic head in the coronary ostia (which always lie within the sinuses) during systole, and thereby aid coronary perfusion.

Since aortic valves normally last for some 70 years in man, and undergo 2800 million cycles without failure, it is likely that the control mechanism provided by the vortices may well be their most important role. The cusps are of different sizes and thicknesses and are not homogeneous. The sinuses differ in size and shape, and the velocity distribution in the ascending aorta is far from uniform. In the absence of a control mechanism, the thin (0.1 mm) cusps would frequently be caught out of position at the end of systole (because of anatomic and flow asymmetries) and would experience huge shock loadings when closed rapidly by reversed aortic flow. Such an uncontrolled closure mechanism would be sure to lead to premature valve failure.

4. CONCLUSION

Decelerating aortic flow, combined with a control mechanism of vortices in the aortic sinuses cause the aortic valve to almost-close by the end of systole. A small amount of reversed flow is required to seal the valve.

When a sinus is blocked completely, the corresponding cusp fails to close in systole.

The geometry of the aortic sinuses has a marked effect on both vortex strength and on valve closure. The vortices scour out the sinuses in systole, preventing stasis and thrombus formation.

The coronary ostia are positioned within the aortic sinuses so that they maximize pressure recovery and therefore coronary artery perfusion in systole, especially in exercise.

SUMMARY

In models of the normal aortic valve, the three cusps open wide early in systole and strong vortices are formed in the aortic sinuses. These vortices help position the cusps during mid-systole. In the latter part of systole, aortic flow decelerates rapidly and a large, adverse pressure-gradient along the axis of the aorta is established. This pressure-gradient and the thrust from the vortices in the aortic sinuses are together responsible for moving the aortic valve cusps towards closure in the latter part of systole, so that the valve is almost closed by the end of systole. A small amount of reversed flow is required to seal the valve.

Since the valve opens wide, it presents negligible obstruction to forward flow. Thus the flow is laminar, and minimal blood trauma is caused. Since the valve moves towards closure during the latter part of systole, there is little backflow and impulsive loading of the valve cusps on closure is minimized.

REFERENCES

1. Schultz DL, Tunstall-Pedoe DS, Lee G de J, Gunning AJ, Bellhouse BJ: Velocity distribution and transition in the arterial system. In: *CIBA foundation symposium on circulatory
   and respiratory mass transport*, London, 1968, p 172.
2. Vinci L da: *Quaderni d'Anatomica* 2:9, 1513.
3. Henderson Y, Johnson FE: Two modes of closure of the heart valves. *Heart* 4:69–82, 1912.
4. Bellhouse BJ, Bellhouse FH: Fluid mechanics of model normal and stenosed aortic valves.
   *Circ Res* 25:693–704, 1969.
5. Bellhouse BJ, Bellhouse FH: Thin-film gauges for the measurement of velocity or skin
   friction in air, water or blood. *J Sci Instr* 1 (series 2):1211, 1968.

## 6.5. MECHANICAL ENERGY LOSSES RESULTING FROM STENOSIS OF SEMILUNAR VALVES

COLIN CLARK

### 1. INTRODUCTION

The reduced area for flow in a stenosed valve results in high blood velocities and correspondingly high kinetic energy. As fluid leaves the valve it encounters a sudden expansion in area, a jet is formed and the high shear at the jet surface results in rapid entrainment of surrounding fluid and turbulent mixing occurs. Because the flow is bounded by an arterial wall (for each of the semilunar valves) a recirculation region is established at the end of which the flow re-attaches to the wall. The resulting energy losses both within and downstream of the valve may be a large fraction of the work output from the ventricle driving the flow.

### 2. *Theory*

Energy losses or, more strictly, the dissipation of mechanical energy in the form of heat by the action of friction, can be studied theoretically by the application of the equations of conservation of mass and energy. In order to determine separately the energy losses occurring within a stenosed valve and in the artery downstream of the valve, these equations will be applied to the two regions illustrated in Figure 1. Each region consists of blood within a volume $V$ which varies with time and which is bounded by a surface $S$. Blood is assumed to be incompressible, which reduces conservation of mass to conservation of volume. Thus, the difference between the volume flow rate entering and leaving through $S$ is the rate of change of volume $V$. This is written:

$$\int_S \mathbf{v} \cdot \mathbf{n} \, dS = -d/dt \int_V dV \qquad [1]$$

where $\mathbf{v}$ is the velocity vector and $\mathbf{n}$ is an outward-pointing unit vector normal to the element of surface $dS$.

Conservation of energy for a region occupied by an incompressible fluid for which gravitational effects are negligible may be stated as follows: the rate at which surface stresses do work on the boundary $S$ plus the difference between the rates of inflow and outflow of kinetic energy across $S$ is equal

J. Baan, A.C. Arntzenius, E.L. Yellin (eds.), Cardiac Dynamics, 497–507.

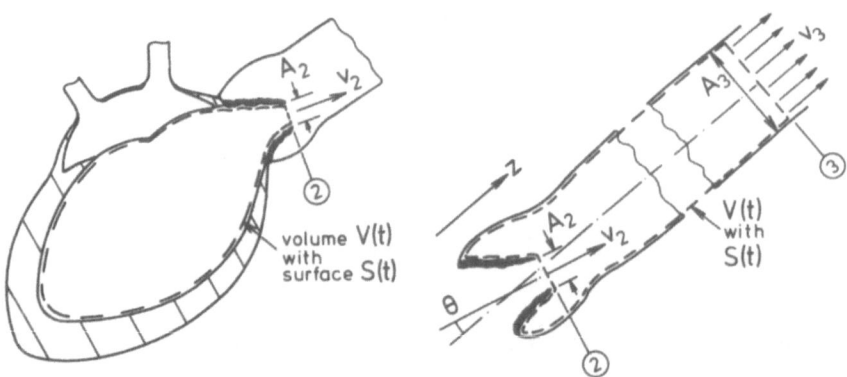

*Figure 1.* The two regions considered in the theory are defined by broken lines: *left*: the ventricle and valve; *right*: the artery downstream of the valve.

to the rate at which kinetic energy (k.e.) changes within the region plus the rate of mechanical energy dissipation. When frictional forces upon $S$ are not included explicitly this may be written as:

$$-\int_S p\mathbf{v}\cdot\mathbf{n}\,dS + \rho\int_S (v^2/2)\mathbf{v}\cdot\mathbf{n}\,dS$$

$$+\rho d/dt\left[\int_V (v^2/2)\,dV\right] + \int_V \phi\,dV = 0 \qquad\qquad [2]$$

where $p$ = pressure, $\rho$ = density and $\phi$ = rate of energy dissipation per unit volume. Equations [1] and [2] are rate equations containing space integrals and they hold at given instants of time. The volume change and energy loss over a period of time may be obtained by integration of the equations with respect to time.

## 2.1. *The ventricle and valve*

The surface $S$ of this region consists of the inner surface of the ventricle and valve cusps $S_1$ and the continuation across the semilunar valve opening $A_2$, which is normal to the direction of outflow (Figure 1, left). The volume $V$ and areas $S_1$ and $A_2$ all vary with time. The direction of outflow from the valve is taken to be inclined in one plane only at an angle $\theta$ relative to the axis of the artery downstream (Figure 1, right). The flow is assumed to have uniform distributions of velocity and pressure across $A_2$. In addition, frictional forces are assumed to act only in the vicinity of the semilunar valve cusps and not within the ventricle. Commonly, the surface of a stenosed valve is quite irregular (due, for example, to calcium deposits) and this may result in local flow separation. For this reason frictional effects will be taken into account by a dissipation term rather then by a surface force acting on $S_1$.

For any instant during ejection [1] becomes:

$$A_2 v_2 = Q_2 = -dV/dt, \qquad\qquad [3]$$

noting that $A_2 = A_2(t)$. Each term in [2] will be considered in turn:

$$\int_S p\mathbf{v}\cdot\mathbf{n}dS = \int_{S_1} p\mathbf{v}\cdot\mathbf{n}\ dS - p_2 A_2 v_2$$

where $S = S_1 + A_2$. The first term in this expression is the rate of work done by the ventricular wall. The second term is the rate of flow work leaving the ventricle. The expression may be simplified to $(p_1 - p_2)Q_2$ where, by analogy with a definition given elsewhere (1),

$$p_1 = \int_{S_1} p\mathbf{v}\cdot\mathbf{n}\ dS/(dV/dt). \qquad\qquad [4]$$

As indicated in (1) this form of definition specifies the only single ventricular pressure which is physically appropriate.

The second term in [2] is the net flux of k.e. across $S$ which is $\rho Q_2 v_2^2/2$. The third term is the rate of change of k.e. within the ventricle. For convenience the integral of the k.e. over volume $V$ is related to the jet k.e. as follows: $\int_V (v^2/2)dV = \alpha(v_2^2/2)V$, where $\alpha$ is a dimensionless number which depends upon the shape and motion of the ventricular wall. If the ventricle remains geometrically similar in time then $\alpha$ is a constant; if this is assumed to be true then:

$$\rho\ d/dt\left[\int_V (v^2/2)\ dV\right] = \alpha\rho[(v_2^2/2)\ dV/dt + Vv_2\ dv_2/dt].$$

The first term in this expression is the rate of k.e. change due to the changing ventricular volume; the second term is due to the changing flow rate. These two quantities are related through [3] and the expression simplifies to:

$$\alpha\rho[Vv_2(dv_2/dt) - Q_2(v_2^2/2)].$$

The last term in [2] is the rate of energy dissipation and may be written $\int_V \phi dV = \Phi_{1,2}$. Thus, when applied to the ventricle and valve [2] becomes:

$$\Phi_{1,2} = Q_2[p_1 - p_2 + (\rho v_2^2/2)(\alpha - 1)] - \alpha\rho Vd/dt(v_2^2/2). \qquad\qquad [5]$$

This is a rate equation which can be integrated to give the energy loss throughout ejection (from time $t=0$ to $\tau$) or over a complete cardiac cycle (from $t=0$ to $T$). For the latter case, to account for filling of the ventricle during diastole, [1] becomes $A_a v_a = Q_a = dV/dt$, where $A_a =$ area of the atrio-ventricular valve normal to the direction of inflow which is assumed to be one-dimensional with velocity $v_a$ and pressure $p_a$. The filling phase introduces additional flow work and k.e. flux terms. The energy loss which now includes wall-frictional effects from distending the ventricle during filling is given by:

$$E_{1,2} = \int_0^T \Phi_{1,2}\, dt = \int_0^T p_1 \, (dV/dt)\, dt + \int_0^T p_a Q_a \, dt$$

$$- \int_0^T p_2 Q_2 \, dt + \rho \int_0^T Q_a(v_a^2\, 2)\, dt - \rho \int_0^T Q_2(v_2^2/2)\, dt \qquad [6]$$

The first term is the work done by and on (during diastole) the ventricular wall. The third term of [2] does not appear because it integrates to zero.if the ventricular volume and residual fluid motions within it (following closure of the atrio-ventricular valve) are the same at $t=0$ and $T$.

Equations [5] and [6] show that both $\Phi_{1,2}$ and $E_{1,2}$ are obtained implicitly by subtraction of mechanical energy terms. Therefore these quantities can only be calculated if all the other terms can be evaluated explicitly. It is possible, however, to gain some idea of how $\Phi_{1,2}$ may vary with time by considering a rigid system and making the approximation of using a nozzle coefficient to characterize frictional effects within the stenosed valve. Such coefficients are used extensively in engineering but are usually defined and measured for steady flows. The use of a nozzle coefficient for theoretical prediction of pressure drop produced by an unsteady flow through a stenosis has been shown to give good agreement with experimental results (2). The coefficient, $C$, is defined for steady flow by:

$$C = [(p_1' - p_2')/(p_1 - p_2)]^{1/2} \qquad [7]$$

where $p_1' - p_2'$ is the pressure drop for frictionless flow, given by application of the Bernoulli equation, as:

$$p_1' - p_2' = \rho (v_2^2/2)[1 - (A_2/A_1)^2]$$

and $p_1 - p_2$ is the actual measured pressure drop. Strictly, $C$ allows for the effects of both friction within the valve and the increase of total momentum flux at the valve exit arising from the development of a viscous boundary layer.

For the rigid system illustrated in Figure 2 the flow rate, $Q$ is a function of $t$ only and does not vary with distance $z$. This simplification means that the third term in [2] can be evaluated without having to introduce the

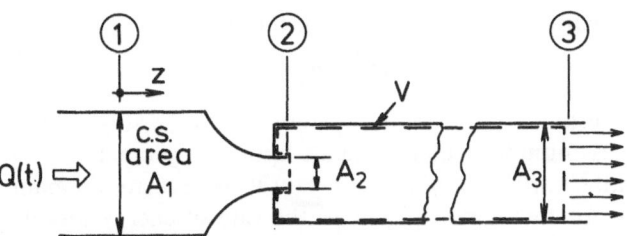

*Figure 2.* Schematic of rigid-walled model: (1) ventricle, (2) valve, (3) artery downstream.

factor $\alpha$, and is given by $\rho Q(dQ/dt)\int_0^z dz/A$. Hence [5] simplifies to give:

$$\Phi_{1,2} = Q\{p_1 - p_2 + \rho(v_2^2/2)[(A_2/A_1)^2 - 1]$$
$$- \rho\, dQ/dt \int_0^{z_2} dz/A\}. \tag{8}$$

Comparison with [5] shows that $(A_2/A_1)^2$ is equivalent to $\alpha$. Thus $\Phi_{1,2}$ can be obtained for a rigid system of known geometry if the pressure difference $p_1 - p_2$ produced by a known flow $Q(t)$ is measured. The measured static pressure $p_1$ is close to the quantity $p_1$ as defined by [4] but not identical because of boundary friction and local flow separation just upstream of the model stenosis. An expression to predict $\Phi_{1,2}$ if $Q(t)$ is known can be obtained by substituting for $p_1 - p_2$ in [8] in terms of $C$. If the losses are treated as quasi-steady, then, for unsteady flow:

$$p_1 - p_2 = (\rho v_2^2/2C^2)[1 - (A_2/A_1)^2] + \rho\, dQ/dt \int_Q^{z_2} dz/A,$$

substituting this expression into [8] then yields:

$$\Phi_{1,2} = \rho\, Q(v_2^2/2)(1/C^2 - 1)[1 - (A_2/A_1)^2]. \tag{9}$$

Thus, predicted values of dissipation rates can be compared with measured values obtained by differencing mechanical energy terms from [8]. The energy loss in one cycle can then be determined by integration as $E_{1,2} = \int_0^T \Phi_{1,2}\, dt$.

### 2.2. *The artery downstream of the valve*

This region (Figure 1, right) extends from the valve sinuses to a position beyond the jet at which the flow is assumed to be approximately uniform. The surface $S$ consists of $S_2$, the inner surface of the artery and facing cusp surfaces, and the continuations $A_2$ and $A_3$ across the valve and artery respectively, such that $S = S_2 + A_2 + A_3$. Frictional forces at the arterial wall will be omitted because energy dissipation in this region is primarily due to turbulent mixing in the main body of the flow. Equation [1] becomes:

$$v_2 A_2 - v_3 A_3 = Q_2 - Q_3 = dV/dt \tag{10}$$

The third term in [2] can be written as $d/dt[\beta\rho(v_2^2/2)V]$ where $\beta$ is a dimensionless number which depends upon the geometry of the artery and the flow pattern within it: $\beta$ is a constant if these factors remain similar with time. Thus, for this region [2] gives the rate of energy loss $\Phi_{2,3}$ as:

$$\Phi_{2,3} = Q_2(p_2 + \rho v_2^2/2) - Q_3(p_3 + \rho v_3^2/2) - \int_{S_2} p\mathbf{v} \cdot \mathbf{n} dS$$
$$- d/dt[\beta\rho(v_2^2/2)V]. \tag{11}$$

The third term on the right-hand side is the rate of work done on the arterial wall.

It is also of interest to apply the equation of conservation of momentum to this region. Written for the $z$-direction (see Figure 1) it is:

$$-\int_S p(\mathbf{i} \cdot \mathbf{n}) \, dS = \rho \int_S (\mathbf{v} \cdot \mathbf{i})(\mathbf{v} \cdot \mathbf{n}) \, dS + \rho \, d/dt[\int_V (\mathbf{v} \cdot \mathbf{i}) \, dV], \tag{12}$$

where $\mathbf{i}$ is a unit vector in the $z$-direction. The first term represents surface forces and may be written as $(p_2'' - p_3)A_3$ where $p_2'' = (1/A_3)\int_{S-A_3} p(\mathbf{i} \cdot \mathbf{n})dS$. This term will be approximated by $(p_2 - p_3)A_3$ where $p_2$ is the average pressure acting on $A_2$. The second term in [12] is the net flux of $z$ direction momentum across $S$ which is given by $\rho(Q_3 v_3 - Q_2 v_2 \cos \theta)$. The last term is the rate of change of $z$-momentum within the region and may be expressed by $\rho d/dt(\gamma v_2 V)$, where $\gamma$ is a dimensionless number which will be constant only if the geometry of the artery and flow pattern within it remain respectively similar with time. Equation [12] then becomes:

$$(p_2 - p_3)A_3 = \rho(Q_3 v_3 - Q_2 v_2 \cos \theta) + \rho d/dt(\gamma v_2 V). \tag{13}$$

At the instant of maximum flow the last term in [13] is approximately zero and, for some range of $\theta$, $Q_2 v_2 \cos \theta$ is greater than $Q_3 v_3$. This means that an increase in pressure occurs downstream of the valve (i.e. $p_3 > p_2$) which is termed pressure recovery. It is due to the reduction of momentum in the direction of flow as the jet decelerates spatially; thus some of the jet kinetic energy is recovered; $\Phi_{2,3}$ can be determined by differencing the mechanical energy terms in [11]. As for $\Phi_{1,2}$ this can only be done if all other terms can be evaluated explicitly, which requires a great deal of information.

It is again possible to obtain some insight into how $\Phi_{2,3}$ varies with time by considering the simpler rigid system shown in Figure 2. For this case $V =$ constant, $Q_2 = Q_3 = Q$ and the momentum equation can be written:

$$(p_2 - p_3) A_3 = \rho Q(v_3 - v_2 \cos \theta) + \rho V \, d/dt(\gamma v_2).$$

Changing signs to give recovered pressure as a positive quantity and normalizing by $\rho v_2^2/2$ yields:

$$(p_3 - p_2)/\rho v_2^2/2 = 2(A_2/A_3)(\cos \theta - A_2/A_3)$$
$$- 2(V/A_3 v_2^2) \, d/dt(\gamma v_2). \qquad [14]$$

The mean value throughout ejection is given by $(1/\tau)\int_0^\tau (p_3 - p_2)dt$ which can be obtained by integration of [14]. For both the mean value and for $\Phi_{2,3}$ at the instant of maximum flow the last term in [14] is approximately zero. Recovered pressure is then given by the first term on the left hand of the equation and this is plotted in Figure 3. It becomes zero if $\theta$ or $A_2/A_3$ increase to the extent that the $z$-component of jet momentum flux drops to become equal to that leaving the region at station 3 (Figure 2). The energy equation, [11], written for the rigid system becomes;

$$\Phi_{2,3} = Q[(p_2 - p_3) + \rho(v_2^2/2 - v_3^2/2)] - \rho V d/dt(\beta v_2^2/2) \qquad [15]$$

$\Phi_{2,3}$ can be obtained for a system of known geometry by differencing the mechanical energy terms in this equation if $p_2 - p_3$ produced by a known flow $Q(t)$ is measured. However, an expression to predict $\Phi_{2,3}$ for a known flow can be obtained by eliminating $p_2 - p_3$ between [14] and [15] and by assuming that $\beta$ and $\gamma$ may be treated as constants, which gives:

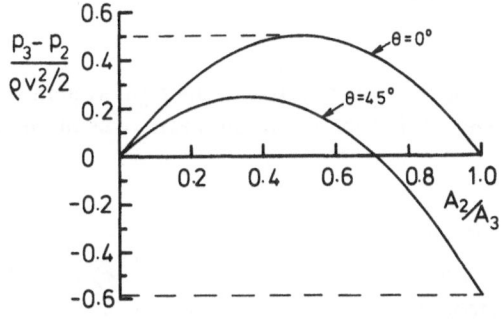

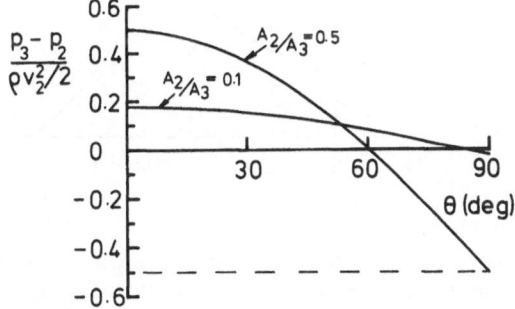

*Figure* 3. Pressure recovery plotted non-dimensionally as a function of area ratio (*top*) and jet angle $\theta$ (*bottom*), from [13].

$$\Phi_{2,3} = \rho Q (v_2^2/2)[(A_2/A_3)^2 - 2(A_2/A_3)\cos\,\theta + 1]$$
$$+ \rho V[(A_2/A_3)\gamma - \beta]\ d/dt(v_2^2/2) \qquad\qquad [16]$$

Values of $\gamma$ as a function of $A_2/A_3$ and $\theta$ can be obtained from [14]. An order of magnitude argument gives $\beta = k(A_2/A_3)\gamma$ and $k$ has been estimated to be about 1.2. Thus, predicted values of $\Phi_{2,3}$ can be compared with measured values obtained from [15]. The energy loss in one cycle, $E_{2,3} = \int_0^T \Phi_{2,3}\ dt$, can be obtained by integration of [15].

The measured total rate of dissipation, $\Phi_T$, is given by $\Phi_T = \Phi_{1,2} + \Phi_{2,3}$ and is obtained from the sum of [8] and [15] for the rigid walled system and from [5] and [13] for the more general case. Integration of these rate equations gives the energy loss over a given time and the total, $E_T$, is given by

$$E_T = E_{1,2} + E_{2,3} \qquad\qquad [17]$$

The fraction of the total energy loss occurring within each region of the rigid system is plotted in Figure 4.


3. APPLICATION OF THE THEORY

The application of these results is illustrated by measurements made during one test with a single flow pulse through the rigid system shown in Figure 2, with $A_2/A_1 = A_2/A_3 = 0.111$. Dynamic similarity was obtained on the basis of

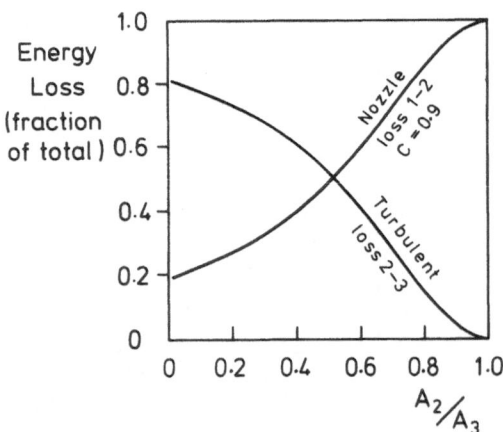

*Figure 4.* Energy loss occurring within the valve ($C = 0.9$, $A_2/A_1 \ll 1$; nozzle loss) and within the artery downstream (turbulent loss) as a fraction of the total loss $E_T$ for a rigid walled system both plotted as a function of area ratio $A_2/A_3$; obtained from [9] and [16] integrated with respect to time and $E_T$ from [17].

the dimensionless groups shown in Figure 5. Values of the groups were chosen to stimulate a heart rate of 64 beats/min (assuming $\tau/T=0.4$) with a stroke stroke volume of 75 ml assuming an aortic or pulmonary artery diameter of 2.8 cm. The flow waveform and measured pressure differences are shown in Figure 5. The recovery of pressure downstream of the stenosis is clearly apparent. The resulting rates of energy loss are shown in Figure 6 on both linear and logarithmic scales; the latter facilitates comparison between predicted and measured values over a wider range. Each measured value of $\Phi_{1,2}$ [8] represents a small difference between terms of much larger magnitude and is, therefore, very susceptible to errors, particularly in the measurement of $Q$. This is illustrated by showing at one instant the effects upon $\Phi_{1,2}$ of a $\pm 2°$ phase shift in the flow signal, which results in changes from $-21\%$ to $+19\%$ of the non-shifted value, but $\Phi_{2,3}$ is a proportionally larger term in [15] and is much less sensitive to this source of error. $A_2/A_3=0.111$ simulates a moderately severe stenosis and for this value most of the energy loss occurs in region 2 (Figure 4). The predicted and measured values of $E_T$ differ by about $1\%$ and they were obtained by measuring areas beneath the appropriate plots of $\Phi$ against time. An indication of corresponding values in the biological system is given by modelling laws which result in the following: pressure differences scale as $\rho v^2$, giving $\Delta p_b = 5.66 \, \Delta p_m$ where $b$ and $m$ refer to the biological and model

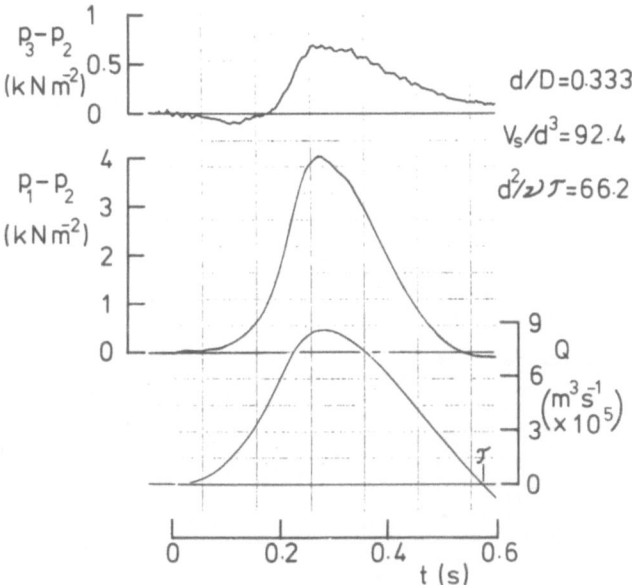

*Figure 5.* Pressure difference measurements during a single flow pulse in the rigid walled model with $A_2/A_1=A_2/A_3=0.111$. Conversion factor 1 kN/m$^2=7.52$ mmHg.

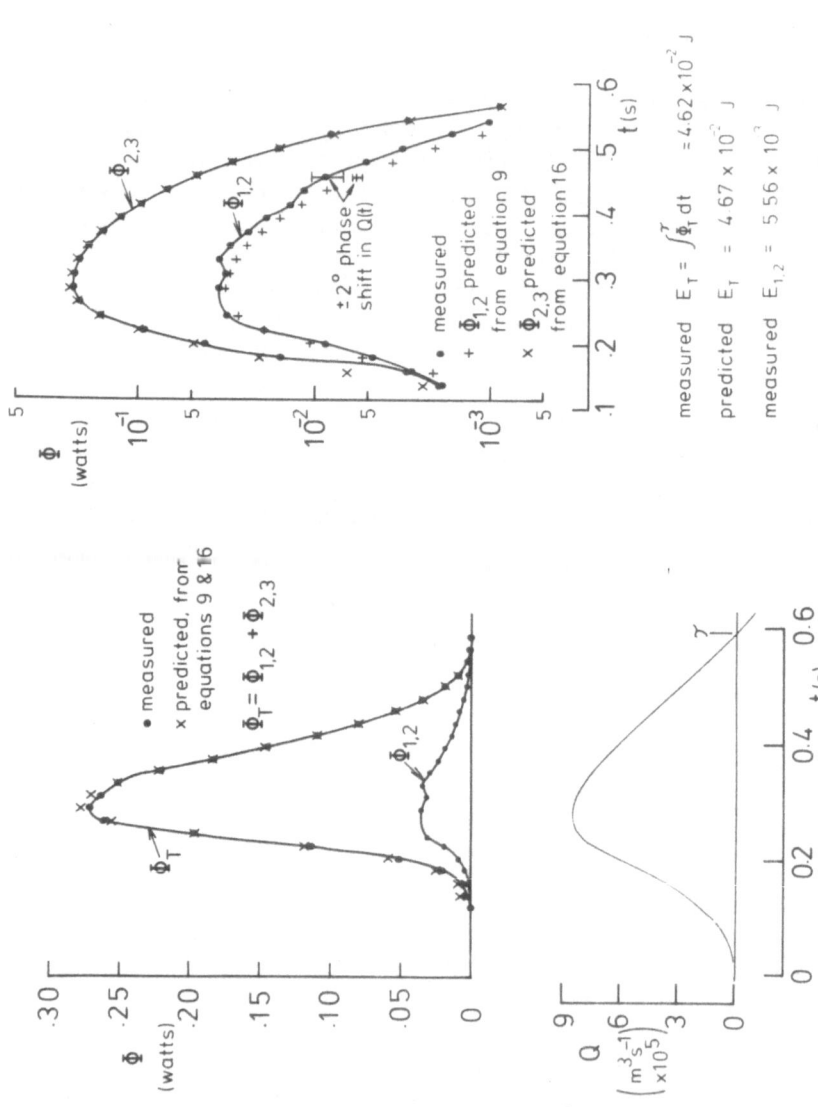

*Figure 6.* Measured and predicted rates of energy loss determined from data in Figure 5, plotted linearly (*left*) and logarithmically (*right*). *Lower left:* flow pulse used.

systems respectively. Energy dissipation rates scale as $\rho Q v^2$, giving $\Phi_b = 29.3$ $\Phi_m$ and dissipated energy scales as $\rho Q v^2 \tau$, giving $E_b = 18.0\ E_m$.

SUMMARY

A theoretical analysis yields equations for the calculation of rates of mechanical energy loss both within a stenosed valve and in the turbulent mixing region downstream. Losses within both regions can be determined implicitly by subtraction of mechanical energy terms, but cannot be obtained explicitly. The simplification of a rigid system allows the derivation of equations to predict rates of energy loss. This gives some insight into the effects upon losses of severity of stenosis, jet angle and post-stenotic dilatation. The theoretical predictions are supported by results from a model study.

REFERENCES

1. Pedley TJ, Seed WA: The fluid mechanics of left ventricular ejection. In: *Cardiovascular and pulmonary dynamics*. Jaffrin MY (ed), INSERM Euromech 92, 1978, vol 71, p 311–320.
2. Clark C: The fluid mechanics of aortic stenosis II: unsteady flow experiments. *J Biomech* 9:567–573, 1976.

# 6.6. PRESSURE-FLOW RELATIONS AND ENERGY LOSSES ACROSS PROSTHETIC MITRAL VALVES: IN VIVO AND IN VITRO STUDIES

Edward L. Yellin, David McQueen, Shlomo Gabbay, Joel A. Strom, Ronald M. Becker, Robert W.M. Frater

## 1. INTRODUCTION

The use of the Gorlin equation (1) to estimate the area of a prosthetic mitral valve has received widespread acceptance despite frequently questionable results. We have found, for example, that intra-operative studies on patients undergoing valve replacement with mitral bioprostheses sometimes yield exceptionally small valve areas during low cardiac output states. This study was designed to analyse the pressure-flow relations across prosthetic mitral valves and to determine the in vivo conditions which would lead to inaccurate area calculations when using the Gorlin equation.

## 2. THEORY

We, as well as others, have determined that the mitral valve apparatus should be treated analogous to an area reduction and hence should be analysed using the equations of motion of flow across an orifice (2, 3). We therefore hypothesize that the pressure-flow relations across the mitral valve are described by

$$\Delta p = (A)dQ/dt + (B)Q^2 \qquad [1]$$

where $\Delta p$ is the pressure difference across the valve (LAP-LVP during diastole); $Q$ is the instantaneous volume flow rate; the first term on the right is the inertial contribution and the second term the dissipative contribution to the pressure difference; $(A)$ and $(B)$ are constants proportional to the valve area.

This equation offers a straightforward approach toward studying the characteristics of prosthetic heart valves. For any given applied pressure gradient, the performance of the valve is determined solely by its flow characteristics, and is independent of the state of the patient's heart, the duration of the filling period or the skill of the surgeon. Difficulties arise only when the equation is incorrectly applied. As will be shown below, in clinical practice this is sometimes unavoidable, but it should not arise under controlled ex vivo conditions.

*J. Baan, A.C. Arntzenius, E.L. Yellin (eds.), Cardiac Dynamics, 509–519.*

From [1], $dQ/dt = 0$ at peak flow (4), therefore

$$\Delta p = (B)Q^2 \qquad [2]$$

The temporal mean of [1] during diastole is

$$\overline{\Delta p} = (B)\overline{Q^2} \qquad [3]$$

since $\int (dQ/dt)dt$ equals 0 integrated over the flow cross-over points. The valve area (MVA) can then be calculated from

$$\text{MVA} = \sqrt{\overline{Q^2}}/(C_d\,51.6\,\sqrt{\overline{\Delta p}}) = \phi_{\text{RMS}}/(C_d\,51.6\,\sqrt{\overline{\Delta p}}) \qquad [4]$$

where $C_d$ is the discharge coefficient and 51.6 is the appropriate conversion factor from mmHg if $Q$ is in ml/sec.

An effective valve area ($A_e$) can be defined (4):

$$A_e = \text{MVA} \times C_d \qquad [5]$$

We prefer this form since it does not require a knowledge of the discharge coefficient and is a suitable figure of merit for valve performance. It will be used in this study. The discharge coefficient is, in fact, equal to $A_e/A_0$, where $A_0$ is the measured valve annulus area.

Equation [4] should be compared to the Gorlin equation:

$$\text{MVA} = (\text{CO}/\text{HR}/\text{DFP})/C_d\,51.6\,\sqrt{\overline{\Delta p}} = Q/C_d\,51.6\,\sqrt{\overline{\Delta p}} \qquad [6]$$

in which CO = cardiac output, HR = heart rate, and DFP = diastolic filling period. While the Gorlin constant ($C_d \times 51.6$) for mitral stenosis has come under revision to accommodate the changes in clinical methodology (5, 6), there has been no evaluation of its use for prosthetic valve function. The basic problem associated with the use of [6] arises from the fact that: $\overline{Q^2} \neq \overline{Q}^2$, or $Q_{\text{RMS}} \neq \overline{Q}$.

In experimental practice:

$$Q_{\text{RMS}} = \sqrt{A_{\text{MiF2}} \times \text{CF}_Q/\text{DFP}} \quad \text{and} \quad \sqrt{\overline{\Delta p}} = \sqrt{A_p \times \text{CF}_p/\text{DFP}}$$

Where $A_{\text{MiF2}}$ is the area under the square of the flow trace, $\text{CF}_Q$ is the calibration factor for flow; $A_p$ is the area of the pressure difference tracing; and $\text{CF}_p$ the calibration factor for pressure (Figure 1). Since the diastolic filling period (DFP) appears as the square root both times, any errors or ambiguity in choosing the correct value for DFP become self-correcting (Figure 1B).

In clinical practice:

$$\overline{Q} = \text{CO}/\text{HR}/\text{DFP} \quad \text{and} \quad \sqrt{\overline{\Delta p}} = \sqrt{A_p \times \text{CF}_p/\text{DFP}}$$

In this approach there are two potentially large sources of error: $\overline{Q}$ may be

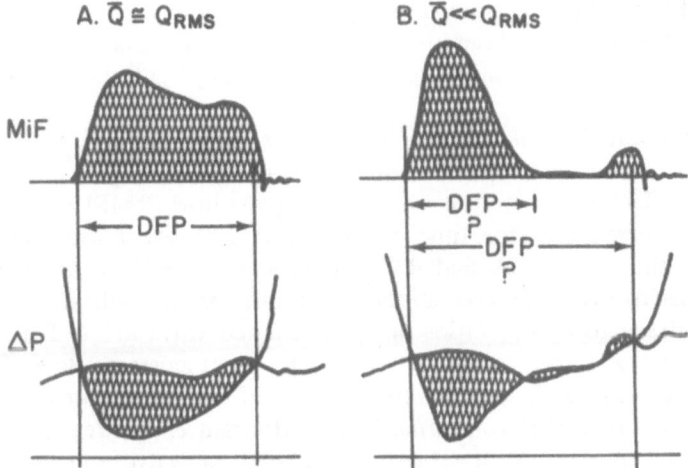

*Figure 1.* Schematic representation of two pressure and flow wave forms. A. A pressure gradient which is sustained throughout diastole and produces a nearly uniform "flat" flow pattern. B. A pressure difference which is not sustained throughout diastole and produces a flow pattern which is not uniform. $\bar{Q}$, $Q_{RMS}$: mean, and root mean square flow, respectively; MiF: mitral flow; $\Delta p$: pressure difference (LAP–LVP); DFP: diastolic filling period.

very much less than $Q_{RMS}$, and the DFP chosen from the pressure cross-over points will be too large (Figure 1B), both of which tend to underestimate the calculated valve area.

This study will focus on those clinical conditions which would lead to large errors in the use of [6]. We will calculate effective valve areas using [4] and [6], modified as in [5], and the results presented in the form of an Area Ratio = MVA from [4]/MVA from [6].

## 3. METHODS

### 3.1. *Animal studies*

Using standard surgical techniques described previously (7, 8), an Ionescu-Shiley 19 bioprosthesis was implanted in series with an electromagnetic flow probe in two open-chest, anaesthetized dogs. Phasic mitral flow was recorded along with high-fidelity, high-gain left atrial and left ventricular pressures. These parameters along with aortic flow, $dp/dt$, aortic pressure and the electrocardiogram were recorded on an oscillographic recorder at paper speeds of 100 mm/sec.

In order to test the equation of motion under a wide variety of conditions, the functional state of the hearts was varied by changing preload, afterload and inotropic state. The duration of the diastolic filling period as well as the wave form of the pressure difference during diastole were further altered by vagal stimulation and induced ventricular premature contractions.

The calibrated pressure and flow curves were digitized with a sonic digitizer coupled to a digital computer programmed to provide the mean pressure difference, mean flow, root mean square flow (RMS), peak flow and pressure difference at the time of peak flow. Effective mitral valve areas based on the mean, peak and RMS approaches were then calculated.

In order to avoid the errors inherent in flow probe calibration, the data were analysed using the ratios of the calculated valve areas. This method also minimizes the error of choosing an incorrect flow baseline. Furthermore, since we are primarily concerned with *analysing* valve performance rather than with *comparing* valve performance, the area ratio method avoids misrepresenting the characteristics of a valve due to surgical problems.

The results were compared for statistical significance with the null hypothesis of 1.0 (a ratio of 1.0 means no difference) using the standard *t*-test with significance accepted at the .05 level. All ratios will be presented as the mean $\pm 1$ S.D. In order to minimize the possibility of flowmeter errors due to random asymmetric flow profiles, more than 100 cycles from each dog were used in the calculations.

### 3.2. *Pulse-duplicator studies*

In order to test the equation of motion under more controlled ex vivo conditions, we used the data of a pulse-duplicator study published separately (9). In that report, three sizes each of four biological and five mechanical prostheses were tested in the "mitral" position of a pulse-duplicator under various conditions of pulse rate and flow rate with approximately sinusoidal flow wave forms (Figure 2).

## 4. RESULTS

### 4.1. *Pulse duplicator*

Figure 2 is an original record from the pulse-duplicator study taken at two pulse rates with similar stroke volumes. Note the nearly sinusoidal flow wave form. Using the data reported by Gabbay et al. (9), for each of the 18 valves tested, we averaged the effective valve areas based on the RMS, peak and steady flow values. This value was divided by the effective valve area

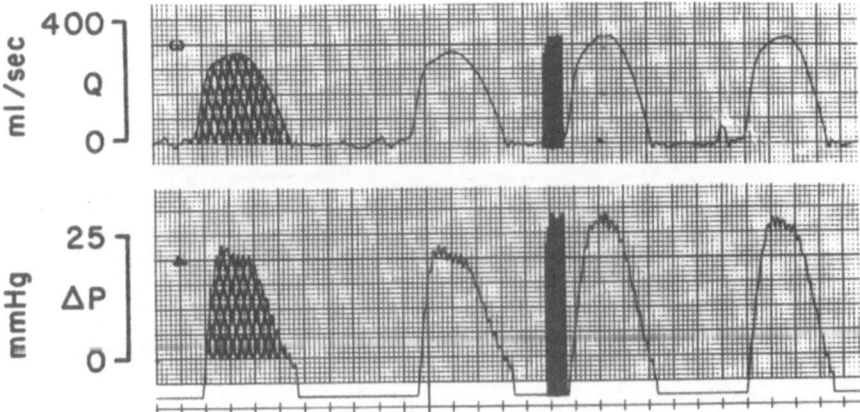

*Figure 2.* Recording of flow (*upper*) and pressure difference (*lower*) across a bioprosthetic valve in the pulse-duplicator. Pulse rate increases, but stroke volume is nearly constant. Note the nearly sinusoidal flow wave form which is characteristic of most pulse-duplicator studies.

using the mean gradient and flow (Gorlin approach). The average ratio for all the valves was $1.12 \pm 0.03$ ($P < .001$). This value is in good agreement with the predicted ratio (1.11) for a nearly sinusoidal flow (Figure 2).

## 4.2. *Animal studies*

For dog 1, Figures 3 and 4 are typical oscillographic records which showed the characteristically "flat" flow and pressure wave forms (Figure 1, left) of mitral stenosis (10) and mitral prostheses (11, 12).

In Figure 3, the diastolic filling period was increased 60% by slowing the heart rate with vagal stimulation. Both the control (left panel) and stimulation (right panel) recordings were taken during the steady state. In Figure 4, three consecutively different conditions of transmitral flow and pressure difference were created by inducing a ventricular premature contraction.

A total of 103 cycles (heart rate range: 100–182) were analysed and the effective valve areas were calculated using the RMS, peak and mean methods for each cycle. Since the RMS and peak values were not statistically different, they were pooled and the area ratio was calculated by dividing by the area based on the mean: Area Ratio $= 1.09 \pm 0.09$ ($p < .001$).

Figures 5, 6 and 7 are selected oscillographic records depicting the various conditions examined in dog 2. Figure 5 is an excerpt from a sequence of sinus arrhythmias with "flat" flow wave forms as in dog 1 (Figure 3). Figures 6 and 7, on the other hand, are taken during periods of mechanical alternans and included biphasic flow wave forms (Figure 6) or

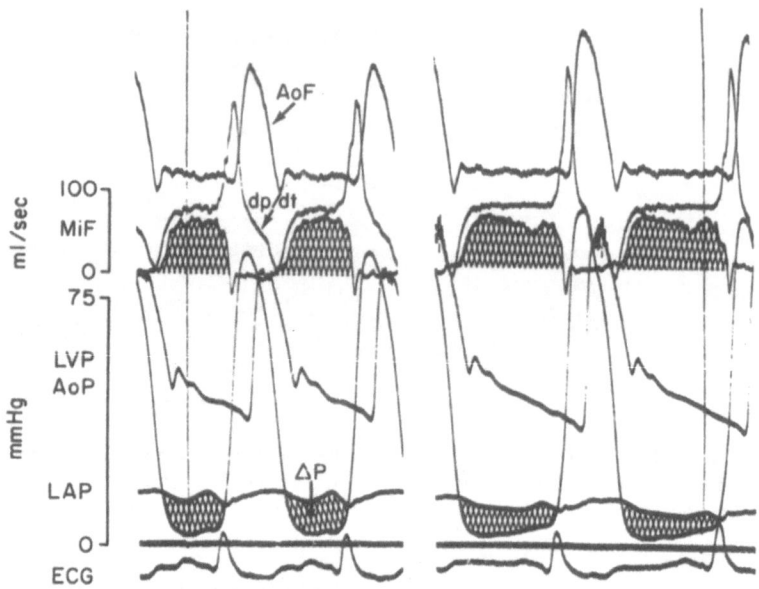

*Figure 3.* Oscillographic record from dog 1 showing its characteristic "flat" flow pattern during control (*left*) and during vagal stimulation (*right*) to slow heart rate and increase diastolic filling period. LVP: left ventricular pressure, AoP: aortic pressure; LAP: left atrial pressure; ECG: electrocardiogram; AoF: aortic flow; *dp/dt*: derivative of left ventricular pressure. MiF and $\Delta p$ are shaded for emphasis. The aortic pressure trace is delayed in time relative to the LAP and LVP because of catheter and pulse transmission delays.

"sinusoidal" wave forms (Figure 7), similar to those shown in Figure 1 (right), in both cases produced by pressure differences which are unlike those in dog 1 and in Figure 5.

One-hundred-and-nine cycles (heart rate range: 90–222) were analysed and the area ratios calculated as above: Area Ratio = $1.27 \pm 0.23$ ($p < .001$). In order to unmask further the effects of pressure-flow patterns on the calculated valve areas using the Gorlin equation, we selected for additional analysis 16 pairs of control and post-extrasystolic cycles.

The diastolic filling period increased twofold during the compensatory pause (166–367 msec), and because this dog tended to have rapid early filling followed by little or no filling (Figures 6 and 7), as predicted above, the valve area based on the mean flow was profoundly less than the combined RMS-peak area, and the error increased as the diastolic filling period increased: Control Area Ratio = $1.24 \pm 0.15$; Post-extrasystolic Area Ratio = $1.58 \pm 0.42$ ($p < .001$). Furthermore, those cycles with a "square root sign" LVP and reversal of the pressure difference during diastole (Figure 7) had mid-diastolic closure of the mitral valve; under such conditions the

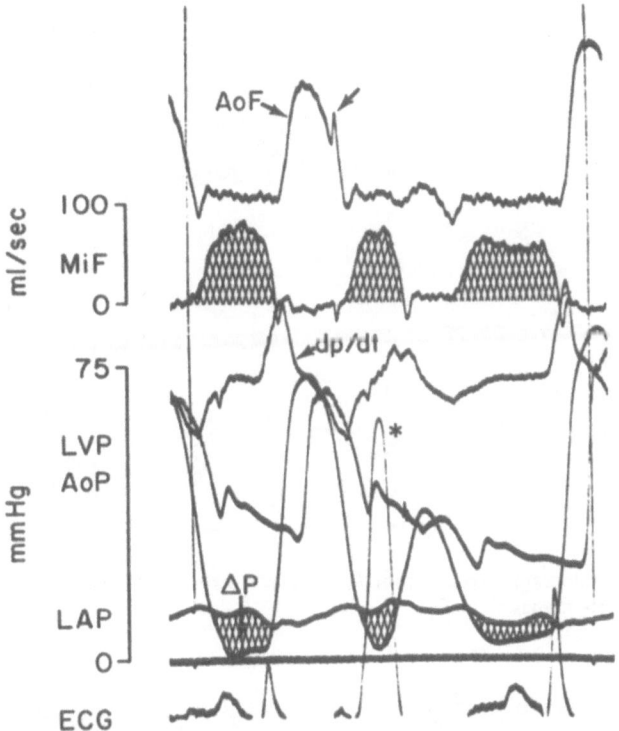

*Figure 4.* As in Figure 3, but illustrating the changing pressure-flow conditions during a ventricular premature contraction. The arrow points to the stimulus artifact, and the asterisk denotes the electrical component of the VPC. Time lines, 1/sec.

calculated diastolic period based on pressure cross-over points and area based on mean flow (Gorlin approach), were increasingly inaccurate.

## 5. DISCUSSION

There seems little question regarding the applicability of [1] to the study of energy losses across mitral prostheses: the analysis of a system with the large time variations of flow found in the heart must include the concept of inertance and all evidence points to the fact that energy losses across prosthetic valves are due to turbulence and vary with the square of the flow (13). Viscous losses are apparently insignificant in comparison to turbulent dissipation. The main problem is in the use of formulae derived from [1]. We have previously shown (10) that the Gorlin equation is a theoretically accurate predictor of the stenotic mitral valve area, in this study we are

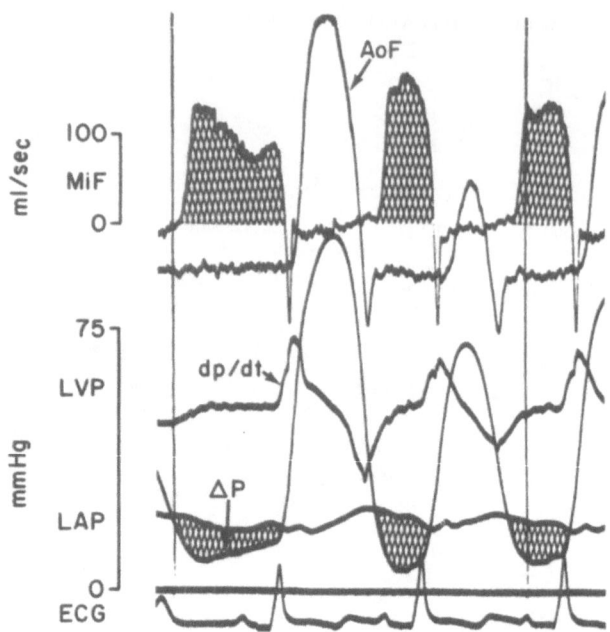

*Figure 5.* An oscillographic record from dog 2 illustrating the changing pressure-flow patterns during sinus arrhythmias.

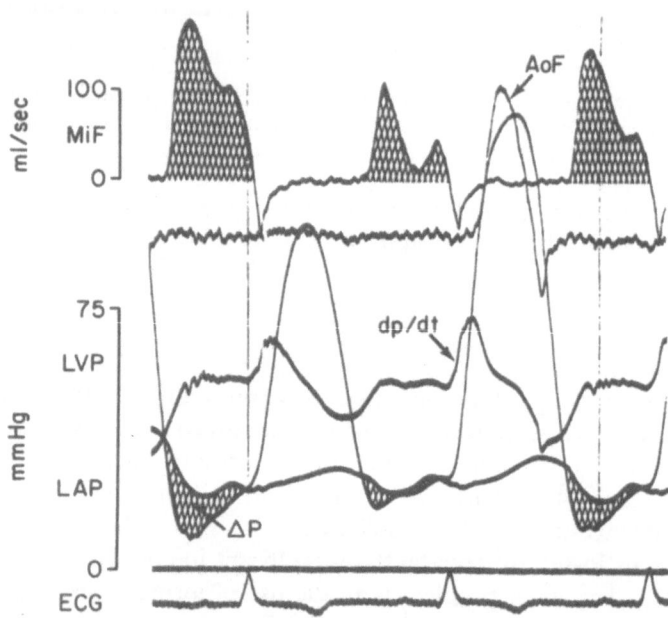

*Figure 6.* As in Figure 5, but during mechanical alternans with markedly different pressure-flow wave forms: biphasic, rather than "flat".

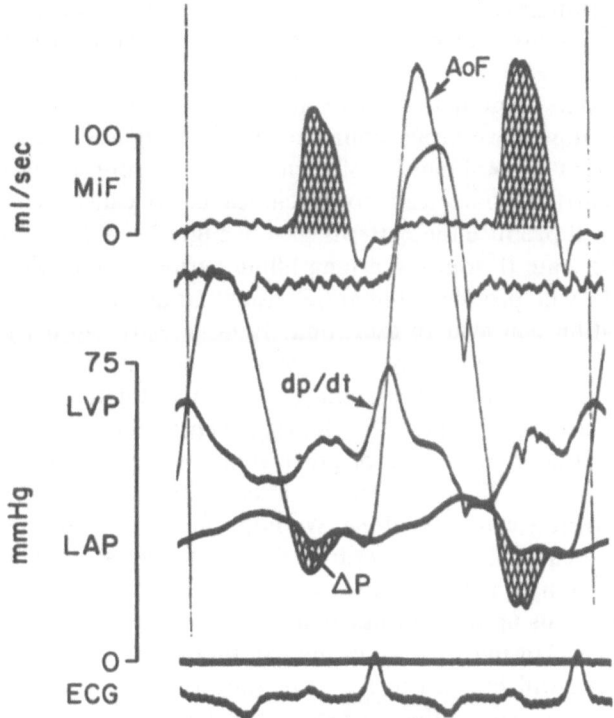

*Figure 7.* As in Figure 6, but with a nearly sinusoidal flow wave form.

particularly concerned with the use of the Gorlin equation for the in vivo evaluation of prosthetic mitral valves.

Since most pulse-duplicators employ nearly sinusoidal flow the error inherent in using the mean, rather than the peak or root-mean-square-based area, is tolerable (10%), particularly since it will be constant for each valve tested. The potential error in clinical studies, however, can be unacceptably large. The main goal of this study was to elucidate those sources of error and help make it possible for the clinician to evaluate his data.

While it is clinically feasible to achieve high-fidelity left atrial and left ventricular pressure recordings (although it is done only rarely), it is not yet possible to measure phasic mitral flow with adequate accuracy in the cath laboratory. As a consequence, much of the discussion which follows is speculative and based on data obtained under experimental conditions in the animal laboratory.

In our opinion the pressure and flow wave forms in patients who have had mitral valve replacement and who are studied under conditions of normal heart rate, cardiac output, ventricular compliance and LVEDP, will probably be similar to those of Figures 1 (left), 3 and 4. Thus, the 10% error in effective valve area calculated from the Gorlin equation will be clinically acceptable.

It is also our opinion that there are clinical conditions which lead to pressure and flow wave forms similar to those of Figures 1 (right), 6 and 7. We believe that a combination of high filling pressure, rapid early filling and a stiff ventricle, which leads to the clinical entity called the "square root sign LVP", will produce the patterns seen in Figure 7. A low cardiac output and low heart rate (leading to a long filling period) in combination with a stiff ventricle will produce similar relations. Under these conditions, the Gorlin equation can lead to exceptionally large errors in calculated valve area. While in the absence of flow measurements in patients we cannot make these statements with certainty, other investigators have measured similar patterns experimentally in the right ventricle of calves (14).

We realize that it would be of great value to the clinician if we could supply him with a simple method of correcting the Gorlin equation. Unfortunately, this cannot be done. We hope, however, that an understanding of the principles and derivation of the Gorlin equation will aid him in the interpretation of patient data.

Finally, when using the Gorlin equation to estimate the area of a stenotic valve, the physician must use an estimated discharge coefficient because the calculated area will be used in the evaluation of the need for surgery. We have found that 0.6 is the correct value (10). The evaluation of the performance of a prosthetic valve, on the other hand, requires the calculation of its effective area. Since we can measure the area of a valve orifice, and since the discharge coefficient can only be determined under controlled ex vivo conditions, we recommend that all prosthetic valves be characterized by an effective area, equation [5] (see 4, 9).

ACKNOWLEDGEMENTS

This work was supported in part by National Institutes of Health Training Grant HL07071–02 and Research Grant HL-19391. It could not have been done without the technical skills of Messrs. Astolfo Leon, Pablo Bon and Felix Rivera.

REFERENCES

1. Gorlin R, Gorlin SG: Hydraulic formula for calculation of the area of the stenotic mitral valve, other cardiac valves, and central circulatory shunts I. *Am Heart J* 41:1–29, 1951.
2. Bellhouse BJ: The fluid mechanics of heart valves. In: *Cardiovascular fluid dynamics*, vol 1, DH Bergel (ed), New York, Academic Press, 1972, p 261–285.
3. Yellin EL, Peskin CS: Large amplitude pulsatile water flow across an orifice. *Journal of Dynamic Systems, Measurement and Control, Trans ASME* 97 (Series G):92–95, 1975.
4. Aaslid R, Levang O, Froysaker T, Skagseth E, Hall DV: In situ evaluation of the aortic pivoting disc valve prosthesis. *Scand J Thorac Cardiovasc Surg* 9:81–84, 1975.

5. Cohen MV, Gorlin R: Modified orifice equation for the calculation of mitral valve area. *Am Heart J* 84:839–40, 1972.
6. Hammermeister KE, Murray JA, Blackmon JR: Revision of Gorlin constant for calculation of mitral valve area from heart pressures. *Brit Heart J* 35:392–96, 1973.
7. Frater RWM, Wexler H, Yellin EL: The in vivo comparison of hemodynamic function of ball, disc and eccentric monocusp artificial mitral valves. In: *Prosthetic heart valves*, Brewer III LA, (ed), Springfield, Ill, Charles C Thomas, 1969, p 262–277.
8. Laniado S, Yellin EL, Miller H, Frater RWM: Temporal relations of the first heart sound to closure of the mitral valve. *Circulation* 47:1006–1014, 1973.
9. Gabbay S, McQueen D, Yellin EL, Becker RM, Frater RWM: In vitro hydrodynamic performance of mitral valve prostheses at high flow rates. *J Thorac Cardiovasc Res* 76:771–785, 1978.
10. Yellin EL, Frater RWM, Peskin CS: The application of the Gorlin equation to the stenotic mitral valve. In: 1975, *Advances in Bioengineering*, Bell AC, Nerem RM, (eds), New York, ASME, 1975, p 45–47.
11. Folts JD, Young WP, Rowe GG: Phasic flow through normal and prosthetic mitral valves in unanesthetized dogs. *J Thorac Cardiovasc Surg* 61:235–241, 1971.
12. Nolan SP, Stewart S, Fogarty TJ, Dixon Jr SH, Morrow AG: In vivo studies of instantaneous blood flow across mitral ball-valve prosthesis: effects of cardiac output and heart rate on transvalvular energy loss. *Ann Surg* 169:551–559, 1969.
13. *Prosthetic heart valves*, Brewer III LA (ed), Springfield, Ill, Charles C Thomas, Springfield, Ill, 1969.
14. Nolan SP, Stewart S, Fogarty TJ, Morrow AG: Instantaneous bloodflow through ball valve prosthesis in the tricuspid position: effects of heart beat rate and atrial contraction, *Arch Surg* 97:696–975, 1968.

## 6.7. BLOOD FLOW VELOCITY IN SUBCLAVIAN ARTERY AND THROUGH MITRAL VALVE MEASURED WITH TRANSCUTANEOUS DOPPLER ULTRASOUND

*The Effects of Exercise and Mitral Valve Disease*

DAN S. TUNSTALL PEDOE

### 1. INTRODUCTION

Measurement of instantaneous blood flow velocity within the heart and great vessels is essential for calculating the mechanical energy losses resulting from heart valve dysfunction and transport of blood through the proximal arterial tree. Direct measurement of local instantaneous blood velocity within the arterial circulation and heart requires invasive instrumentation and is not convenient for the study of blood flow patterns in athletes during exercise, nor for routine use in the study of patients with heart disease.

Doppler ultrasound, a noninvasive technique, which has been regarded as largely qualitative in its measurements of blood velocity (1) can be made quantitative with appropriate care in making the measurements, and with spectral analysis of the Doppler signal.

### 2. METHOD FOR SUBCLAVIAN ARTERY BLOOD VELOCITY MEASUREMENTS

The Doppler equation

$$\Delta f = \frac{2fv \cos \theta}{c}$$

where $f$ = transmitted frequency, $v$ = blood velocity, $\theta$ = angle of ultrasound probe to direction of blood flow, $c$ = velocity of sound in blood, allows an accurate measurement of blood velocity $v$ to be made from a Doppler spectrograph where $\cos \theta$ can be measured and $c$ and $f$ are both known. The $\Delta f$ signal is displayed as a sound spectrograph, which makes a plot of frequency against time, with the amplitude of each frequency being shown by the intensity of the record. A wide range of instantaneous velocities within the sample volume of the Doppler probe is shown by a wide bandwidth of frequencies on the spectrograph; a uniform velocity of blood flow within the sample volume would be shown by a dense high frequency outline to the spectrograph.

Measurements were made from the subclavian arteries of five cross-country runners, at rest and after severe arm and leg exercise on a bicycle ergometer. A 5 MHz Parks Doppler probe was held at 45° to the vessel.

## 2.1. RESULTS

The results from all five subjects were similar. An example is shown in Figure 1. The record obtained before exercise is shown in the upper panel in which the peak velocity was 1 m/sec and the high frequency outline of the spectrograph suggests uniform velocity across the diameter of the

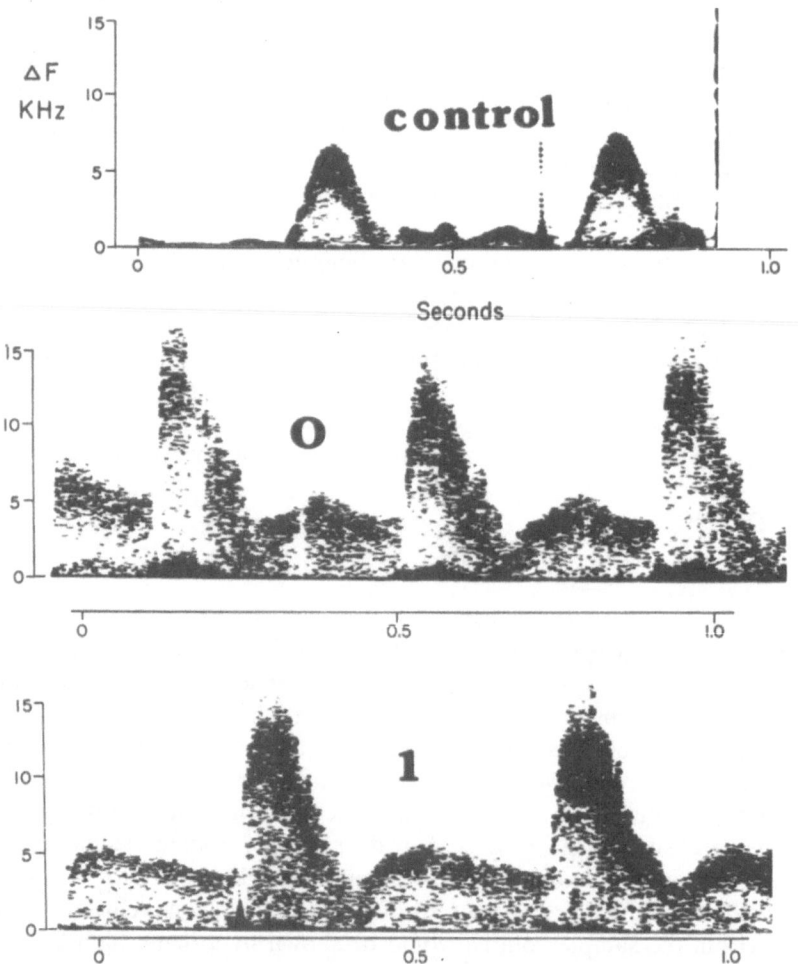

*Figure 1.* Doppler sound spectrograph showing subclavian artery blood flow velocity before (*top*), immediately after (0), and one minute after (1) maximal arm exercise.

artery, characteristic of laminar inlet-length flow. Immediately after three minutes of severe arm exercise (middle panel) and one minute later (lower panel) the blood velocities had increased to over 2.5 m/sec and the wide bandwidth of the signals and the "shaggy" outline of the spectrographs suggest the presence of large vortices in the flow.

## 2.2. DISCUSSION

The records from both arm and leg exercise showed very high blood velocities in the subclavian arteries, but the records obtained after leg exercise showed very little diastolic flow, unlike the massive diastolic flow shown in the lower panels of Figure 1. Cardiac outputs as high as 35 litres/min have been measured in world-class athletes. In a 3 cm-diameter aorta this would give a mean Reynolds number of 5000. It is therefore possible that one of the limits to cardiac output is the development of turbulence in the aorta and major arteries. These Doppler records would be compatible with this hypothesis.

## 3. METHOD FOR INTRACARDIAC MEASUREMENTS

A 2MHz SINTEF PEDOF Doppler instrument (2) was used to measure intracardiac blood velocity transcutaneously from eight patients with rheumatic mitral regurgitation. The Doppler probe was aligned with the transmitral jet (Figure 2). Accurate alignment of the probe with the jet through the mitral valve could be checked by range gating a sample volume but for the peak velocities to be recorded the instrument had to be used in the continuous wave mode. The records were displayed as sound spectrographs with an ECG marker added. The ECG is shown on all the records as a black line at the top of the figures (Figures 3, 4, 5, 6). A directional spectrograph could also be obtained by offsetting zero to 4 kHz. Such a record is shown in Figure 6 where flow towards the probe is shown as a Doppler shift below 4 kHz and flow away from the probe (back into the left atrium) is shown as a Doppler shift of more than 4 kHz.

## 3.1. RESULTS

In seven of the eight patients with mitral regurgitation peak systolic velocities through the mitral valve of more than 4 m/sec were found. An example is shown in Figure 3. This record was from a patient in sinus rhythm. The mitral regurgitant jet S follows the QRS complex of the ECG. It has a peak velocity of 5 m/sec and is followed by diastolic inflow to the

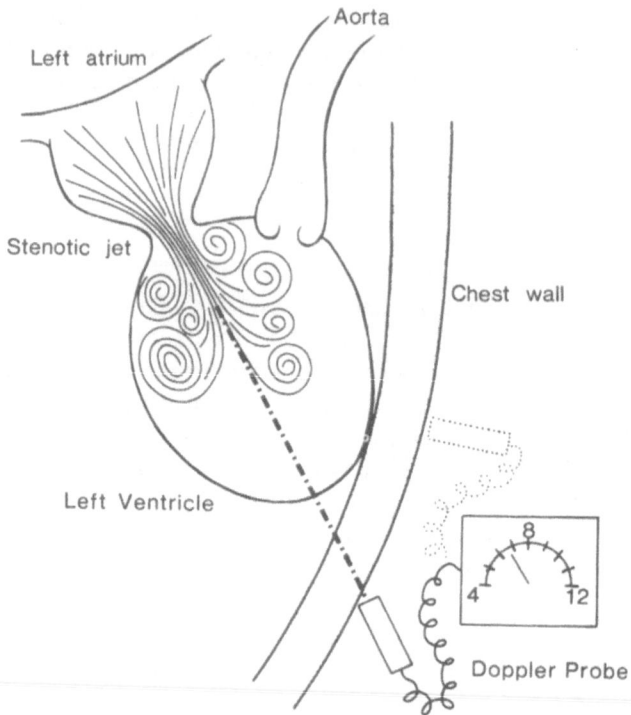

*Figure 2.* Transcutaneous measurement of blood velocity through the mitral valve. Technique of alignment of the Doppler probe with the transmitral jet.

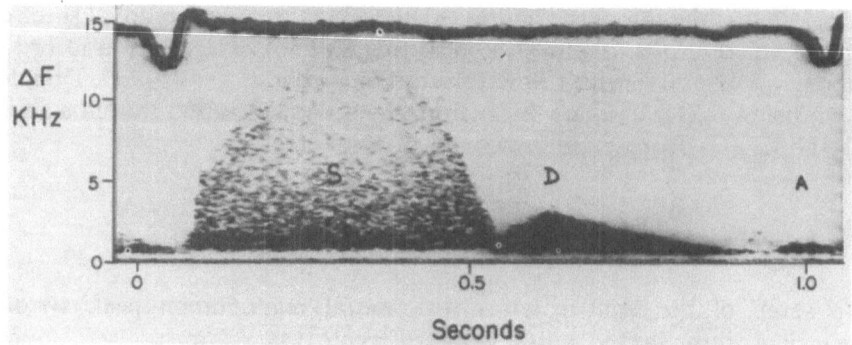

*Figure 3.* Transmitral blood flow velocity in mitral regurgitation. Sinus rhythm. Top tracing: ECG, S: systole. D: diastole, A: atrial contraction.

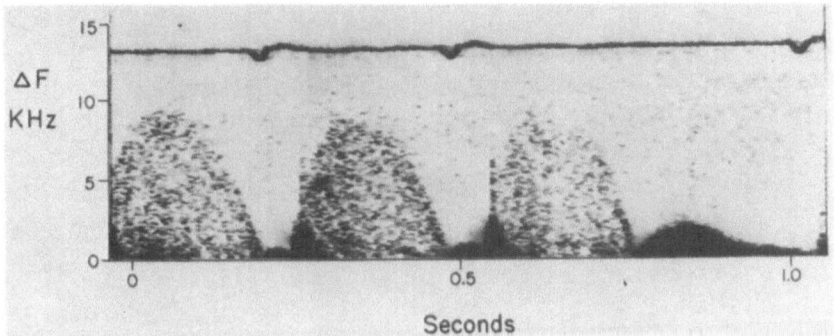

*Figure 4.* Transmitral blood flow velocity in mitral regurgitation. The effect of a ventricular ectopic beat (VEB).

left ventricle. The latter has a much lower velocity, but since the flow is towards the Doppler probe it produces a much more intense signal (D in Figure 3). In late diastole and almost coincident with the QRS of the ECG atrial contraction produces further transmitral flow into the left ventricle (A in Figure 3). Apart from the diagnostic use of this technique in confirming the presence of mitral regurgitation, the effects of dysrhythmias on the mitral regurgitant jet and the diastolic inflow to the left ventricle could be demonstrated.

The record shown in Figure 4 is from a patient with ventricular ectopic beats. The first systolic jet results from a normally conducted beat; it is followed immediately by another systolic jet from a ventricular ectopic beat. The peak velocities are similar but the duration of the second systole is rather less. Even so, from this record it would appear that the amount of regurgitation has almost doubled as a result of the ectopic beat.

Rapid atrial fibrillation is notoriously dangerous to patients with mitral valve disease. The record shown in Figure 5 is from a patient who had

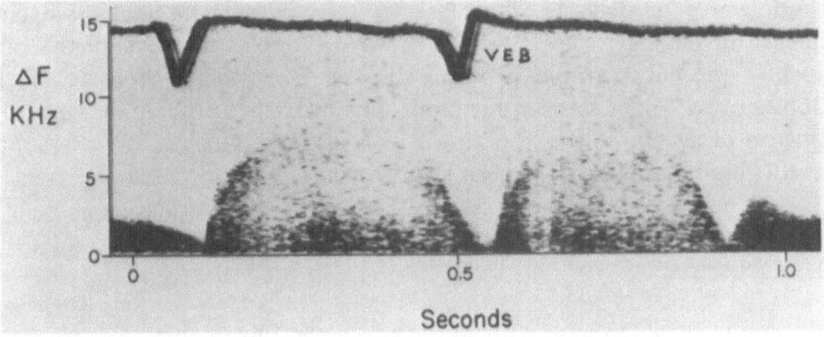

*Figure 5.* Transmitral blood flow velocity in mitral regurgitation. Rapid atrial fibrillation.

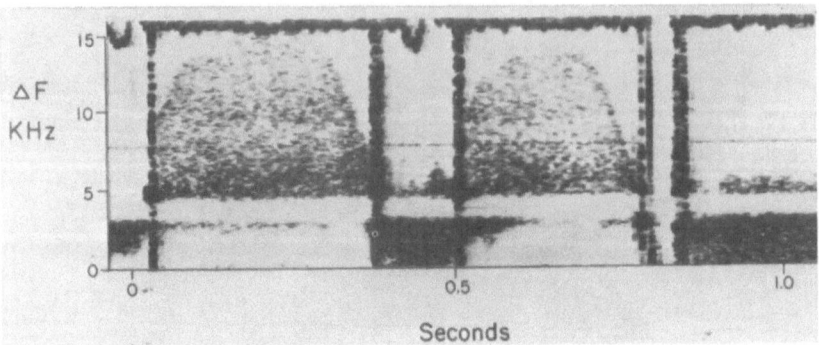

*Figure 6.* Transmitral blood flow velocity in mixed mitral valve disease. This is a directional spectrograph with zero velocity offset to 4 kHz.

occasional runs of beats at a rate of 200 per min. At this very fast heart rate, the regurgitant jets immediately following the QRS complex of the ECG lasted three times longer than the diastolic filling interval between the first three systoles on the trace. With the longer cardiac cycle at the end of the trace diastole was longer and gave the left ventricle a chance to fill. Not surprisingly with the tachycardia potentiating the effect of mitral regurgitation, the patient was hypotensive and in heart failure.

The record shown in Figure 6 is from a patient who had severe stenosis as well as regurgitation of the mitral valve. The spectrograph is directional with the regurgitant jet shown as a Doppler shift of >4 kHz and the flow towards the probe, which is the stenotic jet, shown as a Doppler shift of <4 kHz. In this record the thickened valve produces intense artefacts as it opens and closes. The apparent persistence of the stenotic jet in systole, after the closing artefact of the mitral valve, is probably not the result of transmitral flow towards the transducer, but the result of the slow decay of a large vortex in the left ventricle induced by the 2 m/sec jet through the stenotic valve in diastole. This lack of selectivity is an inevitable consequence of having to use continuous-wave Doppler to measure the high velocities present with heart valve disease. The sample volume of the Doppler probe when used in this mode may introduce ambiguous spectrographs on occasion, as range gating which involves pulsing the ultrasound prevents high blood velocities being recorded.

## 3.2. DISCUSSION

Continuous wave Doppler with sound spectrography enables a noninvasive examination of the function of the diseased mitral valve to be made. Since the malfunction of the valve produces much higher velocities than are usually present in the heart, and since the probe can usually be placed in line with the stenotic and regurgitant jets in rheumatic heart disease, both diagnostic and useful hemodynamic information can be obtained.

## 4. SUMMARY

Measurements of instantaneous blood velocity in the subclavian arteries and through the mitral valve have been made transcutaneously using Doppler ultrasound in two groups of subjects. The blood velocities were displayed in the form of sound spectrographs. In five athletes after maximal exercise the blood flow velocity in the subclavian arteries gave a spectrographic appearance suggestive of transition from laminar to turbulent flow. In a group of eight patients with mitral regurgitation, the transmitral blood flow velocity was measured. The velocity of the systolic jet passing back into the left atrium from the left ventricle exceeded 4 m/sec in seven and the effects of dysrhythmias on the mitral regurgitant jet and on diastolic inflow to the left ventricle was demonstrated.

REFERENCES

1. Franklin DL, Schlegel WA, Rushmer RF: Blood flow measured by Doppler frequency shift of backscattered ultrasound. *Science* 132:564–565, 1961.
2. Angelsen BAJ, Brubakk AO: Transcutaneous measurement of blood flow velocity in the human aorta. *Cardiovasc Res* 10:368–379, 1976.

# CLOSING LECTURE

CLOSING PAGE

# CLOSING LECTURE: APPROACHING THE HEART OF THE MATTER

Abraham Noordergraaf

> *Plusieurs choses certaines sont contredites;*
> *plusieurs fausses passent sans contradiction.*
> *Ni la contradiction n'est marque de fausseté,*
> *ni l'incontradiction n'est marque de verité.*
>
> Blaise Pascal, ~1650

This conference featured approximately 100 presentations in either classical or poster format. The density of presentation, exceeding four presentations per hour for three long working days, guaranteed intense exposure to a large sample of the latest research and clinical developments in the cardiovascular field. These presentations may be categorized in several ways, one of which might recognize the following areas:

1. Exploratory presentations, in which a directed or, more likely, a random search for an "in" is reported;
2. Discovery presentations, which reveal phenomena not previously known or appreciated;
3. Encyclopaedic presentations, which provide an account on wide ranging observations concerning the multiple effects induced by a variety of agents or interventions;
4. Basic presentations, in which fundamental relationships are evolved;
5. Demand presentations, which outline what the clinician needs to know, or should have available, for the purpose of advancing diagnostic or therapeutic faculties.

Even in a single field such as cardiovascular dynamics, progress in any one of these areas is likely to be neither optimal nor even impressive unless there exists extensive cross-fertilization amongst them. Free-ranging discussion among members of a lively, modest-sized group which includes both clinical and basic scientists provides the additional required dimension. It is in this dimension, the full utilization of which is not easily achievable, that many consider a fusion is necessitated by extreme specialization and the resulting trepidation sensed by the members of different specialities. This specialization was initiated by the Renaissance-induced acceleration of scientific growth.

The *theme* "basic and clinical aspects of cardiac dynamics" exerted a powerful focusing influence. The great majority of presentations dealt with the heart itself, its interaction with the receiving arterial trees, and its response to venous return.

Commencing with the last, it is striking that the interaction between the venous system and the receiving atria and ventricles is treated much more superficially than that between the ventricles and their respective arterial circulations. This in spite of the conviction held by many experts that changes in preload affect cardiac behaviour more than do changes in afterload. Undoubtedly this is to be ascribed to the lack of even a simple formulation of the properties and function of the large venous source of blood supply. Brecher's pioneering work with venous return (1) in which he argued for the presence of suction exerted by the relaxing ventricle as an aspirator of blood, appears to have marshalled support at the electronmicroscopic level. Forces exerted by passive elements, defined at the cellular level, are commensurate with a rapidly and vastly increasing compliance of the ventricle beginning at the termination of the contraction phase. (Compliance, $C$, is defined as the instantaneous ratio between a change in ventricular volume $dV_v$ and the accompanying change in pressure $dp_v$ and, with incompressible fluids, implies a precipitous drop in pressure as compliance increases with constant volume.)

Stimulated by available technology, including high-fidelity pressure measurements, ultrasonic fluid velocity and transmitral flow measurements, and ultrasonic distance measurements within the receiving ventricle, a large volume of data is being collected. It includes the influence of heart rate, of circulating volume and of inotropic drugs on duration and magnitude of filling and, indirectly, on the subsequent stroke volume. Determination of velocity patterns within the ventricular cavity are beginning to shed light on mitral leaflet dynamics. Although it is premature to sort out the data collected to date, clinical trials have been initiated to apply preliminary conclusions drawn from these data. The availability of more accurate data also permits, for example, scrutiny of the popular Gorlin formula for the estimation of stenosed valve areas.

It has long been appreciated (2) that the response of the ventricle following A-V nodal triggering depends on both the degree of filling and the contractile properties of the myocardium. It is not surprising, judged by the development of pressure alone during the isovolumic phase, that these variables could play interchangeable roles. McMichael in fact (3) employed this concept in a broad sense in the treatment of patients. He argued that venous congestion tends to serve as a compensatory mechanism for deficient myocardial contractile properties. Such interchangeability of variables emphasizes the difficulty of isolating the pure contractile properties of the ventricle.

As early as 1855 Saint-Venant (4) cautioned that fastening elastic material at its ends for the purpose of determining its elastic properties was likely to produce artifacts. This warning was repeated more emphatically by Timoshenko (5). For active biological material the difficulty may be expected to be more serious and this has proven to be the case (6). Awareness of problems involving end-effects stimulated the introduction of significantly improved techniques for the measurement of properties of isolated heart muscle. New measurements of force-velocity-length relations show the necessity for review of muscle concepts that have come to be accepted. In this context a tendency for extreme, alternate analyses may be discerned. Concepts developed in physics and engineering are currently carried to the muscle area where they may not apply; determination of muscle properties based on the utilization of test frequencies outside the physiological range (up to 1,000 Hz) has been reported. Analysis of systems with time-variant parameters requires considerable judgement to avoid, apparently not so obvious, pitfalls (7).

The abandonment of the operational multiple element model for cardiac muscle (number of elements equal to two, or preferably three, up to at least nine) in favour of the analysis of muscle dynamics at a variety of levels, including at the electronmicroscopic level, signals a liberation from the spiritual domination by skeletal muscle concepts. These achievements open the way towards the elucidation of the particular observed phenomena that are unique to cardiac muscle. Such studies not only expose limitations of the operational models which may have educational value, but also permit basic quantification of the sequence of events, commonly denoted as excitation-contraction coupling. Breaking from skeletal muscle concepts has, interestingly, created both independence for researchers in cardiac muscle and rapprochement with investigators of skeletal muscle regarding fundamental concepts.

With clearer views and improved technology which permits measurements of sarcomere lengths directly, it is possible to address questions pertaining to the interrelationship between inotropic effects and length dependency on force production. It appears that the length-dependent force is governed primarily by the transport of $Ca^{++}$ ions from their stores to active sites within the filament structure, while inotropy influences the supply of $Ca^{++}$ ions in the stores. Whether contractile force is generated as a consequence of linking and disruption of crossbridges or as a result of field effects (8) remains unresolved.

The ventricle, viewed as the major pump in the circuit, receives continual attention in attempts to analyse the complex relationships between preload, afterload, heart rate and the contractile properties of the myocardium itself. Lacking an approach based on a comprehensive theory and with the confusion involving terminology (9), the results of experiments accomplished in different laboratories, even on isolated hearts, are difficult to correlate. Since amassment of experimental data has traditionally preceded the conception of new unifying ideas this should not deter further work.

Heartened by experimentally observed similarity between muscular and ventricular behaviour, designers of ventricular models continue to utilize multiple element models for muscle, or crossbridge concepts for force generation, as building blocks. It is to be expected that newer insight into mechanics of muscle contraction, the organization of muscle bundles, the contribution of wall thickness and the acquisition, by ultrasonic means, of detailed data on wall motion will add further sophistication. The model will then play its rightful role in distinguishing major and minor effects. The history of the development of understanding of the arterial systems repeats itself here. Meanwhile a comparative study of the offerings of the many existing ventricular models should prove instructive.

In contemplating the interaction between the ventricle and its respective arterial trees, for example, with respect to the realization of optimal matching, little attention had been devoted to the interposed valve. This void is now filled for both normal and abnormal conditions. Movement of the leaflets of the normal aortic valve is being scrutinized, in particular to determine whether the vortices, within the coronary sinuses, play a critical role during the closing process, in addition to the breaking of the jet. With respect to valvular stenosis, recent theoretical work indicates that the governing conditions may be such that most of the energy losses occur in the artery beyond the stenosis as a result of turbulent flow, rather than within the stenosis as frictional losses. Analysis is being extended to prosthetic valves, where it is sorely needed, in view of their undesirable effects on blood. There is hope that noninvasive ultrasonic velocity probes will eventually aid in assessing both stenotic and insufficient valves.

Irrespective of the many unsolved basic issues regarding the performance of the heart as a pump, there is a practical need to assess its performance in circumstances of cardiac disease, during treatment, and to evaluate the efficacy of drugs. Consequently the search for indices continues. Although many, once popular, indices have fallen by the wayside, new ones are continually being proposed. Comparative studies of these and older ones are executed regularly. There is some doubt presently as to whether a single index can be found at all. Clinical investigators advocate assessment based on a matrix of clinical data points, although agreement on what constitutes the elements of the matrix does not appear within reach.

Several of the newer indices, measured invasively, either attempt to account for the effect of afterload or circumvent it. Others, currently in the majority, stress noninvasive extraction of information on which the evaluation is based. These include radiography to envision coronary perfusion, ultrasound-based measurements of ejection velocity or flow, and echocardiography to glean information about local wall movement, the last of which is limited to local anatomical information. The electrocardiogram still competes.

As the major supply route for the myocardium, the coronary circulation moves into the limelight in spite of its complex mode of operation. Current studies regarding sensitivity of flow to the presence of stenosed vessels, aggravation of stenoses by platelet plugging, ischaemia as a function of flow reduction, and the quantification of the influence of external forces to provide analytical underpinning all contribute to this move.

It is tempting to look beyond this conference. Indulging briefly in this temptation, we consider the interaction between the left ventricle and the systemic arteries with emphasis on the contractile properties of the left ventricle.

A preliminary series of experiments, executed on pigs (10), indicated that the initial upstroke of the left ventricular ejection curve could be ascribed to a change in compliance of the left ventricle and the characteristic impedance of the receiving arterial tree. In reaching this conclusion it was assumed that the contractile properties of the ventricle during the early ejection phase could be adequately described by a time-varying compliance. Utilizing a newly developed flow-pulse technique, subsequent studies (11, 12) on the beating but not pumping dog heart have demonstrated that the ventricle can indeed be so described during the early part of systole. Later in systole a resistive component gains significance.

Assuming that this characterization will apply as well to the pumping ventricle, at any instant a compliance $C$ can be defined as

$$C = \frac{dV_v}{dp_v} \tag{1}$$

where $dp_v$ denotes the change in ventricular pressure, $p_v$, induced by a change $dV_v$ in ventricular volume $V_v$.

Also, assuming linearity during this phase, for which there is experimental evidence (11), it follows

$$V_v = Cp_v + k \tag{2a}$$

where $k$ is a constant of integration.

The quantities in [2a] are generally functions of time $t$ owing to the progressing contraction phase. Hence

$$V_v(t) = C(t)p_v(t) + k(t) \tag{2b}$$

Suga and Sagawa (13), who assume directly the same relationship with a somewhat different terminology, argue that $k$ may be regarded as independent of time throughout systole. Here it will be assumed only that $k(t)$ does not alter appreciably during the early contraction phase, i.e. from its onset until the peak of ejection. Then, differentiating [2b] with respect to time yields

$$\frac{dV_v}{dt} = C(t)\frac{dp_v}{dt} + p_v(t)\frac{dC}{dt} \qquad [3]$$

in which $dV_v/dt$, the rate of change of ventricular volume, equals $Q$, the instantaneous ejection flow, with a minus sign assigned.

$$Q = -dV_v/dt \qquad [4]$$

Equation [3] relates events while the ventricular musculature contracts against its true afterload (9). With experimentally observed values for $Q$ and $p_v(t)$, $dp_v/dt$ is also known (Figure 1). Equation [3] constitutes a first-order differential equation in $C(t)$ and $dC/dt$ with time-varying coefficients. It has an infinite number of solutions, two of which are plotted in Figure 1. They show a precipitous drop in compliance and concomitant strong changes in $dC/dt$ during the early contraction phase.

The implications of the relationships shown in Figure 1 have direct bearing on the interpretation of indices of contractility proposed earlier (14). During the isovolumic phase of contraction $dV_v/dt = 0$. Hence, from [3]

$$\frac{dp_v}{dt} = -\frac{p_v(t)}{C(t)}\frac{dC}{dt} \qquad [5a]$$

Obviously, its maximum value $(dp_v/dt)_{max}$, usually occurring around the time of aortic valve opening, is not a pure measure of the change is compliance, $dC/dt$, but is also sensitive to ventricular pressure and ventricular compliance. Its companion index $(1/p_v)/(dp_v/dt)$ equals

$$\frac{1}{p_v}\frac{dp_v}{dt} = -\frac{1}{C(t)}\frac{dC}{dt} \qquad [5b]$$

and is seen to depend on both the values of $C(t)$ and of $dC/dt$. In both cases, since the compliance varies continuously, the values for the indices obtained are sensitive to the instant at which $C(t)$ is evaluated.

Rather than depend on arbitrary values in the evaluation of the performance of the left ventricle, it would seem more advantageous and informative to secure both $C(t)$ and $dC/dt$ during the early phase of contraction when these quantities undergo major changes. Additional information will be needed for this purpose as the present analysis indicates that ventricles with totally different contractile properties may produce identical ventricular pressure and ejection flow and hence appear to have the same properties. A broader analysis will be required to identify the appropriate additional parameter. Once this has been achieved, a unique solution for $C(t)$, and hence for $dC/dt$ may be obtained by solving [3] with the aid of a computer.

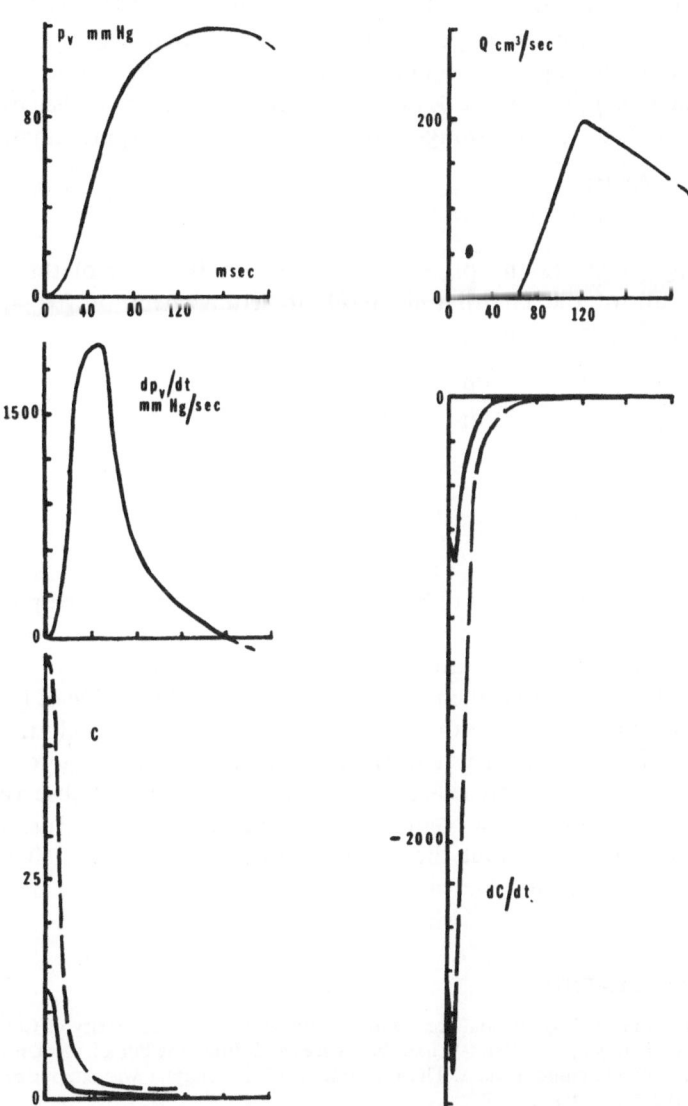

*Figure 1.* Typical curves for ventricular pressure $p_v$, of its time derivative $dp_v/dt$, and of ejection flow, $Q$, during the early part of systole. Two sets of time curves, one in fully drawn lines, the other in broken lines, for ventricular compliance, $C$, and its derivative $dC/dt$ that satisfy [3] are also shown. $C$ is in cm$^3$/mm Hg; $dC/dt$ in c,$^3$/mm Hg sec. (The two sets were computed by choosing different values for $C$ at $t = 120$ msec.) Data used in part based on (11).

The solution for $C(t)$ and $dC/dt$ may be extended into the early ejection phase in one of several ways. The left-hand member of [3] may be secured by measuring ejection flow $Q$, simultaneously with ventricular pressure. Or, recalling that the input impedance of the systemic arterial tree reduces to the characteristic impedance $Z_0$ of the proximal aorta for higher frequency components (14), the following relation holds in good approximation

$$\frac{\Delta p_a(t)}{Q(t)} = Z_0 \qquad [6]$$

where $\Delta p_a(t)$ denotes the pressure increment in the root of the aorta at instant $t$ above the end-diatolic level. Rearrangement of [6] and substitution in [3] results in

$$-\frac{\Delta p_a(t)}{Z_0} = C(t)\frac{dp_v}{dt} + p_v\frac{dC}{dt} \qquad [7]$$

where

$$Z_0 = \frac{\rho c}{\pi r_0^2} \qquad [8]$$

with $\rho$ denoting the density of blood, $c$ the phase velocity of the pulse wave which approximates the wave velocity for higher frequency components, and $\pi r_0^2$ the cross-sectional area of the proximal aorta.

It should be noted that the two terms on the right-hand side of [3] or [7] are of opposite sign during the contraction phase. It is unlikely that either term is negligible with respect to the other in the range of interest.

These considerations provide a foundation for the original observation by Starr et al. (15) and the subsequent argument advanced by Rushmer (16) that key information about the contractile behaviour of the left ventricle can be extracted during the early part of systole.

ACKNOWLEDGEMENTS

The author is indebted to his confreres Don Cunningham of the University of California at Berkeley for identifying the Saint-Venant reference, and Jules Melbin of the University of Pennsylvania for searching debates. The preparation of this chapter was supported by NIH grants HL 10330 and HL 22223.

REFERENCES

1. Brecher GA: *Venous return*, New York, Grune and Stratton, 1956.
2. Starling EH: On the circulatory changes associated with exercise. *J R Army Med Corps* 34:258–272, 1920.
3. McMichael J: The output of the heart in congestive failure. *Q J Med* 7:331–353, 1938.
4. Saint-Venant B de: Mémoire sur la torsion des prismes, avec des considérations sur leur

flexiçon, ainsi que sur l'équilibre intérieur des solides élastiques en général, et des formules pratiques pour le calcul de leur résistance à divers efforts s'exerçant simultanément. *Mémoires des Savants étrangers* 14:233–560, 1855.

5. Timoshenko S: *Theory of elasticity*, New York, McGraw-Hill, 1934, p 31.
6. Pollack GH, Krueger JW: Myocardial sarcomere mechanics: some parallels with skeletal muscle. In: *Cardiovascular system dynamics*, Baan J, Noordergraaf A, Raines J (eds), Cambridge, Massachusetts, MIT Press, 1978, p 3–10.
7. Hunter WC, Noordergraaf A: Can impedance characterize the heart? *J Appl Physiol* 40:250–252, 1976.
8. Iwazumi T: Molecular mechanism of muscle contraction: another view. In: *Cardiovascular system dynamics*, Baan J, Noordergraaf A, Raines J (eds), Cambridge, Massachusetts, MIT Press, 1978, p 11–21.
9. Noordergraaf A, Melbin J: Ventricular afterload: a succinct yet comprehensive definition (editorial). *Am Heart J* 95:545–547, 1978.
10. Noordergraaf A, Meester GT: Hemodynamics and the heart. *Bibl Cardiol* 30:75–85, 1972.
11. Hunter WC: A new approach to ventricular dynamics: the flow-pulse response. PhD thesis, University of Pennsylvania, Philadelphia, 1977 University Ann Arbor, Michigan (University Microfilms).
12. Hunter WC, Janicki JS, Weber KT, Noordergraaf A: The flow-pulse technique; a new way to study ventricular dynamics (in press).
13. Suga H, Sagawa K: Instantaneous pressure-volume relationship and their ratio in the excised, supported canine left ventricle. *Circ Res* 35:117–126, 1974.
14. Noordergraaf A: *Circulatory System Dynamics*, New York, Academic Press, 1978, chapters 7 and 9.
15. Starr I, Horwitz O, Mayock RL, Krumbhaar EB: Standardization of the ballistocardiogram by simulation of the heart's function at necropsy. *Circulation* 1:1073–1096, 1950.
16. Rushmer RF: Initial ventricular impulse: a potential key to cardiac evaluation. *Circulation* 29:268–283, 1964.

# SUBJECT INDEX